SOCCER DISEASES

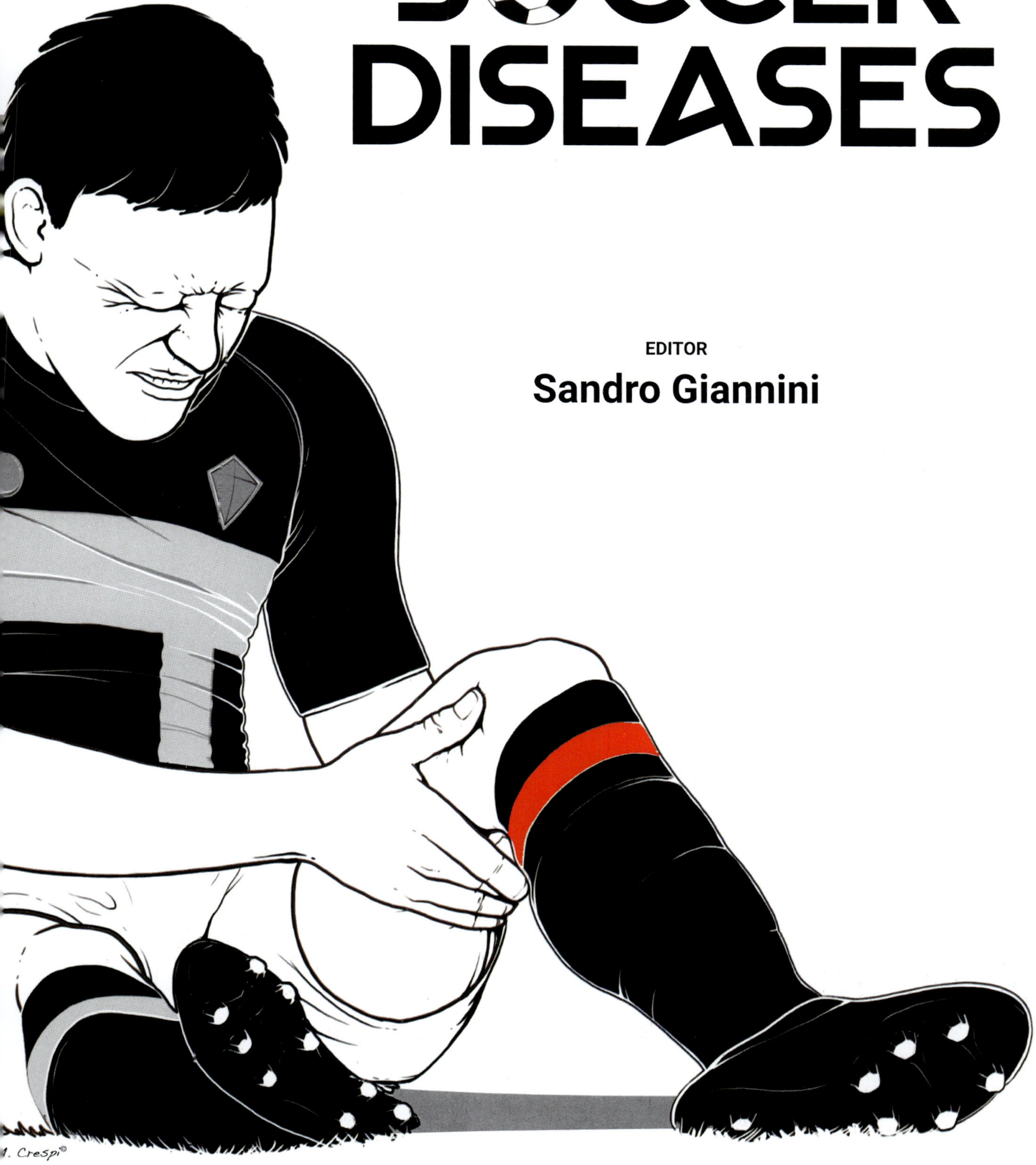

EDITOR

Sandro Giannini

TIMEO

WITH THE PATRONAGE OF

Fondazione C. Rizzoli per le Scienze Motorie

ALMA MATER STUDIORUM UNIVERSITÀ DI BOLOGNA
DIPARTIMENTO DI SCIENZE PER LA QUALITÀ DELLA VITA

ALMA MATER STUDIORUM UNIVERSITÀ DI BOLOGNA
DIPARTIMENTO DI SCIENZE BIOMEDICHE E NEUROMOTORIE

SERVIZIO SANITARIO REGIONALE
EMILIA - ROMAGNA
Istituto Ortopedico Rizzoli di Bologna
Istituto di Ricovero e Cura a Carattere Scientifico

ISOKINETIC MEDICAL GROUP
FIFA MEDICAL CENTRE OF EXCELLENCE

SOCCER DISEASES

Editor: **Sandro Giannini**

Editing: **Andrea Peren**
Proofreading: **Maria Camillo**
Coordination: **David Manco**

Graphics and internal layout: **Massimo D'Onofrio**
Graphics and cover layout: **Marco Redaelli**
Cover painting: **Massimiliano Crespi**

Printing: Starprint srl, Bergamo, Italy
First edition: january 2020

TIMEO DIVISIONE LIBRI
Griffin

PUBLISHER
Griffin srl unipersonale
Via Ginevrina da Fossano 67/A - 22063 Cantù (Como)
Tel. 031.789085 - Fax 031.6853110
customerservice@griffineditore.it
www.griffineditore.it

Preface

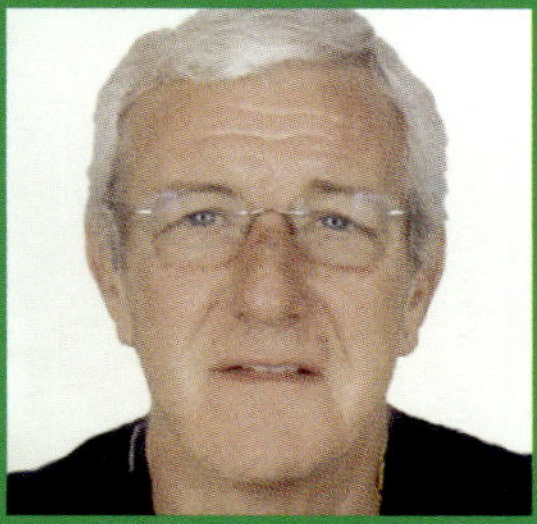

Marcello Lippi
International
Soccer Coach

It is a real pleasure for me and an honor to have been invited to present a book on soccer diseases, for several reasons.
Soccer has always been and still is a very important part of my life, first as a professional player, then as a coach of important Italian and Asian teams. From soccer I have had the maximum professional satisfactions that a coach can hope to achieve in his career. In fact I had the pleasure, in my long activity, of training teams that won their respective national championships, the Champions League, the Asian cup and the World cup.
The theme of the book "Soccer Diseases" takes into consideration not only injuries but also many other pathologies that more frequently affect soccer players. The problem is very important for coaches since, as a consequence, important technical and tactical management problems arise due to the interruption of sport activity for more or less long periods.
These circumstances are particularly frequent in soccer, due to the specific characteristics of this sport. It leads to contrasts capable of involving numerous districts, from head to toe; it takes place at high speed, with repeated shots, sudden changes of direction, jumps, uncoordinated falls, and it is also practiced on grounds that are not always regular with the possibility of loss of motor coordination.
In addition to trauma, some other conditions are much more frequent than in the past, such as pubalgia, inflammation of the Achilles tendon, fasciitis or muscle injuries: these are particularly felt by those coaches with a limited number of players.
I want to point out how, in case of an injury, it is always important to have the player recovered as early as possible while at the same time limiting the possibility of relapse and for this reason I believe a continuous collaboration between doctor-trainer and player is essential to optimize the time to return to sport.
The book was born under the aegis of the Carlo Rizzoli Foundation which promotes and supports educational, scientific and research activities, and is sponsored by important institutions such as: the Department of Life Quality Sciences (QuVi), the Department of Biomedical and Neuromotor Sciences (Dibinem) of the University of Bologna, the Isokinetic rehabilitation center of Bologna and the Rizzoli Orthopedic Institute of Bologna.
Finally, I want to highlight the friendship that binds me to the book Editor and President of the Carlo Rizzoli Foundation, Professor Sandro Giannini, to whom I have been linked since my childhood and with whom I started kicking the ball in the Viareggio pinewood in Tuscany.

Presentation

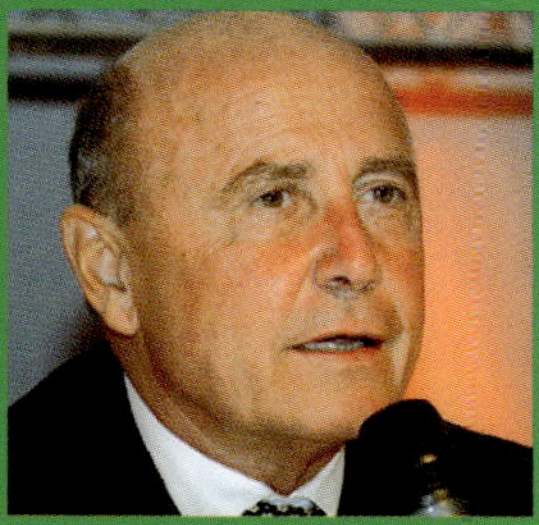

Sandro Giannini
Emeritus Professor
at the University
of Bologna, Italy
President of the Carlo
Rizzoli Foundation

Soccer is one of the most practiced sports in the world, with a growing diffusion due to its progressive extension to all continents, to be increasingly practiced by women, and to the introduction of several variants of the game in addition to traditional soccer.
The typical characteristics of this sport lead to many direct traumas and frequent other types of micro-traumatic pathologies.
The high number of practitioners also, in the case of an accident, needs to be recovered as quickly as possible for the activity resumption.
Soccer is a contact sport in which players clash, kick, shove themselves, hit their heads, hold on, and push on.
Soccer is practiced on soils with sometimes irregular and slippery grounds, which make movements unstable, and is played with a ball of over 400 grams that moves at high speed.
All this leads to frequent direct traumas that can affect the whole body. The most frequent are represented by bruises, wounds, sprains, muscle-tendon injuries and, less frequently, fractures.
In addition to direct trauma, a wrong contrast or movement can cause loss of motor coordination during running and jumping, with uncontrolled falls and abnormal muscle-tendon and joint stress.
Regardless of the contrast, due to the variability of athletic gestures such as running, sprinting, shooting, twisting, turning, jumping, landing, and tackling, various injuries etiologies and types may be present.
Tackling causes injury when the player is unable to respond quickly enough to avoid an uncontrolled movement. Muscle and tendon injuries are more frequent during sprinting. Twisting and turning can cause excessive stress on ligaments. Shooting, due to the contrast with the opponent or with the ball, can cause micro-injuries or sprains. Finally, traumas often occur during jumping and landing due to an incorrect landing technique or a collision after the take-off or before landing.
There are also several micro-traumatic and degenerative lesions favored by repeated stresses or foot deformities. Furthermore, the lesions are more frequent during the official game, together with fatigue conditions and advanced age.
The main sites affected in male players are ankle, foot and knee, while in women knee, ankle and upper limb.

Why a book regarding most common soccer injuries?
There are already several articles in the literature treating these lesions separately but a specific book that completely collects lesions of the whole

body, from head trauma to foot injuries, including clinical features, treatment, and rehabilitation, is still lacking.

Why the title Soccer Diseases?

The word diseases, in addition to traumas, also includes other types of micro-traumatic and degenerative pathologies, often favored by overloads due to pre-existing anatomical alterations or deformities.

What were the reasons why this book has been written?

Soccer has always been one of my great passions and in my youth I was actively involved as a semi-professional player for several years. The interest subsequently matured for Medicine and in particular for Sports Traumatology led me to specialize in Orthopedics and Traumatology and in other related disciplines: Sports Medicine and Physical and Rehabilitative Medicine. Moreover, in my long activity as a Full Professor at the University of Bologna, Alma Mater Studiorum, and during my surgical activity at the Rizzoli Orthopedic Institute, I was able to stay close to the soccer environment by visiting and operating several both amateur and professional athletes.

Finally, my current position as President of the Carlo Rizzoli Foundation, which provides for the development and dissemination of Motor Sciences and supports for the didactic, scientific and research activities of the Motor Sciences courses of the University of Bologna led me to the creation of this book, combining the specific skills of various specialists, in order to understand, divided by topics, the whole body, from the cranial pathology to the foot diseases. Many of these specialists belong to the University of Bologna, the oldest European University, specifically to the Departments of Sciences for the Quality of Life (QuVi) and of Biomedical and NeuroMotorie Sciences (Dibinem) and to the Istituto Ortopedico Rizzoli, one of the main world orthopedics centers founded by Francesco Rizzoli and inaugurated in 1896.

To complete the book, the rehabilitative section was commissioned to a large and famous European center for sports rehabilitation, the Isokinetic of Bologna.

I want to thank Marcello Lippi who agreed to write an introduction for this book, all the colleagues who brilliantly carried out the individual chapters, the Scientific Committee, the Directors Board of the Carlo Rizzoli Foundation, the Griffin-Timeo publishing house, for taking care of the publication, the Bologna University Departments, the Rizzoli Orthopedic Institute and the Isokinetic Center for their patronage, hoping that this book will be useful and easy to consult not only for surgeons, sports doctors and rehabilitators but also for all those interested in the pathology of soccer and in the treatment of its related injuries.

Finally, I hope that any revenue from this publication may help support the purpose of the foundation.

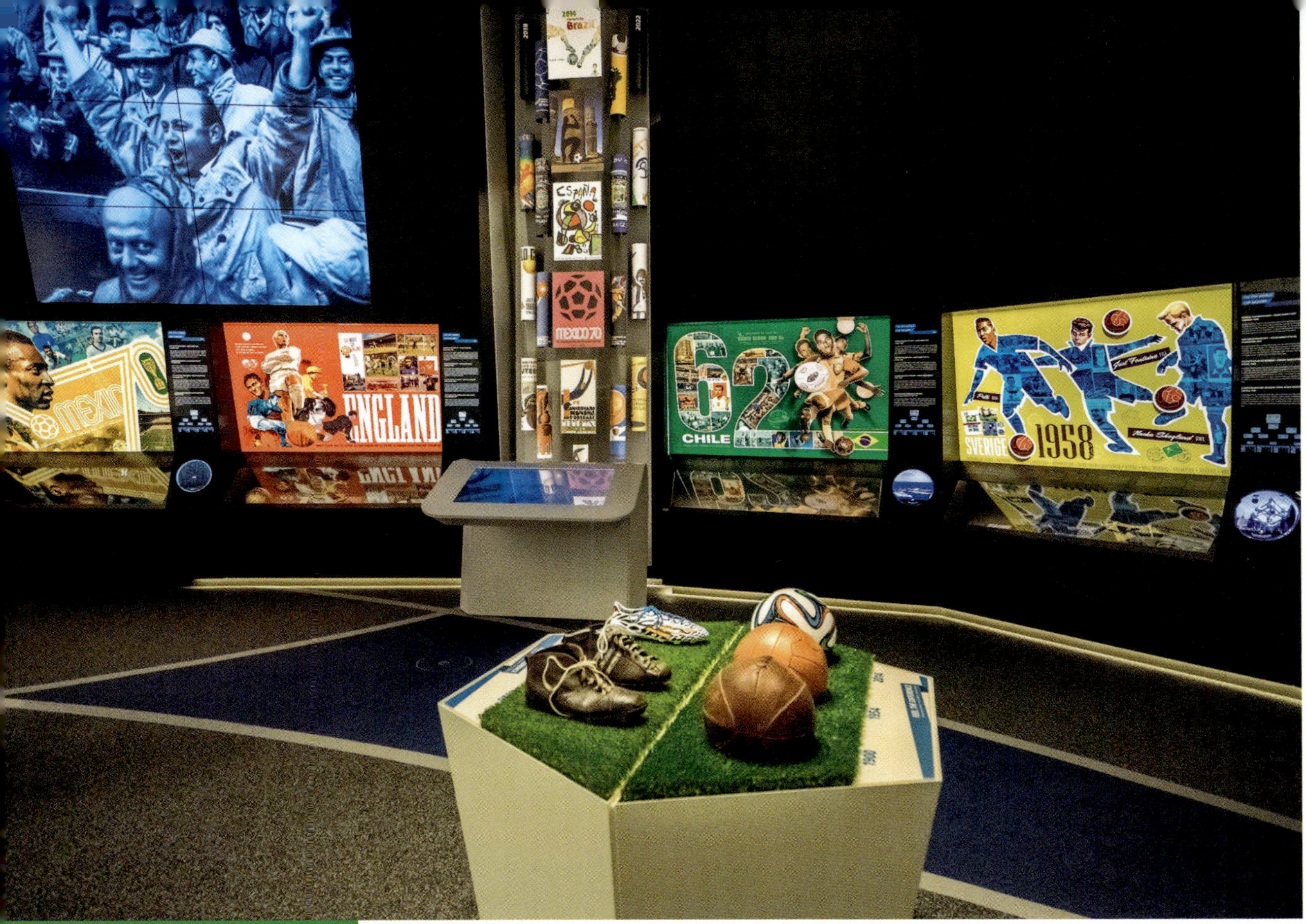

Image of the FIFA World Cup Gallery at the FIFA World Football Museum in Zürich

Brief history of soccer

Soccer is one of the oldest team games in the world, it was already practiced in Asia and Japan in the 11th century BC. In China in the same period the "Tsu Chu" became famous, which meant "leather ball kicked from the foot", a military game in which the ball, filled with feathers and hair, was kicked with the feet in a hole formed by two bamboo canes. Still in Japan, about 500 years later, the Kemari spread, and it is still practiced. In a relatively small space, the players had to pass a leather ball with inside an inflated animal bladder, without let it touching the ground.

Other testimonies come from ancient Greece were the "Episkyros" became widespread in the fourth century BC, but it was not included among the Olympic disciplines of the time.

In Rome a similar game was called "Harpastum". A small ball was used and two teams faced each other on a rectangular field and passages with hands and feet were permitted.

Martial described two types of ball that were used: a ball made of leather and full of feathers and another leather ball named "follis", with an air chamber made up of a bladder. The game was played by legionaries who spread it throughout Europe.

In the Britain islands in the Middle Age, towards the end of the thirteenth century, the term "large-soccer" identified a game with a ball played during the carnival. A century later, in 1388, due to its violent nature, the game was banned with an edict by King Henry V. At the same time in France the "Soule" (or "Choule") was played with a ball made of a pig's bladder. The ball was struck with hands, feet and sticks.
The Vikings practiced the "Knattleikr" with a hard and heavy ball on grass or ice divided into two teams and with a captain.
The Celtic version called "Knappan" used a wooden ball soaked in grease to make it more viscous and elusive. Two teams from one or more villages faced each other with the aim of winning the ball and conquering the opposing field. The unwritten rules of the competition foresaw that the game, if the heat was excessive, could be stopped by the word: "Heddwch!" ("Peace!").
Soccer had a great development in the Medicean Florence where special balloons were used and beaten with a punch armed with a single glove. In the nearby Prato large balloons were created and kicked. These sports included what are now soccer and rugby.
In the modern era soccer was introduced, starting in the 1600s, in universities: the teams were composed of ten students and a teacher as a goalkeeper. From this moment on the classic number of players and the figure of the captain were born.
Initially the game was generally called "dribbling-game", ancestor of both soccer and rugby, and involved the use of both hands and feet.
In 1857 the first Soccer Club, the Sheffield Soccer Club, was founded, and in 1858 the Sheffield Rules were written. However, it was only in 1863 that the Soccer Association was founded in London, whose regulation was a compromise between the primitive soccer and rugby.
Only on October, 26th 1863 soccer as it is today is known born, under the impetus of the English Ebenezer Cobb Morley, and it is then officially written that "no player can run with the ball in his hands or charge the opponent".
At the beginning there was no distinction between the players on the pitch. Then the distinctions between the different players was proposed, then divided between attackers and defenders. To overcome the offensive imbalance forward, three attackers were set back and the figure of the median created.
Only in 1870 the team started proposing a classic line-up with a goalkeeper, two full-backs, three medians and five forwards.
In 1871 the size of the ball was established, and the goalkeeper becomes the only player allowed to touch the ball with hands.
In 1878 a referee used a whistle for the first time to direct a game.
Considerable progress was also made in the materials used for the manufacture of the ball, which, with the advent of rubber introduced by the British from a composition made of pig bladder or canvases filled with corks, became more sophisticated in structure adding a chamber air. This allowed great progress also in the control of the ball.
Some peculiarities are interesting.

Why are players 11? In English colleges the dormitories were composed of 10 students and a tutor and this number has been maintained over time.

How did the offside develop? The first type of offside is from 1863 and refers to the position of the player closest to the opponent's bottom line at the time the ball was kicked. Then, three variations were proposed. In 1866 the player was considered in offside when, at the time of kicking the ball in any area of the field, he did not have at least three opposing players in front of him. From 1907 the player was considered in offside only if in the middle of the opposing field. Since 1925, then redefined in 1990, it is not considered offside who is in line with the penultimate opponent, considering the goalkeeper as the last.

How was the penalty kick born? It appeared in 1891 and could be kicked from any point as long as it was 11 meters away from the goal line. For this purpose a semicircle was drawn in front of the goal line on which the ball could be placed. From 1902 it was definitively established that it could only be pulled from 11 meters on the perpendicular to the goal line.

Why do we say goal when we score? The word indicates the success for the game purpose.
In 1880, the English and Welsh Federation were also joined by the Irish one and in 1886 the International Soccer Association Board (IFAB) was established, consisting of the four British federations (England, Scotland, Ireland and Wales).
In 1886, professional sportsmanship is officially recognized: players are on a par with other categories of workers and must receive a salary for their work.
In 1890 the goal lines are finally equipped with nets.
The diffusion of the discipline quickly reached the whole globe. In 1891 the Football Federation of New Zealand was born, in 1892 the same in South Africa, in 1893 in Argentina, Belgium and Chile, in 1895 in Switzerland, in 1898 in Italy and in 1900 in Germany.
The FIFA, acronym of Fédération Internationale of Soccer Association, was founded, initially without the English one (then added in 1905), on May 21st 1904 on the purpose of France, Switzerland, Netherlands, Belgium, Sweden, Denmark, and Spain. Robert Guérin was elected first President.
The final approval of the game took place with the London Olympics in 1908. In 1914 FIFA recognized the Olympic football tournament as an amateur championship and in 1920, in the first edition recognized by FIFA, Belgium was winner, while in 1924 and 1928 it was Uruguay. In 1930 FIFA decided to establish a world cup for professional national clubs and Uruguay was chosen as the host country and from that moment it was decided to repeat the event every four years.
The international cup was the first competition for international soccer teams played in Europe and it was held from 1927 to 1960.
The UEFA Champions League was born in 1955, an annual European com-

petition, and in 1960 the Copa Libertadores was established, with the same characteristics but reserved for South American teams.
Until 1995, UEFA club teams were bound to have no more than three foreign players in the team. Subsequently the soccer market was liberalized allowing to enter in the team how many foreign players as preferred.
On March, 6th 2016 the International Soccer Association approved the use of the VAR (Video Assistant Referee) which consists of a referee assisted by two competition officials watching the game video. The first of September VAR debuts in Bari (Italy) during the game Italy-France.
On December, 18th 2016 in the final of the club world championship, Real Madrid carries out the fourth replacement for the first time in the history of football, one more than the three previously scheduled.
On August, 3 2017 the most expensive transfer in the history of football took place: Neymar was transferred from Barcelona to Paris Saint Germain (PSG) for euros 222 million.

Female football
The birth of women's football dates back to the time of the First World War in England with the team of "Ladies of Kerr", a group of women who were put to work in a factory for lack of men engaged in war, and who, during work breaks, played soccer. Since then other teams were born and in 1921 the number of teams in England and Scotland was around 150.
However, in December 1921 the English Soccer Association decided to ban this sport: "Complaints have been made to soccer being played by women", the Council felt impelled to express their strong opinion of the game as a whole". This halted the expansion of women's football and delayed its development, not only in England but all over the world. Women's football went on a period of stagnation until World War II, when it began to spread in the European northern countries such as Norway, Sweden, and Germany. From this moment on its development became inexorable; before the 1960s, in the wake of national leagues, several regional federations were created and even international meetings started becoming common.
The first women's world championship was held in China in 1991, and the first Olympics in which women's football enters was in Athens in 1996. From a 2016-2017 UEFA research it appears that the female footballers are over 1,270 million and that over 827 thousand are under 18. The professional players are 2,853 and 52 countries have a dedicated championship.

Other variants
Other variations of traditional football are 5-a-side football born in 1933 and internationally known as "futsal" which differs not only in the number of players but also in the playing field (made of parquet or synthetic ground) and on its rule characteristics.
Another variant is the beach soccer, established in 1992: this includes 5 players, but with the difference that the playing field is made of sand and players are barefoot.

Index

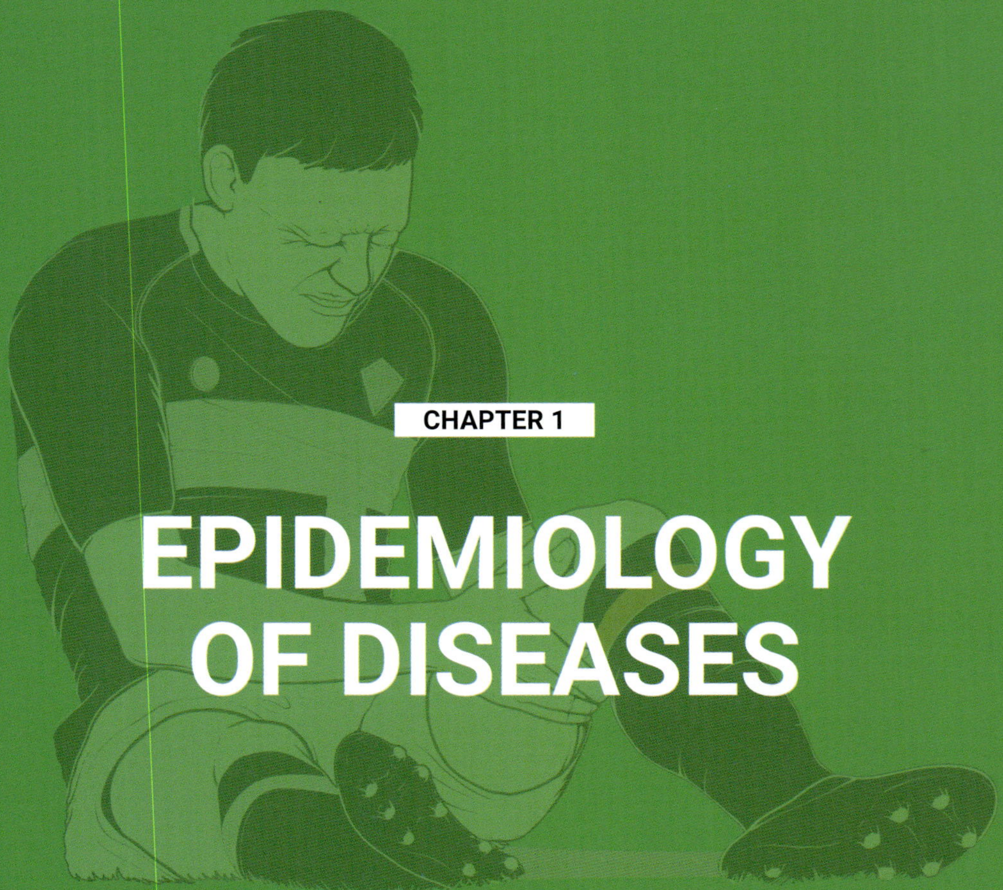

CHAPTER 1

EPIDEMIOLOGY OF DISEASES

Alberto Di Martino
Francesca Barile
Cesare Faldini

1st Orthopaedic and Traumatologic Clinic (Director: C. Faldini)
IRCCS Istituto Ortopedico Rizzoli, Bologna, Italy

Department of Biomedic and Neuromotor Sciences (Dibinem)
Alma Mater Studiorum, University of Bologna, Italy

Introduction

Soccer (or football) is the world's most popular sport and its increasing popularity is leading to faster and more aggressive games than in the past, requiring elevated physical fitness levels. It is also a complex contact sport with high risks and rates of injury [1] and these injuries often lead to long term sequelae [2]. For these reasons soccer related diseases are a composite topic to treat and so it is their epidemiology.

At a professional level, high physiological, psychological, technical, and tactical demands predispose players to a substantial injury risk. This risk is estimated to be about 1,000 times higher compared to industrial jobs [3]. As outlined by Ekstrand and Dvorak (two of the main experts in soccer/football injuries epidemiology), considering professional players as employees, their working condition can equate to eight new injuries each week in a staff of 25 employees working full time [4].

Therefore, international soccer societies are concerned about the increased mental and physical demands leading to injuries [5] and many studies were conducted with the objective of understanding mechanisms and risk factors of those injuries. Epidemiological data were collected on the incidence and characteristics of soccer injuries, and a consensus regarding the methodological standards for epidemiological studies was published [6].

However, differences in study design and in definition of injury itself make analysis of literature difficult [5]; moreover, it is still the smallest fraction of the playing population (adult male professionals) that attracts most of researchers' attention, while the highest proportion of participants (22 million of the 38 million officially registered players) is actually under the age of 18 years [7].

In this chapter we try to present and discuss the current understanding of injuries and pathologies in soccer players at any level and present the epidemiologic information, which provides a composite picture of injuries prevalence and incidence, and we can enable researchers to detect possible susceptibilities to injury in different age groups and across different performance levels.

Definitions

The starting point for any systematic analysis is consensus about definitions.

As a part of the First World Congress on Sports Injury Prevention in 2005, the FIFA Medical Assessment and Research Centre (F-MARC) established injury, severe injury, recurrent injury definitions [8].

- Injury: any physical complaint sustained by a player that results from a soccer match or soccer training, irrespective of the need for medical attention or time loss from soccer activities. An injury that results in a player receiving medical attention is referred to as a "medical attention" injury and an injury that results in a player being unable to take a full part in future soccer training or match play as a "time loss" injury [5, 9].
- Traumatic injury: violent and sudden injury caused by a specific, identifiable traumatic event, such as sprains, lacerations, torn ligaments, pulled muscles or broken bones by a fall. Immediate professional treatment is usually required. Traumatic injuries are divided into contact and non-contact injuries [10].
- Overuse injury: injuries caused by repetitive stress without sufficient time to undergo the natural regenerative process.
- Recurrent injury: an injury of the same type and at the same site as an index injury and that occurs

after a player's return to full participation from the index injury. A recurrent injury occurring within 2 months of a player's return to full participation is referred to as an "early recurrence", one occurring 2 to 12 months after a player's return to full participation as a "late recurrence" and one occurring more than 12 months after a player's return to full participation as a "delayed recurrence".

• Severe injury: the number of days that have elapsed from the date of injury to the date of the player's return to full participation in team training and availability for match selection determines the injury severity.

1. Slight: 0 days lost
2. Minimal: 1-3 days lost
3. Mild: 4-7 days lost
4. Moderate: 8-28 days lost
5. Severe: >28 days lost

How often do soccer players get injured?

The incidence of peculiar injury is defined as the number of injuries occurring during a time period, when the player was at risk of injury. Consequently, the incidence of soccer injuries has most frequently been calculated based on hours played during games and training. This overall incidence among adult male players (tab. 1) has been estimated to be between 10 and 35 per 1,000 game hours, and between 2 and 9 injuries per 1,000 training hours [1, 6].

Dvorak and Junge [11] found that, on average, all players experienced 1 activity-limiting injury per season. However, the overall risk of injury resulted to be highly variable depending on player age, sex, exercise load, level of play, and playing position [12, 13]. Understanding data about different groups of soccer athletes allows us to better outline risk factors for injuries.

Male players of different age and skill levels

Soccer is the fastest growing sport worldwide with approximately 265 million registered soccer players, most of them under the age of 18 [10, 14]. However, with regard to children and young players, comparable data on the frequency and pattern of soccer injuries are missing. What is demonstrated is that the incidence of injuries varies between players of different ages and skill levels [6, 15]. The total incidence in youth players ranges from 2 to 19.4 per 1,000 hours of global exposure (game and training) [5, 10, 16, 17].

Country	Level of play	Injuries per 1000 game hours	Injuries per 1000 training hours
• males			
Sweden	National team	30.3	6.5
Sweden	National top division	25.9	5.2
US	MLS professionals	35.5	2.9
UK	Premiere League, 1st and 2nd division	25.9	3.4
Sweden	1st division 2nd division 3rd division 6th division	21.8 18.7 16.9 14.6	4.6 5.1 7.6 7.5
Denmark	2nd division (high) Series (low)	18.5 11.9	2.3 5.6
• females			
Sweden	Senior players, varius skill levels	14.3	3.7
Sweden	Premier, 2nd division	24	7
• youth (<18y)			
Switzerland	High level males Low level males	18.7 21.7	4.1 8.2
Denmark	Male youth	14.4	3.6

Table 1 - Incidence of soccer injuries in different studies (modified from Dvorak and Junge [6])

	All injuries		Competitions injuries		Training injuries	
Nature of injury	**No**	**%**	**No**	**%**	**No**	**%**
Muscular strain	1141	31	558	29	583	33
Ligamentous sprain	748	20	389	21	359	20
Muscular contusion	299	8	211	11	88	5
Tendinitis	162	5	73	4	89	5
Fracture	145	4	77	4	68	4
Osgood-Schlatter's	112	3	28	1	84	4
Inflammatory synovitis	71	2	30	2	41	2
Meniscal tear	48	1	28	2	20	1
Other overuse	23	1	14	1	9	1
Dislocation	21	1	7	0	14	0
Ligament rupture	19	1	11	1	8	0
Other diagnosis	305	6	152	6	153	9
Total	**3688**	**100**	**1899**	**100**	**1789**	**100**

Table 2 - Nature of injuries sustained during training and competition (modified from Price et al. [15])

Both the F-MARC and other studies [6, 10, 16, 18] outline an increase in incidence of injury with age progression, linking it to enhanced competitiveness and increased player-to-player contact [19]. They also report that players of both sexes aged 17-19 approach the values observed in adults.
In relation to sex differences among youth players, no relevant difference in injury incidence of boys and girls was evident, and the comparison between the injury incidence in elite youth players and sub-elite players suggested that the two groups show a similar risk [6, 10].
The F-MARC study also reports a decrease in injury incidence between youth/adult and professional/amateur players: part of the explanation for this pattern could be related to the amount and quality of training and subsequent level of fitness [6].
Price et al. [15] undertook a prospective epidemiological study of the injuries sustained in English youth academy football over two competitive seasons (tab. 2).
Not only are their results in line with F-MARC (with the highest incidence of injuries in the oldest age group, under 19), but also they added data: first, strains were found to be a significant proportion of injuries (the reasons of this may include incomplete development of muscle in adolescents and limited shock absorption of the developing muscle); on the other hand, they found 5% of injuries being related to growth spurt and musculoskeletal system development (Osgood-Schlatter and Sever's disease).

Female players

Soccer is becoming so popular among girls and women all over the world that FIFA president Joseph S. Blatter once said: "We have seen the future of football and that future is feminine".
It is played officially in more than 100 countries, and the total number of female players worldwide can be estimated at around 30 million [20]. But, despite the increase in participation in women's soccer, the research on women's soccer had lagged behind and only a few studies report epidemiology of soccer diseases among female players [6].
One of those studies was conducted by Faude et al. [21], who analyzed professional female soccer players in German Bundesliga and found no significant difference in injury rates between them and their male colleagues (around 2.8 injuries per 1,000 training hours and 23.3 per 1,000 match hours) [21, 22].
No differences have been found between men and women (the thigh results to be the most frequently injured site, followed by the knee and ankle) regarding injury sites either.
The most interesting finding was an extremely higher risk of ACL rupture in females than in males (2.2 per 1,000 match hours). In fact, even though ACL is the most frequently injured knee ligament in both men and women, females were found to be more prone to suffering its rupture [21, 22].
Many studies tried to explain this; some [23] tried to link it to intrinsic anatomical differences be-

tween men and women such as increased quadriceps angle and increased posterior tibial slope in females; others [24] analyzed the influence of sex hormons on the strength of ligaments. Up to now, further research is needed because no study demonstrated a direct and significant correlation with any of those hypotheses.

The effect of playing position

There is substantially no agreement regarding the effect of player position on general injury in soccer. No study could prove a statistically significant difference in injury rates between players with different position (fig. 1).

However, one consistent trend is the lower risk of injury in goalkeepers compared to outfield players: 12.9 injuries per 1,000 game hours vs 22.6 per 1,000 game hours of outfield positions [13, 25, 26, 27]. Many studies discussed those data and they concluded that the reason of this trend may be due to the uniqueness of goalkeepers' somatotype and the reduced distance covered during the match, as well as less direct contact with opponents [13, 27].

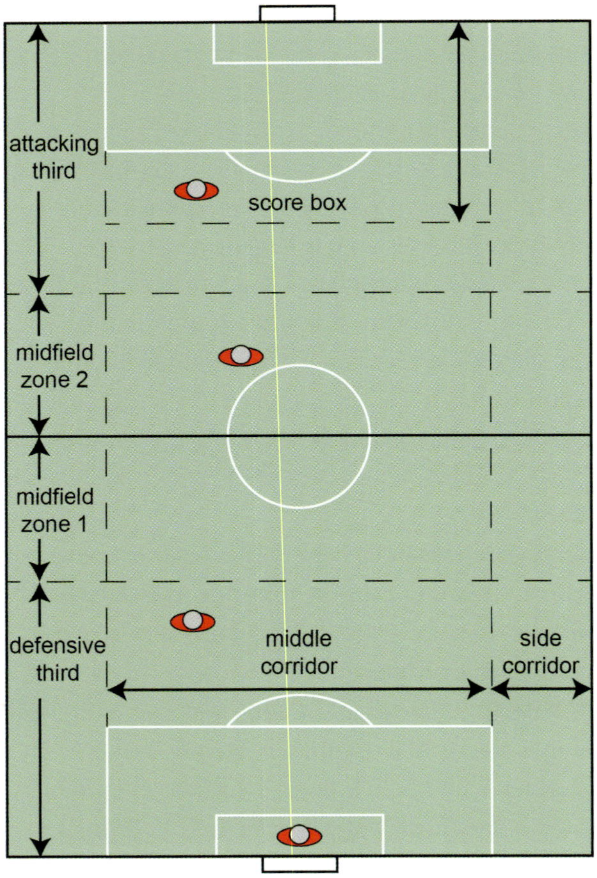

Figure 1 - Different roles and positions in the soccer field are related to different risk to develop specific kind of injuries

Although players with different position have substantially the same risk in terms of injury frequency (except for goalkeepers), the mechanism and pattern of those injuries often changes because of their specific tasks and activities.

Defenders seem to be at higher risk of knee injuries (most of all anterior cruciate ligament lesions); the reason might be that they often takle the opponent with risky maneuvers and with minimal planning time [13, 29].

When considering midfielders, they are generally the players who cover more distance during a match and it is logical to think that they would be predisposed especially to muscle and overuse injuries [31].

In relation to strikers (that usually get injured in the "attacking third"), there is a tendency towards them to have the highest risk of match (but not training) injuries overall; however, this result is not consistent between all the studies [13].

Several hypotheses to explain this have been put forward: first, the clear majority of incidents happen in the defensive zone and in the score box [1]; second, forwards do more acceleration/deceleration and fast kicking activities than other players, which may predispose them for thigh muscle injuries (around 25% on the total time off injuries in soccer) [13].

As regards youth players (<17 years), it is not possible to reach conclusions about field related injuries, because they often change playing position during the season and in different seasons [6].

Is there an intra-seasonal variation of injury pattern?

Injury risk has been reported to vary considerably over the months of the season. According to some studies the difference between the highest (april) and the lowest (september) injury count in the competitive season appears to be 150% [3, 32].

However, Drawer et al. [3] divided the season in periods (pre-season, first part of championship, winter break, second part of championship, final matches), rather than in months, considering it a more effective way of analyzing the intra-seasonal variation of injury pattern: this better reflects the organization of soccer clubs, which divide the season into preparatory and competition periods. Each period has a unique profile in terms of work-recovery ratio, match/training ratio, and friendly/competition match ratio, and this of course is likely to directly influence injury characteristics and frequency.

Preseason and winter break – due to the lower number of matches and the lower intensity – have the lowest rate of traumatic injuries. On the other hand, the rate increases during the last period of seasons: a logical explanation could be the higher frequency of game, the increased competitiveness (more decisive matches are played in the late part of the year), and consequent accumulation of fatigue [4, 32, 33].

Soccer related musculoskeletal diseases and lesions

The pattern of musculoskeletal injury site is neither affected by the age, nor by the gender, suggesting common and constant features for injuries [5, 16, 17, 34, 35].

The most common injury in soccer is thigh strain, typically affecting the hamstrings muscle group. It represents more than 10% of all injuries, meaning that a 25-player team can expect 10 strains each season [20, 22, 36].

Overall, the most frequent non-time-loss injury locations are: hip/groin (17%), knee (14%), ankle (12%). The most common time-loss injury locations are: ankle (22%), knee (18%), hamstrings (11%), thigh (10%), and hip/groin (9%) [6, 36].

Maxillofacial trauma

Soccer generates a great number of maxillofacial injuries, mainly fractures, resulting in esthetic or functional problems. Bobian et al. [37] analyzed 2054 facial traumas occurred during soccer games and they found that laceration was the most common diagnosis (44.2%), followed by contusions and fractures. Fractures can occur from contact between two players (the most common mechanism) or between athletes and their surroundings (including their equipment). Soccer is one of the sports most frequently involved in sport-related facial bone fractures, owing to its competitive and contact nature [38].

In soccer, the most violent impacts between players (that can cause maxillofacial traumas) take place mainly when the ball is played with the forehead: in this moment there can be an elbow-head impact or a head-head impact. Therefore, the most common mechanism of injury is a clash of heads (23%) followed by an elbow to the face (17%) [39, 40]. When considering sex differences, Cerulli et al. considered 329 athletes with maxillofacial injuries and outlined that the male: female ratio was 6.6:1 [40].

Head trauma

Neurological diseases in soccer players are the result of one or more head traumas. Head injuries account for between 3 and 18% (depending on age, sex) of all reported soccer-related injuries and concussions resultant of these injuries have been estimated to account for up to 11% of reported injuries [41, 42, 43]. Head trauma is a common incident observed in both professional and amateur contact sports. When head trauma results in transient neurological impairment, a so-called "sports-related concussion" has occurred. Soccer fulfills the criteria of a contact sport and is therefore characterized by high incidence of concussion (also known as "minor traumatic brain injury"). There is wide evidence that these events cause functional and structural cerebral disorders [44].

Concussion may be caused either by a direct blow to the head, face, neck, or elsewhere on the body with an "impulsive" force transmitted to the head [6]. It results in a graded set of clinical syndromes that may or may not involve loss of consciousness and it is typically associated with normal structural neuroimaging studies [6, 41].

In European professional soccer, concussions show incidence rates ranging between 0.03 and 0.07 concussions per 1,000 player hours. During the last five World Cups of the Fédération Internationale de Football Association (FIFA; 1998-2014), only 12 concussions were reported [41, 42]. There is insufficient evidence to suggest a statistically significant sex-difference in head injury rate but in female players those injuries are usually more severe [43]. Delaney et al. tried to explain it from a physiological perspective, suggesting that a stronger neck in males could better dissipate the energy transmitted from head to the upper body rather than having the skull or brain alone absorbing that impact [45].

Spine disease

Athletic injuries to the cervical, thoracic, and lumbar spine are relatively common in soccer. In most cases, they are secondary to overuse. The most common etiologies are improper mechanics and overuse that affect the stability of the spine through disruption of the spinal support mechanisms [46]. In fact, the osseous, musculo-ligamentous, and neuroanatomical aspects of the spine allow for complex multiplanar movements, and dysfunction of any one of these structural elements can lead to injuries [67].

Injuries can occur from either a direct trauma or from subjective muscle imbalances that prevent optimal kinematics during athletic participation.

Traumatic injury mechanisms and overuse injuries that lead to back diseases have been described.

Additionally, spine injuries can be observed in the same athlete, whom a lower extremity injury occurs, in up to 24% of cases [47].

The overall frequency of spine injuries in soccer is 3% of all musculoskeletal diseases; 45% of the cases occurred in lumbar region, 12% in the erector spinae muscles and 6% in quadratum lumborum region. Event type, mechanism of injury and severity are not different between men and women [46, 47, 48, 49].

An important injury to be mentioned is Spinal Chord Injury (SCI). It is an uncommon event but, even if it is a rare injury, its substantial emotional and physical repercussions make the mention of it fundamental [68].

Other spine diseases (like lumbar or cervical disc herniation and spondylolistesis) may occur in soccer players. Since they are extremely rare (<1% of all injuries), obtaining reliable data about their frequency and risk factors is difficult [6].

As for spinal fractures, 15% of all of them are sports-related. Their frequency in soccer players is relatively low (<1%) but their impact in terms of

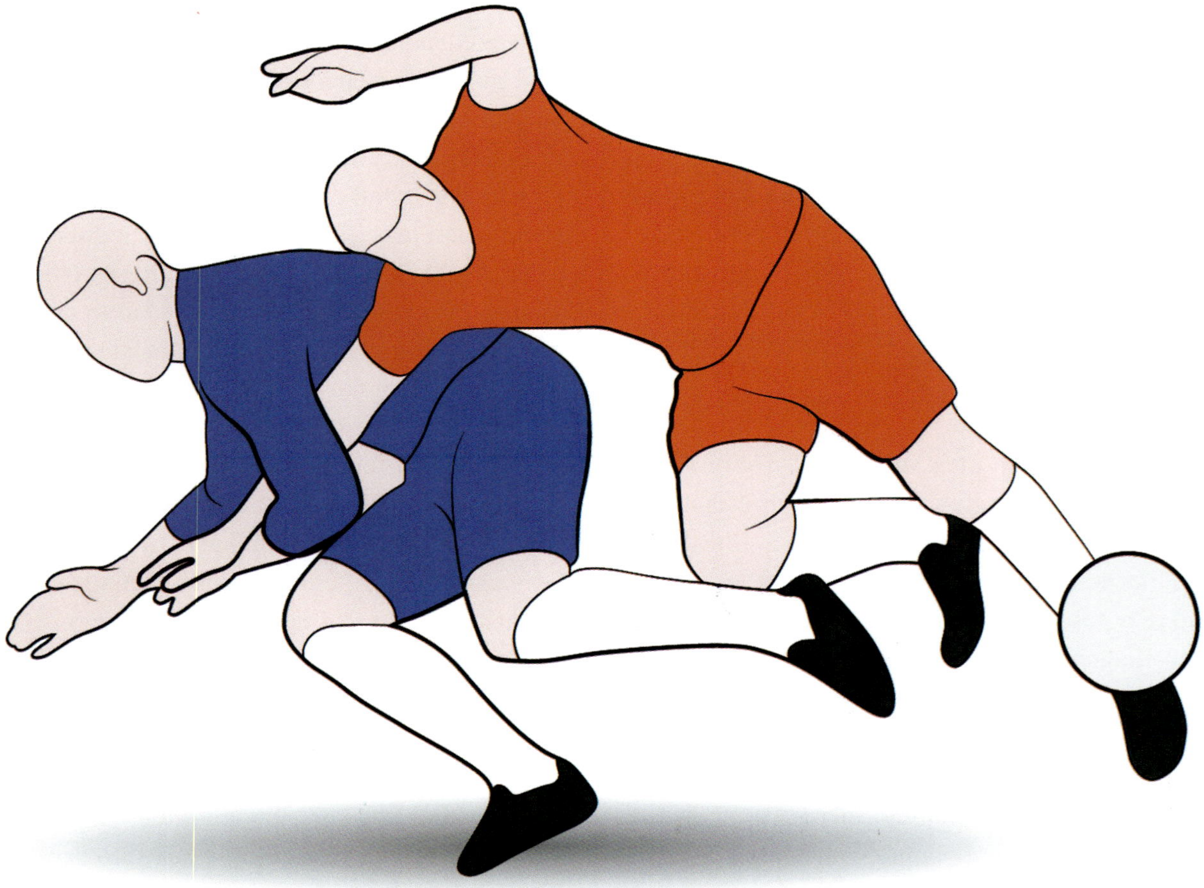

Figure 2 - A drawing of Mohammed Salah's mechanism of shoulder injury during the Champions League final of 2018

time-loss and outcome is often high. Their mechanism is usually a direct trauma (due to a contact with another player or a fall) [6, 47].

Shoulder injury

The majority of upper extremity injuries in professional soccer players are shoulder injuries [50]. Their frequency is approximately 13.20 per 10,000 game hours, most commonly acromioclavicular separation (29.9%), anterior shoulder subluxation (9.0%), shoulder contusion (9.0%), and rotator cuff tear/sprain (8.0%). Competition has an eight times higher incidence than practice [6, 51].

Shoulder instability (with all its different etiologies) comprises 28.1% of all upper extremity injuries; in terms of mechanism, it usually (56% of the cases) occurs with a high energy trauma in the position of combined humeral abduction and external rotation against a force of external rotation and horizontal extension (fig. 2) [51].

The goalkeepers are five-six times more prone to shoulder disorders than other field players [50, 52]. Even if shoulder injuries are not as common as lower limb injuries, a third of them can be classified as severe because the player stops his/her participation in training and games for >28 days [51, 52]. Ekstrand et al. [53] reported that shoulder dislocation represents the most severe upper extremity injury with a mean of 41 days of absence from the field. This absence from full training and games is of course longer (about 150% longer) for goalkeepers than for outfield players.

Elbow injury

The elbow is a complex joint that is crucial for effective transmission of forces from the shoulder to the hand. Although the incidence of elbow instability is low in the general population, such injuries are common in athletes and are frequently observed in contact sports like soccer. Given the complexity and serious implications of elbow injuries, knowing their incidence and risk factors is of crucial importance. It is reported that 10% of all upper extremity injuries in professional soccer players are elbow injuries, of which 19% are considered severe injuries and require more than 28 days of absence from playing soccer [50, 53, 54]. The most common of those injuries is medial collateral ligament (MCL) sprain and olecranon bursitis. The overall incidence of elbow diseases in soccer players is 0.04 per 10,000 game hours [55]. The mechanism is usually player-to-player contact or a fall on the palm of the hand with the arm extended. Posterolateral is the most common type of elbow dislocation [54].

Wrist and hand disease

According to Ekstrand et al. [53], 5% of all upper extremity injuries are wrist injuries; of those, only 2% are considered severe (requiring >28 days of absence from the field). The most common wrist injuries in soccer, which is considered a high-impact sport, are fractures (distal radius, scaphoid, capitate), whilst the less reported ones are dislocations (lunate, perilunate) and ligamentous injuries or tears (scapholunate ligament). A typical injury scenario would be a player falling on an outstretched hand and sustaining a scaphoid fracture during a match or training session [50, 53].

The hand is involved in 25% of upper extremity injuries in professional soccer players. A quarter of them are classified as severe injuries.

Specifically, hand metacarpal and phalanx fractures are the most common reported injuries in sports in general and, alone, they account for 14% of all upper extremity injuries in professional soccer players. The period of absence from soccer is four times longer in goalkeepers respect to outfielders because, of course, goalkeepers require a perfectly functional hand to play, whereas an outfielder can play with protection on the injured area [50, 53].

An example of a common hand injury is the so called "Mallet finger" injury (fig. 3): it can be observed in goalkeepers and it is caused by a flexion force on the tip of the finger while the distal interphalangeal (DIP) joint is extended. This force results in tearing of the extensor tendon and an avulsion fracture at the tendinous attachment on the dorsal lip of the distal phalangeal base. The classic mechanism of injury is an extended finger struck on the tip by a ball [50].

Hip and groin injury

The hip/groin is referred to as "the region between the front of the hip and the inner front of the thigh" [56]. Groin pain causes can be classi-

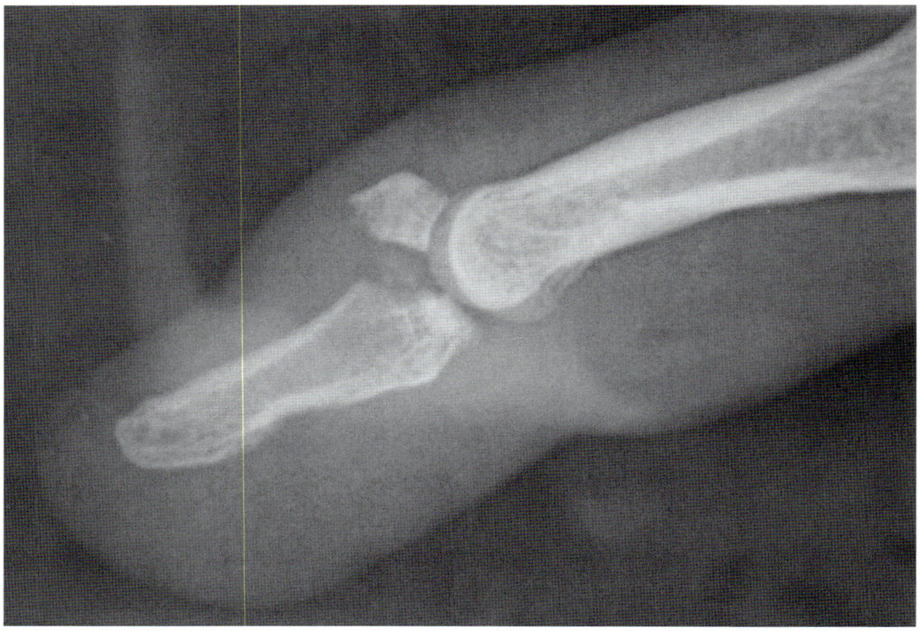

Figure 3 - Classic mallet finger lesion in a goalkeeper

fied into three different categories, based on the Doha agreement [57].

1. Defined clinical entities (adductor-related, iliopsoas-related).

2. Hip-related groin pain (hip morphologic abnormalities, labral tears, chondral injuries).

3. Other causes.

While they are not a cause of groin pain, proximal hamstring and gluteal and piriformis injuries are important causes of posterior and lateral hip pain in soccer players.

The epidemiology of hip/groin diseases in athletes is very complex. We will follow the Doha agreement classification in order to analyze all the injuries and diseases [57, 58].

1. Defined clinical entities. Acute groin pain in soccer players is most commonly caused by muscle strain: 66% of them involve the adductor longus, 25% the iliopsoas, and 9% other muscles. Adductor longus strains in soccer players are typically noncontact injuries (62.5%) and the average playing time lost is 2 weeks. As for the iliopsoas, a strain usually results from an impact that causes eccentric overload while kicking the ball [58, 59, 60]. In the 9% of other causes we find hamstring, rectus femoris, gluteal, and piriformis injuries [59].

2. Hip-related groin pain has previously been an underdiagnosed entity; it is now gaining more and more attention after one study found that practitioners treated groin pain in athletes for 7 months on average before recognizing that the pathology was intra-articular [60]. The most frequent intra-articular causes of groin pain in athletes are: femoral-acetabular impingement (FAI), labral tears, and chondral injuries.

3. Other causes: inguinal or femoral hernia, nerve entrapment, avulsion fracture of anterior superior/inferior iliac spine.

Langhout et al. [36] observed 525 players from 35 teams for one season and they found out that hip and groin injuries had a high preseason (27%) and within season (40%) prevalence. Moreover, more than half of those injuries are recurrent or chronic. They also found out that non-time-loss rates (63%) were almost double that time-loss rates (37%), which is in line with previous studies [6, 30, 31].

All those data make the importance of this pathology clear, because of its high frequency, its recurrence, and the difficult differential diagnosis.

Knee ligament injury

Multiple reports refer that almost one fifth of all soccer-related injuries presenting to the emergency room involve the knee [61, 62]. The majority of these injuries are non-contact injuries and they often involve ligaments or cartilage.

Anterior Cruciate Ligament (ACL) lesions may occur via contact or noncontact mechanisms; noncontact contribute to about 85% of injuries. Typical noncontact mechanism of injury involves

a forceful valgus collapse with the knee near full extension and combined external or internal rotation of the tibia (fig. 4).
Some risk factors for this injury in soccer are non-modifiable (such as age and gender) and others are modifiable (level of conditioning, force, balance, and flexibility). Importantly, gender has been reported to play a significant role as risk factor for ACL injury. In fact, female players have a 3 to 5 times higher risk of significant knee injury, including ACL injuries, than male players [21, 22, 61, 62].
Lateral and Medial Collateral Ligaments (MCL and LCL) injuries are less common than ACL injuries: their frequency is between 2 and 3% of all time-loss soccer-related injuries. Medial Collateral Ligament is more frequently involved (75% of cases) and the injury is usually due to a contact between two players (tackling or being tackled) [6].
Posterior Cruciate Ligament injuries are rare (only 33-40% of these occur during sport, while the others are related to motor vehicle accidents). The mechanism of injury during sport generally involves a fall onto the hyperflexed knee with the foot in plantar-flexion or a direct blow to the anterior tibia in a flexed knee [63, 64].

Foot and ankle lesions

The ankle is the second most commonly injured joint in soccer (the first being the knee). Ankle sprains specifically are a very common occurrence in this sport, followed by bruises/contusions and tendon lesions. Fractures are very rare (1%) in soccer, but when they do occur they impart a much more extended recovery [66, 67, 68, 69].
Soccer places an extremely high demand on both the foot and ankle structures when compared with other sports. Injury to the lateral ligaments of the ankle represents 77% to 91% of all ankle sprains in soccer. The main risk factor for an ankle sprain in soccer players is a history of prior sprain.
Considering the medial side, striking the ball requires the player to abduct and externally rotate the foot, which preloads medial structures. Pronation with eversion and extreme rotational injuries are well known to cause deltoid ligament injury (fig. 5). However, complete rupture of the deltoid ligament is very rare, and it usually occurs in association with ankle fractures [66, 68].

Cartilage and meniscal lesions

Articular cartilage injury in athletes may occur in two separate pathways.
1. Catabolic enzymes and cytokines, fragmentation of collagen and fissuring of the articular surface are the consequences of chronic repetitive loading of the articular cartilage and they lead to

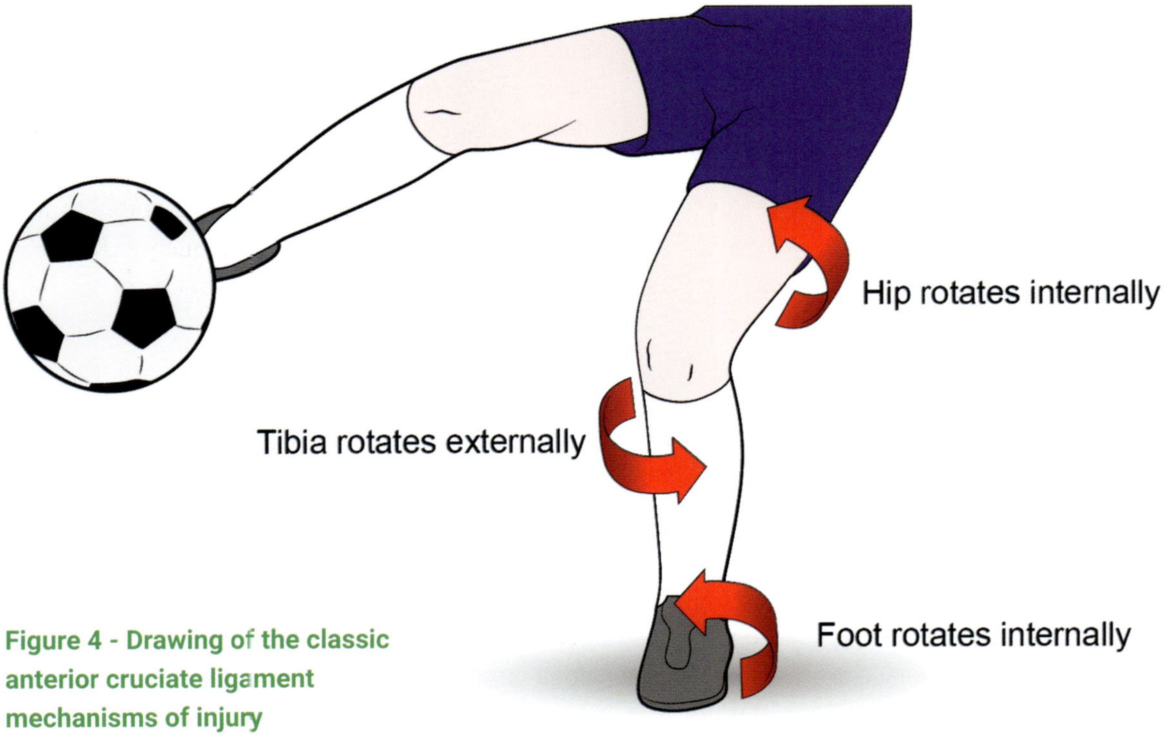

Figure 4 - Drawing of the classic anterior cruciate ligament mechanisms of injury

its degradation [61].
2. Acute traumatic cartilage injuries (often in association with ligament/meniscal lesions or dislocations). They can present with a spectrum of severity (acute chondral and osteochondral defects or ultrastructural injury with disruption of collagen and proteoglycan network).
In soccer, injury to articular cartilage occurs in approximately one third of athletes, which is more of the double of the general population risk [6].
Meniscal tears are the most common acute cartilage injuries; consistent with ACL injuries, female players are at least twice as likely to sustain a meniscal tear. Meniscal damage can occur in isolation or in association with ACL rupture [61].
Osteochondral lesions (OCLs) are the most common ankle articular cartilage injury and they occur in up to 50% of acute ankle sprains; their frequency is 5.2 injuries per 10,000 game hours [6, 71]. They are cartilage-bone defects that are usually located in the talus. They can be due to an acute traumatic event or repetitive microtrauma with no apparent history of trauma (ankle instability).

Tendon lesions

The prevalence of tendinopathies in soccer players has not been well examined so far; the probability of a player to sustain a tendon injury during his career is about 5% in women and 13% in men [71, 72].
One of the most common tendinopathies is Patellar Tendinopathy (PT); although mainly mild in nature, it is often a recurrent complaint (with a high risk to develop a chronic disease). PT is more frequent in youth players than in adults, with a frequency of 16-17% [72, 73].
Considering the ankle, a mechanism of both dorsiflexion and inversion may cause injury to the superior peroneal retinaculum with reflex contraction of the peroneal muscles and subluxation or dislocation of the contained tendons (peroneus brevis and longus) [66].
Another common location of tendon injury is Achilles tendon rupture, with a prevalence of 4% among professional soccer players [73, 74].

Non musculoskeletal soccer injuries

Sudden cardiac death

Though rare, sport-related deaths have considerable public significance and impact [75]. Sudden cardiac death (SCD) is defined as any witnessed death occurring unexpectedly within 1 hour of the onset of symptoms, or any unwitnessed death occurring within 24 hours of having been seen alive and asymptomatic.
Soccer is a demanding sport: during a 90 min game,

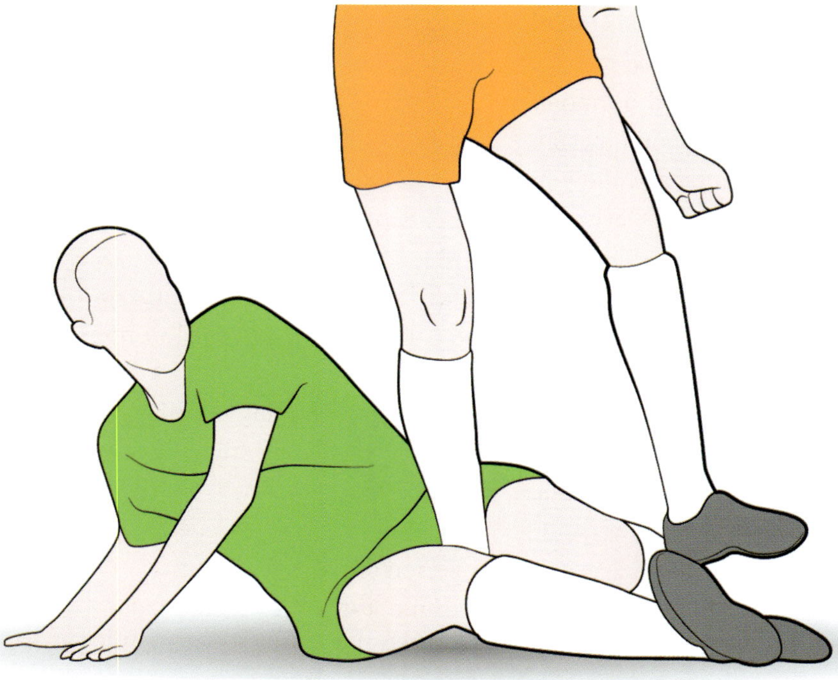

Figure 5 - Typical mechanism of tackle-related ankle injury

professional players run about 10 km at high intensities (close to the anaerobic threshold, at 80% to 90% of maximal heart rate) and with numerous explosive bursts (jumping, sprinting) [76]. Thus, active players with undetected cardiovascular abnormalities may be at risk for exertional SCD.
In fact, coronary artery disease seems to be a leading cause of SCD in young soccer players (<35 years of age). The potential pathophysiological mechanisms include increased catecholamine release and platelet aggregation, electrolyte abnormalities and dehydration [77].
Diseases that are associated with SCD have been identified in 0.38% of adolescent soccer players who underwent cardiovascular screening in the United Kingdom.
The incidence of SCD is estimated to be 1.04 per 100,000 athletes/year and the majority of these cases are due to cardiomyopathies, undetected on screening [78].

Overtraining syndrome and burnout

In sports, the health benefits of regular soccer practice and training have been demonstrated [80]. In addition, early specialization, such as performing only a specific type of sport throughout the year from early elementary school age, is progressing [81, 82]. Early specialization and overtraining increase the risks of overuse injuries and overtraining syndrome.
Overtraining Syndrome may be defined as "series of psychological, physiologic, and hormonal changes that result in decreased sports performance" which can have a detrimental effect on the athlete participating in sports. Its most common symptoms include chronic muscle or joint pain, personality changes, elevated resting heart rate, and decreased sports performance. The athlete may also have fatigue, lack of enthusiasm about practice or competition, or difficulty with successfully completing usual routines.
Burnout should be recognized as a severe sequela of overtraining syndrome. It has been defined to occur as a result of chronic stress that causes an athlete to cease participation in a previously enjoyable activity. Data suggest that athletes who had early specialized training withdrew from their sport due to either an injury or a burnout [83, 84].

Risk factors for injuries

In order to prevent injury, the factors that contribute to it must be identified. Once they have been identified, studies need to test just which of them are significant predictors of injury. After the significant risk factors have been identified, prevention programs can be designed.
As opposed to external influences, the primary player-related risk factors in risk assessment are psychological components. It had been shown that they not only affect the overall performance of a player, but also his/her injury risk [85].
The results reported by all the authors who studied the topic are in general that "life events" can influence the risk of injury in athletes. In most cases, some major life event preceded an injury or was related to the severity of injury [6, 85, 86].
After demonstrating the existence of the psychological component as a risk factor, the F-MARC [6] undertook a prospective project, following 400 elite players for one year. As a result, they identified 17 other player-related risk factors for soccer injuries; the more the risk factors, the more likely the risk of injury (fig. 6).

1. Number of previous injuries
2. Wearing bandages to cure acute injuries
3. Pain in the joints
4. Age of beginning soccer (beginning when >6yrs is considered a risk factor)
5. Did not begin soccer in a club
6. Recently changed to another club
7. Body fat proportion
8. Smoking
9. Drinking alcohol (more than 2 days per week)
10. Reaction time
11. Life-event stress
12. Poor muscular warm-up
13. Endurance (pulse >135 bpm 5 minutes after a 12 min run)
14. Poor self rating in dribbling or passing
15. Being more a "fighter" than technician
16. Exhausted or aching muscles before the game
17. Not enough regeneration during preparation period (1 day/week or less)

While F-MARC focused more on personal and technical history of players, Ekstrand's analysis of risk factors [87] is based on players' age, position and kind of exposition (game vs training hours).

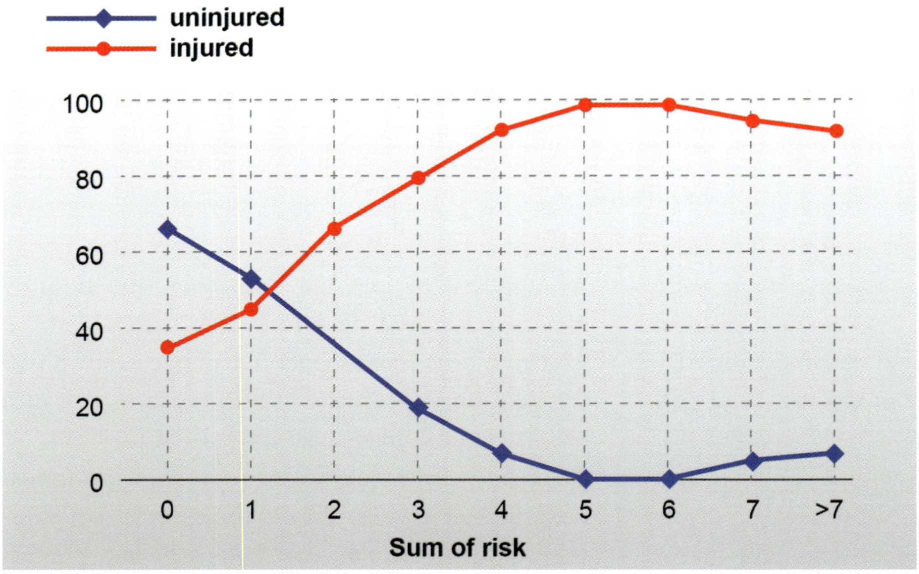

Figure 6 - Proportion of uninjured and injured players in relationship to the sum of risk factors, according to the F-MARC [6]

They reached complementary conclusions, adding five important risk factors to F-MARC study.

1. Match hours [6, 87]
2. End of each half [6, 22, 87]
3. Being a forward [3, 13, 87]
4. Previous injuries [5, 6]
5. Being <17 yrs [88]

It is well known [5, 6, 13, 87] that when a player had previous injuries the risk of subsequent injury becomes higher; some studies say it becomes 4 to 7 times higher [5, 87].

With but a few exceptions, if a player had five or more risk factors, he suffered another injury during season.

Another important aspect to be considered is that the more baseline risk factors, the more severe the injury [6, 13, 87, 88].

From all those data we understand the importance of epidemiology: analyzing the determinants of disease conditions in soccer players can help clubs developing prevention programs in order to have healthier and more performing players.

Long-term sequelae

Osteoarthritis

The prevalence of osteoarthritis (OA) in retired soccer players is higher than in unexposed people. The magnitudes of association are relatively large: those in elite soccer have a 3 to 7 times higher prevalence than in unexposed persons [13, 61, 70].

Articular cartilage degeneration with subsequent OA occurs in up to 32% of soccer players and leads to significant disability and retirement from the sport. High physical demands and concomitant knee injuries probably predispose to the development of posttraumatic OA [2, 61].

Soccer might increase the risk for low extremity OA in two different ways. First, by the increased risk for knee injuries, such as meniscus and ACL injuries, and second, by the high loading on hip and knee joints that occurs in soccer, especially in high-level soccer.

Brain impairment

Acute concussion, repetitive concussions, and cumulative "sub-concussive" head impacts may increase the risk of developing cognitive and behavioral deficits for athletes, as well as accelerated cerebral degeneration. Heading, as a repeat sub-concussive impact, has been linked to structural brain changes and neurocognitive impairment [44, 90].

Rodrigues and colleagues [90] conducted a neuropsychological examination (which included tests of attention, concentration, memory, and judgment) of soccer players' brain compared to controls, and demonstrated that 81% of the athletes had some degree of impairment, compared to 40% of the controls. They hypothesize that their findings probably reflect the cumulative result of repeated traumas from heading the ball.

Bibliography

1. Andersen TE, Tenga A, Engebretsen L, Bahr R. Video analysis of injuries and incidents in Norwegian professional football. Br J Sports Med. 2004 Oct;38(5):626-31.
2. Roos H. Are there long-term sequelae from soccer? Clin Sports Med. 1998 Oct;17(4):819-31.
3. Drawer S, Fuller CW. Evaluating the level of injury in English professional football using a risk based assessment process. Br J Sports Med. 2002 Dec;36(6):446-51.
4. Ekstrand J, Dvorak J, D'Hooghe M. Sport medicine research needs funding: the International football federations are leading the way. Br J Sports Med. 2013 Aug;47(12):726-8.
5. Pfirrmann D, Herbst M, Ingelfinger P, Simon P, Tug S. Analysis of Injury Incidences in Male Professional Adult and Elite Youth Soccer Players: A Systematic Review. J Athl Train. 2016 May;51(5):410-24.
6. Dvorak J, Junge A F-MARC - Football for Health 20 years of F-MARC Research and Education 1994 – 2014.
7. Hawkins RD, Hulse MA, Wilkinson C, Hodson A, Gibson M. The association football medical research programme: an audit of injuries in professional football. Br J Sports Med. 2001 Feb;35(1):43-7.
8. Fuller CW, Ekstrand J, Junge A, Andersen TE, Bahr R, Dvorak J, Hägglund M, McCrory P, Meeuwisse WH. Consensus statement on injury definitions and data collection procedures in studies of football (soccer) injuries. Clin J Sport Med. 2006 Mar;16(2):97-106.
9. Brenner JS; American Academy of Pediatrics Council on Sports Medicine and Fitness. Overuse injuries, overtraining, and burnout in child and adolescent athletes. Pediatrics. 2007 Jun;119(6):1242-5.
10. Nogueira M, Laiginhas R, Ramos J, Costa O. Injuries in Portuguese Amateur Youth Football Players: A Six Month Prospective Descriptive Study. Acta Med Port. 2017 Dec 29;30(12):840-847.
11. Junge A, Dvorak J. Soccer injuries: a review on incidence and prevention. Sports Med. 2004;34(13):929-38.
12. Hägglund M, Waldén M, Ekstrand J. Injury incidence and distribution in elite football: a prospective study of the Danish and the Swedish top divisions. Scand J Med Sci Sports. 2005 Feb;15(1):21-8.
13. Della Villa F, Mandelbaum BR, Lemak LJ. The Effect of Playing Position on Injury Risk in Male Soccer Players: Systematic Review of the Literature and Risk Considerations for Each Playing Position. Am J Orthop (Belle Mead NJ). 2018 Oct;47(10).
14. FIFA Communications Division. FIFA Big Count 2006: 270 million people active in football. Zurich: FIFA; 2007.
15. Price RJ, Hawkins RD, Hulse MA, Hodson A. The Football Association medical research programme: an audit of injuries in academy youth football. Br J Sports Med. 2004 Aug;38(4):466-71.
16. Ergün M, Denerel HN, Binnet MS, Ertat KA. Injuries in elite youth football players: a prospective three-year study. Acta Orthop Traumatol Turc. 2013;47(5):339-46.
17. Junge A, Chomiak J, Dvorak J. Incidence of football injuries in youth players. Comparison of players from two European regions. Am J Sports Med. 2000;28(5Suppl):S47-50.
18. Faude O, Rößler R, Junge A. Football injuries in children and adolescent players: are there clues for prevention? Sports Med. 2013 Sep;43(9):819-37.
19. Giannotti M, Al-Sahab B, McFaull S, Tamim H. Epidemiology of acute soccer injuries in Canadian children and youth. Pediatr Emerg Care. 2011 Feb;27(2):81-5.
20. Fédération Internationale de Football Association (FIFA). Women's Football Survey. Zurich: FIFA; 2014.
21. Faude O, Junge A, Kindermann W, Dvorak J. Injuries in female soccer players: a prospective study in the German national league. Am J Sports Med. 2005 Nov;33(11):1694-700.
22. Del Coso J, Herrero H, Salinero JJ. Injuries in Spanish female soccer players. J Sport Health Sci. 2018 Apr;7(2):183-190.
23. Sutton KM, Bullock JM. Anterior cruciate ligament rupture: differences between males and females. J Am Acad Orthop Surg. 2013 Jan;21(1):41-50.
24. Stijak L, Kadija M, Djulejić V, Aksić M, Petronijević N, Marković B, Radonjić V, Bumbaširević M, Filipović B. The influence of sex hormones on anterior cruciate ligament rupture: female study. Knee Surg Sports Traumatol Arthrosc. 2015 Sep;23(9):2742-9
25. Aoki H, O'Hata N, Kohno T, Morikawa T, Seki J. A 15-year prospective epidemiological account of acute traumatic injuries during official professional soccer league matches in Japan. Am J Sports Med. 2012 May;40(5):1006-14.
26. Andersen TE, Larsen Ø, Tenga A, Engebretsen L, Bahr R. Football incident analysis: a new video based method to describe injury mechanisms in professional football. Br J Sports Med. 2003 Jun;37(3):226-32.
27. Arliani GG, Lara PHS, Astur DC, Pedrinelli A, Pagura JR, Cohen M. Orthopaedics injuries in male professional football players in Brazil: a prospective comparison between two divisions. Muscles Ligaments Tendons J. 2018 Jan10;7(3):524-531.
28. Ekstrand J, Hägglund M, Törnqvist H, Kristenson K, Bengtsson H, Magnusson H, Waldén M. Upper extremity injuries in male elite football players. Knee Surg Sports Traumatol Arthrosc. 2013 Jul;21(7):1626-32.
29. Waldén M, Krosshaug T, Bjørneboe J, Andersen TE, Faul O, Hägglund M. Three distinct mechanisms predominate in non-contact anterior cruciate ligament injuries in male professional football players: a systematic video analysis of 39 cases. Br J Sports Med. 2015 Nov;49(22):1452-60.
30. Deehan DJ, Bell K, McCaskie AW. Adolescent musculoskeletal injuries in a football academy. J Bone Joint Surg Br. 2007 Jan;89(1):5-8.
31. Cloke D, Moore O, Shah T, Rushton S, Shirley MD, Deehan DJ. Thigh muscle injuries in youth soccer: predictors of recovery. Am J Sports Med. 2012 Feb;40(2):433-9.
32. Carling C, Orhant E, LeGall F. Match injuries in professional soccer: inter-seasonal variation and effects of competition type, match congestion and positional role. Int J Sports Med. 2010 Apr;31(4):271-6.
33. Leventer L, Eek F, Lames M. Intra-seasonal variation of injury patterns among German Bundesliga soccer players. J Sci Med Sport. 2019 Jun;22(6):661-666.
34. Junge A, Dvorak J. Soccer injuries: a review on incidence and prevention. Sports Med. 2004;34(13):929-38.
35. Wong P, Hong Y. Soccer injury in the lower extremities. Br J Sports Med. 2005 Aug;39(8):473-82.
36. Langhout R, Weir A, Litjes W, Gozeling M, Stubbe JH, Kerkhoffs G, Tak I. Hip and groin injury is the most common non-time-loss injury in female amateur football. Knee Surg Sports Traumatol Arthrosc. 2018 Jun 2.
37. Bobian MR, Hanba CJ, Svider PF, Hojjat H, Folbe AJ, Eloy JA, Shkoukani MA. Soccer-Related Facial Trauma: A Nationwide Perspective. Ann Otol Rhinol Laryngol. 2016 Dec;125(12):992-996.
38. Romeo SJ, Hawley CJ, Romeo MW, Romeo JP. Facial Injuries in Sports: A Team Physician's Guide to Diagnosis and

Treatment. Phys Sportsmed. 2005 Apr;33(4):45-53.
39. Kim SY, Chan CL, Hyam DM. Facial fractures in football: incidence, site, and mechanism of injury. Br J Oral Maxillofac Surg. 2016 Oct;54(8):936-940.
40. Cerulli G, Carboni A, Mercurio A, Perugini M, Becelli R. Soccer-related craniomaxillofacial injuries. J Craniofac Surg. 2002 Sep;13(5):627-30.
41. McCrory P, Feddermann-Demont N, Dvořák J, Cassidy JD, McIntosh A, Vos PE, Echemendia RJ, Meeuwisse W, Tarnutzer AA. What is the definition of sports-related concussion: a systematic review. Br J Sports Med. 2017Jun;51(11):877-887.
42. Gouttebarge V, Cowie C, Goedhart E, Kemp SPT, Kerkhoffs GMMJ, Patricios J, Stokes KA. Educational concussion module for professional footballers: from systematic development to feasibility and effect. BMJ Open Sport Exerc Med. 2019 Mar 7;5(1):e000490.
43. Chandran A, Barron MJ, Westerman BJ, DiPietro L. Multifactorial examination of sex-differences in head injuries and concussions among collegiate soccer players: NCAA ISS, 2004-2009. Inj Epidemiol. 2017 Oct 25;4(1):28.
44. Hubertus V, Marklund N, Vajkoczy P. Management of concussion in soccer. Acta Neurochir (Wien). 2019 Mar;161(3):425-433.
45. Delaney JS, Lacroix VJ, Leclerc S, Johnston KM. Concussions among university football and soccer players. Clin J Sport Med. 2002 Nov;12(6):331-8.
46. Donatelli R, Dimond D, Holland M. Sport-specific biomechanics of spinal injuries in the athlete (throwing athletes, rotational sports, and contact-collision sports). Clin Sports Med. 2012 Jul;31(3):381-96.
47. Hassebrock JD, Patel KA, Makovicka JL, Chung AS, Tummala SV, Peña AJ, Williams KE, Hartigan DE, Chhabra A. Lumbar Spine Injuries in National Collegiate Athletic Association Athletes: A 6-Season Epidemiological Study. Orthop J Sports Med. 2019Jan 23;7(1):2325967118820046.
48. Chan CW, Eng JJ, Tator CH, Krassioukov A; Spinal Cord Injury Research Evidence Team. Epidemiology of sport-related spinal cord injuries: A systematic review. J Spinal Cord Med. 2016 May;39(3):255-64.
49. Shah T, Cloke DJ, Rushton S, Shirley MD, Deehan DJ. Lower Back Symptoms in Adolescent Soccer Players: Predictors of Functional Recovery. Orthop J Sports Med. 2014 Apr 17;2(4):2325967114529703.
50. Marom N, Williams RJ 3rd. Upper Extremity Injuries in Soccer. Am J Orthop (Belle Mead NJ). 2018 Oct;47(10).
51. Goodman AD, Raducha JE, DeFroda SF, Gil JA, Owens BD. Shoulder and elbow injuries in NCAA football players, 2009-2010 through 2013-2014. Phys Sportsmed. 2018 Dec 4.
52. Terra BB, Ejnisman B, Figueiredo EA, Andreoli CV, Pochini AC, Cohen C, Arliani GG, Cohen M. Arthroscopic treatment of glenohumeral instability in soccer goalkeepers. Int J Sports Med. 2013 Jun;34(6):473-6.
53. Ekstrand J, Hägglund M, Törnqvist H, Kristenson K, Bengtsson H, Magnusson H, Waldén M. Upper extremity injuries in male elite football players. Knee Surg Sports Traumatol Arthrosc. 2013 Jul;21(7):1626-32.
54. Rahman RK, Levine WN, Ahmad CS. Elbow medial collateral ligament injuries. Curr Rev Musculoskelet Med. 2008 Dec;1(3-4):197-204.
55. Goodman AD, Lemme N, DeFroda SF, Gil JA, Owens BD. Elbow Dislocation and Subluxation Injuries in the National Collegiate Athletic Association, 2009-2010 Through 2013-2014. Orthop J Sports Med. 2018 Jan 16;6(1):2325967117750105.
56. Rae K, Orchard J. The Orchard Sports Injury Classification System (OSICS) version 10. Clin J Sport Med. 2007 May;17(3):201-4.
57. Weir A, Brukner P, Delahunt E, Ekstrand J, Griffin D, Khan KM, Lovell G,Meyers WC, Muschaweck U, Orchard J, Paajanen H, Philippon M, Reboul G, Robinson P, Schache AG, Schilders E, Serner A, Silvers H, Thorborg K, Tyler T, Verrall G, de Vos RJ, Vuckovic Z, Hölmich P. Doha agreement meeting on terminology and definitions in groin pain in athletes. Br J Sports Med. 2015 Jun;49(12):768-74.
58. Serner A, Tol JL, Jomaah N, Weir A, Whiteley R, Thorborg K, Robinson M,Hölmich P. Diagnosis of Acute Groin Injuries: A Prospective Study of 110 Athletes. Am J Sports Med. 2015 Aug;43(8):1857-64.
59. Sherman B, Chahla J, Hutchinson W, Gerhardt M. Hip and Core Muscle Injuries in Soccer. Am J Orthop (Belle Mead NJ). 2018 Oct;47(10).
60. Eckard TG, Padua DA, Dompier TP, Dalton SL, Thorborg K, Kerr ZY. Epidemiology of Hip Flexor and Hip Adductor Strains in National Collegiate Athletic Association Athletes, 2009/2010-2014/2015. Am J Sports Med. 2017 Oct;45(12):2713-2722.
61. Roth TS, Osbahr DC. Knee Injuries in Elite Level Soccer Players. Am J Orthop (Belle Mead NJ). 2018 Oct;47(10).
62. Agel J, Rockwood T, Klossner D. Collegiate ACL Injury Rates Across 15 Sports: National Collegiate Athletic Association Injury Surveillance System Data Update (2004-2005 Through 2012-2013). Clin J Sport Med. 2016 Nov;26(6):518-523.
63. Fanelli GC, Edson CJ. Posterior cruciate ligament injuries in trauma patients: Part II. Arthroscopy. 1995 Oct;11(5):526-9.
64. Schulz MS, Russe K, Weiler A, Eichhorn HJ, Strobel MJ. Epidemiology of posterior cruciate ligament injuries. Arch Orthop Trauma Surg. 2003 May;123(4):186-91.
65. Waldén M, Hägglund M, Ekstrand J. UEFA Champions League study: a prospective study of injuries in professional football during the 2001-2002 season. Br J Sports Med. 2005 Aug;39(8):542-6.
66. Feria-Arias E, Boukhemis K, Kreulen C, Giza E. Foot and Ankle Injuries in Soccer. Am J Orthop (Belle Mead NJ). 2018 Oct;47(10).
67. Cloke DJ, Spencer S, Hodson A, Deehan D. The epidemiology of ankle injuries occurring in English Football Association academies. Br J Sports Med. 2009 Dec;43(14):1119-25.
68. Chomiak J, Junge A, Peterson L, Dvorak J. Severe injuries in football players. Influencing factors. Am J Sports Med. 2000;28(5 Suppl):S58-68.
69. Cloke DJ, Ansell P, Avery P, Deehan D. Ankle injuries in football academies: a three-centre prospective study. Br J Sports Med. 2011 Jul;45(9):702-8.
70. Mithoefer K, Peterson L, Zenobi-Wong M, Mandelbaum BR. Cartilage issues in football-today's problems and tomorrow's solutions. Br J Sports Med. 2015 May;49(9):590-6.
71. Shimozono Y, Yasui Y, Ross AW, Kennedy JG. Osteochondral lesions of the talus in the athlete: up to date review. Curr Rev Musculoskelet Med. 2017 Mar;10(1):131-140.
72. Bode G, Hammer T, Karvouniaris N, Feucht MJ, Konstantinidis L, Südkamp NP, Hirschmüller A. Patellar tendinopathy in young elite soccer- clinical and sonographical analysis of a German elite soccer academy. BMC Musculoskelet Disord. 2017 Aug 8;18(1):344.
73. Hägglund M, Zwerver J, Ekstrand J. Epidemiology of patellar tendinopathy in elite male soccer players. Am J Sports Med. 2011 Sep;39(9):1906-11.
74. Docking SI, Rio E, Cook J, Orchard JW, Fortington LV. The prevalence of Achilles and patellar tendon injuries in

Australian football players beyond a time-loss definition. Scand J Med Sci Sports. 2018 Sep;28(9):2016-2022.
75. Kucera KL, Fortington LV, Wolff CS, Marshall SW, Finch CF. Estimating the international burden of sport-related death: a review of data sources. Inj Prev. 2019 Apr;25(2):83-89.
76. Santos-Lozano A, Martín-Hernández J, Baladrón C, Turrado-Sevilla MÁ, Amarás-Flores Á, Villacastín JP, Boraita A, Bueno H, Lucia A. Sudden Cardiac Death in Professional Soccer Players. J Am Coll Cardiol. 2017 Sep 12;70(11):1420-1421.
77. Mavrogeni SI, Tsarouhas K, Spandidos DA, Kanaka-Gantenbein C, Bacopoulou F. Sudden cardiac death in football players: Towards a new pre-participation algorithm. Exp Ther Med. 2019 Feb;17(2):1143-1148.
78. Malhotra A, Dhutia H, Finocchiaro G, Gati S, Beasley I, Clift P, Cowie C, Kenny A, Mayet J, Oxborough D, Patel K, Pieles G, Rakhit D, Ramsdale D, Shapiro L, Somauroo J, Stuart G, Varnava A, Walsh J, Yousef Z, Tome M, Papadakis M, Sharma S. Outcomes of Cardiac Screening in Adolescent Soccer Players. N Engl J Med. 2018 Aug 9;379(6):524-534.
79. Mohananey D, Masri A, Desai RM, Dalal S, Phelan D, Kanj M, Wazni O, Griffin BP, Desai MY. Global Incidence of Sports-Related Sudden Cardiac Death. J Am Coll Cardiol. 2017 May 30;69(21):2672-2673.
80. Krustrup P, Nielsen JJ, Krustrup BR, Christensen JF, Pedersen H, Randers MB, Aagaard P, Petersen AM, Nybo L, Bangsbo J. Recreational soccer is an effective health-promoting activity for untrained men. Br J Sports Med. 2009 Oct;43(11):825-31.
81. Intensive training and sports specialization in young athletes. American Academy of Pediatrics. Committee on Sports Medicine and Fitness. Pediatrics. 2000 Jul;106(1 Pt 1):154-7.
82. Brenner JS; American Academy of Pediatrics Council on Sports Medicine and Fitness. Overuse injuries, overtraining, and burnout in child and adolescent athletes. Pediatrics. 2007 Jun;119(6):1242-5.
83. Patel DR, Omar H, Terry M. Sport-related performance anxiety in young female athletes. J Pediatr Adolesc Gynecol. 2010 Dec;23(6):325-35.
84. DiFiori JP, Benjamin HJ, Brenner JS, Gregory A, Jayanthi N, Landry GL, Luke A. Overuse injuries and burnout in youth sports: a position statement from the American Medical Society for Sports Medicine. Br J Sports Med. 2014 Feb;48(4):287-8.
85. Junge A. The influence of psychological factors on sports injuries. Review of the literature. Am J Sports Med. 2000;28(5 Suppl):S10-5.
86. Dvorak J, Junge A. Football injuries and physical symptoms. A review of the literature. Am J Sports Med. 2000;28(5 Suppl):S3-9.
87. Ekstrand J, Hägglund M, Waldén M. Epidemiology of muscle injuries in professional football (soccer). Am J Sports Med. 2011 Jun;39(6):1226-32.
88. Le Gall F, Carling C, Reilly T, Vandewalle H, Church J, Rochcongar P. Incidence of injuries in elite French youth soccer players: a 10-season study. Am J Sports Med. 2006 Jun;34(6):928-38.
89. Driban JB, Hootman JM, Sitler MR, Harris KP, Cattano NM. Is Participation in Certain Sports Associated With Knee Osteoarthritis? A Systematic Review. J Athl Train. 2017 Jun 2;52(6):497-506.
90. Rodrigues AC, Lasmar RP, Caramelli P. Effects of Soccer Heading on Brain Structure and Function. Front Neurol. 2016 Mar 21;7:38.

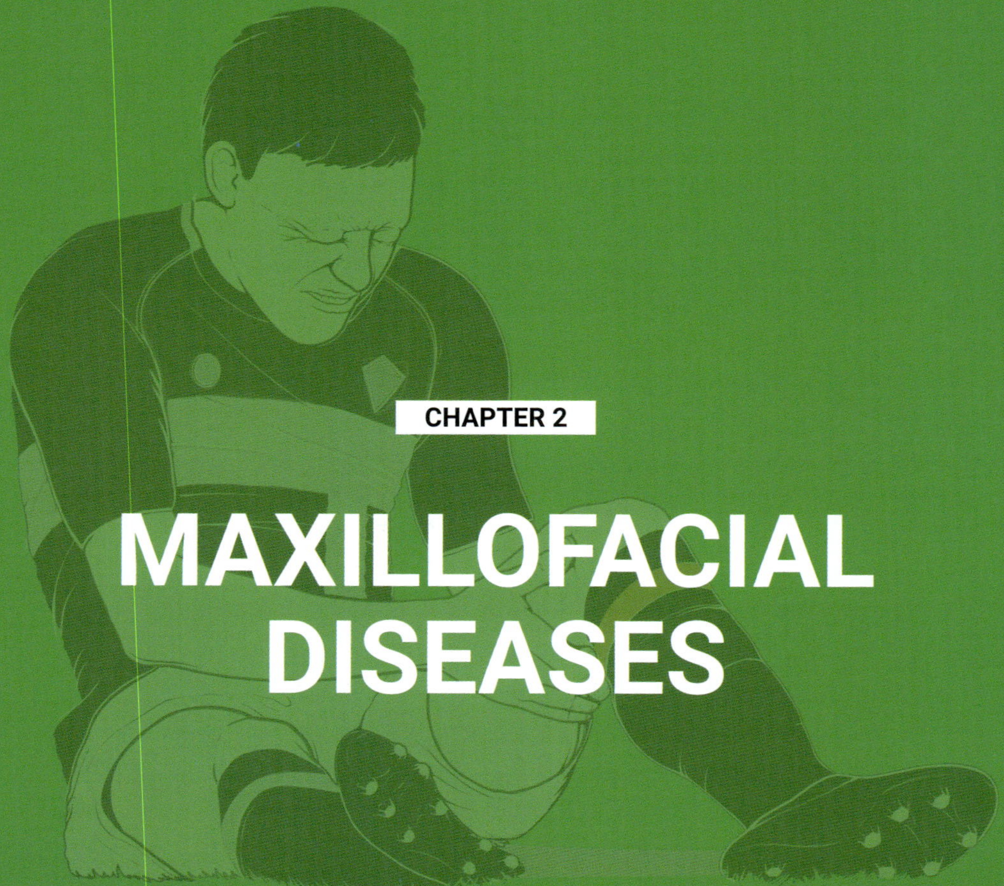

CHAPTER 2

MAXILLOFACIAL DISEASES

Claudio Marchetti
Francesco Ricotta
Liliana Feraboli

Oral and Maxillofacial Surgery Unit (Director: C. Marchetti)
St. Orsola-Malpighi Polyclinic, Bologna, Italy

Introduction

Team contact sports are popular in various cultures and countries. One of the most popular sports is soccer, and several studies have shown it to be a common source of maxillofacial sports-related trauma [1, 2]. Soccer is considered a high-risk game, especially with regard to the maxillofacial area; in fact, some of the main acts of the game (kick and header) are aggressive, repeated and can cause various injuries. It is estimated that, today, there are 120 million participants in this sport and the number is rapidly increasing; consequently also maxillofacial lesions are growing in frequency, influencing soccer in social and financial terms.

Sport-related traumas involving the maxillofacial district are associated in 73.9% of cases with soccer. The trauma in the maxillofacial area is a topic of considerable importance among professional soccer players, being 3% of all traumas [3, 4].

Sports accidents can occur in three ways: falling, impact with sports equipment, and violent contact between the players. The latter is the main cause of fractures, in fact, about 40% of fractures are due to direct impact (video 1).

According to the Peynègre and Strunski classification, there are three main maxillofacial regions that can be involved in traumatic events.

- Lower area: including the mandible and maxillary bone.
- Medial area: including the maxillary process, the nose, the ethmoid and the orbital cavity.
- Side area: including zygomatic body and arch (fig. 1).

In a series of European, Japanese, and Australian studies, the most frequently reported trauma was the fracture of the zygomatic complex [5, 6, 7]. This lesion can occur at the level of the zygomatic body, causing important aesthetic problems, or more commonly at the level of the zygomatic arch, with a higher risk of functional impairments (for example, limitation of the opening of the mouth).

For the mandibular lesions, the most commonly fractured site is the angle, because here the bone is weaker due to the common presence of impacted and semi-impacted third molars.

The head shot mainly causes fractures of the zygomatic complex, a considerable number of mandibular fractures, and most of the oral-facial lacerations. The impact of the elbow on another player's head is responsible for most fractures of the alveolar process (67%), temporomandibular joint (TMJ), and orbito-zygomatic lesions.

Nowadays, thanks to the rigid internal fixation, the healing time has been reduced. However, a period of 12 to 24 weeks should be considered in non-professional players and in all those activities where there is no direct contact between the players. In addition, in the case of professional soccer players, surgeons must give the opportunity to practice competitive sports during convalescence and guarantee adequate protection of the traumatized area.

VIDEO 1

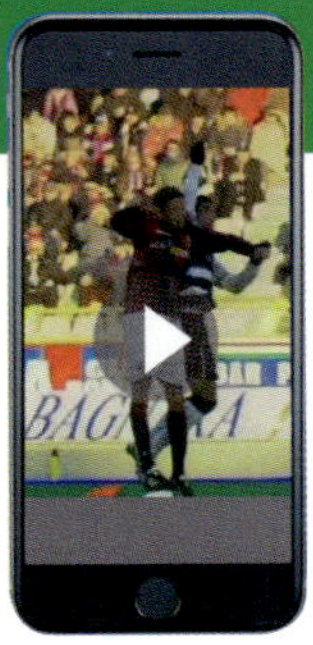

Example of direct trauma between players during a soccer match

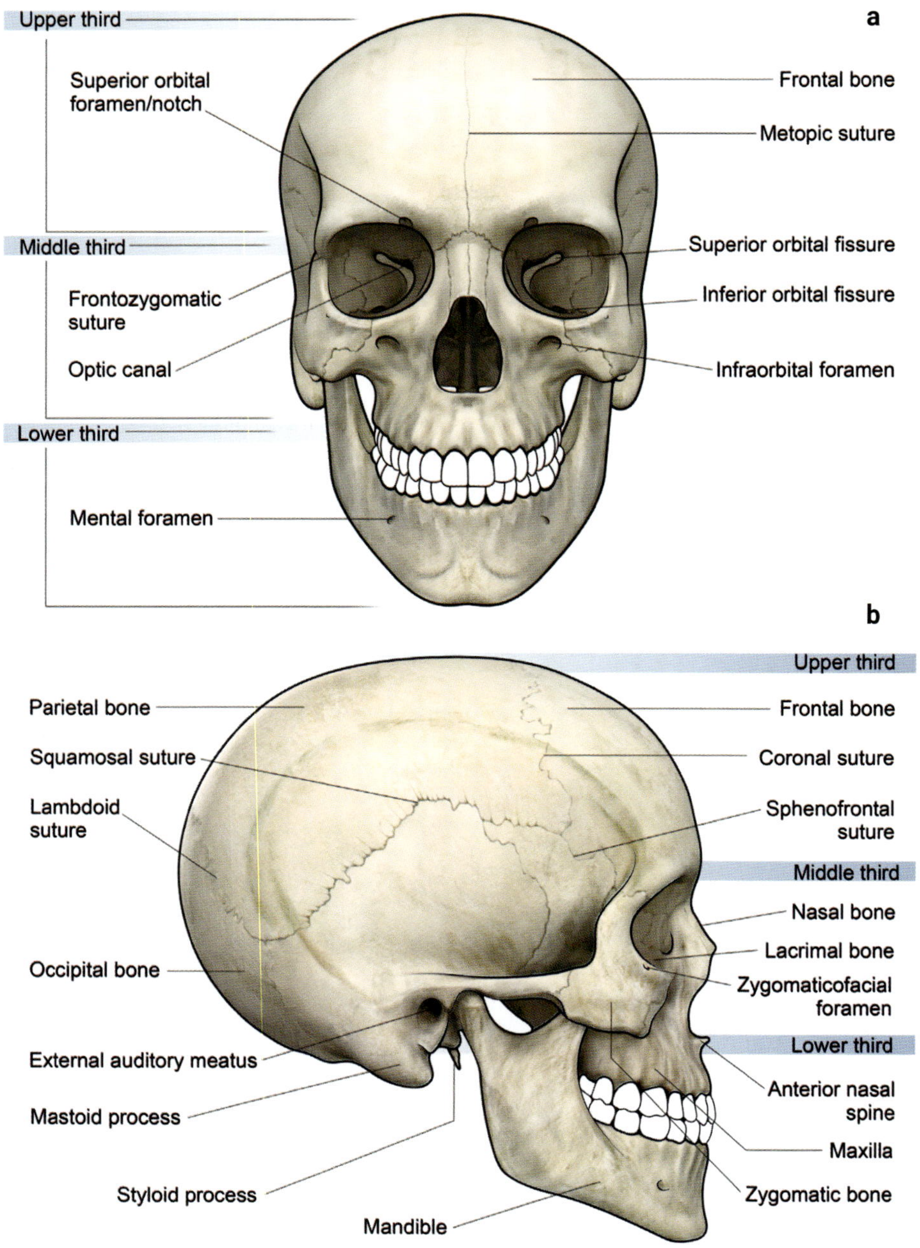

Figure 1 - Anatomy of the Skull. A: skull's frontal view; B: skull's lateral view

Alveolar and dental fractures

Dentoalveolar lesions occur most commonly in pediatric, adolescent, and adult populations. In the adult population, most injuries are caused by contact sports and playground activities. In fact, about a third of all dental trauma is secondary to sports accidents.

In recent years, the use of appropriate mouthguards and headgear has helped reduce sports-related injuries. However, in the case of soccer, this type of habit is not yet present, probably due to the need for a soccer player to use his head in the game.

Alveolar and dental trauma can occur in both anterior and posterior areas.

In the case of direct trauma (i.e. head to head impact, elbow to head impact, falls etc.), maxillary incisors are the most frequently involved teeth, especially if associated with a Class II Division 1 malocclusion.

After a violent blow in the region of the chin one can also have an indirect trauma of the teeth resulting from the violent impact of the two jaws. In the latter case there are often injuries to the posterior teeth.

Classification

The most commonly used classification of dentoalveolar lesions is the one developed by Andreasen and also adopted by the World Health Organization, using the codes of the International Classification of Diseases. This classification can be applied to both permanent and primary dentition and it includes descriptions of teeth injuries, injuries to supporting structures, and to gingival and oral mucosa.

Dental tissues and pulp injuries

- Infraction of the crown (i.e. a crack in the tooth without loss of tooth substance).
- Fracture of the crown, which is limited to enamel, or enamel and dentin, without exposure of the root (uncomplicated).
- Fracture of the crown, which produces an exposure of pulp (complicated).
- Fracture involving enamel, dentin and cement without exposure to the pulp (fracture of the uncomplicated coronary root).
- Fracture involving enamel, dentin and cement with pulp exposure (complicated coronary root fracture).
- Root fracture involving dentin and cement and producing exposure of the pulp (root fracture) (fig. 2).

Periodontal tissue injuries

Periodontal tissue injuries are divided into three categories and include those commonly referred to as subluxations and avulsions.

- Concussion: defined as a lesion of the periodontium producing sensitivity to percussion without loosening or moving of the tooth.
- Subluxation: the tooth is loose but not displaced.
- Dislocation (i.e. lateral, intrusion, and extrusion) or partial avulsion: the tooth is moved without a comminution or fracture of the alveolar socket (fig. 3).

Supporting bone injuries

- Comminution of the alveolus, often with intrusive or lateral dislocation.
- Fracture of a single wall of a socket.
- Fracture of the alveolar process, in a block, in a patient with teeth but without the fracture line that necessarily extends through a tooth.
- Fracture involving the main body of the jaw (fig.4).

Diagnosis

Injuries to the teeth and to the supporting structures must be considered an emergency circumstance that requires a prompt diagnosis and treatment, mainly in case of avulsions and alveolar fractures.

In fact, teeth and alveolar fractures must be reduced as quickly as possible to improve the survival of these structures.

The initial assessment must include an accurate assessment of the patient's general conditions.

A thorough history can provide valuable information on the nature of the lesion and any alteration in the normal occlusion. This should be followed by a careful clinical examination which should include soft tissue inspection to find fragments of teeth or embedded debris. It is important to look for lacerations, abrasions and bruises and investigate the presence of damage to vital structures, such as the parotid duct, submandibular duct,

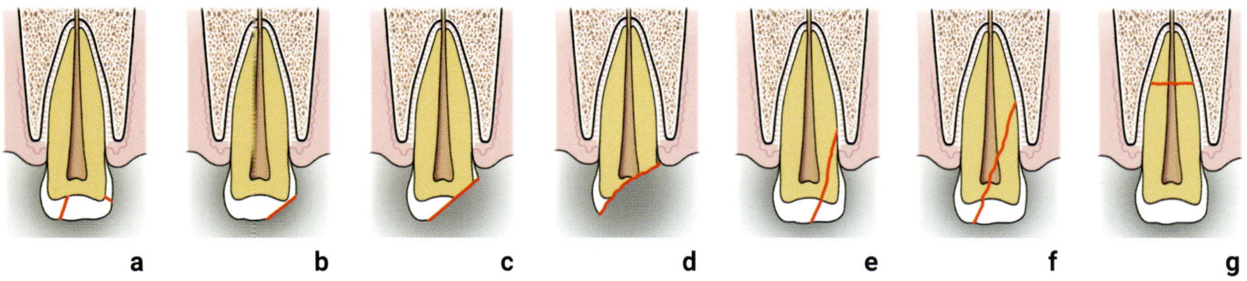

Figure 2 - Hard dental tissue and pulp tissue injuries. A: crown infraction. B-C: uncomplicated crown fracture. D: complicated crown fracture. E: uncomplicated crown-root fracture. F: complicated crown-root fracture. G: root fracture

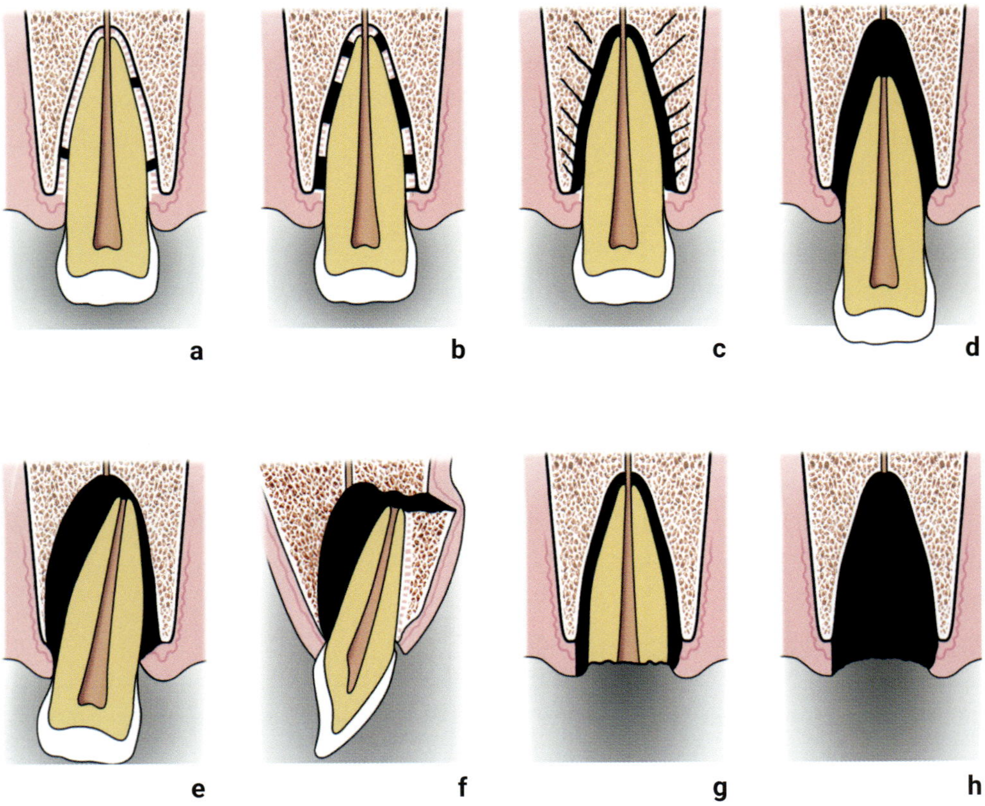

Figure 3
Periodontal tissue injuries.
A: concussion;
B: subluxation;
C: intrusive luxation;
D: extrusive luxation;
E-F: lateral luxation;
H: exarticulation

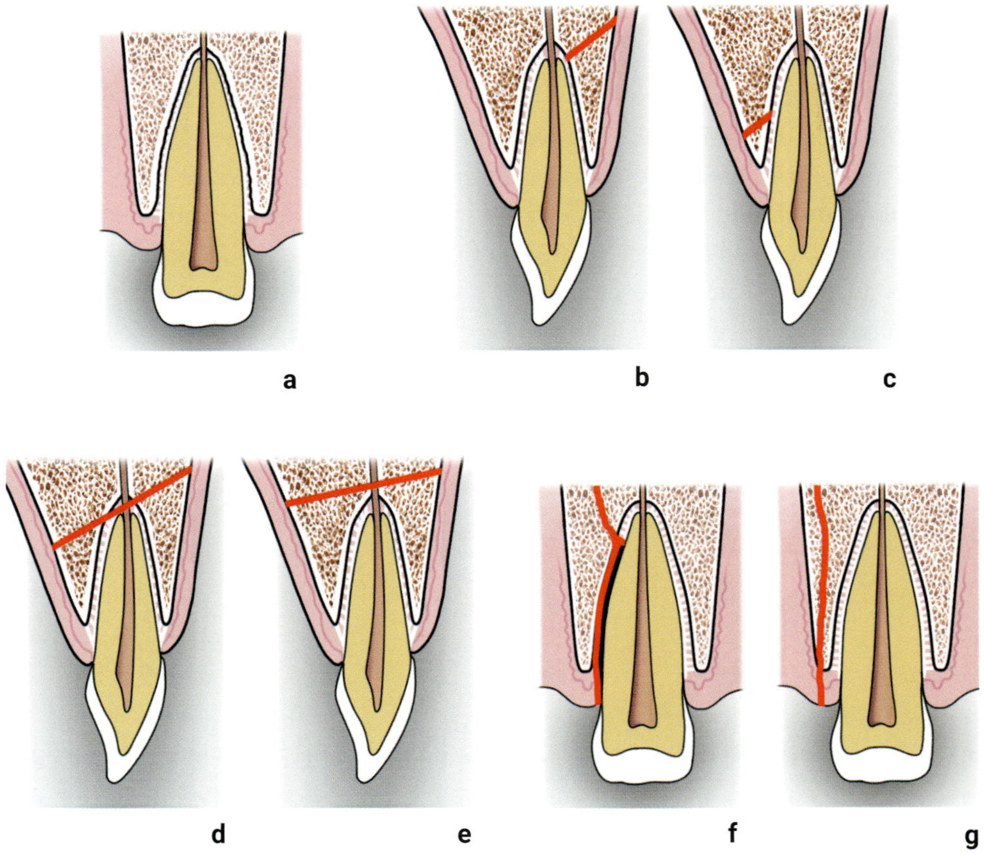

Figure 4 - Supporting bone injuries. A: alveolar comminution;
B-C: alveolar wall fracture;
D-E: alveolar process fracture;
F-G: jaws fracture

nerves and blood vessels, but also underlying dentoalveolar lesions.

All teeth should be tested for abnormal mobility, horizontally and axially, which would suggest luxation of the teeth or alveolar or mandibular fractures. An interruption of the vascular supply to the pulp should be expected when axial mobility is present.

The vitality of the pulp should also be tested but it should be noted that testing it in acutely traumatized teeth is of questionable value because these procedures require the collaboration of a relaxed patient to prevent false-positive reactions. Mechanical stimulation and electrical pulp testing can then be used in an emergency situation to examine the vitality and sensory perception of the dental pulp.

Radiographic evaluation of dentoalveolar lesions should include at least one panoramic radiograph and periapical radiographs of the teeth involved. Computed tomography (CT) and cone beam CT (CBCT) provide more detail and are useful for diagnosing fractures of teeth, roots and supporting bones. Patients who are evaluated in a hospital setting will often have CT performed if there is evidence of head injury and maxillofacial structures.

A complete radiographic examination should therefore provide information on the presence of root fracture, tooth extrusion or intrusion, pre-existing periodontal disease, jaw fractures, size of the pulp chamber and of the root canal, fragments of teeth and foreign bodies into the soft tissues, presence of caries [9] (fig. 5).

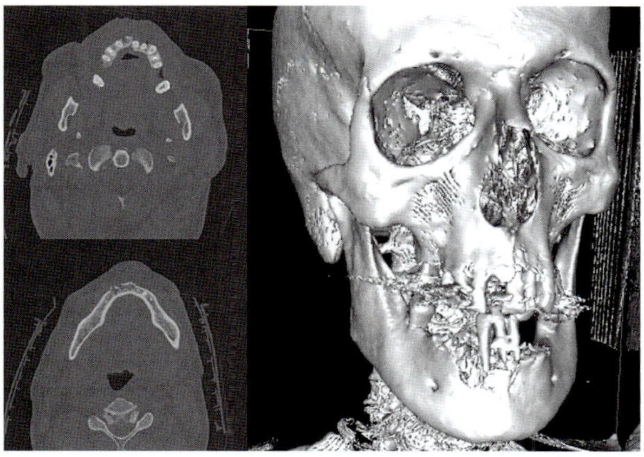

Figure 5 - CT imaging and 3D rendering of a dentoalveolar fracture

Treatment

Treatment depends on the type of injury that has occurred. Surgeons need to analyze this area taking into account all the different components involved.

Teeth

Generally, a violation of the crown does not need any treatment. In the case of an "uncomplicated" crown fracture, the treatment is aimed at protecting the pulp by sealing the dentinal tubules conservatively. On the contrary, in "complicated" crown fractures it is necessary to eradicate the pulp and root canal therapy before crown restoration.

The extraction is recommended when there is a longitudinal fracture that follows the long axis of the tooth or if the coronal fragment constitutes more than a third of the root.

Root fractures in the apical third or middle third are generally not splinted unless there is excessive mobility. The treatment of mobile radical fractures consists in the application on the fractured segments of a rigid splint for 12 weeks.

Treatment for apical fractures of one third of the roots usually involves tooth extraction or orthodontic root extrusion.

Alveolar process

Treatment involves the early reduction and stabilization of the segments involved. It is possible to use the open or closed technique depending on the severity of the fracture. Manipulation and digital pressure, together with the stabilization with a rigid splint, will usually be sufficient in the closed technique.

A gross shift and/or difficulties to the reduction may require the open technique.

Periodontal tissue

The treatments depend on the degree of mobilization of the tooth/teeth involved. In case of dislocation (intrusive, extrusive or lateral), repositioning and endodontic treatment (in presence of pulp necrosis) is necessary, associated with an accurate splinting.

In a complete avulsion, an early or immediate reimplantation should be performed. Teeth that are in poor condition from a hygienic point of view,

with moderate to severe periodontal disease, gross caries involving the pulp, apical abscesses or presenting infection at the site of reimplantation, bone defects and/or alveolar lesions, are not generally reimplanted.
The treatment is more effective when the reimplanting and splinting are performed within the first 2 hours, since the cells of the periodontal ligament become irreversibly necrotic after this period of time.

Mandibular fractures

Jaw fractures are among the most common fractures of the facial skeleton, although they do not occupy the very first positions in soccer maxillofacial traumas. Mandibular fractures are rarely closed fractures and tend to bleed significantly from the overlying oral mucosa. Also, the airways are affected by the integrity of the jaw, as it is connected to numerous muscles important for the patency of the upper airways. Mandibular fractures, and in particular fractures with multiple parts, allow posterior displacement of these muscle origins and airway loss can occur [10, 11].

Classification

Mandibular fractures can be classified according to the present fracture pattern (simple, compound, greenstick, comminuted etc.) and by anatomical location (fig. 6).

- Symphysis fracture: any fracture in the region of the incisors that goes from the alveolar process through the inferior margin of the mandible in vertical direction.
- Parasymphysis fracture: a fracture localized between the mental foramen and the distal aspect of the lateral mandibular incisor extending from the alveolar process through the lower margin.
- Body fracture: any fracture localized in the region between the mental foramen and the distal portion of the second molar and extends from the alveolar process through the lower margin.
- Angle fracture: any distal fracture with respect to the second molar, which extends from any point of the curve formed by the junction of the body and branch in the retromolar area at any point of the curve formed by the lower edge of the body and by the posterior edge of the branch of the jaw.
- Ramus fracture: a fracture in which the fracture line extends horizontally across the anterior and posterior edges of the branch or which runs vertically from the sigmoid mark to the lower edge of the mandible.
- Condylar process fracture: a fracture that goes from the sigmoid notch to the posterior margin of the mandibular branch along the superior aspect of the branch. Fractures that affect the condylar area can be further classified as extracapsular or intracapsular, depending on the relationship between the fracture and the capsular attachment.
- Coronoid fracture: a fracture that involves only the coronoid process of the mandible.

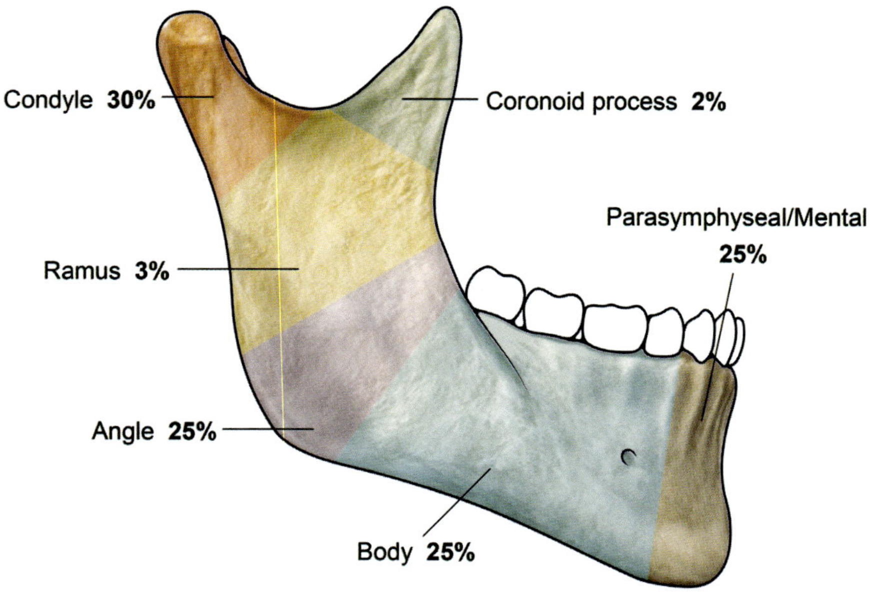

Figure 6 - Mandibular fractures, frequency by location

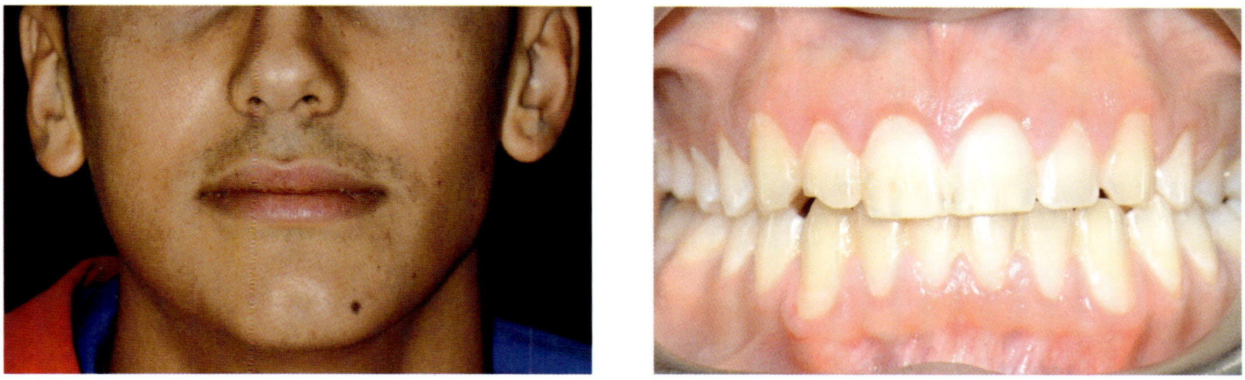

Figure 7 - Signs of mandibular fracture. On the left, extraoral view of a mandibular angle fracture with swelling of the right cheek. On the right, intraoral view of the dentition showing an ipsilateral openbite

Diagnosis

Knowing the type and direction of traumatic force can be extremely useful for diagnosis and can help the doctor to diagnose concurrent fractures.

The object that caused the fracture can also influence the type and number of fractures.

For example, an anterior blow directly to the chin can cause bilateral condylar fractures and an angulated murmur of the parasymphysis can cause a condylar or contralateral angular fracture.

However, the jaw must be evaluated after the patient has been stabilized and more life-threatening injuries have been addressed (fig. 7).

The signs and symptoms of mandibular fractures are listed below.

- Change in occlusion. Any change in occlusion is highly indicative of the mandibular fracture. The clinician should ask the patient if his bite feels different. A change in occlusion can result from fractured teeth, fractured alveolar process, fractured mandible in any location, and TMJ trauma and mastication muscles. For example, post-traumatic premature dental contact or an anterior open bite may result from bilateral mandibular or angle condyle fractures and maxillary fractures with lower posterior maxilla displacement.
- Anesthesia, paresthesia or dysesthesia of the lower lip. The numbness in the distribution of the inferior alveolar nerve after the trauma is almost pathognomonic of a distal fracture with respect to the mandibular foramen.
- Abnormal mandibular movements. Most patients with fractured mandibles have a limited opening and trismus due to the protection of the chewing muscles. However, some mandibular fractures lead to predictable abnormal movements, such as the deviation while opening the mouth towards the side of a condylar fracture.
- Change of the facial contour and the shape of the mandibular arch (it might be difficult to notice if masked by swelling).
- Lacerations, hematomas and ecchymoses. A trauma that is significant enough to cause loss of skin or continuity of the mucosa or submucosal subcutaneous hemorrhage can cause trauma to the underlying jaw. Tears must be carefully checked before closing.
- Teeth and rattles loose on palpation. A thorough examination of the teeth and supporting bone can help diagnose alveolar process, body, and symphyseal fractures.

The initial diagnostic examination for all patients with suspected mandibular bone injury is an orthopantomography (OPG). This radiograph, in some cases, is sufficient to allow not only a definitive diagnosis, but also a definitive treatment. CT can be used as first choice, if it is not possible to carry out an OPG, or more commonly as a second level exam. In fact, it can integrate the results of normal radiographs and is particularly useful in case of fractures in the mandibular branch region and in the condylar process, since these fractures can have more variable degrees of displacement and the results on CT imaging can have significant implications on the definitive management. Furthermore, many patients with mandibular fractures need to be evaluated for closed head injuries with CT imaging [10] (fig. 8).

Obviously, considerations on radiation exposure

should be balanced against the convenience of obtaining CT images on any suspected facial fracture. Magnetic resonance imaging is of very limited use, with the exception of patients with suspected soft tissue structure lesions around the temporomandibular joint, since MRI is superior to the CT for the detection of lesions of the articular cartilage and associated ligament structures.

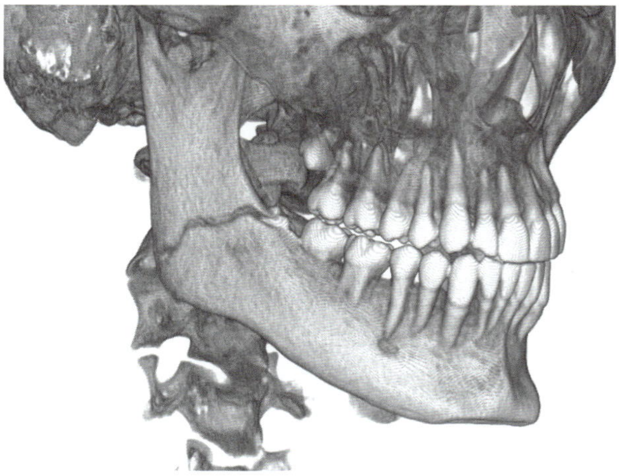

Figure 8 - OPG and 3D rendering of a fracture at the level of the right mandibular angle

Treatment

The definitive management of mandibular fractures depends on many factors, including the fracture pattern(s), and patient factors including age, comorbidity, other maxillofacial lesions, and expected compliance.

The treatment can be very variable.

- Observation with dietary and functional restrictions.
- Closed "reduction" followed by immobilization with various forms of fixation between the fractured mandible and the non-fractured maxilla (intermaxillary fixation).
- Open reduction and immobilization.
- Open reduction with rigid or non-rigid internal fixation (through various trans-oral and/or transcutaneous approaches) [1].

In the case of professional soccer players, internal fixation surgery is usually the best solution, even in those cases with compound fractures, as it allows players to resume sports faster (fig. 9) (video 2).

VIDEO 2

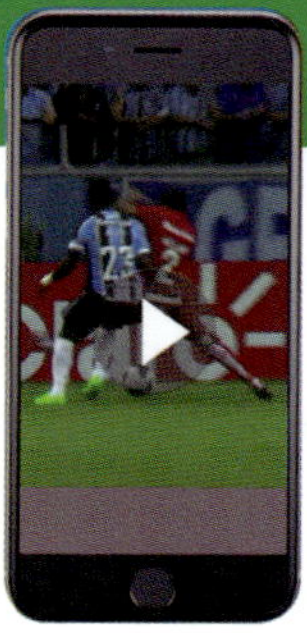

Mandibular fracture due to elbow on the jaw shot

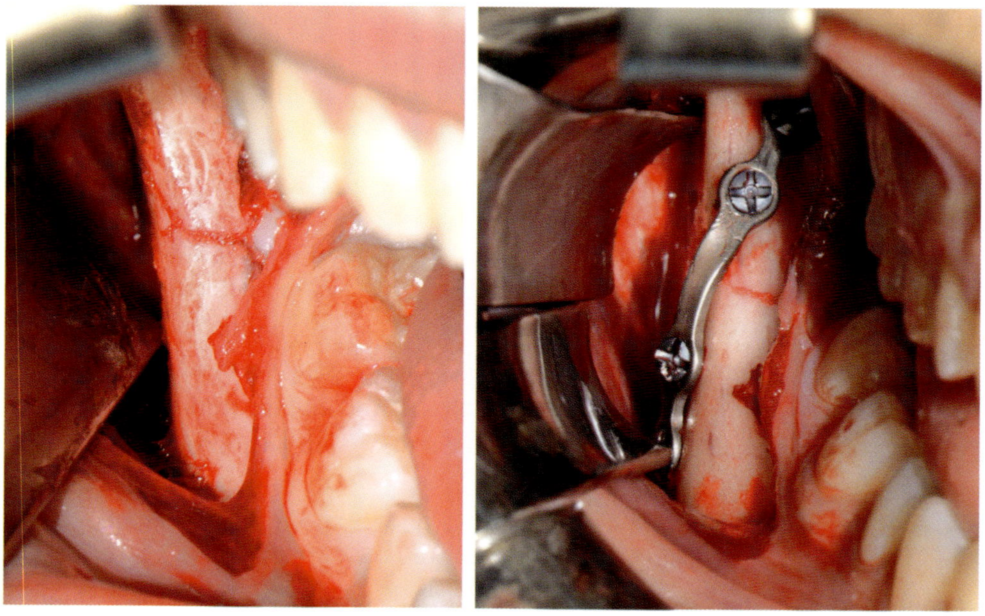

Figure 9 - On the left, intraoperative image of a fracture of the mandibular ramus. On the right, open reduction and internal fixation with a Champy mini-plate

Maxillary fractures

Maxillary fractures often occur in conjunction with other facial fractures and are often associated with lacerations, orthopedic, or neurological lesions [1]. However, it is very rare to find these lesions during a soccer match.

The midface complex consists of a series of vertical pillars that mainly provide protection from vertically directed forces. These include naso-maxillary (nasofrontal), zygomaticomaxillary, and pterigo-maxillary reinforcements. These vertical pillars are supported by horizontal buttresses: the super orbital or frontal bar, the infraorbital edges, and the zygomatic arches.

Behind this buttress system we have the medial and lateral pterygoid plates inferiorly and the cranial base superiorly. This structure results in some anatomical sites of weakness, resulting in predictable fracture patterns (fig. 10).

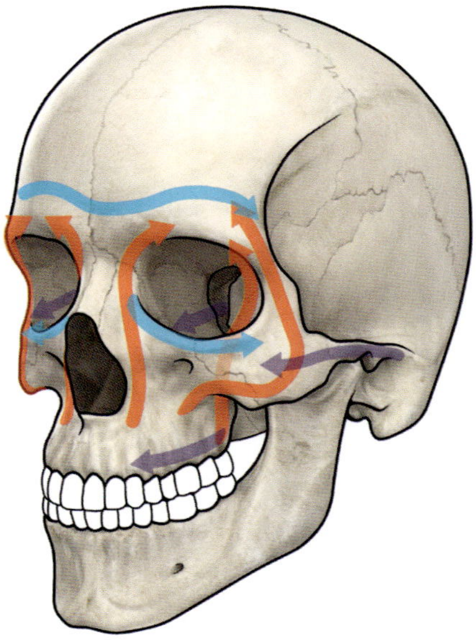

Figure 10 - The maxillary vertical (red arrows) and horizontal (blue and purple arrows) buttresses

Classification

At the beginning of the 20th century Rene Le Fort's corpse studies defined the three weakest levels of the complex when attacked from a frontal direction. He defined the three most common "linea minoris resistentiae", which are classified as the fractures of Le Fort I, Le Fort II and Le Fort III (fig. 11).

- Le Fort I fracture derives from a force directed above the maxillary teeth, resulting in a floating palate.
- Le Fort II fracture derives from a force delivered at the level of the nasal bone, with consequent mobility of the median area through the orbits and the mid-facial region.
- Le Fort III fracture derives from a force directed to the orbital level, with consequent craniofacial disjunction or separation of the entire middle third of the craniomaxillofacial skeleton from the base of the skull.

Diagnosis

Advanced trauma life support protocols must be followed for all traumatized patients. The detailed examination of maxillofacial fractures is completed in the secondary survey, after the primary investigation and successful resuscitation have been completed. The clinical examination should begin with the initial observation of the patient, followed by palpation of the fractures [15, 16].

Periorbital bruising and facial edema must be noted and are very typical of these fractures. Epistaxis with any evidence of cerebrospinal fluid leakage (clear fluid mixed with blood in a "tramline" mod-

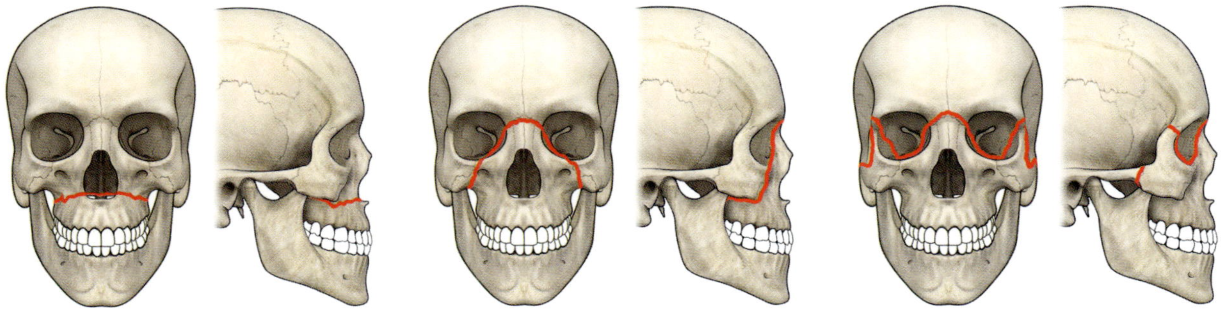

Figure 11 - Le Fort classification of maxillary fractures

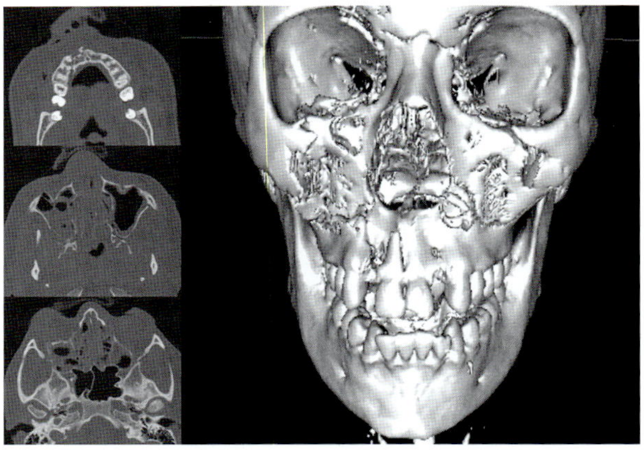

Figure 12 - CT images and 3D reconstruction of a comminuted Le Fort II fracture

el) must be investigated. Other identifiable features are nose asymmetry, traumatic telekinesis, a flat nasal bridge and a dish-shaped face, fracture of the teeth, ecchymoses and vestibular edema, palatal ecchymoses, lacerations and mucosal bleeding, misalignment or diastema in the maxillary teeth and malocclusion.
The skeletal structure of the face must be carefully palpated. As far as the jaw is concerned, the alveolus must be palpated and fractures or mobility must be noted. The doctor must also observe the jaw for movement as a unit, while palpating the forehead, the nasal bridge, and the frontal zygomatic sutures.
Fractures are then confirmed radiographically. In the past, some 2D radiographic examinations (for example water vision and lateral facial radiographs) have been used, but with these radiological examinations the fine details of the fracture sites are very difficult to visualize. Today, CT is the first choice imaging technique and both axial and coronal CT scans should be obtained. In fact, high quality CT scans are essential also for optimal surgical planning (fig. 12).

Treatment

As for all traumas, initial attention must be directed to establish the airway patency and control bleeding (e.g. nasal septum, ethmoid region, internal maxillary artery, etc.).
Isolated maxillary fractures involving only the dentoalveolar process must be reduced manually and rigidly fixed with arch and ligature wires.
In larger lesions the treatment of maxillary fractures largely depends on the associated injuries. Nasotracheal intubation is preferred when it is not contraindicated by the need for complicated repairs of the nasal lesions. In these cases a submental intubation technique with the method decided by Hernandez Altemir in 1986 can be used, which allows to keep the mouth and nose free from any encumbrance (fig. 13).
Tracheotomy is necessary only in a few cases.
Although many wiring techniques have been described, rigid internal fixation is the standard and more effective of care.
The maxilla must be stabilized at the next higher stable face structure, which varies with the Le Fort fracture level.

Zygomatic complex fractures

The zygomatic bone represents the main structure of the lateral midface. Its shape approximates a four-sided pyramid. It has a temporal, orbital, maxillary and frontal process, and articulates with four bones: the frontal, sphenoidal, maxillary, and temporal bones (fig. 14).
Zygomatic fractures represent the most common facial fractures [17] or the second in frequency after nasal fractures [18]. The high incidence of these fractures is probably due to the prominent position of the zygomatic bone inside the facial skeleton, which often exposes it to traumatic forces. During a soccer match, direct trauma (e.g. elbow, head, etc.) is the most common cause of injury (video 3). Because the shape of the face is largely influenced by the underlying bone structure, the zygoma plays an important role in the contour of the face.

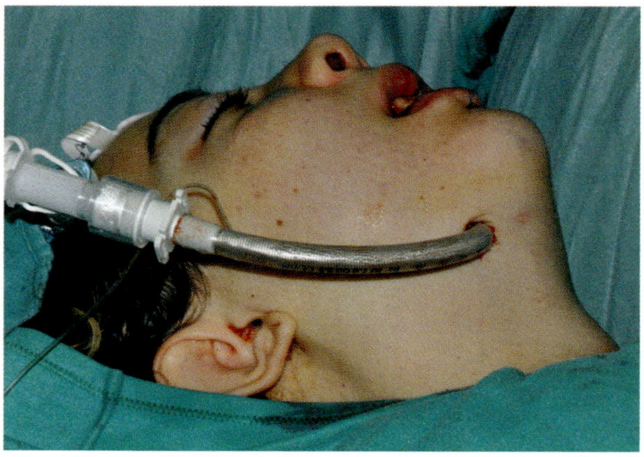

Figure 13 - Altemir submental intubation technique

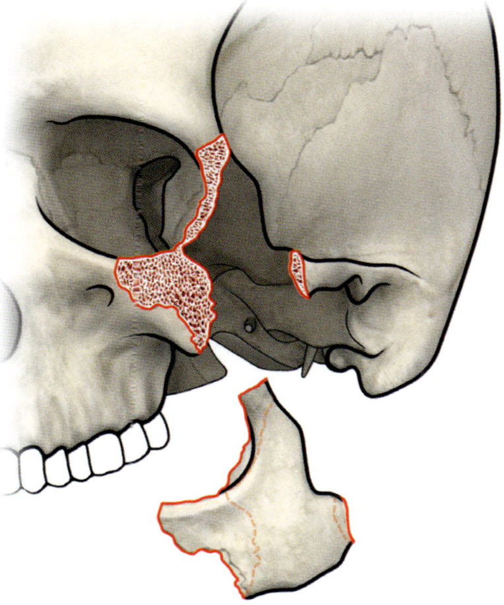

Figure 14 - Illustration of the zygomatic complex

Figure 15 - Common patterns of ZMC fractures. A: medial fracture to the zygomaticomaxillary suture and along the zygomaticosphenoid suture within orbit. B: fractures going through a frontozygomatic suture and posterior to a zygomaticotemporal suture. C: fractures going from the inferior orbital fissure through the zygomaticosphenoid suture and through the zygomatic buttress of the maxilla. D: triple fracture through the zygomatic arch

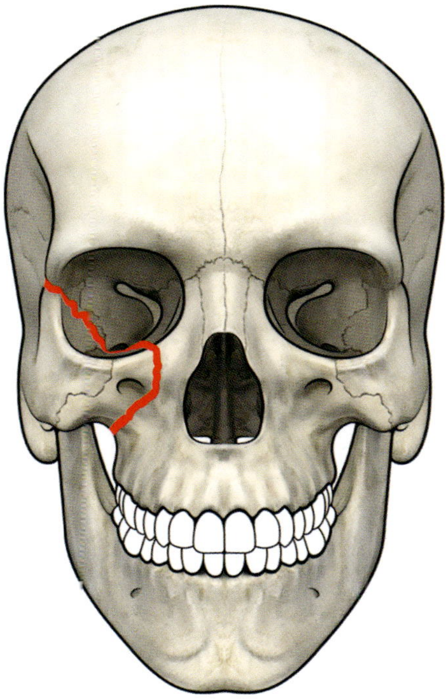

a

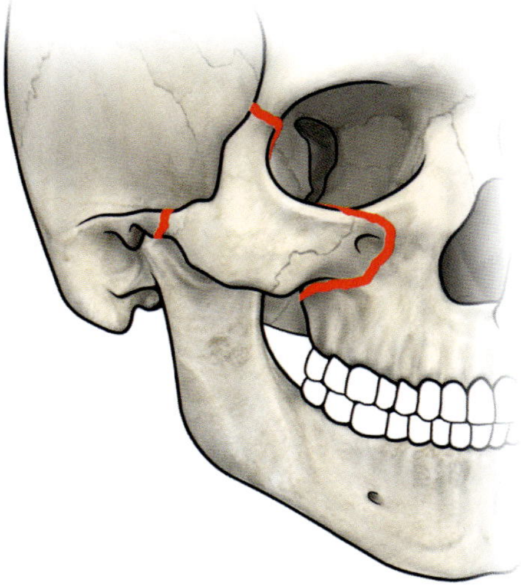

b

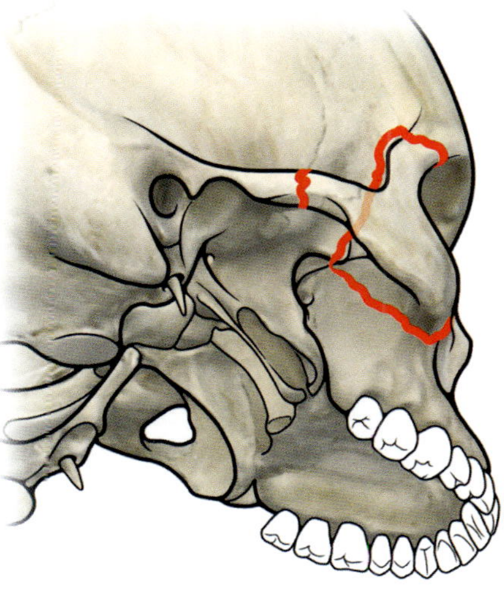

c

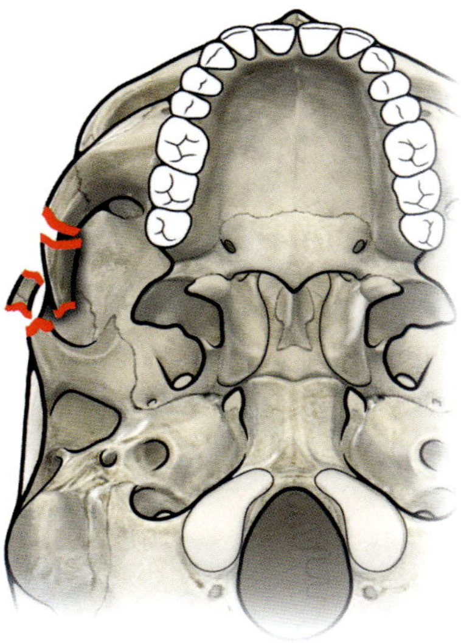

d

VIDEO 3

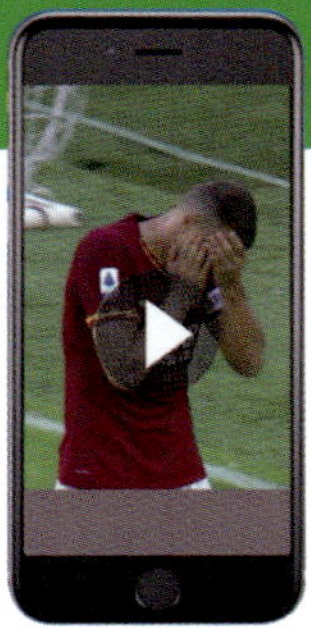

Zigomatic complex fracture due to an head shot on the zygomatic body

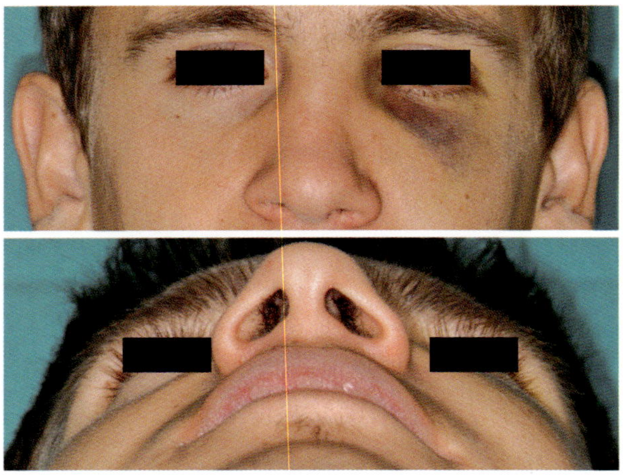

Figure 16 - Downward displacement of the zygoma producing swelling and ecchymosis, enophthalmos, and accentuation of the supratarsal fold of the upper eyelid

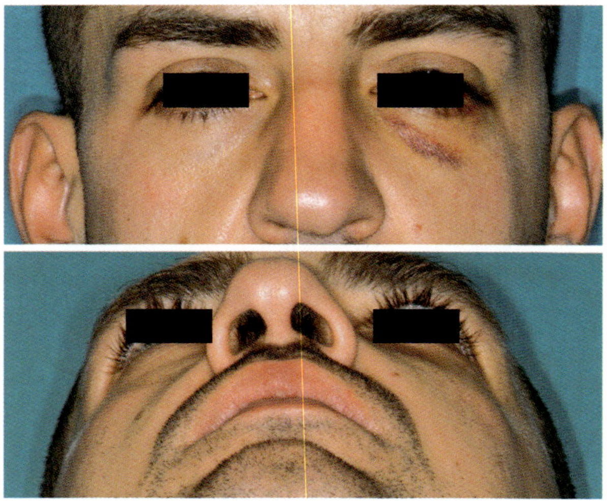

Figure 17 - Isolated zygomatic arch fracture causing a visible depression, anterior to the left tragus

Furthermore, the interruption of the zygomatic position also has a great functional significance because it causes an impairment of the occlusal and mandibular function. Therefore, both for aesthetic and functional reasons, it is important that the zygomatic lesions are correctly diagnosed and adequately treated.

Classification

The type of fracture of any bone depends on several factors, including the direction and extent of the force. First of all, it is necessary to distinguish fractures involving the zygomatic and adjacent bones (defined as zygomatic-maxillary) from fractures of isolated zygomatic arch (zygomatic fractures) (fig. 15).

Historically, the classification of zygomatic fractures is used to predict which fractures would remain stable after reduction. From the clinical point of view, this would allow the surgeon to identify those fractures that would require open reduction and fixation.

In 1990, Manson and colleagues proposed a classification method based on segmentation and displacement of bony segments.

- Low energy fractures have little or no movement. Incomplete fractures of one or more joints may be present.
- Medium-energy fractures present a complete fracture of all joints with mild to moderate displacement. The comminution may be present.
- High energy fractures are characterized by comminution in the lateral orbit and lateral displacement with segmentation of the zygomatic arch.

Diagnosis

The initial evaluation of the patient with zygomatic fracture includes the documentation of the bone lesion and the state of the surrounding soft tissues (eyelids, lacrimal apparatus, cantonal tendons, and globe) and cranial nerves II to VI. An ophthalmologist must be consulted in case of suspicious or questionable ophthalmic lesions.

The patient with a complex zygomatic fracture complains of pain, periorbital edema, and ecchymosis. There may be paraesthesia or anesthesia on the cheek, lateral nose, upper lip, and anterior maxillary teeth resulting from lesions to the zygo-

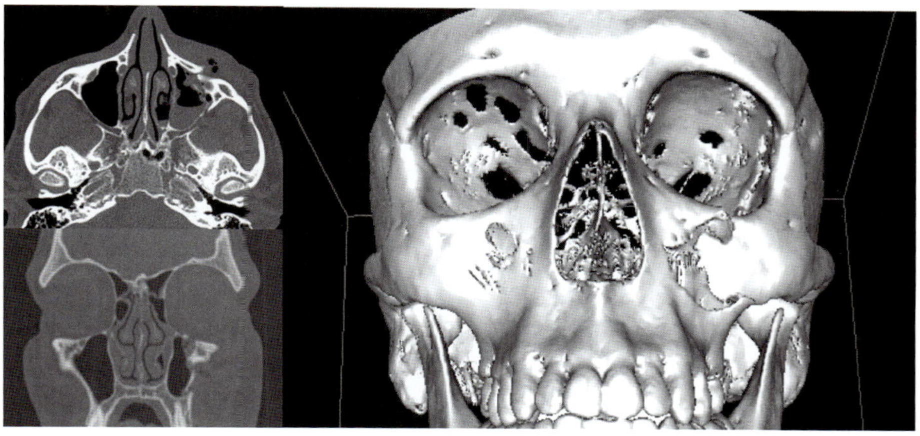

Figure 18 - CT scan and 3D reconstruction of a fracture of the left zygomatic complex

maticotemporal or infraorbital nerves.

The most common early clinical signs are ecchymosis and edema and these are present in about 60% of all zygomatic lesions [19]. The depression of the malar eminence and the infraorbital edge produce the flattening of the cheek.

The downward shift of the zygoma produces an antimongoloid inclination to the lateral canthus, enophthalmos, and accentuation of the supratarsal fold of the upper eyelid (fig. 16).

In isolated fractures of the zygomatic arch a depression is observed and palpated anteriorly to the tragus (fig. 17).

In the case of orbital involvement, it's important to evaluate the extraocular movements to exclude the mechanical entrapment or paresis, which usually manifest with diplopia.

It's recommended the use of Hess screen to objectify the extent of diplopia.

CT scan of facial bones, in axial and coronal planes, is the gold standard for all patients with suspected zygomatic fractures. Specifically, CT scans allow detailed visualization of the skeleton of the medial face: nasomascellar, zygomatic-vascular, infraorbital, zygomatic-frontal, zygomatic-phosphenoid, and zygomatotemporal (fig. 18).

The best plain radiograph to evaluate complex zygomatic fractures is the Waters view. It is a posteroanterior projection with the head positioned at an angle of 27° with respect to the vertical plane and the chin resting on the X-ray cassette. This one projects the petrous pyramids from the maxillary sinuses, allowing the visualization of the sinuses, lateral orbits, and borders infraorbital.

Treatment

Management of zygomatic complex and zygomatic arch fractures depends on the degree of dislocation and the consequent aesthetic and functional deficits. The treatment can therefore vary from simple observation to open reduction and internal fixation.

Zygomatic arch fractures

The standard technique for treating zygomatic arch fractures was first described by Gillies, Kilner and Stone in 1927. This is a temporal incision (2 cm in length) that is performed behind the hairline. The dissection continues through the temporal planes and the bone is lifted outward and forward with an elevator, being careful not to force the temporal bone. The arch should be continuously palpated as a guide for proper reduction. Alternatively, a J-shaped curved hook elevator can be used which is inserted just below the anterior zygomatic arch towards the articular eminence through a preauricular incision. The tip of the hook is directed under the shifted fragments and the reduction is obtained with controlled lateral traction (fig. 19).

Zygomatic complex fractures

Undisplaced or minimally displaced complex low-energy fractures may not require any correction. The patient must be periodically checked to identify any signs of dislocation, extraocular muscle dysfunction and enophthalmos after the swelling resolves.

Zygomatic complex displaced medium-energy fractures require reduction and internal fixation. If the reduction is unstable or if there are problems

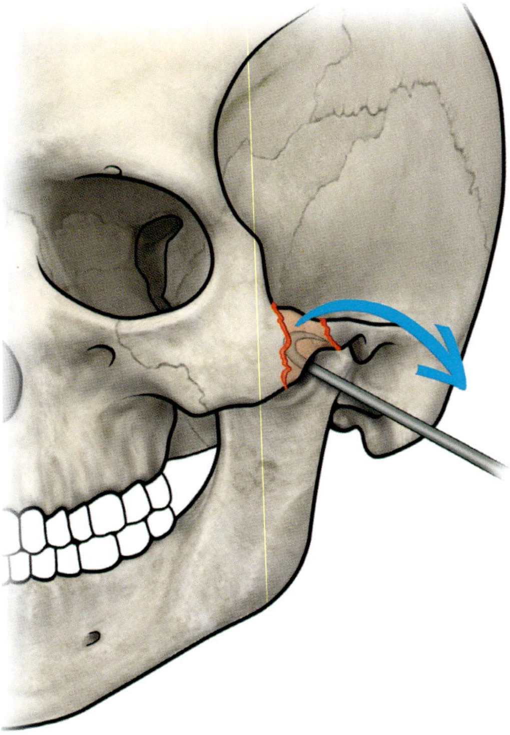

Figure 19 - A percutaneous hook is placed through the skin around the depressed zygomatic fracture segments and pulled laterally

in the accuracy of the reduction, it is advisable to proceed with open reduction and internal fixation. In this case, the zygomatic-maxillary buttress is exposed first and stabilized with a plate; the zygomatic frontal buttress is subsequently exposed and stabilized with a plate if necessary.
A more aggressive surgical approach should be planned to treat high-energy fractures.
There is often significant comminution of the anterior buttresses, making anatomical reduction difficult. Furthermore, these fractures often require orbital reconstruction.
To restore the correct projection, exposure of the zygomatic arch and of the orbital plane in addition to the exposure of the front buttresses is often required. In these cases, a coronal flap is used to access the zygomatic arch while a transcutaneous or transconjunctival incision is used to explore and reconstruct the internal orbit.

Orbital floor fractures
Patients with complex zygomatic lesions of medium energy and no clinical or radiographic evidence of orbital interruption do not require exploration.
Medium energy injuries with displacement of the orbital edge or floor or herniated soft tissue in the sinus should be explored. Clinical indications for orbital exploration include enophthalmos, limitation of extraocular muscle function with positive forced duction test and persistent diplopia.
High energy fractures require a more aggressive approach and the orbital edge and plane should be explored and reconstructed.
Access to the floor is performed by a trans-cutaneous or trans-conjunctival incision. Simple linear fractures may only require the removal of trapped tissue, while major defects require soft tissue reduction and floor reconstruction with a bone graft or implant.

Nasal fractures

Nasal fractures are the most common facial fractures and occur more frequently in males compared to females [20, 21]. The high frequency of nasal fractures can be attributed to the prominent position of nasal bones in the facial skeleton and to the little force required to produce a fracture compared to the other facial bones.
Athletic injuries, scuffles, falls, and motor vehicle accidents account for most of the causes. In children and adolescents, sports and falls are the main causes of isolated nasal bone fractures.
A study on sports-related fractures in US high schools found a fracture rate of 10.1% with the highest rate in soccer, basketball, and soccer [22].

Classification
In clinical practice it is essential to analyze all the components of the nose, evaluating the bones (nasal bones, frontal bone, frontal jaw process, ethmoid bones, tear bones) and cartilages (septum, lateral cartilage septum, major alar cartilage) (fig. 20).
Typically, the so-called "nasal fractures" are those that involve only the nasal structures, while complex fractures that also involve other adjacent bone structures are called "ethmoid nasal-orbital fractures".

Diagnosis
A detailed history that takes into account the trauma mechanism may help distinguish isolated

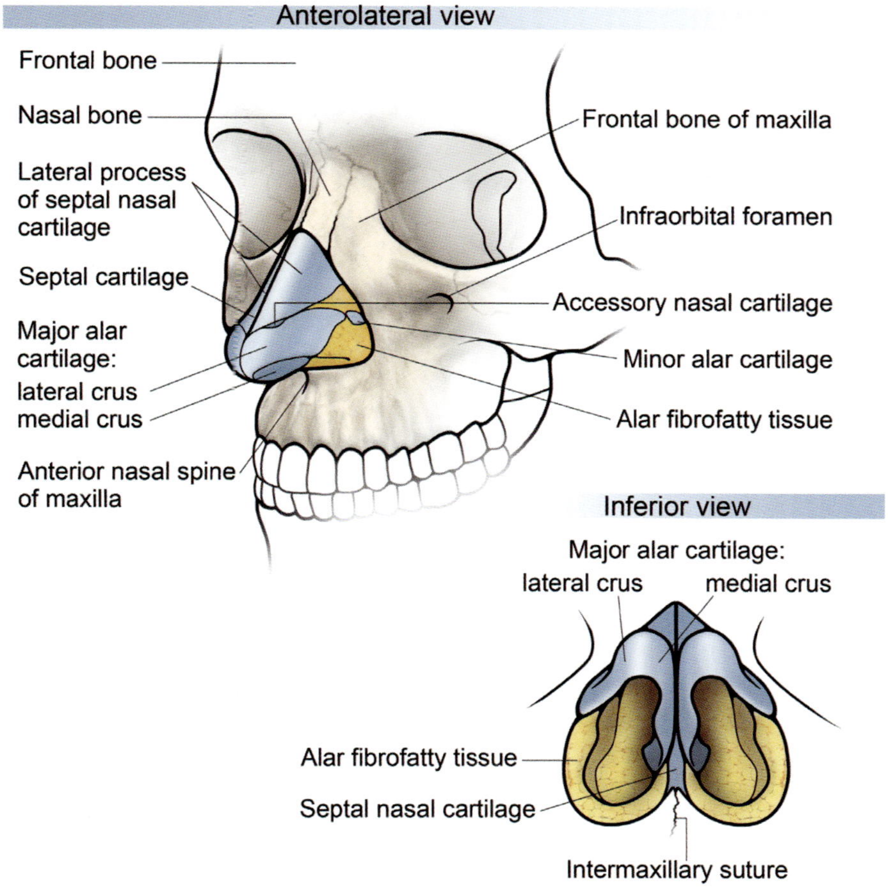

Figure 20 - Anatomy of the nose

nasal fractures from those that could be associated with other injuries. Any history of previous nasal trauma and/or septal trauma and/or surgery should also be investigated.

It is important to properly recognize and manage any symptoms of head injury such as headache, nausea or vomiting, dizziness, disorientation or lethargy.

During the examination, it is necessary to look for any nasal and septal deviation and gross deformity. The observation of the nasal back from different points of view will help the clinician to appreciate any external nasal deformity (fig. 21). Intranasal examination with a nasal speculum, appropriate illumination and vasoconstrictors, if necessary, is important for assessing the state of the cartilaginous and bony nasal septum, to exclude the septum hematoma and to determine the origin and extent of epistaxis and/or cerebrospinal fluid (CSF) loss. In some cases, it may be useful to use fiber optic nasoendoscopy to evaluate

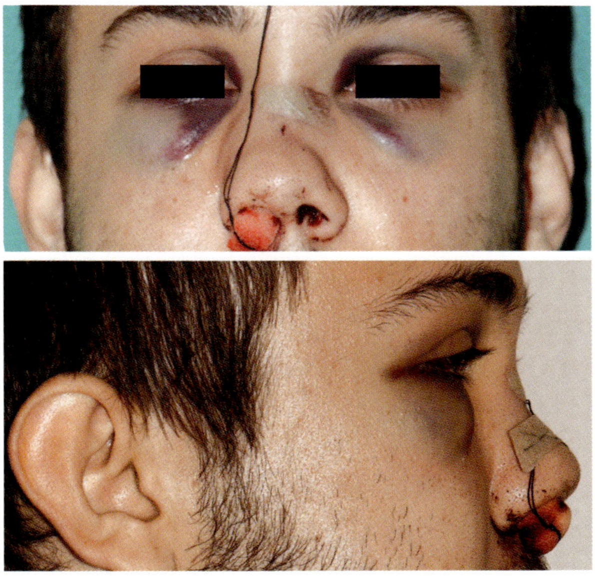

Figure 21 - Clinical presentation of a typical fracture of the nose and maxilla, with bilateral orbital swelling and ecchymosis, clinically evident deviation of the nasal septum and bones, and epistaxis managed with the positioning of an anterior packing

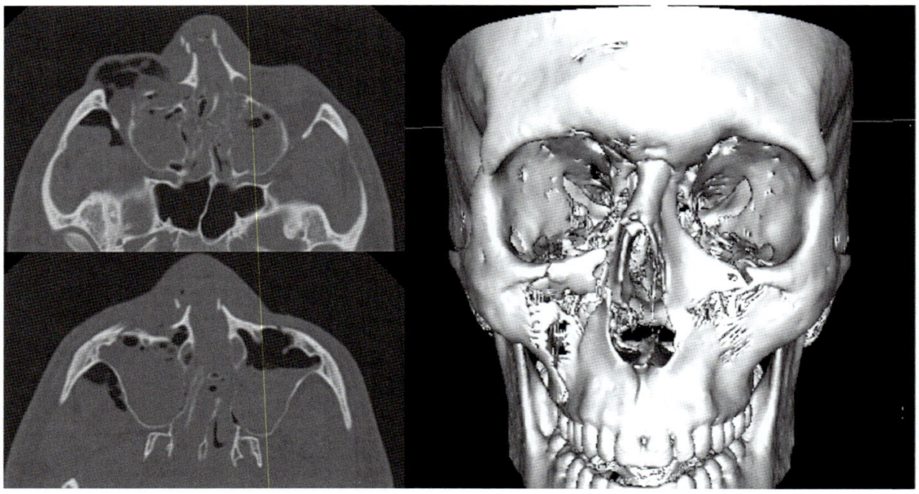

Figure 22 - CT scan and 3D reconstruction of a nasal and maxillary comminuted fracture

the posterior nasal complex and the nasopharynx. A detailed examination of the face, including the evaluation of visual acuity, the movement of extraocular muscles, the size and reactivity of the pupil, the intercantal distance, the position of the medial cantonal tendon, the range of the mandibular movement and occlusion, is also important. Simple X-ray films can be adapted to assess the extent and displacement of nasal bone fractures when no other lesion is suspected; however, nowadays, with the advent of CT, they are used less frequently (fig. 22).

Furthermore, due to the proximity of other anatomical structures, some nasal fractures cannot be completely visualized with plain films. In these cases CT provides excellent details and can more easily identify concomitant fractures such as orbital, ethmo-orbital, naso-orbital, zygomatic, maxillary and frontal fractures, or cribriform plate fractures.

Treatment

Routine management of nasal fractures requires consideration of timing, anesthesia, treatment setting, and details of the operative approach [23]. Although immediate treatment is possible, sometimes, it may be preferable to let the swelling decrease. The delay should be no more than 1 week, otherwise fibrinization and fibrosis occur and the fracture becomes increasingly difficult to treat with a closed reduction alone.

Therefore, treatment in the early days facilitates the healing process, limits the patient's disability and decreases the time spent by the patient away from daily activities.

Most nasal fractures are treated with closed reduction and external stabilization, with or without packaging materials for the inner nose.

The nasal bones can be repositioned with digital manipulation using the maxillary and frontal bones for anchoring and guiding or using an elevator. The adequacy of the reduction is determined by palpation and visual inspection from different points of view.

Nasal packs and splints help stabilize comminuted fractures and prevent internal collapse of bone fragments. The pack can also allow the control of bleeding and prevent the formation of hematoma of the septum. Nasal packets are usually removed 1 to 3 days after surgery, while the septum splint can be maintained for 1 week or more if necessary.

In the case of complex nasal fractures, an open approach with coronal access is usually required, as these fractures are usually associated with other related fractures such as the frontal sinus and the nose-orbital-ethmoid complex (NOE).

When facing nasal fractures, it is of fundamental importance to know their possible complications. A septal hematoma is a rare complication and can present itself as a complaint of nasal obstruction, pain or fever when infected. This collection of blood separates the cartilage of the septum from its perichondrium and must be treated promptly to prevent necrosis of the cartilage of the septum. The treatment consists of incision and drainage, nasal packing to prevent the accumulation of blood and to promote intimate contact between

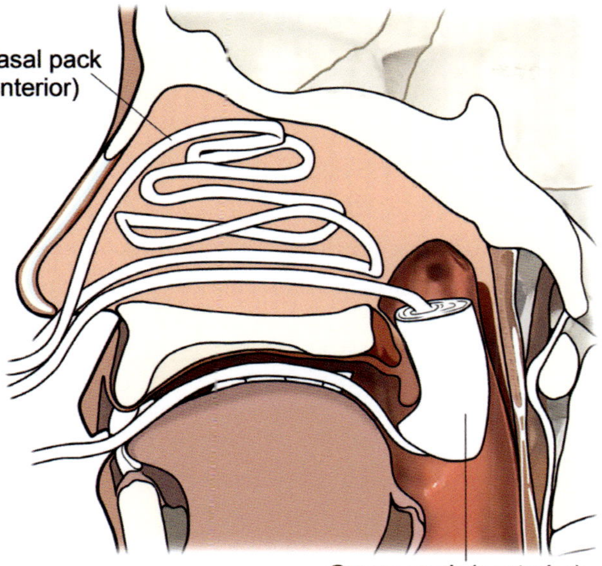

Figure 23 - Examples of anterior nasal pack and posterior gauze pack

perichondrium and nasal septum, and antibiotic coverage.

Epistaxis is another potential complication and may be anterior or posterior. Significant bleeding can compromise the respiratory tract. These cases usually resolve with the placement of a front or back packing, depending on where the bleeding starts (fig. 23).

Complications

Late complications may arise because of many different reasons: delayed or inadequate treatment, poor patient constitution, or poor post-operative care. On the contrary, acute complications are the result of trauma itself. Intermediate complications are those caused during surgery while the advanced ones arise immediately after surgery. The overall complication rate is 3 times higher if the fracture is treated more than 10 days after the initial injury.

Delayed union and nonunion

Delayed union and lack of consolidation occur in about 3% of fractures.

The delayed union is a temporary condition in which bony union occurs in more time than it's usually necessary.

Failure to heal indicates a lack of bone healing and it's characterized by abnormal pain and mobility between the segments that persists indefinitely with no evidence of bone healing, unless surgery is undertaken another time [24].

Radiographs show no evidence of healing and in later stages they even show rounding of bone ends.

The most probable cause of delayed union and pseudoarthrosis is poor reduction and immobilization, followed by infection of the surgical site. Another possible cause is excessive stripping of the periosteum, which leads to a reduction in blood supply, especially in comminuted and edentulous fractures.

Infection

Both local and systemic factors can contribute to the development of an infection. Local factors include poor reduction and fixation, fractured teeth in the fracture line, and comminuted fractures.

Systemic factors include alcoholism, immunocompromission, and lack of proper antibiotic coverage.

When an infection is present, it must be managed with debridement, drainage, and antibiotic therapy before going to the actual surgery.

Malunion

The malunion is defined as an inaccurate alignment of the healed bone segments.

It should be noted that not all malunions are clinically significant, but when a toothed portion is involved, malocclusion can occur. These malocclusions can be treated orthodontically or with osteotomies after complete bone union has occurred.

In the case of involvement of the central portion, it may be necessary to perform additional osteotomies or perform a Cad/Cam surgical procedure to restore an acceptable morphology.

In the case of fractures of the orbital floor, the most common complications are entrapment of the lower rectus muscle and enophthalmos. In these cases a surgical revision is mandatory.

Nerve injury

The inferior alveolar nerve and its branches are the most commonly injured nerves. The primary sign of damage to the inferior alveolar nerve is numbness or other sensory changes in the lower lip and chin.

Damage to the marginal mandibular branch of the facial nerve is rare and appears as paresis of the innervated structures with depression of the ipsilateral lip angle.

It's more commonly seen in case of trauma in the condyle region, but also at the level of the mandibular branch and angle and in case of lacerations along its course.

The infraorbital nerve is often involved in orbital and zygomatic complex fractures. It is usually enough to reduce the fracture to get nervous recovery.

In general, most of the sensory and motor functions of these nerves improve and return to normal over time.

Root damage

The fixing screws may inadvertently damage teeth roots. However, only minimal adverse consequences result from an involuntary transfixion of the tooth root using osteosynthesis screws [25].

Computer assisted surgery in facial trauma

Over the years, the development of reconstructive surgical techniques and technology has helped to improve surgical outcomes. Although surgical techniques are well defined, the problem relating to human error remains. The development of new materials and the advancement of technology have allowed us to address this problem, thus improving surgical outcomes [26].

The three-dimensional complexity of facial anatomy requires accurate three-dimensional reconstruction to ensure a good aesthetic result as well as functional recovery. At present, computer-assisted maxillofacial surgery, when it's possible, is recommended in traumatology [27].

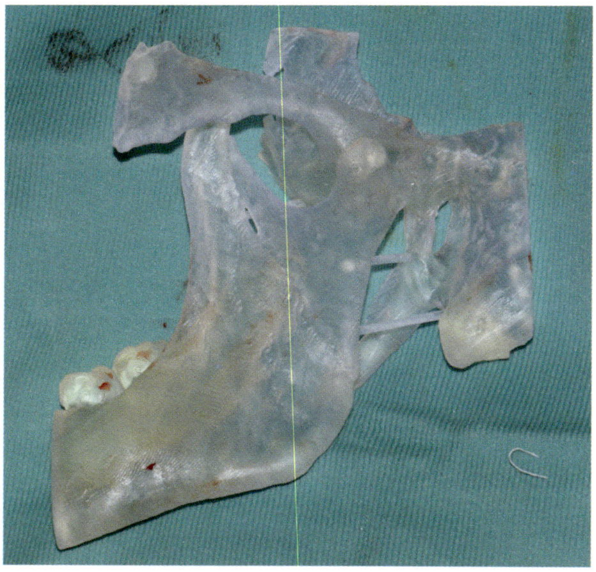

Figure 24 - Stereolithographic model of a subcondylar mandibular fracture

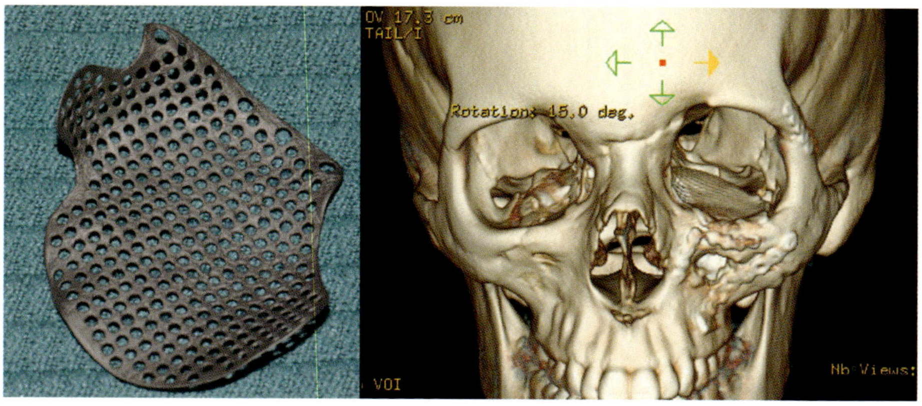

Figure 25 - On the left, custom-made orbital floor grid; on the right, surgical planning with 3D imaging

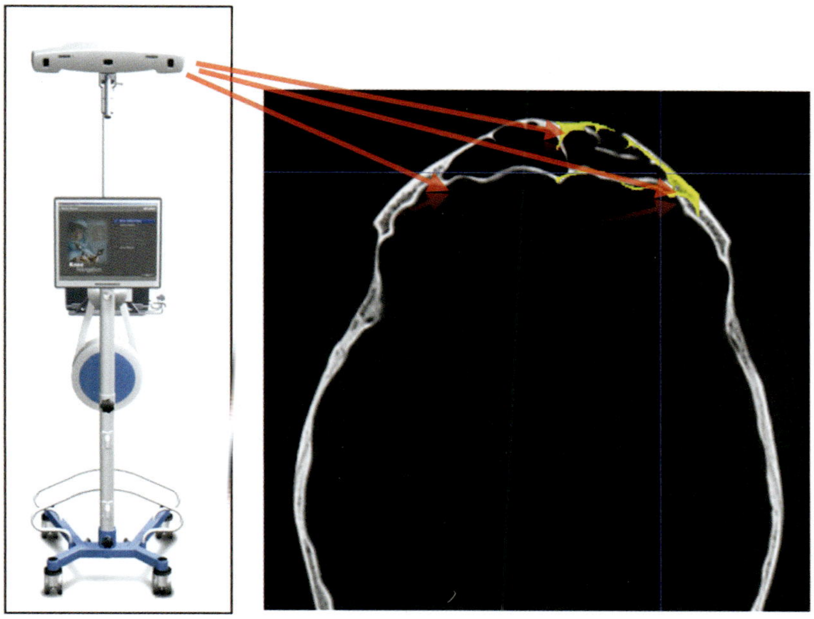

Figure 26 - Navigation system and preoperative planning of a frontal sinus fracture using the mirroring technique to restore the native anatomy

Technological development has covered four areas: image management and processing software, reconstruction materials, stereolithographic technology, and surgical navigation. Presurgical planning has become possible through the development of image management software. Specifically, the use of stereolithographic models in maxillofacial surgery introduces the possibility of three-dimensional presurgical planning directly on the model (fig. 24).

The introduction of preformed titanium meshes for orbital reconstruction makes it possible to manufacture custom-made structures which facilitate the correct restoration of the orbital anatomy (fig. 25).

Finally, the introduction of surgical navigation in cranio-maxillofacial surgery radically changed the surgical approach to facial and orbital diseases (fig. 26).

Facial protective shield

Usually, patients who undergo surgery for a maxillofacial fracture do not need any special postoperative treatment, but professional soccer players need to return quickly to their sport activities. Returning to sport practice early after surgery presents a high risk of refracture and can jeopardize sport performances causing fear in the athlete and even in his opponents [28].

Actually, the use of a facial protection mask after a facial fracture treatment is suggested for these reasons, and is already been reported in a lot of scientific studies [29].

A facial protection mask should be characterized by a light, flexible structure that even provides a complete peripheral vision. Only this kind of mask can give a soccer player the opportunity to quickly return to his professional activity, maintaining his own level of performance (fig. 27). Two layers form the mask structure: the outer layer is responsible for the impact energy transmission to the skull; then, its structure should be made of a material able to be stiff and flexible at the same time.

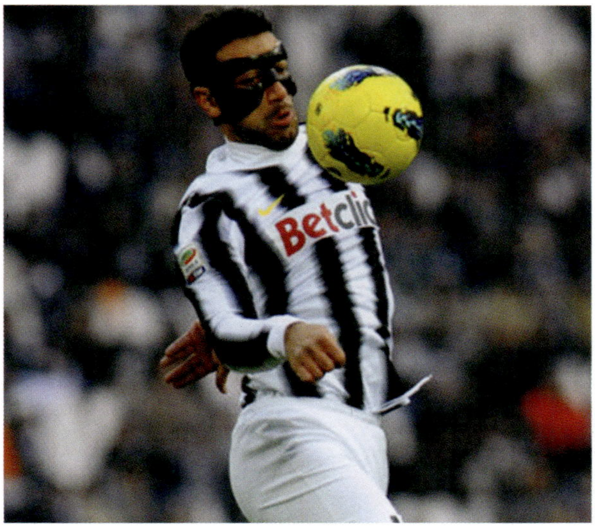

Figure 27 - Soccer player wearing a facial protective shield (sport.sky.it)

The project of an individual protection facial mask has the same purpose as that of a conventional face guard. In case of nasal bone fractures, the mask should protect the nasal structure, especially from direct frontal contact. The mask is x-shaped to obtain, in case of frontal impact, a simultaneous load discharge to both zygomatic buttress and frontal zygomatic process bilaterally. Protection of orbit-maxillary-zygomatic fractures presents many difficulties. The load dispersion force can be complicated, given the absence of a discharge vector to neighboring bones. Nevertheless, the mask should not only be trimmed as large as possible to obtain the maximum force transmission to frontal and temporal bones but also be realized as large as possible to increase the attenuation effect due to the inner layer capable of deformation.

Patients should use individual facial protection mask for 1 month after surgery while bone healing process should be completed.

Bibliography

1. Carroll SM, Jawad MA, West M, O'Connor TP. One hundred and ten sports related facial fractures. Br J Sports Med. 1995 Sep;29(3):194-5.

2. Tanaka N, Hayashi S, Amagasa T, Kohama G. Maxillofacial fractures sustained during sports. J Oral Maxillofac Surg. 1996 Jun;54(6):715-9; discussion 719-20.

3. Waldén M, Hägglund M, Ekstrand J. UEFA Champions League study: a prospective study of injuries in professional football during the 2001-2002 season. Br J Sports Med. 2005 Aug;39(8):542-6.

4. Nielsen AB, Yde J. Epidemiology and traumatology of injuries in soccer. Am J Sports Med. 1989 Nov-Dec;17(6):803-7.

5. Delilbasi C, Yamazawa M, Nomura K, Iida S, Kogo M. Maxillofacial fracturessustained during sports played with a ball. Oral Surg Oral Med Oral Pathol Oral Radiol Endod. 2004 Jan;97(1):23-7.

6. Cerulli G, Carboni A, Mercurio A, Perugini M, Becelli R. Soccer-related craniomaxillofacial injuries. J Craniofac Surg 2002;13:627–30.

7. Lim LH, Moore MH, Trott JA, David DJ. Sports related facial fractures: a review of 137 patients. Aust N Z J Surg 1993;63:784–9.

8. Lephart SM, Fu FH. Emergency treatment of athletic injuries. Dent Clin North Am 1991;35:707.

9. Assael LA, Ellis EE. Soft tissue and dentoalveolar injuries. In Peterson LJ, et al. Contemporary oral and maxillofacial surgery, St. Louis, 1988, CV Mosby.

10. Viozzi CF. Maxillofacial and Mandibular Fractures in Sports. Clin Sports Med. 2017 Apr;36(2):355-368.

11. Murphy C, O'Connell JE, Kearns G, et al. Sports-related maxillofacial injuries. J Craniofac Surg 2015;26(7):2120–3.

12. Cienfuegos R, Cornelius CP, Ellis E III, Kushner G. AO - mandible surgery reference. AO Foundation.

13. Haug RH, Prather J, Indresano AT. An epi- demiologic survey of facial fractures and concomitant injuries. J Oral Maxillofac Surg 1990;48:926–32.

14. Iida S, Kogo M, Sugiura T, Mima T, Matsuya T. Retrospective analysis of 1502 patients with facial fractures. Int J Oral Maxillofac Surg. 2001 Aug;30(4):286-90.

15. Blair VP. Surgery and diseases of the mouth and jaws. St. Louis (MO): C.V. Mosby Co. 1914;p.603.

16. Rowe NL, Killey HC. Fractures of the facial skeleton. Edinburgh and London: E. & S. Livingstone Ltd. 1955;p.923.

17. Dawson RL, Fordyce GL. Complex fractures of the middle third of the face and their early treatment. Br J Surg. 1953 Nov;41(167):255-68.

18. Middleton DS. Management of injuries of the nose and upper jaw. Proc R Soc Med. 1953 Jul;46(7):476-9.

19. Matsunaga RS, Simpson W, Toffal PH. Simplified protocol for treatment of malar fractures. Based on a 1,220-case eight-year experience. Arch Otolaryngol 1977;103:535.

20. Perkins SW, Dayan SH, Sklarew EC, Hamilton M, Bussell GS. The incidence of sports-related facial trauma in children. Ear Nose Throat J. 2000 Aug;79(8):632-4, 636, 638.

21. Schultz RC. One thousand consecutive cases of major facial injury. Rev Surg. 1970 Nov-Dec;27(6):394-410.

22. Swenson DM, Yard EE, Collins CL, Fields SK, Comstock RD. Epidemiology of US high school sports-related fractures, 2005-2009. Clin J Sport Med. 2010 Jul;20(4):293-9.

23. Staffel JG. Optimizing treatment of nasal fractures. Laryngoscope. 2002 Oct;112(10):1709-19.

24. Ostrander BT, Wang HD, Cusano A, Manson PN, Nam AJ, Dorafshar AH. Contemporary management of mandibular fracture nonunion-a retrospective review and treatment algorithm. J Oral Maxillofac Surg. 2018 Jul;76(7):1479-1493.

25. Borah GL, Ashmead D. The fate of teeth transfixed by osteosynthesis screws. Plast Reconstr Surg. 1996 Apr. 97(4):726-9.

26. Schramm A, Suarez-Cunqueiro MM, Rücker M, Kokemueller H, Bormann KH, Metzger MC, Gellrich NC. Computer-assisted therapy in orbital and mid-facial reconstructions. Int J Med Robot. 2009 Jun;5(2):111-24.

27. Novelli G, Tonellini G, Mazzoleni F, Sozzi D, Bozzetti A. Surgical navigation recording systems in orbitozygomatic traumatology. J Craniofac Surg. 2012 May;23(3):890-2.

28. Morita R, Shimada K, Kawakami S. Facial protection masks after fracture treatment of the nasal bone to prevent re-injury in contact sports. J Craniofac Surg. 2007 Jan;18(1):143-5.

29. Procacci P, Ferrari F, Bettini G, Bissolotti G, Trevisiol L, Nocini PF. Soccer-related facial fractures: postoperative management with facial protective shields. J Craniofac Surg. 2009 Jan;20(1):15-20.

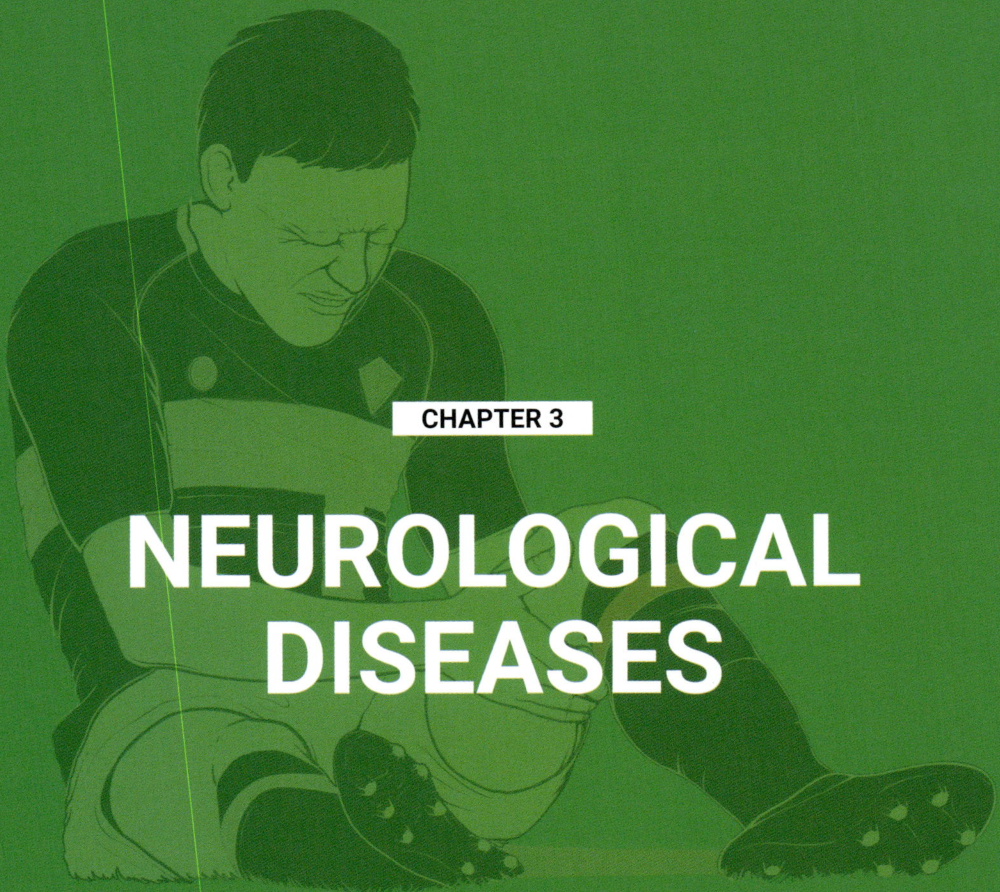

CHAPTER 3

NEUROLOGICAL DISEASES

Pietro Cortelli [1]

Umberto Pensato [2]

[1] Clinica Neurologica Rete Neurologica Metropolitana (NeuroMet) IRCCS Istituto delle Scienze Neurologiche, Bologna, Italy

[2] Department of Biomedic and Neuromotor Sciences (Dibinem) Alma Mater Studiorum, University of Bologna, Italy

Introduction

Soccer is one of the most popular sports worldwide, played by over 250 millions people, followed by many more. Numerous aspects of human health are positively influenced by soccer and physical activity in general, including neurological health. We will discuss about these benefits, particularly as a powerful strategy to prevent and ameliorate neurodegenerative processes. Also patients who have a neurological disease may enjoy the same health benefits when they play soccer with the right precautions.

We will discuss the example of individuals suffering from multiple sclerosis and epilepsy, two common neurological diseases among young people, who may play soccer.

Nonetheless, soccer, like all sports that expose to repetitive head impacts, may result in acute brain damage and possible neurological sequelae. Particularly important in this field are the emerging data about chronic traumatic encephalopathy (CTE), a neurodegenerative disease that specifically affects athletes exposed to head injury risk. Although soccer may seem to expose less to head injury compared to other sports, such as American football or boxing, it has a unique move that is the heading of the ball, whose possible cumulative damage effects have been studied only over the last few years.

Furthermore, we will review the correlation between amyotrophic lateral sclerosis and soccer, which seems to be soccer-specific, leading to the hypothesis that head trauma may not be the main putative factor.

Finally, we will discuss about sleep in soccer players life and how ameliorating its quality may be of benefit not only for the athletes' health, but also for their performance on the soccer field.

Head traumas

Contact sports athletes are exposed to many head injuries during their careers. Sports-related concussions are increasingly recognized as a public health problem [1, 2], not only because of their immediate effects, but in particular because of the increasing literature reporting associations with later neurological symptoms [3]. Head injuries may cause neurological damage after a single trauma or as a consequence of repetitive minor head traumas.

Soccer, despite not being a mainly physical contact sport such as boxing or American football, exposes to the risk of repetitive head injuries regardless of the soccer player's field position.

Soccer players are exposed to two different types of head impacts.

1. Unintentional head impacts (head to head contact or elbow/other body part against head) occur frequently in soccer matches. During the 2014 FIFA World Cup, the second most injured body part was the head, accounting for 18% of all traumas [4].

2. Intentional head impacts (e.g. heading) could cause micro traumas that can account for small but frequent sub-concussions. Among other sports, soccer is unique in its purposeful use of the head (heading), thus soccer players are the only athletes exposed to these intentional head impacts. Even if headings do not have a role in neurological symptoms after a single head trauma (they cannot cause a concussion), they may have a role in cumulative sub-concussive impacts that affect cognitive functions. It has been estimated that an average soccer player heads the ball 6-12 times per game and performs at least 2,000 headers during a 20-year career in addition to repetitive heading drills at training [5].

A recent study included 22 amateur soccer players who completed baseline and serial questionnaires covering soccer practice, head impacts (both intentional and unintentional) and frequency/severity of CNS symptoms. After the 2-week reported period, a median of 38 headers and 0.7 unintentional head impacts were reported. The authors found that both headers and unintentional head impacts were independently associated with CNS symptoms [6]. Moreover, participants reported a median of 4 outdoor practices per 2 weeks and 2 outdoors games, which would be comparable to many amateur soccer players around the world [7].

Classification

Many individuals who are exposed to an external force suffer a trauma limited to the cranial structure, without the involvement of the brain. Instead, whenever a patient presents with a loss of consciousness or the onset/worsening of a neurological sign or cognitive impairment, they had a traumatic brain injury (TBI).

The pathophysiology of such injuries consists in functional damage that cannot be seen with classic brain CT or MRI imaging, which are able to detect only structural damages.

TBIs are usually subdivided at onset on the basis of the Glasgow Coma Scale (GCS) into: mild (GCS 13-15), moderate (GCS 9-12), and severe (GCS <9). Severe TBIs are usually associated with structural damage, but also mild-moderate TBIs can rarely be associated with intracranial lesions. Many authors speak about concussion whenever an individual suffers from any neurological symptom/sign after a head trauma with the brain appearing normal on CT/MRI, so the term concussion may be synonymous with mild-moderate TBI. However, a patient's brain may be damaged even in the absence of any symptoms, because the neurological damage may have been too mild to be clinically appreciated. The term sub-concussions is used in these cases.

Single and repetitive head impacts may cause different neurological sequelae (tab. 1).

Assessment

Sport-Related Concussion (SRC) is a traumatic TBI occurring during a sport activity. The acute assessment of SRC in soccer is similar to that performed in other sports, with emphasis on early recognition, which is particularly important in order to recognise severe TBI that can cause structural damage and needs to be addressed in a hospital environment in order to perform neuroimaging evaluations. Sub-concussive events are not addressed in this section because they cannot be recognised nowadays.

A key component in side-line assessment is the rapid screening for a suspected concussion, rather than the definitive diagnosis.

Players manifesting clear on-field signs of concussion (e.g. loss of consciousness, tonic postur-

	Onset and progression	Type of trauma	Histology
Post-concussion syndrome	Acute onset * (usually resolved within 10 days)	Single concussion (usually mild to moderate)	Unknown
Chronic post-concussion syndrome	Acute onset *	Single concussion ** (usually moderate to severe)	Unknown
Post-traumatic dementia or parkinsonism	Acute onset *	Single concussion ** (usually moderate to severe)	Unknown
Chronic traumatic encephalopathy	Insidious onset and progressive course	Repetitive concussive and sub-concussive blows	Characteristic tau deposition

Table 1 - Neurological complications of head impacts
*** temporally related to an acute concussion**
**** athletes may have a history of previous multiple TBI**

Step 1 (red flags)	Neck stiffness/tenderness, vomiting, double vision, motor/sensory deficits of the extremities, severe/increasing headache, seizure, loss of consciousness, deterioration of conscious state, increasingly restless/agitated behaviour
Step 2 (observable signs)	Lying motionless on the playing surface, balance or gait difficulties, confusion, blank or vacant look
Step 3 (Maddocks' Questions)	
Step 4 (GCS and spine assessment)	

Table 2 - SCAT-5 four steps
SCAT-5: Sport Concussion Assessment Tool-5
GCS: Glasgow Coma Scale
(Modified from Echemendia RJ et al. [8])

ing, balance disturbance) should immediately be removed from sporting participation. Players with a suspected concussion following a significant head impact or presenting with symptoms can undergo a side-line screening with appropriate assessment tools.

A side-line evaluation should assess state of consciousness, orientation, cranial nerve function, balance as well as detect warning symptoms for severe injury.

The suspected diagnosis of concussion includes the following: somatic (headache), cognitive or emotional (lability) symptoms, physical signs (loss of consciousness, amnesia, neurological deficits), balance impairment, behavioural changes, sleep/wake disturbances (somnolence).

Sport Concussion Assessment Tool (SCAT) 5 currently represents the most well established and rigorously developed instrument available for side-line assessment [8].

SCAT-5

The SCAT-5 includes four steps to follow for on-field assessment (tab. 2).

The first two steps involve the identification of red flags and observable signs, which are warning signs of a serious injury (structural damage) requiring further evaluation using brain CT and/or MRI.

Step 3 consists in a side-line cognitive function evaluation: administration of Maddocks' Questions, a brief neuropsychological test with batteries that assess attention and memory function [9].

The fourth and last step consists in an evaluation specifically using the Glasgow Coma Scale and a cervical spine assessment.

Evolving and delayed-onset symptoms of concussion are well documented and highlight the need to consider a follow-up with serial evaluations after a suspected concussion, regardless of a negative side-line screening test.

Ideally SCAT-5 side-line evaluations should be complemented with a SCAT-5 baseline evaluation at the beginning of the season, aiming at the possibility to compare the individual baseline performance with post-injury performance, thus further improving the reliability of the individual assessment.

If, according to SCAT-5, a concussion cannot be definitively ruled out, the athlete should be removed from playing and not be allowed to continue the activity on the same day.

Although these recommendations have been well established, a recent assessment after head collision events during the FIFA 2014 World Cup showed that they were not followed in the majority of cases. Indeed, of 81 identified head collisions with two or more concussion signs, only 19 were officially reported. Eighty-six percent of the players who displayed three or more concussion signs returned to play during the same game although they should have been removed from participating [10].

One problem with SCAT-5 that may explain its low compliance rate is the need to isolate the affected athlete for about 10 minutes. This might be feasible in American football, as the game time can be paused, in soccer, however, the game time keeps running, the athlete is eager to play, and therefore a standardized neurological assessment is not routinely performed, increasing the risk of missing concussions.

Early and appropriate treatment

Soccer players, regardless of the level of participation (professional or not) should be treated using the same management principles noted above.

There is no specific treatment for SRC. After removal from play and medical and neurological clearance, a resting phase should follow. The basis for recommending physical and cognitive rest is that rest may ease discomfort during the acute recovery period by mitigating post-concussion symptoms and/or that rest may promote recovery by minimising brain energy demands following concussion. So far, the exact duration and amount of rest has not been well defined.

Following the first resting phase (usually 24-48 hours), a gradual return-to-play strategy should be followed (tab. 3). This stepwise approach includes designated time periods with increasing activity levels that the athletes must complete without worsening symptoms before moving on. First, the athlete is allowed minimal activity following the initial resting phase. Subsequently, training intensity increases until full performance.

Generally each step should take 24 hours, with downgrading to the previous stage if symptoms occur, so that athletes would take a minimum of one week to proceed through the full rehabilitation protocol once they are asymptomatic at rest.

Ensuring a sufficient period of absence from sports participation protects the athlete from the aggravating consequences of repetitive concussions.

Ongoing or persistent symptoms data support intervention including psychological, cervical and vestibular rehabilitation.

Concerning pharmacotherapy, currently there is limited evidence to support its use. If pharmacotherapy is used, concussed athletes should not only be free from concussion-related symptoms to return to play in the field, but they also should not be taking any pharmacological agents that may mask or modify such symptoms.

Recovery time

Clinical recovery encompasses a resolution of post-concussion-related symptoms and a return to clinically normal balance and cognitive functioning.

Post-concussion syndrome is largely a time-limited injury with clinical recovery occurring in 7-10 days for most of the professional players. Research on predicting recovery duration is limited. The most predictable variable associated with prolonged recovery is the immediate symptoms burden [11, 12, 13]. Other potential variables include history of prior concussion, younger age, prior history of headache or migraine or both, and prior mental health history [11, 12, 14]. These factors may potentially lead to chronic post-concussion syndrome.

No specific differences in recovery from SRC in

Stage	Aim	Activity	Goal of each step
1	Symptom-limited activity	Daily activities that do not cause symptoms	Gradual reintroduction of work/school activity
2	Light aerobic exercise	No resistance training	Increase heart rate
3	Sport-specific exercise	No head impact activities	Add movement
4	Non-contact training drills	Possible start of progressive resistance training	Exercise, coordination and increased thinking
5	Full contact practice	Participating in normal training activities	Restore confidence and assessment of functional skills by the coaching staff
6	Return to sport	Normal game playing	

Table 3 - Gradual return-to-play strategy for soccer players (Modified from McCrory P et al. [109])

Reduced total number of head impacts	- Soccer laws
Reduced intensity of head impacts	- Headgear - Neck muscle strength - Properties of the ball and playground surface
Early recognition of concussion	- Reduce barriers - Education - Spotters - Biomechanical sensors

Table 4 - Strategies to reduce the risk of neurological complication due to head impacts

soccer players compared with athletes of other sports have been found [15].
It is important to note that the physiological time of recovery may outlast the time for clinical recovery. Consequently, the athletes may be exposed to additional risks by returning to play.
Persistent symptoms are defined as symptoms that persist beyond the expected time frames (>10-14 days in adults and >4 weeks in children).

Prevention

No established treatment exists for head trauma chronic sequelae, thus prevention is paramount. Limiting the athlete's exposure to concussive and sub-concussive head impacts is the first approach. There are two main strategies: first preventing any kind of trauma and second reducing the trauma intensity so that it is less likely that a trauma will cause a concussion (tab. 4).
In order to prevent traumas, one of the possible solutions is to enforce more severe punishment (such as a red card and suspension for several matches) for players causing avoidable trauma to an opponent's head [16]. Studies reported a lower incidence of head-to-head and elbow-to-head incidents after granting the referee the authority to punish intentional elbow-to-head with immediate red cards [17, 18]. Thus, enforcement of existing rules can limit concussive injury.
The use of headgear can protect against severe traumatic brain injury. Soft-shelled headgear has been developed under the hypothesis of preventing concussion through the use of energy absorbent padding designed to reduce head impact force and subsequent acceleration. Laboratory testing has shown that headgear is effective in reducing impact force at high speeds in simulated head-to-head impacts [19, 20, 21], but not during heading [22]. The effect of soccer headgear on reducing cumulative effects of repetitive head trauma is unknown as there is a paucity of high-quality field research to date. Furthermore, it would be very challenging to propose it to soccer players rather than to combative sports athletes, because heading is an integral part of soccer. Finally, wearing headgear may also change the athlete's playing behaviour, giving them a false sense of protection and potentially inducing them to play more aggressively [23].
Strength imbalance in the neck contributes to greater head acceleration, thus strengthening the neck muscles should be protective against head injury. It is well known that the neck muscles are amenable to training and short-term training (5 weeks, twice per week in professional rugby players) can increase neck strength by nearly 20%. There is some evidence showing reduced concussion after neck muscle strengthening, however so far data are still conflicting and further studies are necessary.
Finally, the properties of the ball as well as the playing surface are areas that potentially have implications for injury prevention. The former is particularly important for young players who should play with an appropriately sized ball and attend to the inflation pressure of the ball. Instead, whether different playing surfaces are associated with different risks for injury is at this time unclear, but it is an area of future research [24].
A central feature of any successful concussion management programme is the accurate and timely identification of possible injury. Education to be recognised by the referee, who is the one who decides to stop the game, is pivotal to injury identification. However, it is important that also other figures be educated in this area, such as athletes,

athletic trainers, sports medicine physicians and coaches because they can potentially alert the referee [15].

The use of in-game spotters who review live game play can help recognize unnoticed injuries [25]. The 2018 FIFA World Cup in Russia was the first tournament using spotters to assist and communicate possible injuries to the medical teams on the field [15]. However, the institution of such programmes is complex and expensive, placing them out of reach for most non-professional or non-elite organisations.

Another possible measure is the use of biomechanical sensors, both in helmeted sports and non-helmeted sports (e.g. mouthguard, earpiece, retainer). They can potentially work as radiation sensors work for radiologists, alerting when a dangerous threshold has been exceeded. However, they did not show a specific "concussion threshold" (impact magnitude is an insufficient predictor of concussion) [26] and none have been validated in soccer so far.

Finally, there are many barriers to identifying head injuries during a soccer game. Indeed, soccer is a fast moving game with many players spread out across a large playing surface. Players are competitive and often reluctant to report to coaches and medical staff that they are experiencing symptoms because of the fear of being removed from the play. Furthermore, additional challenges are delayed symptom onset, if any (sub-concussion), only two halves and no time-outs with few stoppages of play, substitution rules and inadequate time to evaluate injured athletes.

Chronic post-concussion syndrome

Chronic post-concussion syndrome refers to a condition in those athletes in whom post-concussion symptoms do not appear to resolve, lasting longer than one year. Common symptoms may include headache, dizziness, impaired attention, poor memory, executive dysfunctions, irritability, and depression [27]. Unlike CTE, chronic post-concussion syndrome and post-traumatic dementia/parkinsonism have an acute onset that is temporally related to a single concussive event and does not occur insidiously following a latent period, which is characteristic of CTE.

Chronic traumatic encephalopathy

Chronic traumatic encephalopathy (CTE) is a progressive neurodegenerative disorder caused by repeated concussive or sub-concussive head injuries. It has a unique neuropathological finding distinct from other neurodegenerative disorders. It is characterised by perivascular accumulations of phosphorylated tau (p-tau) in neurons and astrocytes at the depth of the sulci. It was described for the very first time in 1926 in some retired boxers who developed behavioural, cognitive and mood symptoms. Thus the syndrome was called "punch-drunk syndrome" [28] and later "dementia pugilistica" [29]. In the following years, CTE has been recognised in the brains of many other contact sport athletes, mainly in American football [30], but also in many other sports including soccer [31].

The very first documented case of CTE in a retired soccer player occurred to be a very famous one. Bellini, the captain of the Brazilian team that won the first Football World Cup for Brazil in 1958, was initially diagnosed with presumed Alzheimer's disease. However, after his death, a neuropathological examination showed macroscopic and microscopic alterations of CTE [32]. The case was published only in 2016 and his story was also published in a book written by his wife entitled "Bellini: the first captain champion" [16].

In the following years, further cases of CTE confirmed pathology in retired soccer players were published [33, 31].

Epidemiology

The true incidence and prevalence of CTE is unknown because of a lack of epidemiologic data. However, an anatomopathological study among 202 deceased individuals who had a significant history of repetitive head trauma related to either contact sport or military service found CTE in 87% of cases [30]. Furthermore, a recent retrospective epidemiological analysis comparing 7,476 former Scottish professional soccer players, found a 3.45 higher risk of mortality with neurodegenerative diseases compared with controls [110]. No anatomopathological data was available, thus the true incidence of CTE among neurodegenerative diseases in this population remains unknown.

Duration of exposure to soccer
Years since retirement from soccer
Increasing age
High number of concussions
High number of sub-concussions
Apolipoprotein E (APOE) ε4 genotype

Table 5 - Possible risk factors for developing CTE in soccer players
CTE: Chronic Traumatic Encephalopathy

Risk factors

Exposure to head injuries is a necessary yet not sufficient factor in developing CTE. The frequency, severity, and total exposure to head trauma necessary to cause the condition and how other factors, such as genetics and modifiable lifestyle factors, may contribute to it is still not known (tab. 5). Some associations have been found between APOE ε4 and risk of worse outcome [34]. Also a correlation between exposure to sports, years since retirement, and age at death has been found [35].

Clinical presentation

CTE is characterized by a clinical constellation of usually progressive cognitive, behavioural and mood changes. Cognitive symptoms are the most common at clinical presentation, involving mainly attention, executive functions, and impaired memory [36]. Also behavioural and mood disorders are very common, presenting as depression or aggressive behaviour (emotional explosiveness, physical or verbal aggressiveness, impulse and control problems) [36]. These symptoms may lead to very important social problems such as substance abuse, bankruptcy and failed relationships. Motor symptoms are much more subtle in the disease as they are present in less than one third of patients at presentation. However, clinicians should always evaluate signs of motor neuron disease, parkinsonism, and cerebellar signs as they have been associated with head injuries [37].

Diagnosis

Similarly to other neurodegenerative conditions, neuropathological findings are the gold standard for diagnosis, therefore a definitive diagnosis of CTE in a living person is not yet possible. Currently, no clinical diagnostic consensus criteria for CTE exist, but only research diagnostic criteria have been validated [38]. In these criteria the term traumatic encephalopathy syndrome (TES) is used to refer to the clinical syndrome associated with repetitive blows to the head. Thus, the criteria allow a TES diagnosis. The proposed TES diagnostic criteria include general criteria and core/supportive features (tab. 6).

General criteria specify a minimum amount of head traumas and exposure. In particular in contact sports, such as soccer, a minimum of a 6-year exposure is required.

The research diagnostic criteria describe also four TES subtypes based on the presence of the core clinical features.

1. A behavioural/mood variant that represents 28% of cases at the initial clinical presentation and occurs in young patients (average age of onset 34 years).

2. A cognitive variant that represents 32% of cases at the clinical presentation and occurs in older patients (average age of onset 59 years).

3. A mixed variant (40% of cases).

4. TES dementia form, which is the natural history of all the previous subtypes and is defined as presence of severe cognitive/behavioural symptoms interfering with usual activities.

There are some peculiar neuroradiological features that can support the diagnosis: cortical thinning and atrophy and a cavum septum pellucidum. Indeed, during a trauma, fluid waves may produce fenestrations within the septum and allow the entry of fluid between the leaflets creating a separation within the structure. However, this sign can be present in up to 15% of healthy individuals [39]. PET and single-photon emission computed tomography (SPECT) scans may also be useful in the investigational evaluation. Glucose hypometabolism and hypoperfusion in the frontal-parieto-occipital lobes, posterior cingulate cortex, and cerebellum among the referred population exposed to repetitive head injuries [40, 41] has been observed.

A very recent study used flortaucipir PET and florbetapir PET to measure deposition of tau and amyloid beta in living CTE patients showing a higher tau level and not elevated level of amyloid beta. In particular three regions were associated with a

General criteria (all three criteria must be met)	Core clinical features (at least one must be present)	Supportive clinical features (at least two must be present)
History of multiple impacts to the head *	Cognitive difficulties	Impulsivity
Absence of other neurological disorders that could account for all clinical features	Behavioural changes (in particular aggressiveness)	Anxiety
Clinical features must be present for a minimum of 12 months	Mood changes (in particular depressive symptoms)	Apathy
		Paranoia
		Suicidality
		Headache
		Motor signs
		Documented progressive decline of symptoms
		Delayed onset after head impact exposure (usually at least two years after the period of maximal exposure)

Table 6 - Research diagnostic criteria for traumatic encephalopathy syndrome
*** minimum of four mild traumatic brain injuries or moderate/severe traumatic brain injury or sub-concussive trauma. A minimum of 6 years involvement in soccer is required**
(Modified from Montenigro PH et al. [38])

higher tau deposition compared to matched controls: bilateral superior frontal, bilateral medial temporal, and left parietal [42].

All potential useful biomarkers are illustrated on the following table (tab. 7) [38].

Further research diagnostic criteria exist for CTE based on clinical and biomarker evaluation (tab. 8).

Therapy

Treatment in CTE is currently supportive and several classes of medications that are commonly used in other neurodegenerative diseases can be tried. Medications to consider include acetylcholinesterase inhibitors for cognitive issues, selective serotonin reuptake inhibitors (SSRI) for depression and anxiety, memantine for attentional issues in those with TES dementia and, with caution, antipsychotics for aggressive behaviour [37].

Amyotrophic lateral sclerosis and soccer

Amyotrophic lateral sclerosis (ALS) is a neurodegenerative disorder characterized by the loss of lower and upper motor neurons and a progressive and fatal course. Its cause is unknown, although several putative pathogenetic mechanisms have been proposed: excitotoxicity, oxidative stress, damage of axonal flux, and protein aggregation. The mean age of onset is 56 years in individuals without a known family history and 46 years in individuals with familial ALS. The spinal form of ALS (onset in a distal limb) is the most common. However, 20-30% of patients present with bulbar onset and a very small percentage of patients present with respiratory onset or frontotemporal dementia. The prevalence is estimated as 5 per 100,000 people [43, 44].

A higher risk of developing ALS has been reported in a cluster of professional soccer players in Italy. In particular, the latest epidemiological study enrolled 7,325 male professional soccer players who were active between 1970 and 2001, observing a 6.5 higher risk of developing ALS compared to the calculated risk (8 observed risk vs 1.24 expected cases) [45]. Furthermore, these 8 patients showed unique peculiarities such as a higher prevalence of bulbar onset (5 out of 8 cases), an over-representation of midfielders, whose physical activity characteristics differ from those of other soccer players (a higher maximal oxygen uptake – VO2max – rel-

Brain MRI findings	- Cavum septum pellucidum, cavum vergae or fenestration - Evidence of increased cortical thinning consistent with neurodegeneration - Evidence of cortical atrophy (particularly in the frontal, hippocampal, thalamic, and amygdala regions)
Cerebrospinal fluid (CSF) findings	- Normal CSF amyloid beta levels - Increased phosphorylated tau to total tau ratio
PET findings	- Negative PET amyloid imaging - Positive PET tau imaging

Table 7 - Potential biomarkers for chronic traumatic encephalopathy
MRI= Magnetic Resonance Imaging; CSF= Cerebrospinal Fluid; PET= Positron Emission Tomography

ative to body mass, a marker of aerobic power, and a higher proportion of lean body mass [46]), and younger age of onset. The authors also compared the prevalence of ALS in a basketball cohort and a road cyclists cohort, who have some possible common risk factors such as drug abuse and physical activity, without finding any case of ALS, leading to the hypothesis that the unknown risk factor may be soccer specific.

Two possible explanations have been proposed: (i) an absolute risk of developing ALS for soccer players or (ii) an anticipation effect (earlier development of ALS in subjects who, without specific triggers, would have developed ALS at an older age). In any case, Italian soccer players must have been exposed to some potential risk factors.

The apparent relation between ALS and Italian soccer reflects the attention paid by local neurologists following the report by a prosecutor who investigated the early deaths from ALS of more than 40 former soccer players, driven by concerns about illegal drug use. There have been occasional reports of soccer players elsewhere in Europe, but the association between ALS and professional soccer has never been extensively investigated in countries outside Italy.

Here we review all the possible risk factors to which soccer players who have developed ALS may have been exposed.

Head traumas and ALS

The hypothesis that ALS may be caused by antecedent trauma dates back to 1911 or earlier. This was driven by observations that the clinical onset of ALS occasionally follows trauma. After it was accepted that trauma in general did not occur in excess prior to the biological onset of ALS [47], attention shifted to head trauma. In support of this hypothesis an apparent excess of ALS cases was found not only in soccer players, but also in US

Probable CTE (all the following)	- Any type of TES - Does not meet criteria for another disorder more consistently than TES - Has at least one positive potential biomarker for CTE
Possible CTE (all the following)	- Any type of TSE - No presence of potential biomarkers - Meets diagnostic criteria for another disorder that on its own could account for the clinical presentation
Unlikely CTE (either of the following)	- Does not meet TES diagnostic criteria - Negative tau PET imaging

Table 8 - CTE Diagnostic Classification
CTE: Chronic Traumatic Encephalopathy; TES: Traumatic Encephalopathy Syndrome; PET: Positron Emission Tomography
(Modified from Montenigro PH et al. [38])

footballers [48], in whom a risk factor as high as 40-fold was found in a retrospective study [49], and not among other athletes such as road cyclists and basketball players who do not share exposure to head injury [45]. A recent meta-analysis showed a moderate association among persons with previous head injuries and risk of ALS; in particular, in persons with multiple head injuries, the risk was more than 10-fold higher [50]. It has been proposed that ALS may in some instances be a complication of CTE, although this has been vigorously disputed [51].

Exercise and ALS

The mechanisms underlying the adverse effects of physical activity include oxidative stress and glutamate excitotoxicity. Increased physical activity has given conflicting results in ALS mice models and humans. Most studies showed no evidence of any real association, but a recent study provided class one evidence for a positive association between the history of physical activity and risk of development of ALS and showed an increased linearity with increasing physical activity [52]. However, possible confounding factors such as the additional effect of trauma exposure may have contributed. Furthermore, the cumulative effects of vigorous exercise cannot be established with precision in humans, thus all the findings must be interpreted in the light of these difficulties.

Although it is intuitive that physical activity is linked to the onset of ALS since it is a disorder long recognised to be associated with neuronal excitotoxicity, so far, there are no strong data to confirm it.

Substance overuse and ALS

The abuse of drugs, both therapeutic drugs and illegal substances, has also been proposed to explain the observed risk in soccer players. Consistently, some professional soccer players make excessive use of medications and nutritional supplements and exposure to anti-inflammatory medications is extensive among patients with ALS compared to the general population. The most frequent medications use by soccer players are non-steroidal drugs (NSAIDs) [53]. However, a large study investigating 708,000 participants, 708 of whom later developed ALS, did not find any association [54]. In summary, at present, there is no clear evidence that any drug is related to ALS.

Dietary supplements and ALS

It has been proposed that branched-chain amino acids (BCAAs), commonly used as dietary supplements by athletes to stimulate muscle growth and recovery after intense exercise, lead to an increased incidence of ALS among professional soccer and US football players. BCAAs can accelerate the progression of the disease in patients with ALS and there has been excess mortality in patients randomized to BCAAs in a multicentre study in Italy [55]. High BCAAs doses for a long period induced hyperexcitability in cultured cortical neurons and pyramidal neurons from motor cortex slices of mice. The data seem to indicate a similar phenotype of neurons treated with BCAAs and neurons from the G93A mouse model of ALS [56]. However, in vivo studies are needed to investigate behavioural and electrophysiological changes and the neuroprotective action of compounds reversing hyperexcitability [57].

Exposure to pesticides and ALS

A distinctive feature of soccer players, compared to other sports, is the continuous contact with grass, an environmental exposure that links them to farmers, a population group that has an increased risk for ALS [58].

Exposure to pesticides used in soccer field is an alternative explanation of the possible association between ALS and soccer. The pesticides used in agriculture have been reported to be associated with ALS, sometimes with evidence of dose-response effects [59, 60, 61]. However, no association with ALS and gene polymorphism of paraoxonase (an enzyme detoxifying organophosphate pesticides) was found in a meta-analysis [62]. In summary, contact with pesticides as a risk factor for ALS in soccer players cannot be excluded but the extent of exposure cannot be calculated, thus leaving the question of a possible association unanswered.

In conclusion, evidence from epidemiological studies on the association of soccer and ALS remains inconclusive and larger more focused studies are needed. Furthermore, the specific soccer-related trigger could not be determined so far and it is likely that the susceptibility of soccer players to develop ALS has derived from a complex interplay between a genetic predisposition for physical endurance and external factors such as drugs and herbicides.

Soccer players are a small proportion of all Italian cases of ALS (about 0.25% of prevalent cases), but this subgroup may help to uncover the pathophysiology and risk factors of this fatal neurodegenerative disease.

Sleep and soccer

Sleep has a pivotal function for surviving and enhancing cognitive and motor performances as shown by prolonged and partial deprivation of sleep in healthy controls, although its exact physiological mechanism is still largely unknown.

A body of evidence showed that a partial sleep disturbance, defined as compromised intermittent periods of less than required sleep, has mostly psychological effects (mood alterations, confusion, anger) and increases reaction time. These effects have a secondary negative impact on physical performance such as what has been demonstrated in swimmers and weightlifters [63].

A recent study outlined the negative effect of a single night sleep deprivation also on specific soccer skills (e.g. ball control, kicking, dribbling) [64].

Interestingly, in partial sleep disturbances, extended sleep time or brief naps programmed during the day (for example before afternoon and evening training sessions) can improve cognitive and motor performance.

Conditions interfering with sleep

Regular physical activity improves the quality and quantity of sleep and this has been shown also in a soccer players cohort [65].

However, elite soccer players are often exposed to various conditions that can interfere with sleep, potentially leading to sleep restriction, both after a soccer match and chronically (tab. 9). Indeed, a survey involving UEFA Europa League soccer players indicated worse sleep following night matches and this is related to acute conditions that are related with night matches [66]. Practising physical activity in the evening or, more accurately, close to sleep time, is commonly discouraged, but different studies did not show any related clear alteration [67]. Thus, other environmental and match-related behaviour may have a role.

Soccer players are exposed to night light during the match (stadiums are very brightly lit) and after the match (e.g. use of tablets, smartphones). Night light exposure decreases the physiological melatonin release by the hypothalamic suprachiasmatic nucleus, which is fundamental in sleep onset.

Night matches are also usually the most important matches (e.g. Champions League matches or national league big matches) resulting in excitement/stress and an important post-match outcome-related mood [68]. Light exposure and hyperadrenergic state may lead to difficulties in initiating sleep.

Furthermore, soccer players take activating substances (caffeine, energy drinks) that impact on sleep onset, and alcohol, which worsens sleep quality.

Soccer teams are asked to arrive at the place of the competition the day before the match, resulting in a night spent in a hotel before a game for the away team. The first-night effect is a well-known phenomenon that is thought to result from an individual's lack of adaptation to the unfamiliar environment [69]. Moreover, travelling across differ-

Potential (acute) match-related stressors	Potential chronic stressor
Bright light exposure at night	Travelling (jet lag)
Match outcome-related mood	Individual chronotype
Night physical activity	Inconsistency in match schedules
Pre and post-match substance use (caffeine, energy drinks, alcohol)	
First night effect	

Table 9 - Potential conditions that may lead to sleep deprivation in soccer players ent time zones may result also in a jet-lag effect. Finally, the individual chronotype (predisposition to sleep at a certain time of the day) may be in conflict with the demands of the soccer club [70].

Sleep and recovery post-exercise

Sleep provides also physiological functions that are critical for recovery after prolonged exercise [68], thus it is even more paramount for an athlete to have good quality sleep.

Sleep deprivation among professional soccer players may be detrimental to the post-match recovery time course. The time necessary to fully recover after a soccer match is estimated at 2-3 days, but can be as long as 4 days when the schedule is particularly congested (e.g. two matches per week) [71, 72, 73]. It has been demonstrated that sleep deprivation prolongs the necessary time to recover due to decrease in glycogen synthesis, potentially leading to an increase in injury risk. Finally, sleep is pivotal to recover also from mental fatigue, which, chronically, may lead to persistent fatigue [74].

Possible interventions to improve sleep benefits

Kick-off time is often out of synchrony with the typical time for training during the week leading to the match. This lack of synchrony might affect both performance in competition and internal circadian rhythm synchronization. It has been shown that reduced physical performance due to expression of circadian variation can be partially ameliorated by training at that particular time of day [75]. Consequently, professional soccer players may potentially benefit from training in the night under floodlights in anticipation of playing night soccer matches [68].

Overall, it is very common among athletes to have lower total sleep time or efficiency of sleep; thus, obtaining a detailed sleep history is pivotal because improving sleep has the potential to improve an athlete's overall physical performance.

Neuroprotective effects of physical activity

It is widely recognised that physical activity as a lifestyle represents a pivotal issue for the enhancement and preservation of body and brain well-being during all stages of life. Indeed, physical activity and running highly diminish several diseases through neurogenesis, which is paramount in preventing neurodegenerative diseases and rescuing from brain damage.

The beneficial effects of exercise may be mediated by multiple factors: (i) improving brain blood flow, (ii) enhancing subventricular zone (SVZ, the niche of neuronal progenitors) cell proliferation and migration, and (iii) increasing levels of neurotrophic factors such as the brain-derived neurotrophic factor (BDNF).

The influence of exercise in brain functioning may be directly fixed into human evolution; indeed, physical activity is correlated with survival and individuals who exercise might show a biological advantage over sedentary individuals [76].

Benefits on cognitive functions

The effect of running during adolescence, compared to later stages of life, might exert a more persistent benefit on brain functioning. This is likely related to the reorganization, both morphological and functional, that occurs at this stage of life, when the transiently higher neuroplasticity may promote enduring changes in response to environmental stimuli (including exercise) [77].

The beneficial effect on this stage of life is also confirmed in a study investigating exercise benefits in adolescent and adult rats, which showed significant age-related differences in the duration of the effect of running [78]. These data are also supported by studies in humans that showed a superior ability in cognitive functions in high levels of aerobic fitness in childhood and larger bilateral hippocampal volume measured on brain MRI compared to less fit controls [79, 80]. In this regard, it is important to note that, recently, children have become increasingly sedentary and typically adult-onset diseases, such as cardiovascular ones, are becoming more prevalent during childhood.

Benefits on depression symptoms

It has been suggested that defective adult neurogenesis may result in depression disorders. In fact, following stress paradigms, adult neurogenesis is altered in rodents. It is thought that in depression disorders the brain is unable to respond with appropriate adaptive plasticity and decreased neurogenesis is a factor contributing to such reduction of plasticity. This has been called "neurogenesis hypothesis" and has some supporting evidence: (i) depressed patients showed a volumetric reduction of hippocampi [81] (likely due to impaired neurogenesis because neurodegeneration should not occur in these patients), (ii) antidepressant medications enhance neurogenesis in adult mice [82], (iii) the time of maturation of newly generated neurons equals the latency to the onset of therapeutic effects of antidepressant medications (around 4 weeks) [83]. In line with this, several epidemiological studies showed that individuals who followed different programmes of exercise displayed milder depressive symptoms and were less likely to develop major depressive disorders and this anti-depressive effect may be mediated by the exercise-induced neurogenesis [84].

Benefits after traumatic brain injury

Evidence showed that pre-traumatic brain injury (TBI) exercise improves the recovery of sensorimotor and cognitive performances after a TBI compared to sedentary controls. Moreover, in the early aftermath of TBI, exercise increases the number of endogenous stem cells around the damaged area. These results support the idea that exercise may represent an important aid for neuroprotection against TBI [85, 86].

Benefits on aging and neurodegeneration

Normal aging is characterized by morphological and functional brain changes, leading to cognitive weakening. The main mechanisms are inflammatory process, oxidative stress, reduced synaptic plasticity, which lead to an irreversible loss of neurons and white matter volume, and progressive decrease of neurogenesis, particularly in the hippocampi.

Several lines of evidence suggest that physical activity counteracts the cognitive decline occurring in adulthood [87] and randomized clinical trials have revealed that aerobic exercise can lower the rate of cognitive decline in the elderly [88]. Indeed, the greater extent of physical activity is prognostic of larger hippocampal volume in healthy elderly individuals [89].

Exercise also favours brain health attenuating influences on atherosclerotic cerebrovascular disease. In fact, it has been observed that regular exercise during old age is able to enhance hippocampal volume up to 2% and to ameliorate performance in spatial and episodic memory tasks [90, 91], as well as attention [92].

Alzheimer's disease

Epidemiological data suggest that physical activity is correlated with decreased frequency of Alzheimer's disease (AD) [93] and higher rate of survival in patients diagnosed with AD [94]. Other clinical evidence indicates that regular exercise reduces amyloid plaques deposition and preserves from brain atrophy and temporal lobe volume loss [95]. Finally, a recent study has confirmed that 30 min of daily physical training in AD patients significantly decreases depressive symptoms and improves their quality of life [96]. In mice models of AD, running has shown conflicting evidence regarding the amyloid plaques depositions and load, suggesting that benefits mediated by exercise in humans may be related also to an increment of the cognitive reserve [84].

Parkinson's disease

Accumulating evidence suggests that physical exercise may have a neuroprotective effect in Parkinson's disease (PD), beyond the general salutary effects on age-related afflictions.

Moderate to vigorous exercise habits in midlife significantly reduced the risk of later developing PD in three large cohorts [97, 98, 99]. The PD risk reduction was significant even when restricted to periods well before PD. A meta-analysis of prospective studies documented a risk reduction with odds ratio 0.67 [98]. There is also increasing evidence that exercise not only prevents but also slows down the progression of the disease. In keeping with this, exercise has been associated with better cognitive and motor scores, improved corticomotor excitability, and longevity in PD patients [100].

However, it must be taken into account that reverse causality cannot be excluded in the studies of exercise and subsequent neurodegenerative risk because no randomized clinical trials have been carried out. Indeed, preclinical PD or AD may manifest years earlier due to reduced activities or aversion to exercise. Also, health-conscious people who exercise may be more likely to consult physicians and have PD diagnosed.

In conclusion, data available so far indicate that physical activity may have a positive effect on brain function throughout the lifespan. Even if there are no specific studies on soccer, studies about aerobic exercise and running may largely be extended for soccer playing, suggesting that soccer may have a positive effect on neuroprotection.

Neurological patients who practise soccer

When athletes have a neurological disease, many believe that the correct approach is to keep them off the playing field. Instead, these athletes may enjoy the same health benefits as others, such as improved cognition, sleep, mood, and life satisfaction. Furthermore, a meta-analysis substantiated that exercise improves depression symptoms in individuals with neurological disorders [101].

At the same time, concern has been expressed that soccer participation may place individuals with a neurological disease at risk. Of course, the level of risk is disease specific. Healthcare practitioners and athletic trainers should be aware of the evidence associated with these risks. We will discuss the possible contraindications in two common neurological diseases among young individuals: multiple sclerosis and epilepsy.

Multiple sclerosis patients

No formal exercise or sport participation guidelines exist for athletes with multiple sclerosis (MS). The common myth that MS patients should not exercise may date back to 1890, when Wilhelm Uhthoff first described the relapse of symptoms in patients with MS after increased physical activity. He thought that physical exercise made the symptoms come back and he determined that these patients should not be allowed to exercise. Later, increased core body temperature was revealed as the cause of symptom relapse after physical activity (Uhthoff's phenomenon) [102] and new publications began to show benefits of aerobic exercise in MS management [63]. Indeed, exercise improves pulmonary function and the immune system through increasing vitamin D levels [103] and is generally considered safe. In order to avoid the relapse of symptoms, a core body temperature cooling protocol has been suggested: these athletes should gradually perform a routine warm-up until they reach their maximum activity level, followed by a cool-down period and several hours of recovery [102].

Epileptic patients

In adolescents with epilepsy, regular exercise decreases seizure frequency and it also provides a psychosocial benefit, as epileptic individuals are not isolated from their peers [104].

First of all, it is important to note that one seizure is not enough to define an athlete as suffering from epilepsy.

The International League Against Epilepsy (ILAE) defines epilepsy as any of the following conditions: (i) at least two unprovoked (or reflex) seizures occurring more than 24 hours apart; (ii) one unprovoked (or reflex) seizure and an at least 60% probability of further seizures over the following 10 years (similarly to the general recurrence risk after two seizures); or (iii) diagnosis of an epilepsy syndrome. Epilepsy is considered resolved if the epilepsy syndrome is age dependent and the individual passes that age or the individual is seizure free for 10 years and is off seizure medications for at least the last 5 years of seizure freedom [105].

The ILAE established a task force specifically for sports and epilepsy. In 2016, they published a statement that summarized recommendations and research. Recommendations included the following: (i) a neurologist must be directly involved to determine the risk for an athlete with seizures; (ii) before an athlete participates in sports, a neurologist should obtain a full seizure history, including seizure type, frequency, semiology, aura presence, severity, provoking factors, compliance with therapy, and previous injuries related to seizures; (iii) a neurologist must ensure that the athlete will be fully supervised by family members or the athletic team staff during competitions [106].

The ILAE categorizes sports into different groups based on potential injury or death to persons with

≥ 1 symptomatic seizures	Permitted
Single unprovoked seizure	Permitted
Seizure free ≥ 12 months	Permitted
Sleep-related seizures only	Permitted
Seizures without impaired awareness	Permitted
Seizures with impaired awareness	Permitted at neurologist's discretion; it applies when seizures are precipitated by a specific activity
Epilepsy resolved (no seizures >10 years and off anti-epilepsy drugs >5years)	Permitted
Medication withdrawal	Permitted at neurologist's discretion; it applies when seizures are precipitated by a specific activity

Table 10 - Recommendations for soccer participation for people with epilepsy or with other seizure disorders
(Modified from Capovilla G et al. [106])

epilepsy, and possible harm to other players. Soccer is categorized among collective sports on the ground, which is the safest group (there are no additional risks for epilepsy patients playing soccer) and then can be sub-categorized based on the athlete's seizure frequency and semiology [106] (tab. 10).

Injury rates during competition are equal or lower in athletes with seizures compared to players without seizures. The hospitalization rate for comparable injuries is higher in athletes with seizures than in others, but this rate is most likely caused by a more cautious approach in athletes with seizures [104]. Healthcare practitioners and athletic trainers must be familiar with sports-related factors that may lower the seizure threshold. Common electrolyte imbalances occurring in sports include hyper- and hypoglycaemia, hyponatremia, hypocalcemia, and hypomagnesemia [107]. Since electrolyte changes are common in all athletes after exercise, athletes with seizures must be advised to maintain proper nutrition and hydration to prevent such changes [108]. Poor sleep hygiene and sleep disruption also lowers the seizure threshold, and athletes must maintain proper sleep hygiene daily [63].

Given the numerous medications and substances that may lower the seizure threshold, athletes should have their physician evaluate seizure risk for any prescribed medications.

Multiple medications are used to treat seizures. Studies show that exercise does not affect anticonvulsant pharmacokinetics [104]. However, if athletes decrease or eliminate seizure medications as part of a planned overall reduction of seizure therapy, the ILAE guidelines suggest that they take a 6-month break from sport participation to determine whether sport activity was worsening seizures [106]. If seizures worsen during a period of medication reduction, the ILAE guidelines suggest that athletes take an additional 3-month break from sport participation, resume medications, and then be re-evaluated.

Finally, athletes should be counselled on the potential side effects of seizure medications that may impair performance. Such effects include decreased hand-eye coordination, reflex speed, mental clarity, nausea, vomiting, diarrhoea, constipation, changes in vision, weight, appetite or personality, somnolence, bone density loss, tooth decay, hair loss, and hyponatremia.

Bibliography

1. Faul M, Xu L, Wald MM, Coronado VG. Traumatic Brain Injury in the United States. Emergency Department Visits, Hospitalizations and Deaths 2002-2006. March 2010, Centers for Disease Control and Prevention - National Center for Injury Prevention and Control.
2. Centers for Disease Control and Prevention. Nonfatal traumatic brain injuries related to sports and recreation activities among persons aged ≤19 years--United States, 2001-2009. MMWR Morb Mortal Wkly Rep. 2011 Oct 7;60(39):1337-42.
3. Guskiewicz KM, McCrea M, Marshall SW, Cantu RC, Randolph C, Barr W, Onate JA, Kelly JP. Cumulative effects associated with recurrent concussion in collegiate football players: the NCAA Concussion Study. JAMA. 2003 Nov 19;290(19):2549-55.
4. Junge A, Dvořák J. Football injuries during the 2014 FIFA World Cup. Br J Sports Med. 2015 May;49(9):599-602.
5. Spiotta AM, Bartsch AJ, Benzel EC. Heading in soccer: dangerous play? Neurosurgery. 2012 Jan;70(1):1-11; discussion 11.
6. Stewart WF, Kim N, Ifrah CS, Lipton RB, Bachrach TA, Zimmerman ME, Kim M, Lipton ML. Symptoms from repeated intentional and unintentional head impact in soccer players. Neurology. 2017 Feb 28;88(9):901-908.
7. Lingsma H, Maas A. Heading in soccer: More than a subconcussive event? Neurology. 2017 Feb 28;88(9):822-823.
8. Echemendia RJ, Meeuwisse W, McCrory P, et al.The Sport Concussion Assessment Tool 5th Edition (SCAT5): Background and rationale. Br J Sports Med. 2017 Jun;51(11):848-850.
9. Maddocks DL, Dicker GD, Saling MM. The assessment of orientation following concussion in athletes. Clin J Sport Med. 1995;5(1):32-5.
10. Cusimano MD, Casey J, Jing R, Mishra A, Solarski M, Techar K, Zhang S. Assessment of Head Collision Events During the 2014 FIFA World Cup Tournament. JAMA. 2017 Jun 27;317(24):2548-2549.
11. Iverson GL, Gardner AJ, Terry DP, Ponsford JL, Sills AK, Broshek DK, Solomon GS. Predictors of clinical recovery from concussion: a systematic review. Br J Sports Med. 2017 Jun;51(12):941-948.
12. Morgan CD, Zuckerman SL, Lee YM, King L, Beaird S, Sills AK, Solomon GS.
Predictors of postconcussion syndrome after sports-related concussion in young athletes: a matched case-control study. J Neurosurg Pediatr. 2015 Jun;15(6):589-98.
13. Putukian M, Echemendia R, Dettwiler-Danspeckgruber A, Duliba T, Bruce J,Furtado JL, Murugavel M. Prospective clinical assessment using Sideline Concussion Assessment Tool-2 testing in the evaluation of sport-relatedconcussion in college athletes. Clin J Sport Med. 2015 Jan;25(1):36- 42.
14. Zemek R, Barrowman N, Freedman SB, et al. Clinical Risk Score for Persistent Postconcussion Symptoms Among Children With Acute Concussion in the ED. JAMA. 2016 Mar 8;315(10):1014-25.
15. Putukian M, Echemendia RJ, Chiampas G, et al.D. Head Injury in Soccer: From Science to the Field; summary of the head injury summit held in April 2017 in New York City, New York. Br J Sports Med. 2019 Nov;53(21):1332.
16. Nitrini R. Soccer (Football Association) and chronic traumatic encephalopathy: A short review and recommendation. Dement Neuropsychol. 2017 Jul-Sep;11(3):218-220.
17. Beaudouin F, Aus der Fünten K, Tröß T, Reinsberger C, Meyer T. Match Situations Leading to Head Injuries in Professional Male Football (Soccer)-A Video- based Analysis Over 12 Years. Clin J Sport Med. 2018 Jan 19.
18. Bjørneboe J, Bahr R, Dvorak J, Andersen TE. Lower incidence of arm-to-head contact incidents with stricter interpretation of the Laws of the Game in Norwegian male professional football. Br J Sports Med. 2013 May;47(8):508-14.
19. Broglio SP, Ju YY, Broglio MD, Sell TC. The Efficacy of Soccer Headgear. J Athl Train. 2003 Sep;38(3):220-224.
20. Hrysomallis C. Impact energy attentuation of protective football headgear against a yielding surface. J Sci Med Sport. 2004 Jun;7(2):156-64.
21. Naunheim RS, Ryden A, Standeven J, Genin G, Lewis L, Thompson P, Bayly P. Does soccer headgear attenuate the impact when heading a soccer ball? Acad Emerg Med. 2003 Jan;10(1):85-90.
22. Withnall C, Shewchenko N, Wonnacott M, Dvorak J. Effectiveness of headgear in football. Br J Sports Med. 2005 Aug; 39.
23. Hagel B, Meeuwisse W. Risk compensation: a "side effect" of sport injury prevention? Clin J Sport Med. 2004 Jul;14(4):193-6.
24. Emery CA, Black AM, Kolstad A, et al. What strategies can be used to effectively reduce the risk of concussion in sport? A systematic review. Br J Sports Med. 2017 Jun;51(12):978-984.
25. Echemendia RJ, Broglio SP, Davis GA, Guskiewicz KM, Hayden KA, Leddy JJ, Meehan WP 3rd, Putukian M, Sullivan SJ, Schneider KJ, McCrory P. What tests and measures should be added to the SCAT3 and related tests to improve their reliability, sensitivity and/or specificity in sideline concussion diagnosis? A systematic review. Br J Sports Med. 2017 Jun;51(11):895-901.
26. Mihalik JP, Lynall RC, Wasserman EB, Guskiewicz KM, Marshall SW. Evaluating the "Threshold Theory": Can Head Impact Indicators Help? Med Sci Sports Exerc. 2017 Feb;49(2):247-253.
27. King NS, Kirwilliam S. Permanent post-concussion symptoms after mild head injury. Brain Inj. 2011;25(5):462-70.
28. HS M. Punch drunk. J Am Med Assoc. 1928;91(15):1103-1107.
29. Corsellis JA, Bruton CJ, Freeman-Browne D. The aftermath of boxing. Psychol Med. 1973 Aug;3(3):270-303.
30. Mez J, Daneshvar DH, Kiernan PT, et al. Clinicopathological Evaluation of Chronic Traumatic Encephalopathy in Players of American Football. JAMA. 2017 Jul 25;318(4):360-370.
31. Ling H, Morris HR, Neal JW, Lees AJ, Hardy J, Holton JL, Revesz T, Williams DD. Mixed pathologies including chronic traumatic encephalopathy account for dementia in retired association football (soccer) players. Acta Neuropathol. 2017 Mar;133(3):337-352.
32. Grinberg LT, Anghinah R, Nascimento CF,et al. Chronic Traumatic Encephalopathy Presenting as Alzheimer's Disease in a Retired Soccer Player. J Alzheimers Dis. 2016 Jul 29;54(1):169-74.
33. Hales C, Neill S, Gearing M, Cooper D, Glass J, Lah J. Late-stage CTE pathology in a retired soccer player with dementia. Neurology. 2014 Dec 9;83(24):2307-9.
34. Deng H, Ordaz A, Upadhyayula PS, et al. Apolipoprotein E Epsilon 4 Genotype, Mild Traumatic Brain Injury, and the Development of Chronic Traumatic Encephalopathy. Med Sci (Basel). 2018 Sep 14;6(3).
35. McKee AC, Stern RA, Nowinski CJ, et al. The spectrum of disease in chronic traumatic encephalopathy. Brain. 2013 Jan;136(Pt 1):43-64.
36. Stern RA, Daneshvar DH, Baugh CM, et al. Clinical presentation of chronic traumatic encephalopathy. Neurology. 2013.

37. Turk KW, Budson AE. Chronic Traumatic Encephalopathy. Continuum (Minneap Minn). 2019 Feb;25(1):187-207.
38. Montenigro PH, Baugh CM, Daneshvar DH, et al. Clinical subtypes of chronic traumatic encephalopathy: literature review and proposed research diagnostic criteria for traumatic encephalopathy syndrome. Alzheimers Res Ther. 2014 Sep 24;6(5):68.
39. Gardner RC, Hess CP, Brus-Ramer M, Possin KL, Cohn-Sheehy BI, Kramer JH, Berger MS, Yaffe K, Miller B, Rabinovici GD. Cavum Septum Pellucidum in Retired American Pro-Football Players. J Neurotrauma. 2016 Jan 1;33(1):157-61.
40. Amen DG, Newberg A, Thatcher R, et al. Impact of playing American professional football on long-term brain function. J Neuropsychiatry Clin Neurosci. 2011 Winter;23(1):98-106.
41. Provenzano FA, Jordan B, Tikofsky RS, Saxena C, Van Heertum RL, Ichise M. F-18 FDG PET imaging of chronic traumatic brain injury in boxers: a statistical parametric analysis. Nucl Med Commun. 2010 Nov;31(11):952-7.
42. Stern RA, Adler CH, Chen K, et al. Tau Positron-Emission Tomography in Former National Football League Players. N Engl J Med. 2019 May 2;380(18):1716-1725.
43. Tiryaki E, Horak HA. ALS and other motor neuron diseases. Continuum (Minneap Minn). 2014 Oct;20(5 Peripheral Nervous System Disorders):1185-207.
44. Goutman SA. Diagnosis and clinical management of amyotrophic lateral sclerosis and other motor neuron disorders. Continuum (Minneap Minn). 2017 Oct;23(5, Peripheral Nerve and Motor Neuron Disorders):1332-1359.
45. Chiò A, Calvo A, Dossena M, Ghiglione P, Mutani R, Mora G. ALS in Italian professional soccer players: the risk is still present and could be soccer-specific. Amyotroph Lateral Scler. 2009 Aug;10(4) 205-9.
46. Al-Hazzaa HM, Almuzaini KS, Al-Refaee SA, et al. Aerobic and anaerobic power characteristics of Saudi elite soccer players. J Sports Med Phys Fitness. 2001 Mar;41(1):54-61.
47. Armon C. An evidence-based medicine approach to the evaluation of the role of exogenous risk factors in sporadic amyotrophic lateral sclerosis. Neuroepidemiology. 2003 Jul-Aug;22(4):217-28.
48. Lehman EJ, Hein MJ, Baron SL, Gersic CM. Neurodegenerative causes of death among retired National Football League players. Neurology. 2012 Nov 6;79(19):1970-4.
49. Abel EL. Football increases the risk for Lou Gehrig's disease, amyotrophic lateral sclerosis. Percept Mot Skills. 2007 Jun;104(3 Pt 2):1251-4.
50. Chen H, Richard M, Sandler DP, Umbach DM, Kamel F. Head injury and amyotrophic lateral sclerosis. Am J Epidemiol. 2007 Oct 1;166(7):810-6.
51. Armon C, Albert SM. A blow to the head trauma--ALS hypothesis. Neurology. 2015 Apr 28;84(17):1728-9.
52. Visser AE, Rooney JPK, D'ovidio F, et al. Multicentre, cross-cultural, population-based, case-control study of physical activity as risk factor for amyotrophic lateral sclerosis. J Neurol Neurosurg Psychiatry. 2018 Aug;89(8):797-803.
53. Tscholl P, Junge A, Dvorak J. The use of medication and nutritional supplements during FIFA World Cups 2002 and 2006. Br J Sports Med. 2008 Sep;42(9):725-30.
54. Fondell E, O'Reilly ÉJ, Fitzgerald KC, et al. Non-steroidal anti-inflammatory drugs and amyotrophic lateral sclerosis: results from five prospective cohort studies. Amyotroph Lateral Scler. 2012 Oct;13(6):573-9.
55. Beghi E. Are professional soccer players at higher risk for ALS? Amyotroph Lateral Scler Frontotemporal Degener. 2013 Dec;14(7-8):501-6.
56. Contrusciere V, Paradisi S, Matteucci A, Malchiodi-Albedi F. Branched-chain amino acids induce neurotoxicity in rat cortical cultures. Neurotox Res. 2010 May;17(4):392-8.
57. Manuel M, Heckman CJ. Stronger is not always better: could a bodybuilding dietary supplement lead to ALS?. Exp Neurol. 2011;228(1):5–8.
58. Morahan JM, Yu B, Trent RJ, Pamphlett R. A gene-environment study of the paraoxonase 1 gene and pesticides in amyotrophic lateral sclerosis. Neurotoxicology. 2007 May;28(3):532-40.
59. Morahan JM, Pamphlett R. Amyotrophic lateral sclerosis and exposure to environmental toxins: an Australian case-control study. Neuroepidemiology. 2006;27(3):130-5.
60. Govoni V, Granieri E, Fallica E, Casetta I. Amyotrophic lateral sclerosis, rural environment and agricultural work in the Local Health District of Ferrara, Italy, in the years 1964-1998. J Neurol. 2005 Nov;252(11):1322-7.
61. Furby A, Beauvais K, Kolev I, Rivain JG, Sébille V. Rural environment and risk factors of amyotrophic lateral sclerosis: A case-control study. J Neurol. 2010.
62. Wills AM, Cronin S, Slowik A, et al. A large-scale international meta-analysis of paraoxonase gene polymorphisms in sporadic ALS. Neurology. 2009.
63. Guidry A, Crutchfield K. Athletes with neurologic disease. In: Handbook of Clinical Neurology; 2018.
64. Pallesen S, Gundersen HS, Kristoffersen M, Bjorvatn B, Thun E, Harris A. The Effects of Sleep Deprivation on Soccer Skills. Percept Mot Skills. 2017.
65. Brand S, Beck J, Gerber M, Hatzinger M, Holsboer-Trachsler E. Evidence of favorable sleep-EEG patterns in adolescent male vigorous football players compared to controls. World J Biol Psychiatry. 2010.
66. Nédélec M, Dawson B, Dupont G. Influence of Night Soccer Matches on Sleep in Elite Players. J strength Cond Res. 2019.
67. Kredlow MA, Capozzoli MC, Hearon BA, Calkins AW, Otto MW. The effects of physical activity on sleep: a meta-analytic review. J Behav Med. 2015.
68. Nédélec M, Halson S, Abaidia AE, Ahmaidi S, Dupont G. Stress, Sleep and Recovery in Elite Soccer: A Critical Review of the Literature. Sport Med. 2015.
69. Suetsugi M, Mizuki Y, Yamamoto K, Uchida S, Watanabe Y. The effect of placebo administration on the first-night effect in healthy young volunteers. Prog Neuro-Psychopharmacology Biol Psychiatry. 2007.
70. Samuels C. Sleep, Recovery, and Performance: The New Frontier in High-Performance Athletics. Phys Med Rehabil Clin N Am. 2009.
71. Krustrup P, Ortenblad N, Nielsen J, et al. Maximal voluntary contraction force, SR function and glycogen resynthesis during the Wrst 72 h after a high-level competitive soccer game. Eur J Appl Physiol. 2011.
72. Skein M, Duffield R, Edge J, Short MJ, Mündel T. Intermittent-sprint performance and muscle glycogen after 30 h of sleep deprivation. Med Sci Sports Exerc. 2011.
73. Jacobs I, Westlin N, Karlsson J, Rasmusson M, Houghton B. Muscle glycogen and diet in elite soccer players. Eur J Appl Physiol Occup Physiol. 1982.
74. Ndlec M, McCall A, Carling C, Legall F, Berthoin S, Dupont G. Recovery in Soccer: Part I-post-match fatigue and time course of recovery. Sport Med. 2012.
75. Edwards BJ, Edwards W, Waterhouse J, Atkinson C, Reilly T. Can cycling performance in an early morning, laboratory-based cycle time-trial be improved by morning exercise the day before? Int J Sports Med. 2005.
76. Vaynman S, Gomez-Pinilla F. Revenge of the "sit": How lifestyle impacts neuronal and cognitive health through molecular systems that interface energy metabolism with neu-

ronal plasticity. J Neurosci Res. 2006.
77. Keshavan MS, Giedd J, Lau JYF, Lewis DA, Paus T. Changes in the adolescent brain and the pathophysiology of psychotic disorders. The Lancet Psychiatry. 2014.
78. Hopkins ME, Nitecki R, Bucci DJ. Physical exercise during adolescence versus adulthood: Differential effects on object recognition memory and brain-derived neurotrophic factor levels. Neuroscience. 2011.
79. Chaddock L, Erickson KI, Prakash RS, et al. A neuroimaging investigation of the association between aerobic fitness, hippocampal volume, and memory performance in preadolescent children. Brain Res. 2010.
80. Herting MM, Nagel BJ. Aerobic fitness relates to learning on a virtual Morris Water Task and hippocampal volume in adolescents. Behav Brain Res. 2012.
81. Mervaala E, Föhr J, Könönen M, et al. Quantitative MRI of the hippocampus and amygdala in severe depression. Psychol Med. 2000.
82. Malberg JE. Implications of adult hippocampal neurogenesis in antidepressant action. In: Journal of Psychiatry and Neuroscience; 2004.
83. Miller BR, Hen R. The current state of the neurogenic theory of depression and anxiety. Curr Opin Neurobiol. 2015.
84. Saraulli D, Costanzi M, Mastrorilli V, Farioli-Vecchioli S. The Long Run: Neuroprotective Effects of Physical Exercise on Adult Neurogenesis from Youth to Old Age. Curr Neuropharmacol. 2017.
85. Itoh T, Imano M, Nishida S, et al. Exercise increases neural stem cell proliferation surrounding the area of damage following rat traumatic brain injury. J Neural Transm. 2011.
86. Zhao Z, Sabirzhanov B, Wu J, Faden AI, Stoica BA. Voluntary Exercise Preconditioning Activates Multiple Antiapoptotic Mechanisms and Improves Neurological Recovery after Experimental Traumatic Brain Injury. J Neurotrauma. 2014.
87. Hillman CH, Erickson KI, Kramer AF. Be smart, exercise your heart: exercise effects on brain and cognition. Nat Rev Neurosci. 2008.
88. Castillo-Garzón MJ, Ruiz JR, Ortega FB, Gutiérrez A. Anti-aging therapy through fitness enhancement. Clin Interv Aging. 2006.
89. Erickson KI, Miller DL, Roecklein KA. The aging hippocampus: Interactions between exercise, depression, and BDNF. Neuroscientist. 2012.
90. Erickson KI, Raji CA, Lopez OL, et al. Physical activity predicts gray matter volume in late adulthood: The Cardiovascular Health Study. Neurology. 2010.
91. Klusmann V, Evers A, Schwarzer R, et al. Complex mental and physical activity in older women and cognitive performance: A 6-month randomized controlled trial. Journals Gerontol - Ser A Biol Sci Med Sci. 2010.
92. Valenzuela M, Sachdev P. Can cognitive exercise prevent the onset of dementia? systematic review of randomized clinical trials with longitudinal follow-up. Am J Geriatr Psychiatry. 2009.
93. Hamer M, Chida Y. Physical activity and risk of neurodegenerative disease: A systematic review of prospective evidence. Psychol Med. 2008.
94. Scarmeas N, Luchsinger JA, Brickman AM, et al. Physical activity and alzheimer disease course. Am J Geriatr Psychiatry. 2011.
95. Burns JM, Cronk BB, Anderson HS, et al. Cardiorespiratory fitness and brain atrophy in early Alzheimer disease. Neurology. 2008.
96. Teri L, Gibbons LE, McCurry SM, et al. Exercise Plus Behavioral Management in Patients With Alzheimer Disease. JAMA. 2003.
97. Chen H, Zhang SM, Schwarzschild MA, Hernán MA, Ascherio A. Physical activity and the risk of Parkinson disease. Neurology. 2005.
98. Xu Q, Park Y, Huang X, et al. Physical activities and future risk of Parkinson disease. Neurology. 2010.
99. Thacker EL, Chen H, Patel A V., et al. Recreational physical activity and risk of Parkinson's disease. Mov Disord. 2008.
100. Ahlskog JE. Does vigorous exercise have a neuroprotective effect in Parkinson disease? Supplemental data at www.neurology.org. Neurology. 2011.
101. Adamson BC, Ensari I, Motl RW. Effect of exercise on depressive symptoms in adults with neurologic disorders: a systematic review and meta-analysis. Arch Phys Med Rehabil. 2015 Jul;96(7):1329-38.
102. Döring A, Pfueller CF, Paul F, Dörr J. Exercise in multiple sclerosis -- an integral component of disease management. EPMA J. 2011 Dec 24;3(1):2.
103. Waschbisch A, Wenny I, Tallner A, Schwab S, Pfeifer K, Mäurer M. Physical activity in multiple sclerosis: a comparative study of vitamin D, brain-derived neurotrophic factor and regulatory T cell populations. Eur Neurol.2012;68(2):122-8.
104. Knowles BD, Pleacher MD. Athletes with seizure disorders. Curr Sports Med Rep.2012 Jan-Feb;11(1):16-20.
105. Fisher RS, Acevedo C, Arzimanoglou A, Bogacz A, Cross JH, Elger CE, Engel JJr, Forsgren L, French JA, Glynn M, Hesdorffer DC, Lee BI, Mathern GW, Moshé SL, Perucca E, Scheffer IE, Tomson T, Watanabe M, Wiebe S. ILAE official report: a practical clinical definition of epilepsy. Epilepsia. 2014 Apr;55(4):475-82.
106. Capovilla G, Kaufman KR, Perucca E, Moshé SL, Arida RM. Epilepsy, seizures, pysical exercise, and sports: a report from the ILAE Task Force on Sports and Epilepsy. Epilepsia. 2016 Jan;57(1):6-12.
107. Beghi E, Carpio A, Forsgren L, Hesdorffer DC, Malmgren K, Sander JW, Tomson T, auser WA. Recommendation for a definition of acute symptomatic seizure. Epilepsia. 2010 Apr;51(4):671-5.
108. Shirreffs SM, Sawka MN. Fluid and electrolyte needs for training, competition,and recovery. J Sports Sci. 2011;29 Suppl 1:S39-46.
109. McCrory P, Meeuwisse W, Dvořák J, Aubry M, Bailes J, Broglio S, Cantu RC, Cassidy D, Echemendia RJ, Castellani RJ, Davis GA, Ellenbogen R, Emery C, Engebretsen L, Feddermann-Demont N, Giza CC, Guskiewicz KM, Herring S, Iverson GL, Johnston KM, Kissick J, Kutcher J, Leddy JJ, Maddocks D, Makdissi M, Manley GT, McCrea M, Meehan WP, Nagahiro S, Patricios J, Putukian M, Schneider KJ, Sills A, Tator CH, Turner M, Vos PE. Consensus statement on concussion in sport-the 5(th) international conference on concussion in sport held in Berlin, October 2016. Br J Sports Med. 2017 Jun;51(11):838-847.
110. Mackay DF, Russell ER, Stewart K, MacLean JA, Pell JP, Stewart W. Neurodegenerative Disease Mortality among Former Professional Soccer Players. N Engl J Med. 2019 Nov 7;381(19):1801-1808.

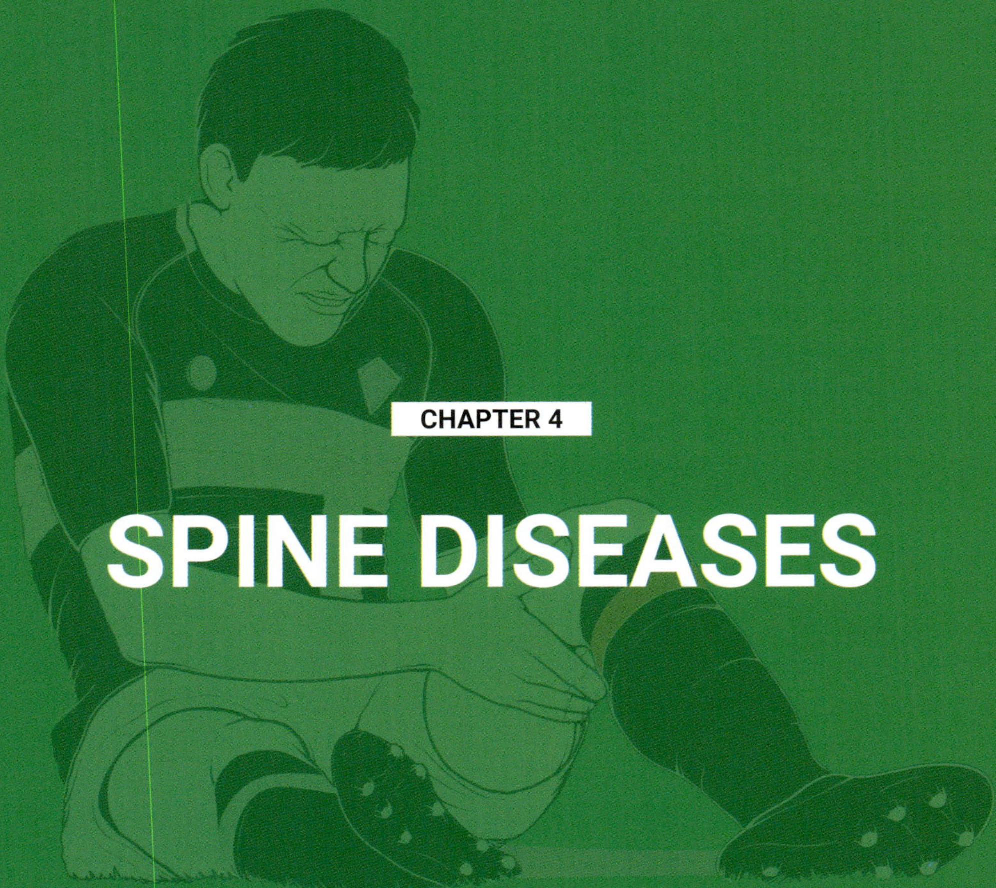

CHAPTER 4

SPINE DISEASES

Cesare Faldini [1]
Fabrizio Perna [2]
Alberto Di Martino [1]
Alberto Ruffilli [1]

[1] 1st Orthopaedic and Traumatologic Clinic (Director: C. Faldini)
IRCCS Istituto Ortopedico Rizzoli, Bologna, Italy

[2] General Orthopedics (Director: G. Pignatti)
IRCCS Istituto Ortopedico Rizzoli, Bologna, Italy

Introduction

Elite athletes like soccer players represent a category at risk of spine trauma and spinal related diseases secondary to a sudden damage or a chronic sufferance of the spinal elements. The consequences of spinal injuries or diseases are vast and can be of great personal and financial cost for both the player and the team.

Adequate training, rules respect, and the conduct during the game controlled by the referees all, serve to reduce the risk of injury related to the sport activity.

Roughly, spine diseases in soccer players can be divided into two broad categories: traumatic and overuse conditions. Soft tissue injuries and fractures belong to the first group and are mostly located at the cervical spine and thoraco-lumbar junction. Conversely, overuse conditions include: spondylolysis, spondylolisthesis, lumbar disc disease with degeneration and lumbar disc herniation, stress fractures and hyper-kyphosis.

Spinal trauma

General assessment

The spine is composed by 7 cervical, 12 thoracic, 5 lumbar vertebrae, the sacrum, and the coccyx. The cervical spine, together with the thoraco-lumbar junction are more commonly involved in traumas. The cervical spine indeed, is both highly mobile and easily exposed to external events. The thoracic spine, on the contrary, is a very stable segment due to its closed relationship to the ribs; hence, it is rarely involved in trauma unless in case of high energy events. The lumbar segment, similarly to the cervical one, is very mobile, but it is surrounded by many muscles which make it less susceptible to severe trauma. The thoraco-lumbar junction, which is located between a very stable and rigid and a very mobile segment, is the second most common location of spine trauma [1].

Following a trauma, regardless of the cause, the player's assessment must be done as quickly and as completely as possible. A systematic approach must be used in order to evaluate the extent of the damage and its severity. In case of spinal trauma, it is essential to identify potential injured sites, protect the spine and provide a safe and fast transport to the hospital while maximizing the hemodynamic and respiratory status of the athlete [1, 2].

Adherence to the Advanced Trauma Life Support (ATLS) remains imperative with a primary survey including the ABCDE evaluation.

- A: Airway maintenance and cervical spine protection.
- B: Breathing and ventilation.
- C: Circulation with hemorrhage control.
- D: Disability and neurologic assessment.
- E: Exposure and nvironmental control of patient.

The airway can be compromised by the initial trauma or secondary by the decreased conscious level induced by trauma and can be evaluated through the Glasgow Coma Scale (GCS). In order to maintain airway clearance, the first possible maneuvers are the jaw-thrust and the neck extension; however, care should be taken in case of suspected cervical spine trauma wherein neck extension may further worsen the vertebral or medullary trauma. Airways aids such like Guedel oropharyngeal cannula, laryngeal mask, and endotracheal intubation may also be used in more severe cases [1, 3].

Breathing evaluation can be initially performed through the assessment of thoracic movements. It is essential to hear the athlete's respiratory sounds, see the thoracic movements and palpate the tho-

racic structures in order to evaluate possible asymmetries or anomalies. Dyspnea, bradypnea and tachypnea should always be carefully evaluated since they can be associated to airway compromise. Pneumothorax can be present in case of severe spinal trauma when the chest is involved, and special assessment of this rare contingency must be performed to avoid further deterioration [4].
Restoring and maintaining a normal circulation is essential to avoid hypo-perfusion to vital organs, and potential sources of bleeding must be promptly recognized since hemorrhage is considered one of the main causes of preventable death. Initial circulation evaluation requires the check of the player's paleness, cardiac frequency, capillary filling, and arterial pressure. It is also of the utmost importance to assess for any hidden source of bleeding, like in the event of associated femur or pelvic fractures or abdominal trauma.
Disability and neurological status assessment starts with the evaluation of the player's status of consciousness, pupils' conditions including size, symmetry and reaction to stimuli, and lateralizing sins on the upper and lower limb [2].
Generally, soccer players trauma occurs during practice and sports competitions, and environmental control can be easily performed. However, trauma patients usually experience loss of temperature, hence as soon as the initial clinical evaluation is completed, it is crucial to warm up the athlete to prevent a possible hypothermia.

Cervical strains

Cervical strain is a common injury routinely seen in the emergency department. Frequently, it is the result of trauma from falls or motor vehicle accidents; however, even high intensity sport activities and sports related trauma can determine such kind of injury. Cervical strains affect the musculotendinous structures of the neck, and in the majority of the cases these are the result of overuse syndrome or whiplash of the head. Despite this condition can cause remarkable distress to the patients, it usually has few long-term sequelae when appropriately managed [4].
The lead diagnostic challenge in the emergent or urgent setting is to differentiate a cervical strain from other causes of neck pain that may result in morbidity or mortality to the patient, hence the most important issues surrounding cervical spine injury involve an accurate diagnosis.
Correct assessment of the mechanism of injury gives significant clues to the relative risk of strain versus a more serious cervical spine injury [5].
Pain, cervical tenderness, and limited range of motion are the typical complains. Following a cervical strain injury, patients may report varying degrees of muscle spasms. Moreover, the assessment of the active range of motion of the cervical spine can help the examining physician to clinically exclude more severe injuries and conditions [2].
Clinically, athletes may present with edema of the cervical tissues, palpable bogginess of the posterior cervical musculature, mild warmth over the involved tissues, and neck stiffness with limited range of motion. At the same time a complete neurological evaluation is performed to exclude potential secondary damage to the spinal cord and nerve roots.
Radiographs are the first line imaging modalities, and they can rule out fractures and dislocations in case of persistent neck pain and symptoms. In case of clinical suspicion of a more severe injury, or radiological doubt, MRI or CT scan are required [4, 6].
Despite the initial presentation may seems serious, the majority of cases resolve with rest and conservative treatment alone. The pharmacology of cervical strains management involves pain control and palliation. Ice packs, nonsteroidal anti-inflammatory drugs (NSAIDs) and painkillers are the mainstays of treatment, and muscle relaxants may be useful to reduce muscle contracture and stiffness. A cervical collar can be used for 7 to 10 days to promote musculotendinous structures recovery. Neuromuscular electrical stimulation, isometric strengthening and mobilization exercises should be part of the rehabilitation program, and are started after resolution of the acute phase [7].

Stinger

Stinger, also known as burner or nerve pinch injury, is a clinical condition characterized by burning pain and numbness in the arm often accompanied by weakness of the upper arm or shoulder muscles after an injury [8]. Stinger occurs when nerves of

the brachial plexus are stretched or compressed after an impact, and it is mostly seen in athletes who play soccer, ice hockey, rugby, or American football. Many athletes playing contact sports have suffered stinger, but they are often unreported because the symptoms are short-lived or they fear being removed from play.
The mechanism of injury is mainly neck flexion to the contralateral side with the shoulder in downward displacement; this can cause brachial plexus lengthening and compression. The upper trunks of the plexus are the most commonly involved with musculocutaneous, axillary, radial, and median nerves involvement [9].
In the majority of cases players experience severe impairment and need to hold the affected arm with the contralateral unaffected limb. Burner and stinger symptoms typically occur in only one arm, and usually lasts only few seconds or minutes. The player reports a burning or an electric shock sensation with numbness and weakness on one arm followed by a warm sensation [10, 11].
Repeated trauma can cause recurring stingers with chronic pain and muscle weakness, while recovery can take weeks to months in these cases [11, 12].
Treatment includes rest, restriction of movement, ice and, in severe cases, a cervical collar in combination with anti-inflammatory medication and painkillers. Return to sport activities can be considered after full recovery from symptoms [13].

Spinal cord neuropraxia
Spinal cord neurapraxia is a clinical condition characterized by pain and neurological symptoms in both arms and/or legs, and it is often associated to transient quadriplegia. Symptoms typically resolve within few minutes or hours, in some cases up to 48 hours. Due to the severe initial clinical presentation, players should be assumed to have a major cervical spinal trauma until proven otherwise [14].
The mechanism of injury is generally the acute stenosis of the spinal cord caused by either a hyperflexion or a hyperextension of the neck that causes a pincer effect between the vertebral bodies, the spinolaminar margin, and the ligamentum flavum. In most patients a pre-existing cervical stenosis is present and predisposes to damage [15].
Players typically complain of temporary paralysis, numbness, tingling, and loss of muscular strength. Neck pain, on the contrary, is usually not present. Usually, the severity of the injury is related to the duration of symptoms, and therefore it is classified as: grade I if symptoms resolve within 15 minutes; grade II if between 15 and 24 hours, and grade III if symptoms last over 24 hours.
Imaging examination must include both a radiographic and MRI evaluation to exclude possible fractures, dislocation, and spinal cord lesion.
Aim of the treatment is to restore a complete function as soon as possible, with a pain free range of motion and complete recovery of the neurological symptoms.
Return to sport activities should be carefully evaluated with the player, considering the anatomic condition of the spinal canal. If complete recovery is achieved and there are no signs of cervical stenosis, full sport activities return without restriction can be permitted. On the contrary, if canal stenosis is present, a return to play soccer should be restricted.

Low back pain

Low back pain (LBP) is the leading cause of disability worldwide, with a lifetime incidence ranging from 50% to 85%. However, less then 3% of patients need surgical treatment. LBP is a symptom that can be generated by multiple diseases and conditions which are not always easy to identify, sometimes leading to an ineffective treatment and risk of chronic evolution [16]. LBP can be classified according to the distribution of pain, as axial or radicular, and it is frequently associated with working conditions or sport activities that cause repetitive functional overload on the lumbar spine. LBP in the athlete is also a common feature, but it is associated to a wide range of variability in relation to the type of sport activity which is performed, with estimated prevalence ranging from 1% to 30%.
As in the general population, LBP is the most common cause of suspension of training and competitive practice; however, most of the players tend not to report mild episodes of LBP, therefore underestimating the real prevalence. Moreover, most of the episodes are of low intensity, and

the players usually continue to compete despite symptoms [17].
Despite the fact that most episodes of acute axial LBP will resolve, a small number of patients will develop recurrent or chronic LBP especially in case of older age, greater baseline pain, depression, and fear of possible future acute events.
Most of the LBP are non-specific and are mainly related to mechanical causes and overload. For this reason, top-level athletes present a major risk due to the repetitive high load exercises required during training, commonly started from a very young age. Moreover, soccer players are often subjected to long training session with high intensity, variety, and inadequate recovery [18].
Despite LBP can be clinically severe, the majority of episodes are self-limiting with a good response to conservative treatment. A specific disorder that requires a more thoughtful evaluation and management can be infrequently found.

General assessment

When considering an athlete with LBP it is essential to evaluate all the possible causes including the less frequent pathologies. Past medical history and the potential injury mechanism must be accurately collected together with the site of pain, irradiation, and associated symptoms. Pain should be characterized asking for its quality, progression, provocative, and relieving factors and movements. Particular attention should be paid in case of associated fever, history of recent infection, immunosuppression, history of cancer, weight loss, night or rest pain, or pain resisting to an appropriate pharmacological treatment, and, in case of severe or progressive neurological impairment like sensory alteration or weakness, bladder or perineal dysfunction. Furthermore, psychological factors like patient's belief, emotional status, familiar, and professional conditions must be assessed. Indeed, the psychological behavior can increase the risk of progression to chronic pain and discomfort leading to a severe professional impairment [19].
The most common sport-related causes of LBP are sprains and soft tissue injuries, discogenic back pain, lumbar disk herniation, spondylolysis and spondylolisthesis, stress fractures, and Scheuermann disease.

The identification of the correct cause of LBP is essential for the physician in order to establish the appropriate rehabilitation therapy. It is often necessary to discontinue or to modify the sport activity with relative rest, and to avoid end-range spine mobility with sparing of spinal excessive lateral bend, flexion, and extension. The management of LBP also includes modifications during training since many of the episodes of LBP can be secondary to repetitive trauma, overuse and fatigue accumulation of musculoskeletal structures. A specific training program should be planned with the coach to work out a period of activity modification and technique adjustment to prevent the occurrence of relapsing events, and the possible chronic evolution of pain and disabilities [20].

Low back pain, specific injuries

Soft tissue injuries

Soft tissue injuries at the lumbar spine are the main cause of LBP in the general population and in elite athletes. However, elite athletes are less frequently exposed to lumbar spine strains and sprains because of their developed musculature and improved proprioceptive control. Nevertheless, at the beginning of the season, in case of inadequate conditioning or after a period of relative inactivity, acute LBP, secondary to soft tissue injury, can easily develop [21].
"Sprains" are lesions involving muscles, tendons, or the musculotendinous junction. These structures may be injured to a varying degree, but their anatomical continuity is maintained. In lumbar strains, the most commonly involved structure is the interspinous ligament.
Instead, "strains" are conditions where the muscle fibers within the muscle belly or at the musculotendinous junction are interrupted. The pain is more severe than in sprains, and lasts longer; it is often associated with muscle spasms and limited function [7]. Most of the times the athlete does not remember a specific traumatic episode and pain and symptoms start without a specific identifiable cause. Symptoms are typically limited in duration. Pain is generally more intense for the initial few hours or days after trauma, and it is typically worse with certain movements and positions, such as bending forward, backward or

during upright posture. Ongoing moderate swelling with pain and rigidity are usually experienced for one or two weeks up to muscles healing. Neurological symptoms are usually not reported; however, if a spasm of the lumbosacral fascia extending to the tensor fascia lata is present, pain can radiate to the hip, mimicking a mild radiculopathy. When the muscle contracture is severe, the player may experience spasmodic scoliosis with local bruising and swelling.

When the traumatic event is violent, symptoms may be more noticeable with severe impairment of the walking ability, and difficulty in keeping an upright posture. In these cases, the physician should always consider potential underlying factors like transverse or spinous process fractures, or even kidney lesions, particularly if hematuria is present [17, 19].

In most cases, in the absence of the suspect of serious injury, specific diagnostic images are not necessary.

Conservative treatment with adequate rehabilitation program is the mainstay of treatment. Treatment of the acute phase includes: ice or heat depending on the time of injury, deep tissue massage, nonsteroidal anti-inflammatory drugs (NSAIDs); painkillers and muscle relaxants may be useful to reduce muscle contracture and stiffness. It is also important to improve spinal function by a rehabilitation protocol including targeted muscle strengthening, recovery of flexibility, and range of motion enhancement.

Usually, complete recovery is achieved within few weeks, and the player can return to sport activities, symptom free and fully functional. When symptoms last beyond two weeks or when conservative treatment seems to be ineffective, a deeper investigation is mandatory [22].

Spondylolysis and spondylolisthesis

Spondylolysis is a pathologic condition consisting on a pars interarticularis defect of the vertebrae. It represents one of the most common causes of low back pain in young athletes.

Spondylolysis is often seen in adolescents because the pars interarticularis has not been fully matured, and it is more prone to overuse injury [23]. The etiology is multifactorial including hereditary, hormonal, and mechanical factors. Elite athletes can be affected because of the repetitive hyperextension of the lumbar spine causing stress lesion of the pars interarticularis. With an incidence of 4.4% at the age of 6, and of 6% in adults, spondylolisthesis is one of the most frequent causes of chronic low back pain [24].

The pars articularis of L5 is the most commonly affected segment, accounting for 90% of cases, followed by L4 accounting for the remaining 10%. Most of these are asymptomatic; however, sometimes players complain of low back pain exacerbated by hyperextension, pain radiating to the buttocks, and hamstrings tightness. Neurological signs and symptoms are usually absent. In the majority of cases, conservative treatment provides satisfactory results, avoiding the need for a more invasive approach. Once this injury is caused by vertebral overloading, the first step is to discontinue the inciting activity, and to use a semirigid or rigid brace for 4 to 6 weeks. At the same time, rest from the sport activity together with muscle strengthening is effective in support healing. If the complete resolution of pain is achieved within 4 to 6 weeks then the player can progressively resume his sport activities, aided by brace for another 4 weeks [23]. In case of pain persistence or recurrence, progression of spondylolysis to spondylolisthesis may be inferred, and the patient is proposed the suspension of sport activities and even surgery of "pars articularis repair".

Spondylolisthesis is the forward slippage of a vertebral segment of the spine on the underlying spinal segment, which typically occurs at the lumbar region. However, despite the segmental involvement, this pathology affects the whole biomechanical balance of the spine. The most frequently affected site is the L5-S1 level because of the L5 pars defect (fig. 1). Less commonly, a L4 pars defect can be present leading to a L4-L5 slippage [25].

Contrary to spondylolysis, spondylolisthesis is more commonly symptomatic with LBP as the main symptom. Often pain radiation to the buttocks or the back of the thigh is present because of hamstring tightness or L5 radiculopathy. Pain is generally exacerbated by extension of the lum-

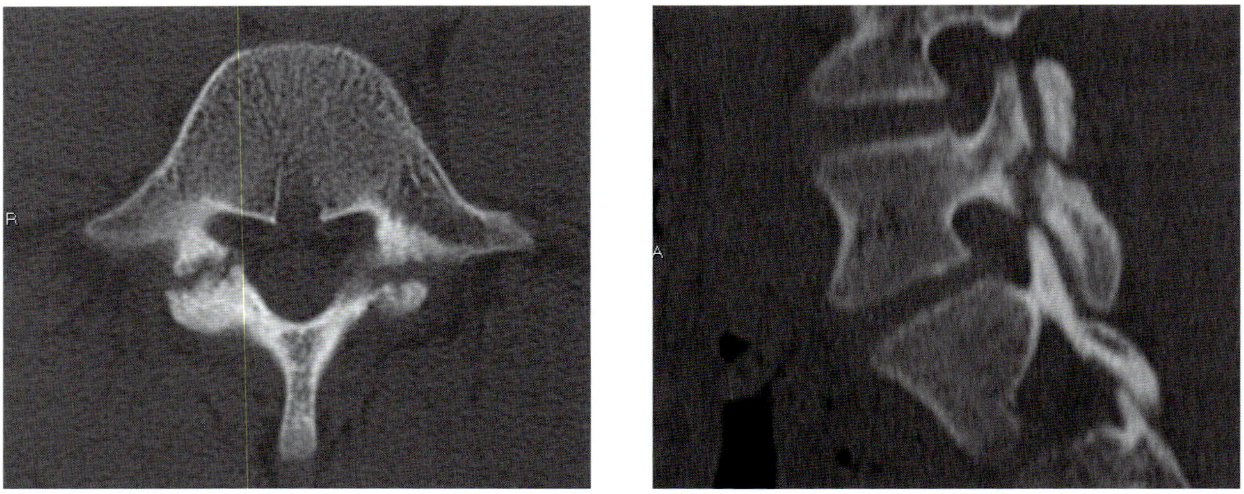

Figure 1 - Axial and sagittal CT scan of 15 years-old male soccer player showing the bilateral pars interarticularis defect of the L5 vertebra

bar spine which is often triggered during physical examination. An increased lumbar lordosis can be demonstrated at inspection with the buttocks in heart-shaped appearance and a midline step-off between the spinous process that can be palpated in more severe slippage. Point tenderness on palpation of the spinous process can occur, together with hamstrings tightness at the straight-leg raising test. Neurological examination is usually normal; however, during the progression of the slippage and in case of acute onset of symptoms, radiculopathy with mild neurological deficit may be encountered [26, 27].

A diagnosis is made by matching clinical symptoms together with diagnostic imaging. These include a series of plain radiographs: anteroposterior, lateral, and bilateral oblique view. A fifth of the spondylolysis are unilateral, hence a bilateral oblique view is imperative. Flexion-extension X-rays help in the determination of segmental instability. Due to the bone nature of the disease, CT scan represents the most sensitive and specific imaging modality to assess the pars interarticularis defect. Moreover, it helps to stage the chronicity of the lesion and to help the planning of an eventual surgical treatment. The MRI scan is reliable for lesions with a secondary slippage. It has the advantage of the absence of radiation exposure, and shows the state of the interposed disc and other possible causes of LBP [28].

Most spondylolisthesis respond well to conservative treatment, and only in few cases surgery is required.

In the acute setting, treatment includes rest, sport activities suspension, brace, and drugs prescription. It is important to achieve a pain free spine before the start of a physical rehabilitation protocol and program a return to play.

The use of brace is useful for both the initial acute phase and for the rehabilitation period and return to sport. The aim of the brace is to support body weight and to limit lumbar hyper-extension.

When conservative treatment fails, the surgical treatment can be considered. Indications for surgery are as follows:

- progression of spondylolisthesis demonstrated by serial radiographic controls. The higher the degree of spondylolisthesis, the greater the chance that it evolves and becomes symptomatic or unresponsive to conservative treatments;
- presence of high grade spondylolisthesis associated with lumbosacral kyphosis and spino-pelvic imbalance;
- occurrence of low back pain and /or sciatica unresponsive to conservative treatment;
- presence of associated neurological deficits.

Surgical options include: decompression, in situ fusion, instrumented fusion with slippage reduction (fig. 2). Despite surgical treatment is completely successful in most cases in term of pain relief and neurological symptoms recovery, return to high level sport activities may be difficult and in most cases the future performance will be affected by the underlying disease and surgery [25].

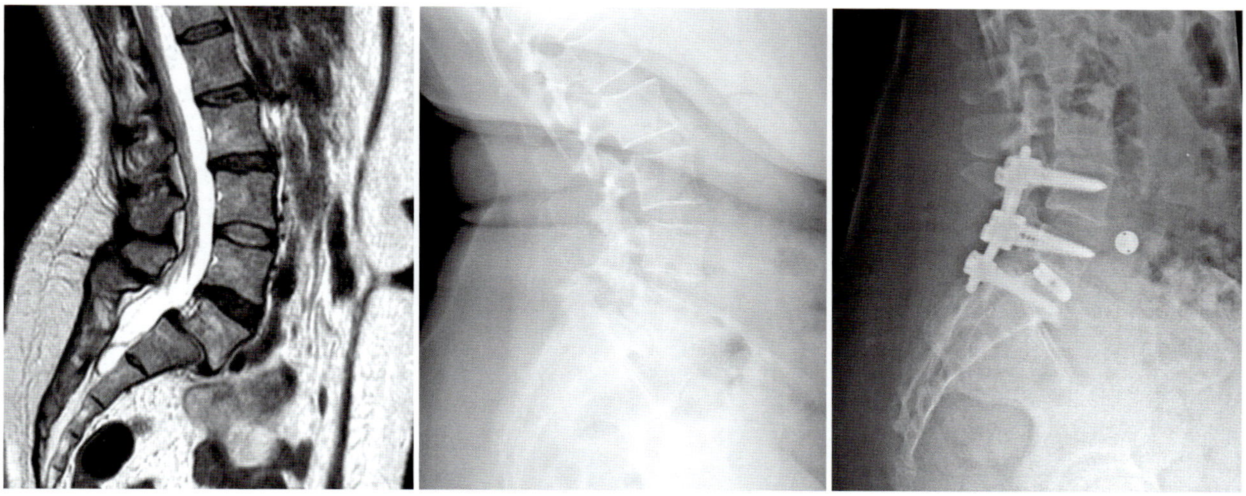

Figure 2 - Preoperative MRI and X-ray of a high-grade isthmic spondylolisthesis of L5 shows the slippage of L5 vertebra on S1 secondary to pars interarticularis defect and disc structural failure. Post-operative X-ray shows the slippage correction and lordosis restoration with posterior pedicle screw and interbody fusion

Lumbar disc disease and herniation

Lumbar degenerative disc disease (DDD) and lumbar disc herniation (LDH) are the most prevalent lumbar conditions causing LBP in professional athletes [19].

Lumbar DDD refers to the progressive degenerative changes of the intervertebral disc which may determine LBP and neurological symptoms. The main characteristic of DDD is the progressive loss of hydration and the occurrence of fibrotic changes at the disc level leading to disc space narrowing and annular tear, culminating in the ankylosing of the spinal segment. The altered biomechanics of the lumbar disc creates a functional overload of the facet joints facilitating facet arthropathy and further deterioration of the segmental lumbar spine function, the main determinants of segmental degenerative instability and slippage in case of anatomically normal pars interarticularis (degenerative spondylolisthesis) [29].

Even though genetic predisposition is the most important risk factor, aging, occupational hazards, smoking, and repetitive microtrauma have been associated with DDD development.

The clinical presentation of lumbar DDD is similar to non-specific LBP. Discogenic pain is exacerbated by movements and loads and is typically relieved by rest and supine position.

The radiographic assessment consists of standard lumbar radiographs that show the narrowing of the disc space, presence of subchondral cysts, osteophytes, and facet degeneration. However, in the majority of cases these findings are generally missing, since these are characteristic of the advanced stages of the disease. MRI has a higher sensibility for the detection of disc disease. Typically, MRI findings include the loss of signal intensity on T2-weighted images, presence of annular tears, and associated bone marrow changes at the vertebral end-plates (fig. 3) [30].

Conservative non-operative treatment is generally successful in the majority of cases using a combination of physical therapy and anti-inflammatory drugs. Physical therapy includes protocols for long term treatment with core strengthening, lumbar mobilization, and stretching. In more severe cases, epidural spinal injections and facet joints injections may be helpful for pain refractory to conventional systemic drugs.

Surgery is rarely required and is performed only in selected athletes with inability to play because of severe and unresponsive pain. It consists of lumbar discectomy and in most cases to segmental fusion.

Indications are: failure of at least six months of conservative therapy, single level DDD on imaging and localized midline tenderness at the same level. However, despite these recommendations and proper player selection, the clinical success of the surgical management of lumbar DDD in these

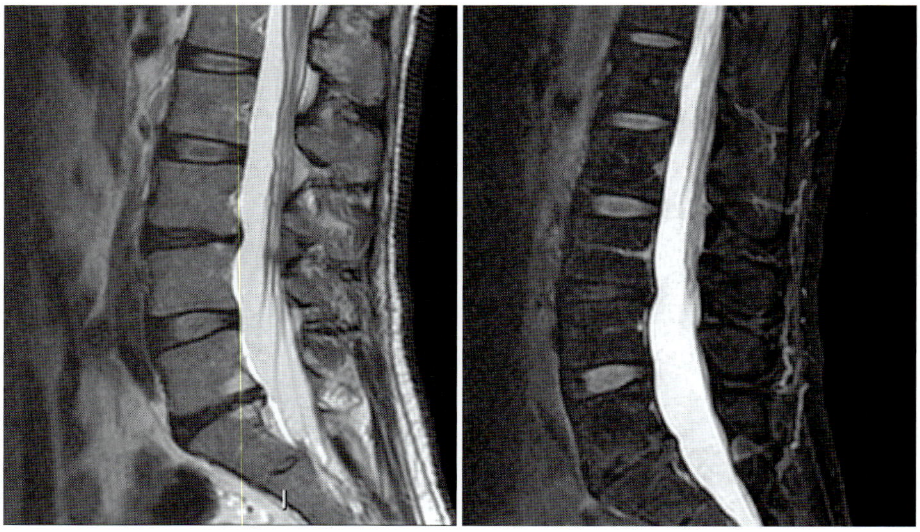

Figure 3 - MRI imaging of a 21 years-old professional soccer player suffering from L3-L4 and L5-S1 DDD. It is possible to evaluate disc narrowing and dehydration together with bone marrow edema at vertebral end-plates

patients is unpredictable. The main concern of the surgical treatment of segmental fusion is the risk of adjacent segment disease secondary to overload and local biomechanical changes [31, 32].

LDH occurs as a consequence of nucleus pulposus migration through a broken anulus fibrosus of the intervertebral disc. It is one of the more common sources of LBP and radiculopathy in the general population. Moreover, in elite athletes, including soccer players, the rigorous activity demand can set up for LDH. At the end of growth, the intervertebral disk has not vascular supply, and is nourished only by diffusion through the endplates. Therefore, similarly to articular cartilage, it has limited ability to self-repair and response to injury. In this contest, repetitive microtraumas, like axial loading and torsion, may not be adequately restored by the normal regenerative process, and determine anulus fibrosus damage and breakage: this is the passage door for nucleus pulposus to herniate. When this event occurs, the nucleus pulposus is estruded into the spinal canal and can compress the emerging nerve roots determining LBP and radiculopathy [33].

Approximately, up to 95% of LDH occurs at L4-L5 or L5-S1 level. Players typically complain about pain in the lumbar spine radiating down a lower limb which can reach up to the foot along the course of the sciatic nerve. For more proximal lumbar sites of herniations, pain radiates along the anterior aspect of the tight following the course of the femoral nerve.

Depending on the affected nerve root, different clinical presentations can develop. Motor examination typically is normal, but weakness may be present according to the rapidity and gravity of nerve root compression. Sensory examination generally shows pain, numbness, and dysesthesia radiating down the leg in the corresponding neural dermatome. Reflexes are typically normal, but hyporeflexia may be present in case of severe and prolonged compression [34].

LDH evaluation should always exclude two surgical urgencies: the cauda equina and the conus medullaris syndromes, and acute paralysis of the L5 nerve root determining footdrop. In cauda and conus syndroms, examination reveals saddle anesthesia, autonomic nervous system dysfunction such like overflow incontinence and sexual impotence associated with LBP radiating along one or both the lower limbs. As in the case of L5 paralysis, the time to surgery is the only determinant to functional recovery.

Diagnostic imaging includes conventional lumbar plain radiographs in order to rule out any associated disease and may show indirect signs of herniation or DDD, like loss of disk eight, loss of lordosis, antalgic scoliosis, or vacuum signs. MRI however, represents the gold standard for diagnosis because of its ability to comprehensively address the location and the characteristics of the herniation, and its relationship with the spinal cord and roots (fig. 4) [29, 34].

In the general population, approximately 90% of patients improve within six months of conservative treatment. Anti-inflammatory medications

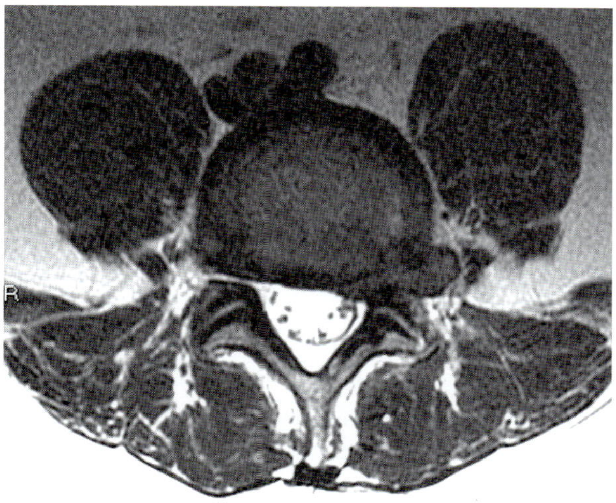

Figure 4 - MRI axial reconstruction of L4-L5 left extra-foraminal LDH causing irritation secondary to conflict with both L4 and L5 roots

like NSAIDs and corticosteroids reduce symptoms by supporting the reduction of inflammatory cytokines. Physical therapy plays a key role during the non-surgical management of LDH with the aim of improve core and back muscles strengthening and flexibility.

When conservative treatment fails, or in case of acute presentation with neurological impairment, surgical treatment may be considered. Surgery consists of partial laminotomy with herniated fragment removal and discectomy. Good to excellent clinical results may be expected in most patients in the general population. However, specific clinical evidence of its efficacy in soccer players is currently lacking because of the number of external variables which are present in elite athletes in terms of biomechanics and type of training in this specific population group [35, 36].

Scheuermann disease

Scheuermann disease (SD) is one of the most common causes of thoracic and thoraco-lumbar hyperkyphosis in adolescence and it is the second most common deformity of the spine after idiopathic scoliosis (fig. 5). The typical onset age is between 12 and 15 years and the main features are the presence of a body wedging, irregularity of the vertebral end-plate, and the presence of Schmorl's nodes. Despite the etiology and the evolution of the disease are still debated, it is considered a form of osteochondrosis of the spine

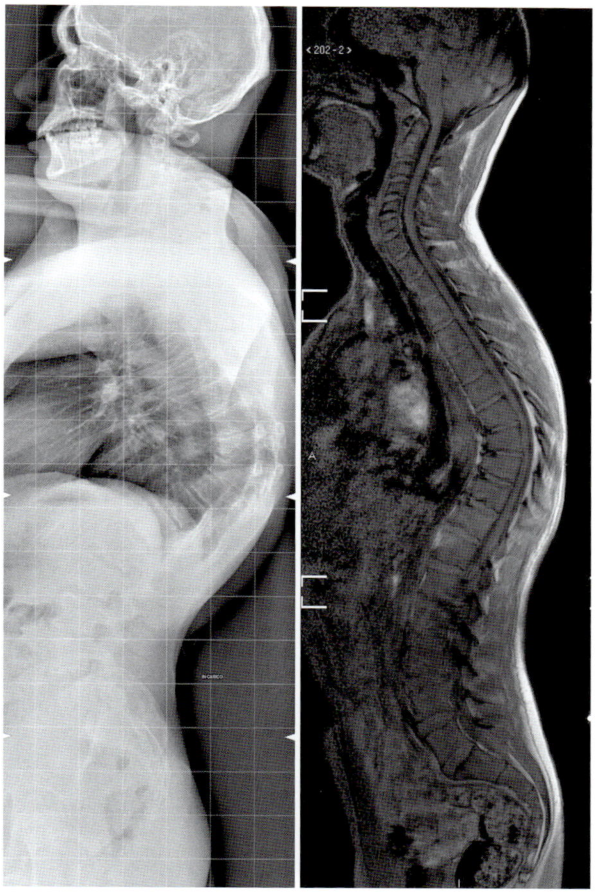

Figure 5 - Full length lateral X-ray and MRI of a 19 years-old soccer players and swimmer shows severe thoraco-lumbar Scheuermann kyphosis. Body wedging, irregularity of the vertebral end-plate and the presence of Schmorl's nodes are easily visible

with both genetic and environmental causes.

Two main types of SD have been described. The thoracic or type 1 pattern is more frequent in young adults and typically patients' major complain is about the cosmetic aspect. The type 2 pattern or thoraco-lumbar pattern, on the contrary, is more frequent in athletic adolescents who practice weight lifting and is typically not associated with a clinical kyphosis. Both the thoracic and the thoraco-lumbar patterns are associated with LBP. The treatment is generally conservative and symptoms resolve with rest and activity modifications [37, 38].

Growth plate fractures of the spine

Growth plates fractures of the spine are frequent causes of low back pain in adolescents and in young athletes due to the presence of growth cartilage and undeveloped ossification centers. The most commonly involved sport activities are: weight lifting, gymnastics, soccer, throwing, and rowing. Reiterative lumbar extension and rotations are the movements of the spine that place the athletes most at risk. This is especially true in the younger athletes, where the bone is immature and the growth plates are still present leading to a greater sensitivity to damage. In particular, at the junction between the vertebral body and the apophysis in the outer annulus fibrosus there is an area of force transfer which can lead to vertebral end-plate fractures. The symptoms, when the avulsed fragment invades the spinal canal, are similar to those of LDH.

Growth plates fractures of the spine are more frequent in the female athlete than in the male, even if precise epidemiological data does still not exist. Diagnosis is not easy since in most cases imaging is not decisive. Plain radiographs are mostly normal and MRI often has not enough sensitivity to identify this type of lesions. The gold standard for the diagnosis of growth plates fractures of the spine is bone scintigraphy, although CT scan has shown to be a reliable alternative with good sensitivity reported in the literature. Conservative treatment with rest and rehabilitation are generally effective to completely resolve pain within 1-3 months [19, 37, 39].

Bertolotti's syndrome

Bertolotti's syndrome is a condition characterized by low back pain associated with the presence of a transitional vertebra in the lumbo-sacral junction. The transitional vertebra can be either secondary to an incomplete segmentation of the lower lumbar vertebra or of the upper sacral vertebra. This vertebra can present a larger transverse process compared to normal lumbar vertebrae generating a mechanical conflict with the sacrum or the ileum that is the origin of pain. This anatomical anomaly was first described by Bertolotti in 1917, it has a prevalence that varies from 4 to 8% in the general population, and is classified into 4 groups based on the development of the transverse process. The clinical presentation is similar to spondylolysisand, in addition to LBP symptoms of L4-L5,degenerative disc disease and L5 radiculopathy can be encountered.

Conservative treatment is generally successful using a combination of anti-inflammatory drugs and physical therapy including protocols for long term treatment with core strengthening, lumbar mobilization and stretching [29, 39].

Bibliography

1. Silva L, de Freitas JMP, Mineiro J. First Aid and Cares in Spine Trauma. Inj Health Probl Footb What Everyone Should Know 2017;259–264.
2. Parizel PM, Gielen JL, Vanhoenacker FM. The Spine in Sports Injuries: Cervical Spine. Imaging Orthop Sports Inj 2007;377–389.
3. Austin N, Krishnamoorthy V, Dagal A. Airway management in cervical spine injury. Int J Crit Illn Inj Sci. 2014 Jan;4(1):50-6.
4. Bragg KJ, Varacallo M. Cervical (Whiplash) Sprain. In: StatPearls. Treasure Island (FL): StatPearls Publishing; 2019 Jan.
5. Drakos MC, Feeley BT, Barnes R, Muller M, Burruss TP, Warren RF. Lower cervical posterior element fractures in the National Football League: a report of 2 cases and a review of the literature. Neurosurgery 2011;68:E1743-1748; discussion E1748-1749.
6. Ben Ayed H, Yaich S, Trigui M, Ben Hmida M, Ben Jemaa M, Ammar A, Jedidi J, Karray R, Feki H, Mejdoub Y, et al. Prevalence, Risk Factors and Outcomes of Neck, Shoulders and Low-Back Pain in Secondary-School Children. J Res Health Sci 2019;19:e00440.
7. Farahbakhsh F, Akbari-Fakhrabadi M, Shariat A, Cleland JA, Farahbakhsh F, Seif-Barghi T, Mansournia MA, Rostami M, Kordi R. Neck pain and low back pain in relation to functional disability in different sport activities. J Exerc Rehabil 2018;14:509–515.
8. Ahearn BM, Starr HM, Seiler JG. Traumatic Brachial Plexopathy in Athletes: Current Concepts for Diagnosis and Management of Stingers. J Am Acad Orthop Surg. 2019 Sep 15;27(18):677-684.
9. Kawasaki T, Ota C, Yoneda T, Maki N, Urayama S, Nagao M, Nagayama M, Kaketa T, Takazawa Y, Kaneko K. Incidence of Stingers in Young Rugby Players. Am J Sports Med 2015;43:2809–2815.
10. Quong WL, Hynes SL, Arneja JS. Pediatric Stinger Syndrome: Acute Brachial Plexopathy After Minor Trauma. Plast Reconstr Surg Glob Open 2015;3:e560.
11. Hakkaku T, Nakazato K, Koyama K, Kouzaki K, Hiranuma K. Cervical Intervertebral Disc Degeneration and Low Cervical Extension Independently Associated With a History of Stinger Syndrome. Orthop J Sports Med. 2017 Nov 2;5(11):2325967117735830.
12. Greenberg J, Leung D, Kendall J. Predicting chronic stinger syndrome using the mean subaxial space available for the cord index. Sports Health 2011;3:264–267.
13. Zaremski JL, Horodyski M, Herman DC.Recurrent stingers in an adolescent American football player: dilemmas of return to play. A case report and review of the literature. Res Sports Med Print 2017;25:384–390.
14. Bernsen HJ, Koetsveld A, Frenken CW, van Norel GJ.Neuropraxia of the cervical spinal cord following cervical spinal cord trauma: a report of five patients. Acta Neurol Belg 2000;100:91–95.
15. Torg JS, Pavlov H.Cervical spinal stenosis with cord neurapraxia and transient quadriplegia. Clin Sports Med 1987;6:115–133.
16. Bono CM. Low-back pain in athletes. J Bone Joint Surg Am. 2004 Feb;86(2):382-96.
17. Farahbakhsh F, Rostami M, Noormohammadpour P, Mehraki Zade A, Hassanmirazaei B, Faghih Jouibari M, Kordi R, Kennedy DJ.Prevalence of low back pain among athletes: A systematic review. J Back Musculoskelet Rehabil 2018;31:901–916.
18. Malliaropoulos N, Bikos G, Meke M, Tsifountoudis I, Pyne D, Korakakis V.Mechanical Low Back Pain in Elite Track and Field Athletes: An observational cohort study. J Back Musculoskelet Rehabil 2017;30:681–689.
19. Mortazavi J, Zebardast J, Mirzashahi B. Low Back Pain in Athletes. Asian J Sports Med 2015;6:e24718.
20. Patel DR, Kinsella E. Evaluation and management of lower back pain in young athletes. Transl Pediatr 2017;6:225–235.
21. Moreno Catalá M, Schroll A, Laube G, Arampatzis A. Muscle Strength and Neuromuscular Control in Low-Back Pain: Elite Athletes Versus General Population. Front Neurosci 2018;12:436.
22. Nowotny AH, Calderon MG, de Souza PA, Aguiar AF, Léonard G, Alves BMO, Amorim CF, da Silva RA. Lumbar stabilisation exercises versus back endurance-resistance exercise training in athletes with chronic low back pain: protocol of a randomised controlled trial. BMJ Open Sport Exerc Med 2018;4:e000452.
23. Selhorst M, Fischer A, MacDonald J. Prevalence of Spondylolysis in Symptomatic Adolescent Athletes. An Assessment of Sport Risk in Nonelite Athletes. Clin J Sport Med Off J Can Acad Sport Med 2017.
24. Warner WC, de Mendonça RGM. Adolescent Spondylolysis: Management and Return to Play. Instr Course Lect 2017;66:409-413.
25. DeWald CJ, Vartabedian JE, Rodts MF, Hammerberg KW. Evaluation and management of high-grade spondylolisthesis in adults. Spine 2005;30:S49-59.
26. Tatsumura M, Gamada H, Ishimoto R, Okuwaki S, Eto F, Ogawa T, Mammoto T, Hirano A. Prevalence of curable and pseudoarthrosis stages of adolescent lumbar spondylolysis. J Rural Med JRM 2018;13:105-109.
27. Faldini C, Martino AD, Perna F, Martikos K, Greggi T, Giannini S. Changes in spino-pelvic alignment after surgical treatment of high- grade isthmic spondylolisthesis by a posterior approach: A report of 41 cases. Eur Spine J 2014;23:S714–S719.
28. Lonstein JE. Spondylolisthesis in children. Cause, natural history, and management. Spine 1999;24:2640–2648.
29. Fett D, Trompeter K, Platen P. Back pain in elite sports: A cross-sectional study on 1114 athletes. PloS One 2017;12:e0180130.
30. Dodwad SNM, Dodwad SJM, Savage JW. Lumbar Discectomy Review. Oper Tech Orthop 2015;25:177–186.
31. O'Sullivan K, O'Sullivan PB, Gabbett TJ, O'Keeffe M. Advice to athletes with back pain-get active! Seriously? Br J Sports Med 2019;53:324-325.
32. Raabe ME, Chaudhari AMW. Biomechanical consequences of running with deep core muscle weakness. J Biomech 2018;67:98-105.
33. Omidi-Kashani F, Hejrati H, Ariamanesh S. Ten Important Tips in Treating a Patient with Lumbar Disc Herniation. Asian Spine J 2016;10:955-963.
34. Deyo RA, Mirza SK. Herniated Lumbar Intervertebral Disk. N Engl J Med 2016;374:1763–1772.
35. Reiman MP, Sylvain J, Loudon JK, Goode A. Return to sport after open and microdiscectomy surgery versus conservative treatment for lumbar disc herniation: a systematic review with meta-analysis. Br J Sports Med 2016;50:221-230.
36. Faldini C, Perna F, Chehrassan M, Borghi R, Stefanini N, Traina F. Surgical tricks for open lumbar discectomy. Eur Spine J 2017;1–2.
37. Gurd DP. Back pain in the young athlete. Sports Med Arthrosc Rev 2011;19:7-16.
38. d'Hemecourt, PA, Hresko MT. Spinal Deformity in Young Athletes. Clin Sports Med 2012;31:441-451.
39. Hasler CC. Back pain during growth. Swiss Med Wkly. 2013 Jan 8;143:w13714.

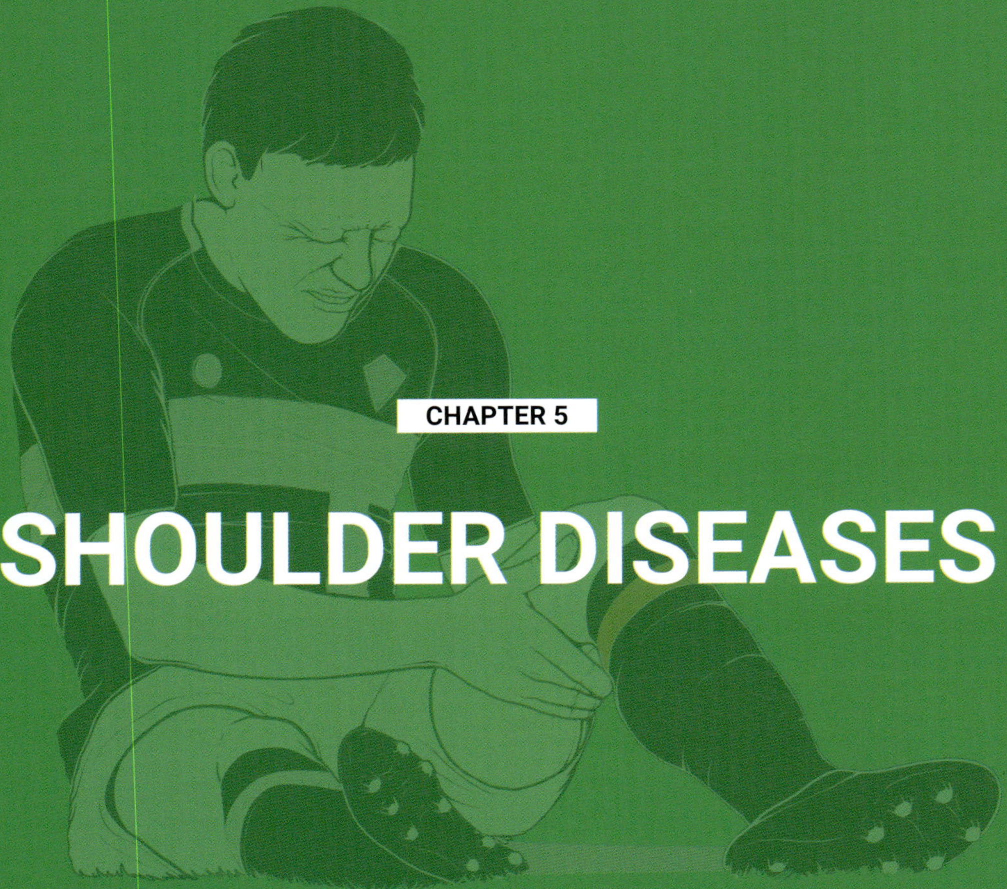

CHAPTER 5

SHOULDER DISEASES

Roberto Rotini
Gerardo Diaz Quiros
Marco Cavallo

Shoulder and elbow Surgery (Director: R. Rotini)
IRCCS Istituto Ortopedico Rizzoli, Bologna, Italy

Introduction

The shoulder does not represent the most commonly injured site in soccer players, but the impact of shoulder lesions on the career can be very important as they are often associated with a prolonged absence from the field. Literature reports different case series, ranging from 2% to 12% of shoulder injuries in elite players' international tournaments and approximately one third of these injuries (28%) are defined as "severe", since they cause over 28 days of absence from trainings and matches [1, 3].

Shoulder injuries in the soccer player are considered an increasing issue, probably due to the greater demands of modern soccer, characterized by high speed, pressures and marking.

Goalkeepers are the players with the highest risk of shoulder injury, collecting 18% of the total. This is due to the use of the hands for repetitive and intense overhead activities like ball stopping and throwing, to multiple falls, and to the high risk of colliding against the poles or other players. In addition, the influence of the same lesions in goalkeepers has a higher impact in sports performance: instability, for example, is much less tolerable than in a field player, who can withstand the eventuality of a shoulder instability without seriously impairing its activity. Field players experience shoulder girdle injuries most commonly after direct traumas, when lesions produced by repetitive microtraumas are very infrequent, being limited to launching mechanisms with both hands in throw-in play phases.

Acute shoulder injuries are generally determined through two mechanisms.

Indirect mechanism:

- by fall on the hand or the elbow, mainly causing sprains or dislocations of the acromioclavicular joint and disorders of the gleno-humeral joint, labral injuries or rotator cuff tears;
- by contact with an opponent, producing gleno-humeral dislocation.

Direct mechanism: direct trauma against an opponent or against a firm obstacle such as the ground or the goal poles, generally causing contusions, fractures or acromio-clavicular dislocation.

In this chapter the most common shoulder injuries in soccer players will be examined.

Contusions

Contusions, along with muscle sprains or strains, represent the most frequent muscular injury, consisting in 90% of all sports injuries. Soccer is a contact sport, where often game actions lead to direct impact on the athlete's shoulder.

Clinic

Contusion consists in the typical direct trauma. The clinical presentation is local pain, inflammation, functional limitation or impotence, palpable mass, and sometimes hematoma.

Several clinical factors can influence the severity of the lesion. The muscular fatigue, coldness (previous superficial muscle warming up or due to outer low temperature), use of bandages or compression devices that may favour the appearance of the bruise or the muscular contraction.

The diagnosis is eminently clinical. Imaging procedures are used to visualize and quantify the hematoma (ultrasound) or the extension of the lesion (MRI). These imaging tools are often used to monitor the recovery from the injury.

The treatment usually consists in immobilization, cryotherapy and compression with the muscle

stretched at least 24-48 hours to avoid the formation of the hematoma. The early and progressive physiotherapy helps to recover the sport practice and to avoid complications, such as calcifications and stiffness. Adjunctive and helpful treatment is NSAIDs for the first 72 hours. Surgical treatment is indicated in few severe cases, in order to evacuate a massive hematoma or to fix a partial muscular rupture. Postoperative treatment is similar to the conservative.
Complications of contusions are infrequent, usually consequence of the more severe cases.
Hereafter the main complications are described.
• Muscle hematoma: in general, evacuation is not indicated because of the risk of infection. If massive or chronic and not reabsorbed it can evolve to pseudocyst, requiring surgical treatment.
• Fibrous nodule: it consists in proliferation of disorganized fibrous tissue in the contest of muscle mass. The treatment is conservative with physiotherapy, ultrasound, stretching, and massage.
• Muscle hernia: quite common at the level of the brachial biceps. If not painful it is usually conservatively treated.
• Compartment syndrome, extremely infrequent but requiring immediate surgical treatment.
• Myositis ossificans: it consists in the formation of osseous tissue in the muscle mass. It is an unfrequent but specific complication of muscular contusions. The clinical presentation is pain, persistent swelling with limited mobility. It can be diagnosed with a simple radiograph, although CT scan represents the gold standard for diagnosis, quantification and precise localization of the etherotopic tissue. Preventive treatment with NSAIDs (indomethacin), ionophoresis, or low-dose radiation may be performed in predisposed patients (with a personal history of the same disease). When the etherotopic tissue is formed, limiting the player's activities, the treatment is surgical with a slow and progressive sport recovery.

Glenohumeral instability

Introduction and epidemiology

The shoulder is the articulation with the highest range of mobility in the whole body, which implies a lower intrinsic biomechanics stability. In fact, the most frequent dislocation is shoulder anterior dislocation.
The stability of this articulation is the result of a complex relationship between the static stabilizers (ligaments, capsules, labarum, bony structures) and dynamic (muscles and joints such as scapulathoracic, sterno-clavicular and acromion-clavicular). Glenohumeral instability accounts for about 25% of the total shoulder sports injuries. As in the general population, in soccer the most frequent shoulder instability is the anterior dislocation, although it can occur also inferior or posterior [4, 5].

Causes of instability

The main reasons why one shoulder becomes unstable are:
• structural causes (injuries to the capsulolabral complex due to trauma);
• capsular injuries;
• labrum injuries (SLAP, Bankart, ALPSA);
• glenoid lesions (bony Bankart);
• injuries to the humerus (tuberosity fractures, Hill-Sachs injury);
• rotator cuff and long head of the biceps injuries;
• muscular imbalances that cause displacement of the humeral head over the glena, when associated to ligament laxity.

Types of instability

Nowadays, despite several attempts to classify the instabilities, two main groups are widely accepted to classify shoulder instability: TUBS (traumatic unilateral lesion with Bankart injury and usually requiring surgery) and AMBRI (atraumatic, multidirectional, bilateral frequently, responds to rehabilitation and rarely requires an inferior capsular shift). In the last years a third group was added, related to shoulder overuse (acquired, instability, overstressed, shoulder, AIOS). Nevertheless, shoulder instability consists in a wide spectrum of diseases, that often cannot be clearly identified in one of these three groups.
In soccer the most frequent form of shoulder instability is represented by the anterior-inferior one, especially affecting goalkeepers. Its origin is generally post-traumatic, most of the time accompanied from the first episode by anatomical lesions as Bankart (bony or soft tissue) and Hill-Sachs injuries, causing recurrent dislocations. For

this reasons, it is important to early detect and correctly classify these injuries, in order to perform the best treatment to provide early return to full sports activity.

Anterior instability

Anterior instability is extremely frequent in soccer players as in general population. After a first episode of traumatic anterior dislocation, it is possible to identify a series of lesions which dramatically reduce the shoulder stabilizing function up to 65%, highly increasing the risk of recurrent dislocations.

The most affected structures are:

- glenoid labrum (Bankart lesion);
- anterior-inferior portion of the glenoid (bony Bankart);
- anterior capsule and inferior glenohumeral ligament;
- posterior aspect of the humeral head (Hill-Sachs lesion);
- rotator cuff (extremely rare in soccer players, but still possible in recreational older players).

Clinic

Unidirectional anterior instability is usually post-traumatic and requires a proper reduction manoeuvre. These lesions occur more frequently when the arm is forced in abduction and maximum external rotation: in soccer it mainly happens in goalkeepers after a strong fall on the hand or elbow or after an impact between the goalkeeper and an opponent player, considering the position of the arm typical of this role. When main shoulder stabilizers are already injured, it is possible to observe shoulder dislocation with low impact trauma, or in regular actions like lifting hands to put on or take off the shirt. The first important key to properly assess and treat an anterior instability is to perform an accurate anamnesis, in order to identify the dislocation mechanism and to look for the possibly injured stabilizers.

The clinical tests are essential.

First of all the patient must be checked for hyperlaxity, looking for the thumb and hand fingers hyper mobility, elbow or knee recurvation, spine hyperflexion and so on.

All the maneuvers must be performed bilaterally in order to compare the injured shoulder to the baseline of the patient.

The first exam is to observe active and passive range of motion of the patient, being able to detect if there are movements that are blocked or that the patient does not want to perform because he feels that the shoulder can dislocate. To assess it we have:

- Gagey test;
- sulcus sign;
- posterior drawer test;
- apprehension/relocation and/or anterior release tests.

Lesions of the axillary nerve must be carefully excluded.

Imaging

Conventional X-ray prior to shoulder reduction is important in order to detect the position of the dislocated shoulder and to exclude fractures. Then, a post-reduction control is still mandatory to confirm the effectiveness of the maneuver.

MRI is essential for the study of labrum, capsule, glenohumeral ligaments, rotator cuff, and articular cartilage. Arthro-MR is still more sensitive and specific, especially for labrum pathology and SLAP lesions detection. In acute lesions Arthro-MRI may be not necessary, since the intra articular fluid acts as a natural enhancing tool.

CT scan is mandatory for surgical decision making and planning. It is able to better highlight bone lesions (humeral or glenoid) and allows the surgeon to quantify them in case it is necessary to perform surgical procedures on bone or ostehchondral portion of the shoulder (figg. 1, 2).

Treatments

There is a strong debate in the scientific community on the surgical indication after the first episode of dislocation of the shoulder, since the lowest rates of recurrent dislocation are described after performing an open or arthroscopic surgical treatment if compared to conservative treatment with shoulder immobilization.

Therefore, the conservative treatment after the first episode of dislocation still remains the gold standard, with joint rest and progressive sports recovery after an appropriate period of rehabilitation. Never-

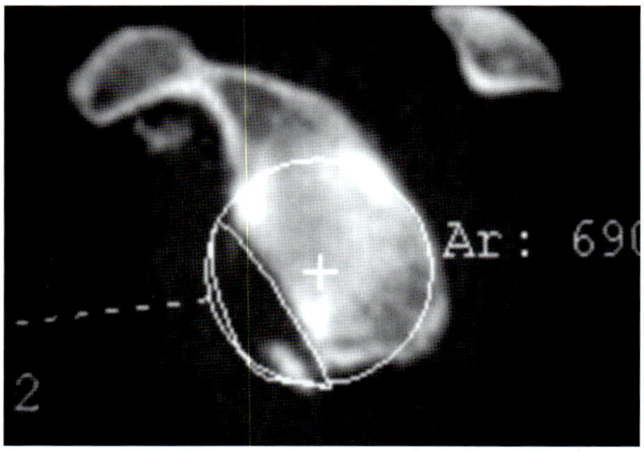

Figure 1 - Bony Bankart lesion of the anterior-inferior margin of the glenoid, causing anterior shoulder instability

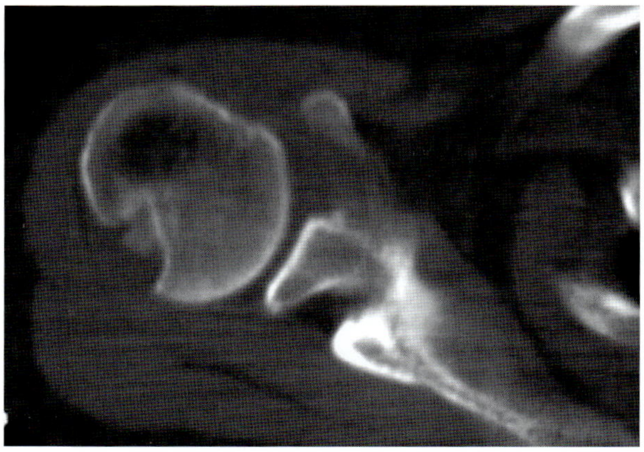

Figure 2 - Hill-Sachs lesion of the humera head following anterior shoulder dislocation and causing anterior shoulder instability

theless, some authors recommend immediate surgical repair in patients who practice contact sports, as in the case for soccer players, especially goalkeepers who are much more exposed to new injuries with recurrent shoulder instability. In case of multiple episode of dislocation, the surgical treatment is mandatory to continue the sports activity.
The surgical indication strictly depends on the presence of bony lesions, such as bony Bankart or Hill-Sachs lesions. In case of their absence (or small size lesions and a low number of recurrences, 3 to 5 episodes), arthroscopic stabilization with capsulolabral reconstruction and tension is the technique of choice, possibly reinforced by rotator cuff remplissage in case of non-engaging small Hill-Sachs lesion.
The loss of 25% or more of the bone stock of the glenoid (straight pear or inverted pear in sagittal plane CT-scan reconstruction) will indicate the necessity of a bone graft, either a coracoid grafting according to the Latarjet technique, the placement of iliac crest autograft on the anterior side of the glenoid (Hebinette procedure), or a cadaver bone graft (fig. 3). On the other hand, the presence of a

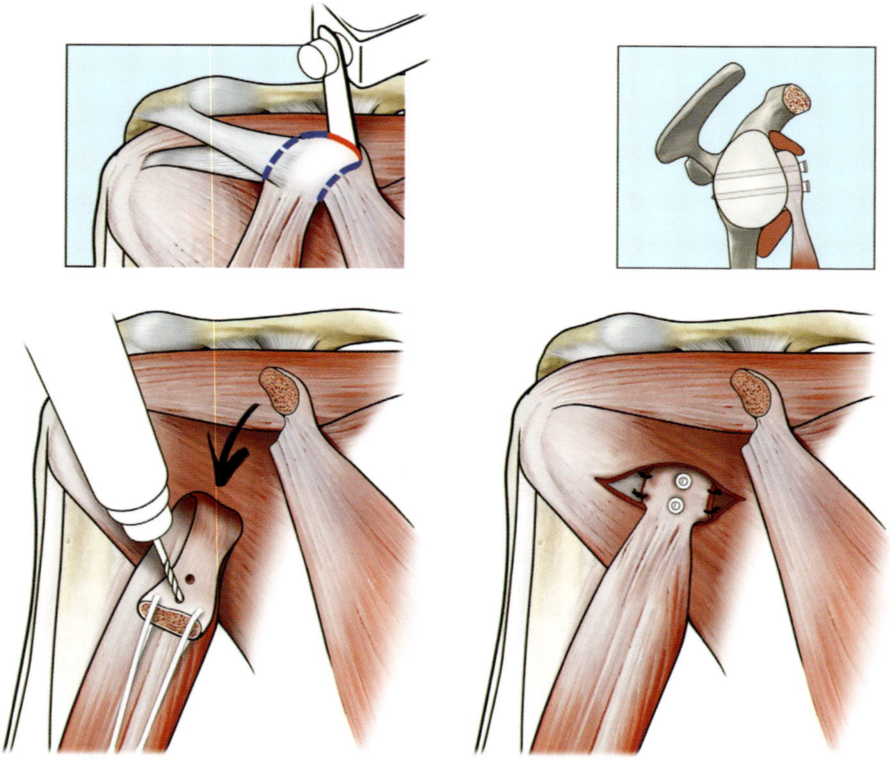

Figure 3 - Illustration of the Latarjet procedure: the coracoid process is resected and fixed to the anterior glenoid portion through a subscapularis split by two parallel screws

Hill-Sachs lesion with affection of more than one third of the articular surface may require a osteochondral graft technique.

Results

Recurrence rates of both arthroscopic and open repairs are below 5%. Boileau developed the Instability Severity Index Score (ISIS) to assess the risk of symple Bankart arthroscopic procedure surgery failure, indicating the risk of 3% recurrence for scores less than or equal to 3 points; 10% for patients with a score less than or equal to 6 points and 70% when they had more than 7 points. Nowadays the current trend is to reinforce Bankart surgery with different procedures, as remplissage (arthroscopic tenodesis of infraspinatus into the Hill-Sachs lesion), arthroscopic bone block under the glenoid labrum, arthroscopic tenodesis of subscapularis at the glenoid (ASA technique) (tab. 1) [6-8].

PROGNOSTIC FACTORS	Points
Age at surgery	
≤ 20	2
> 20	0
Degree of sports participation	
Competitive	2
Recreational	0
Type of sport	
Contact or forced overhead	2
Other	0
Shoulder hyper-laxity	
Antero-inferior	1
Normal	0
Hill-Sachs lesion on AP radiograph	
Loss of contour	2
No lesion	0
Total	**10**

Table 1 - Instability Severity Index Score (ISIS) score, described to assess the risk of symple Bankart arthroscopic procedure surgery failure

Posterior instability

Posterior shoulder instability is much less frequent than the anterior one, both in sports practice and in the general population. It may appear in the context of multi-directional instability or as isolated posterior instability.

The isolated posterior instability in soccer players is usually post-traumatic (after a posterior dislocation, by falling with the arm in full extension or by direct trauma on the anterior aspect of the shoulder) and it is very rarely caused by muscular contractions, as in the case of epileptic crisis. It is necessary to exclude lesions to the axillary nerve that can occur.

MRI and CT scan usually detect a posterior labrum lesion (inverted Bankart, possibly inverted bony Bankart in case of posterior glenoid bone damage) and an anterior humeral head injury (inverted Hill-Sachs).

Treatment algorythm of posterior dislocation (either in acute or chronic phase) usually follows the same rules of anterior dislocation, with similar arthroscopic surgical repair techniques to those used in anterior instability. If it is necessary to fill a humeral head bone defect (reverse Hill-Sachs), it can be done with an osteochondral allograft or a remplissage with the tendon of the subscapular.

Multidirectional instability

Multidirectional shoulder instability usually affects soccer players who have a clinical story of asymptomatic laxity on both shoulders (usually, also other joints are affected), that becomes clinically painful associated with recurrent episodes of subluxation or even complete dislocation, usually autoreduced.

The diagnosis is mainly clinical, with MRI and CTscan showing normal anatomic components of the shoulder. Usually, patients respond positively to rehabilitation and specific neuro-muscular reinforces.

When conservative treatment fails, surgical treatment is indicated, usually performed reducing the redundant antero-inferior and posterior capsule by arthroscopic capsular plication. Attention must be paid in performing this procedure: the risk is to convert a multi-directional instability into a persistent anterior or posterior dislocation by unbalanced overtensioning a single compartment of the gleno-humeral joint. Overtensioning of the capsule may also result in early osteoarthritic degeneration by increasing the pressure on gleno-humeral cartilage surfaces.

Rotator cuff injuries

Rotator cuff injuries are a disabling cause of pain and functional limitation for the player, especially in goalkeepers due to repetitive work performed with the arm above the shoulder level (overhead position). Rotator cuff pathology must be considered as a wide spectrum of diseases, ranging from mild subarcomial impingement syndrome, through partial rupture, complete rupture, massive rupture, and finally rotator cuff arthropathy in older age. Most of the sports injuries of the rotator cuff are the result of progressive microtraumas, although they can sometimes be the result of acute trauma. The typical age of presentation of rotator cuff lesions is in players over 40 years, since in younger age the tendons' elasticity and strength avoid injuries that, in post traumatic events, most likely affect the bones where the tendons are inserted (i.e. avulsion fractures of the proximal humerus tuberosities). Progressively with age, the tendons become thinner and weaker, being more prone to rupture following acute traumatic events or repetitive microtraumas.

Subacromial compression syndrome

This disease is characterized by pain when elevating the arm, especially in internal rotation position, that produces a compression of some elements of the shoulder including supraspinatus tendon, the long head of the biceps tendon, and the subacromial bursa.

Although it is a pathology that mainly affects patients older than 40 years, it can be seen in younger soccer players, who are exposed to repetitive minor trauma and efforts that demand a repetitive overload of the shoulder, as it happens when performing line outs or predominantly in the demanding overhead training of goalkeepers.

In young athletes multi-directional instability with secondary subacromial compression must always been excluded.

Pathogenesis

Symptomatology begins with inflammation or degeneration of soft tissues (very often the supraspinous tendon) which causes an increase in volume in the subacromial space. This causes compression of the tendons and coracoacromial ligament, especially when performing shoulder abduction.

The main function of the rotator cuff is to stabilize the humeral head in the glenoid fossa. In subacromial pain syndrome, when this function is compromised, the deltoid muscle pushes the humerus upward, which leads to a progressive worsening of the symptomatology. Shoulder function will also be limited by decreasing the range of active mobility and altering the scapulohumeral rhythm.

Subacromial syndrome begins with tendinitis or tendons that can progress to severe cuff degeneration and sometimes tear.

Clinical

The pain is unspecified at the beginning and then it is focused on the anterolateral region of the acromion and the acromioclavicular articulation. Also typical is the nocturnal pain when lying on the shoulder affection.

The typical painful arc is between 70-130º of abduction and there is often a weakness in active and passive mobilization.

Diagnosis

The diagnosis is based on a complete physical examination that evaluates the stability of the glenohumeral joint. We can find multiple findings but in a constant way pain is described in the area of insertion of the separator tendon in the greater tuberosity of the humerus. The amplitude of the movement is usually limited, especially abduction, internal rotation, and flexion.

The compression signs of Neer and Hawkins are a diagnostic aid especially if negativizing after subacromial infiltration of local anaesthetic.

Ultrasound or MRI allows us to make a differential diagnosis between compression and degenerative tear of rotator cuff.

Treatment

It is essentially conservative, based on NSAIDs, steroids, and rehabilitation programs, aimed at improving the function of the rotator cuff and the musculature that stabilizes the scapula. The results are satisfactory in 80% of patients. In case of therapeutic failure it would be indicated the surgical evaluation for the eventual realization of a bursectomy or acromioplasty.

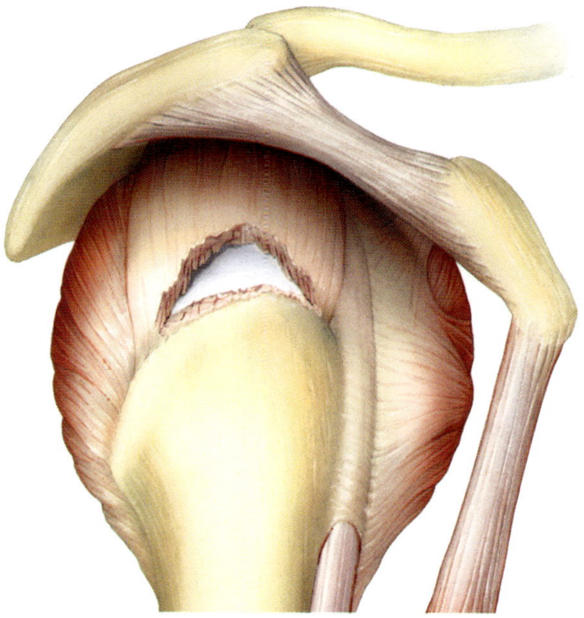

Figure 4 - Illustration of a crescent lesion of the supraspinatus tendon of the rotator cuff

Rotator cuff tears

Lesions of the rotator cuff tendons, expecially of supraspinatus (fig. 4), are an infrequent cause of subacromial pain and functional limitation, affecting mostly middle-aged soccer players. The pathological degeneration process usually begins in the supraspinous tendon due to the inferior blood supply at this level and to the wearing action of the long head of the biceps at the level of the rotator interval. Over time, degeneration and tearing may extend posteriorly also affecting the infraspinatus tendon. The rupture of the upper portion of the subscapular is less frequent, occurring with the same mechanism. In massive ruptures of the cuff the long head of the biceps tendon is often affected, either broken or dislocated. During the launching movements, as frequently performed by the soccer goalkeepers, an eccentric load is rapidly produced, that after several times can cause partial tears of the supraspinous tendon. This type of trauma is associated with rotator cuff tear that is usually located on the lower surface of the tendon, configuring the partial tears on the articular side of the tendons (PASTA lesion of the pitcher).

Diagnosis: physical examination

The patient usually reports insidious pain that is exacerbated by moving the arms above the head, usually causing nocturnal discomfort. As in compression syndrome, the pain is reported in the deltoid region, with muscle weakness and the decrease in the range of motion due to pain limitation. Passive range of motion is usually complete. In case of acute traumatic event, the player complains acute pain and weakness.

At the moment of clinical examination clinical specific test should be performed, in order to assess the validity of the rotator cuff tendons [9].

Main tests for sopraspinatus and infraspinatus:

- Jobe test;
- Patte test;
- External rotation lag sign;
- Drop arm test.

Main tests for subscapularis:

- Napoleon test;
- Belly press;
- Bear-hug test;
- Lift-off test and passive lift-off test.

Main test for teres minor:

- Hornblower's sign.

Diagnosis: imaging

Imaging plays a key role in rotator cuff tears detection. Dynamic ultrasound examination allows to detect partial or complete tears. MRI, especially high resolution MRI with at least 1,5 tesla magnetic field, is the most sensitive tool to detect the tears, whether partial or complete, along with associated lesions. The conventional X-ray study can be useful in chronic massive rotator cuff tear, showing the classic degenerative changes such as upper humeral head migration and diffuse glenohumeral osteoarthritic changes. The CT arthrography is able to reveal a leak through the rotator cuff to the subacromial space, but it is not a routine examination for these problems.

Treatment

In non-traumatic cuff lesions, conservative treatment is generally able to achieve good results in a high percentage of cases. The treatment consists in rest and dedicated physiotherapy, especially with hydrotherapy performed in dedicated pools. Nevertheless it is possible that a progression of the lesion or muscular atrophy will occur over time, especially with sports practice. In this case the surgery is advised.

There are predictive factors that guide towards the need for a surgical intervention.
- Lesion size > 1 cm^2.
- Duration of symptoms of more than six months despite conservative treatments.
- Severe dysfunction in the first presentation.
- Competitive and high level sports activity (small lesions in elite soccer players with high physical demand may not be tolerated).
- Patient expectation of sports activity (in end-career sports players a conservative treatment might be considered, while it is not in a younger player).

The current trend is to perform early surgical treatment on soccer players under the following circumstances:
- acute cuff tears larger than 1 cm^2, with imaging studies showing the acute nature of the lesion;
- acute lesions onto a previous chronic small cuff tear. An athlete with pain or weakness prior to trauma with acute injury, worsening the clinical complains and increasing the lesion size;
- acute rupture involving the subscapular tendon or chronic subscapular lesions associated with biceps instability.

New trends in treatment

The main complication after rotator cuff repair is re-tear of the repaired tendon. For this reason several biological adjuvant (Platelet Rich Plasma, multipotent autologous cells, and so on) for surgical repair of rotator cuff tears have been evaluated in the last years, with controversial results. Nowadays, despite promising lab results, no clinical advantage has been proved with the use of these biological augments. Therefore, it is still early to know whether these therapies will have an effective role in the treatment of this pathology and an intense research activity is still ongoing.

Labrum pathologies

The lesions of the upper labrum glenoid (also defined as SLAP: superior labral avulsion from anterior to posterior) are lesions involving the upper labrum and long head of the biceps tendon origin at the upper part of the glenoid, although it can extend and involve both the anterior and posterior labrum, as well as the surrounding structures [10]. The glenoid labrum is one of the main static stabilizers of the shoulder; it is formed by a peripheral fibrous layer and a transitional fibrocartilage area. The area where the SLAP lesion occur is an area of reduced vascular supply; this explains the unsatisfactory cases of non healing with or without surgery. In soccer players this lesion is usually caused by a fall on the extended arm (usually with the shoulder in abduction and slight flexion) or by repetitive microtraumas suffered during launching movements. So, as well as many other shoulder soft tissue injuries, it is more frequent in goalkeepers than in field players. In addition to the post-traumatic form, the SLAP may be associated with other shoulder pathologies like instability or rotator cuff diseases.

Classification of SLAP injuries

An initial classification of SLAP lesions was proposed by Snyder in 1990, with the identification of four main types. This system, however, was not comprehensive of all cases, and was modified by Maffet et al. introducing types V-VII, but still nowadays most of the surgeons still use Snyder's classification in common practice (fig. 5).
- Type I: degeneration of the upper labrum with

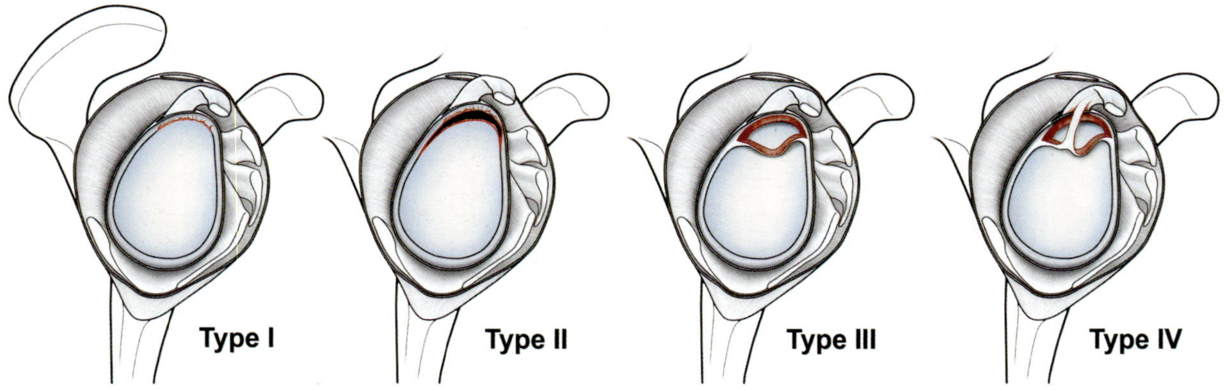

Figure 5 - Classification of superior labral avulsion from anterior to posterior (SLAP) lesions by Sneyder

insertion of the tendon of the normal biceps.
• Type II: (the most frequent in soccer players and also in the general population) detachment of the labrum and the insertion of the biceps of the upper glenoid margin (IIA: anterior; IIB: posterior; IIC: anterior and posterior).
• Type III: vertical breakage of the analogy labrum to a tear in a bucket handle. Anchorage of the normal biceps.
• Type IV: tear of the labrum extended towards the inside of the biceps tendon.

It is important to consider a series of anatomical variants such as the upper sublabral recess, the Buford complex, and the sublabral foramen as they can be confused with real injuries.

Diagnosis

Usually the athlete comes to the clinician's attention complaining progressive and intense shoulder pain, related to a previous shoulder trauma. Sometimes a single trauma is not reported by the athlete, which in this cases usually reports frequent microtraumas in overhead activities (i.e. goalkeepers). Active mobility may be decreased because of pain, but passive range of motion is complete.

There are various clinical tests to check for a SLAP lesion, even if Kibler et al. has recently published a systematic review highlighting the poor clinical validity of all of them. The best known are the O'Brien maneuver and Speed test.

Habermeyer et al. described the maneuver of supine flexion resistance test which reaches a 69% specificity, although its use is limited to detecting type II SLAP injuries.

Arthro-MR or artroCT can be very helpful, also in order to classify the type of lesion. Conventional MRI can help in diagnosing especially in the presence of abundant joint fluid, otherwise it is very difficult to detect these lesions. Conventional radiography and ultrasound are not useful to detect SLAP injuries.

Treatment

Surgical management of SLAP lesions remains controversial. Whereas simple debridement is generally advocated in the treatment of lesions type I and type III, the treatment of the more common type II lesions is more controversial. Management options include isolated debridement, isolated SLAP repair, tenotomy or tenodesis of the long head of the biceps, and a combination of these techniques. Some authors indicate that there are two subgroups of type II lesions that may benefit from tenodesis over labral repair: an older group of patients with poorer quality, degenerate labrum and a younger group with high overhead functional demands. In case of surgical repair it must be performed arthroscopically. In the subgroups of elite athletes, Boileau et al. showed better results performing tenodesis compared to those treated by suture.

Snyder et al. proposed the treatment algorithm for SLAP injuries as in figure 6. Based on this algorithm, the presence of significant pathology in the biceps tendon (degenerative rupture, SLAP IV) or associated pathology (complete rotator cuff rupture, degenerative arthropathy) is an indication to perform a tenodesis instead of a SLAP suture.

The best candidates for the SLAP repair are young patients affected by type 2 subgroup, with traumatic history, a positive physical examination and an Arthro-MR that confirms the lesion.

Although most studies indicate the opportunity to perform arthroscopic repair of SLAP injuries, there is a high variability in results, with a negligible index of failures. Brockmeier et al. described that only 75% of the patients could recover the sport activity level prior to the injury, even if this value increased to 92% when the SLAP recognized a certain traumatic origin [11].

Biceps tendon pathology

The tendon of the long head of biceps (LHB) has its origin in the upper portion of the glenoid and the supraglenoid tubercle. In its intra-articular portion, it presents a wide and flat shape turning more cylindrical when, entering the bicipital groove, it becomes extra-articular passing through the rotator interval. This strucure is the triangular space between the superior border of the subscapularis tendon and the anterior border of the supraspinatus tendon. The groove is bounded by a structure called biceps pulley. The pulley, or "sling", is a capsuloligamentous complex that acts to stabilize the long head of the biceps tendon in the bicipital groove. The pulley complex is mostly composed

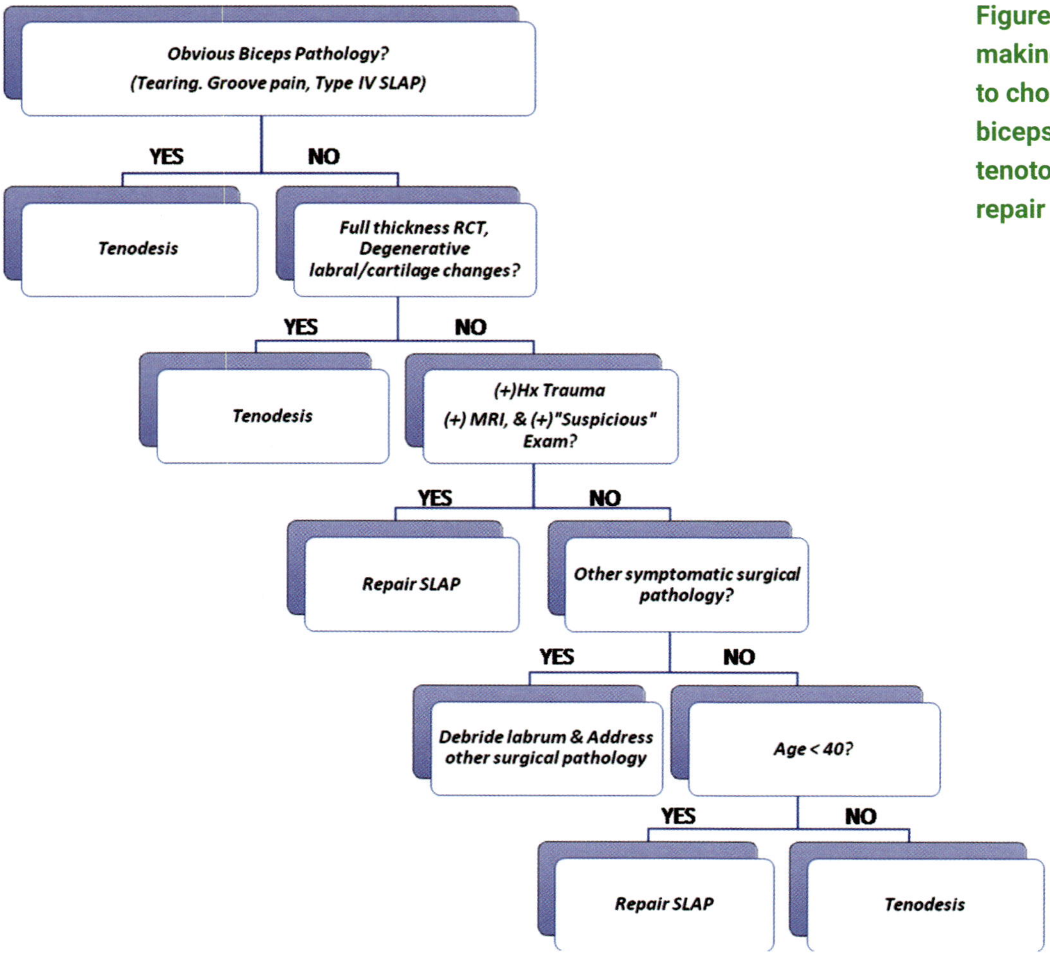

Figure 6 - Decision-making algorithm to choose between biceps tenodesis/ tenotomy or SLAP repair

by two fibrous pillars: the lateral pillar formed by fibers of the supraspinatus tendon, the medial pillar formed by fibres of the coraco-humeral ligament, the upper gleno-humeral ligament and the upper portion of the subscapular tendon and covered mostly by the transverse ligament and coraco-humeral ligament.

Biomechanical studies show a LHB intra articular mobility of approximately 18 mm with the different movements of the arm, also relating the function of the LHB tendon to glenohumeral stability in all directions. Like for other shoulder conditions, goalkeepers are the most affected patient population among soccer players.

Pathology of the LHB

LHB diseases can be classified into three main groups: traumatic, inflammatory, and instability [12-15].

• Traumatic pathology (tendon rupture). Ruptures usually occur at the origin of the LHB tendon or in the bicipital groove. The muscular mass is shifted inferiorly, creating the well-known "Popeye sign". This occurrence is more frequent in patients older than 50 years, even recognizing in its pathogenesis a progressive weakening due to degenerative process, which precipitates with a trauma (fig. 7).

This group also includes the already discussed SLAP injuries. It is important to underline that no direct relationship has been found between bicipital pulley lesions and SLAP injuries.

• Inflammatory pathology (tendinitis). Primary LHB tendinitis is rare, representing approximately 5% of shoulder pathology. More frequently in athletes, this disease is associated with other shoulder conditions, such as subacromial syndrome, rotator cuff ruptures, or pathology of the bicipital groove.

• Tendon instability. This group of diseases is intimately associated with the lesions of the pulley, that usually coincide with rotator cuff ruptures at this level, mostly regarding the subscapular tendon. However, isolated dislocations of the biceps tendon without rotator cuff injuries (although rare) have also been reported. Walch et al. defined bi-

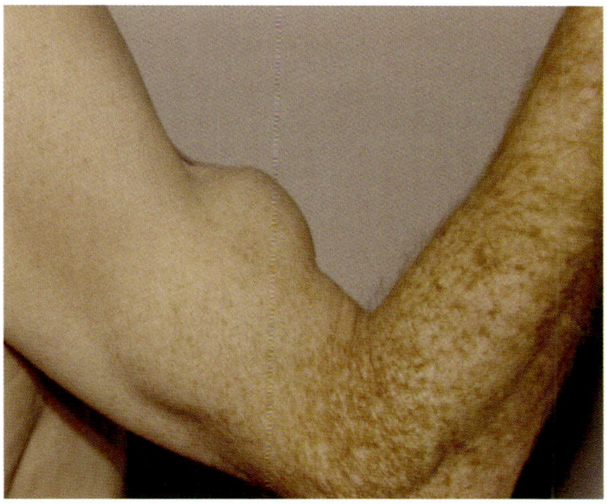

Figure 7 - Popeye sign, indicating a subcutaneous rupture of long head of the biceps

ceps tendon dislocation as "the total and permanent loss of contact between the tendon and the bicipital groove". Many classifications are described, in particular Walch et al. grouped biceps dislocation into four types: (a) dislocation inside the subscapularis tendon, with integrity of the anterior fascia intact; (b) intra-articular dislocation with complete tear of all the insertions on the lesser tuberosity but intact anterior fascia (in this case the lesion is hidden in the joint space); (c) intra-articular dislocation with complete tear of all the insertions on the lesser tuberosity and anterior fascia; (d) dislocation over an intact subscapularis tendon (rupture of the supraspinatus tendon and corcao-humeral ligament) . All dislocations are associated with tears of the ligamentous pulley.

LHB subluxation is more difficult to define because partial or transitional loss of contact between the biceps tendon and the bicipital groove is generally not easy to define.

Diagnosis

The patient usually reports pain in the anterior aspect of the shoulder, that increases with the movement of abduction and external rotation. The patient may also refer crackling sensation.

Clinical tests for diagnosis of biceps tendinopathy are not specific and must be completed by a whole shoulder examination. The most common tests are:

- Tenderness over bicipital groove;
- Speed test;
- Yergason test;
- O'Brien test (active compression test).

The most frequently used imaging tools are ultrasound, MRI and Arthro-MRI. Ultrasound easily detects complete ruptures and dislocations of the tendon but does not well describe partial ruptures. Conventional MRI and Arthro-MR allow more easily a correct diagnosis. Arthroscopy is the gold standard for the detection of pathology of the LHB tendon, allowing also the proper treatment.

Treatment

For the inflammatory pathology the treatment is usually conservative, unless it is accompanied by associated injuries that require a specific treatment. In the young athlete the rupture of the tendon of the LHB of acute origin (post-traumatic) usually has surgical indication especially in those who carry out overhead activities, as goalkeepers. The degenerative rupture of the LHB is usually treated conservatively, because the functional limitation is minimal and the tendon quality is not optimal, increasing the possibilities of rupture recurrence after surgery.

The most used surgical options in case of painful and degenerated LHB are tenotomy or tendon tenodesis. Tenotomy usually leads to pain resolution, with around 30% of the cases associated with aesthetic difference in the anterior aspect of the arm, especially in thin patients due to muscular drop. Tenodesis is generally preferred in young athletes, because of the ability to maintain the biceps muscle length-tension relation, as well as elbow flexion and supination strength, and to achieve improved cosmesis by avoiding a Popeye deformity. Tenodesis can be performed with multiple different techniques, both open or arthroscopic. There is an intense ongoing debate about the type of fixation to be used and about optimal tenodesis location: into the bicipital groove, suprapectoral or subpectoral.

Results

The different studies and reviews reveal the lack of evidence as to whether it is better to perform a tenotomy or a tenodesis, as well as the fact of doing it by open technique or arthroscopy.

Based on the latest data, the current recommendations are to perform tenotomy in elderly patients who have a sedentary life. Tenodesis is recommended in young patients, athletes, patients with thin arms or patients unconfortable with alteration of the cosmetic aspect.

Acromioclavicular joint injuries

Lesions of the acromioclavicular (AC) joint are very common in athletes who practice contact sports activities, like soccer.

AC is a diarthrosis, stabilized by some ligaments: the coracoclavicular (conoid and trapezoid) and acromioclavicular that stabilize the joint and prevent from superior and anterior-posterior dislocation.

Injury mechanism

- Direct: it is the most common form and occurs after a fall or a violent contact, where the shoulder experiences a direct trauma.
- Indirect: this form is generated by falling on the hand or by pulling the arm. Both mechanisms are less frequent than the previous form.

Classification

Rockwood provided the most widely accepted classification of AC joint injuries, considering the entity and direction of displacement, ligament injury, and integrity of the deltoid fascia and trapezius (fig. 8).

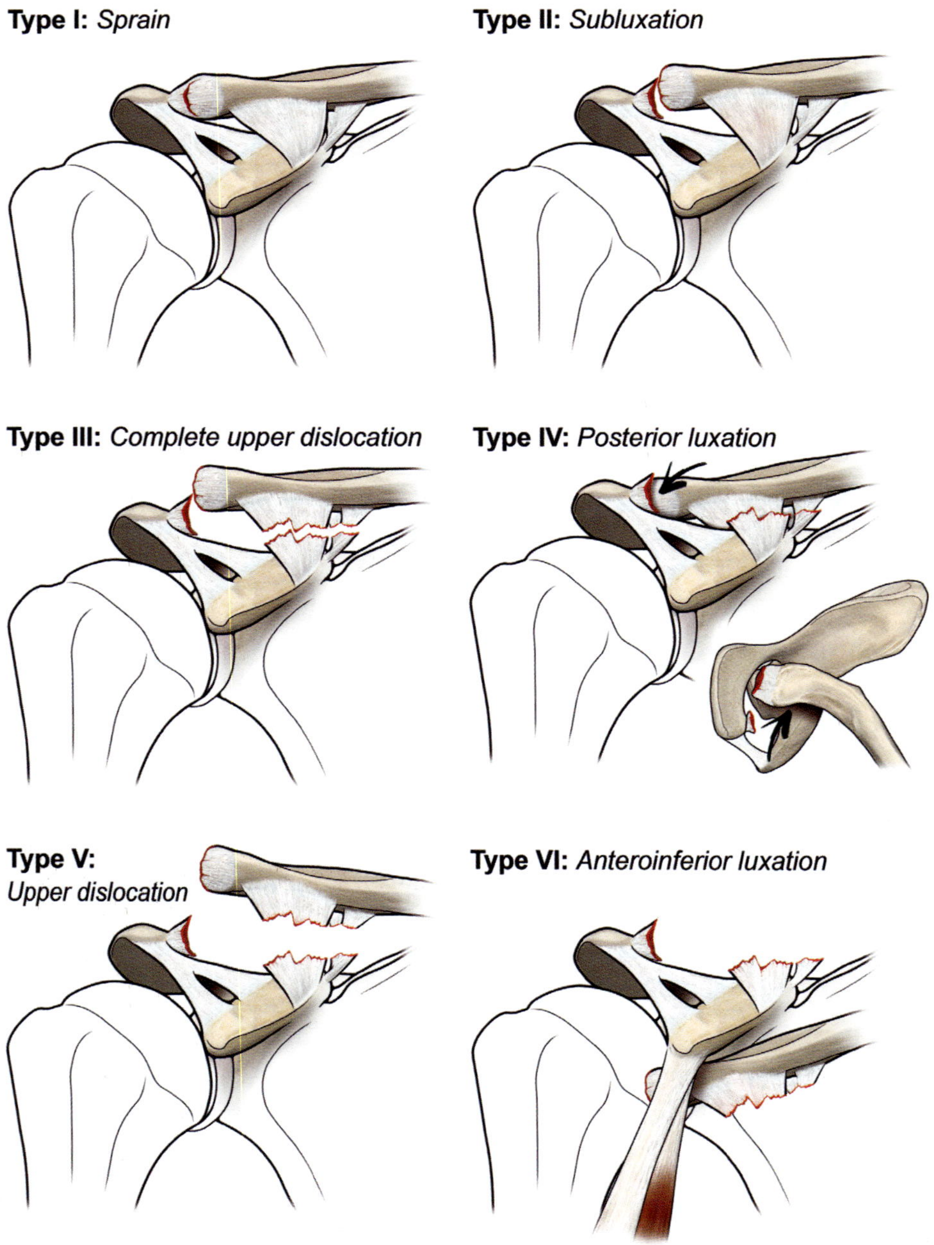

Figure 8 - Rockwood classification of acromion-clavicular joint injuries

• Type I: sprain. There is no loss of the joint relationship, this consists only in a ligamentous sprain. Radiologically, no alterations can be observed.
• Type II: subluxation (incomplete dislocation). Rupture of the acromioclavicular ligaments, with partial capsular rupture and sprain of the coracoclavicular ligaments. Radiologically, there may not be upper displacement of the lateral clavicular margin, or in case of displacement it is inferior to the clavicular thickness.
• Type III: complete upper dislocation. The AC joint is completely dislocated and there is complete rupture of the ligaments acromioclavicular and coracoclavicular. Trapezius and deltoids are partially disinserted. Radiologically it can be observed an elevation of the clavicula over the acromion.
• Type IV: posterior luxation. Dislocation of the AC joint with complete rupture of acromioclavicular and coracoclavicular ligaments, along with injury of the deltoid and trapezium with posterior displacement of the clavicle. The clavicle can perforate the muscular fibers and may not be able to be reduced in place. Radiologically in the axillary projection, the posterior displacement of the distal end of the clavicula can be observed.
• Type V: upper dislocation. It is equivalent to type III, with complete detachment of the trapezius from the outer third of clavicula. Radiographically the coracoclavicular distance is > 100% (100-300%).
• Type VI: anteroinferior luxation (subacromial or sub coracoid). This form is rare, usually with the clavicle irreducible because locked under the coracoid or the acromion.

Diagnosis

After the trauma, the athlete presents pain located in the anterior and upper face of the joint, which can irradiate to the neck and trapezium. A local deformity might be visible, depending on the type of dislocation. If the deformation is reducible with simple pressure on the clavicular lateral edge, the Piano key sign is present.

At physical examination a fundamental test is the Cross body adduction test, which consists in a forced maneuver made by the examinator of adduction and crossing of the arm to the contralateral shoulder, producing a painful compression in the joint.

A correct radiological study is fundamental, in order to correctly classify the lesion and properly treat it. X-rays must be performed in upright position in order to better visualize an eventual AC joint dislocation, that might reduce in supine position. Special projections must be performed, such as the Stringer (10º-15º cephalic inclination), Stryker (helps in visualizing coracoid fractures) or more important the stress X-rays, with a weight held by the hand. In doubtful cases CT and RM scan also have an important role.

Treatment

Type I and II: the treatment is usually conservative, with cryotherapy, NSAIDs, and immobilization with Kenny-Howard sling or the figure-of-8 bandage. The player must rest and avoid contacts or to force the joint for a period of 3 to 6 weeks.

Type III: The ideal treatment for this group is very debated, with different opinions and results presented in the available literature. Currently, the trend is to treat conservatively these lesions, some categories are addressed to surgery in order to avoid complications like persistent pain, muscular impairment, altered shoulder kinematic. Athletes and young heavy workers are usually surgically treated. In case of associated fracture of coracoid the treatment can be also conservative, but in the athlete a open field reduction and fixation coracoid is often performed.

Type IV, V, VI: these lesions are usually addressed to surgery.

Surgical procedure

the surgical procedure consists in an open reduction of the AC joint, that must be held in place by a coraco-clavicolar ligament reconstruction. Multiple techniques have been described, including reconstruction with allograft or multiple different devices. A trans-AC K wire can be positioned in order to temporarily stabilize the joint while the scar tissue begins to form, and must be removed within one month. A hook plate is not necessary in acute cases, but it is often required if the surgery is performed in a chronic setting, in order to provide a stronger stabilization of the joint. The plate must be removed within 6 months, in order to avoid erosions of the inferior margin of the acromion or possible rotator cuff injuries due to hook impingement (even if modern plates are designed with the hook going posteriorly, avoiding contacts with rotator cuff, still concerns remain in case of trauma occurred with plate in situ).

Complications
The AC joint, especially after conservatively treated grade 1-2 dislocation, can undergo a progressive degeneration process due to the overloading and recurrent traumas during gym training and during matches in soccer players. This may also cause osteolysis of the lateral aspect of the clavicle. In both cases, if conservative treatment fails, there is indication to perform the resection of the lateral portion of the clavicle according to Mumford or Weaver-Dunn.

Nerve pathology (neural impingement)

Pain and inability of the shoulder may be due to compression of the peripheral nerves around the shoulder. This injury can occur in soccer players and must be considered in those players who present a shoulder weakness or pain not explained by common causes.

Suprascapular nerve compression
Suprascapular neuropathy is uncommon, being responsible of 1%-2% of shoulder pain in the athlete. It is also the second most affected nerve after gleno-humeral dislocation, following the axillary nerve [16-18].
Due to its anatomical position, it is susceptible to being compressed at the level of the transverse ligament of the scapula or the spino-glenoid ligament. It may also be affected by direct trauma or secondarily injured by fractures of the scapula. Nevertheless the major cause of compression in sports practicing people is by a cyst originating by a lesion of the posterior labrum or a SLAP lesion, growing in dimension with a valve-mechanism.
Nerve compression produces weakness and atrophy of the supraspinous (proximal lesions) and infraspinatus, detectable with the specific clinical test already mentioned for rotator cuff pathology. Patients also report pain in the posterior region of the shoulder.
MRI and elettromiography confirm the diagnosis and lead to the proper treatment.
The cases produced by overuse and dynamic compression against the transverse ligament usually benefit from conservative treatment with rest and NSAIDs. Other cases of nerve compression are generally successfully treated by surgery, that might be arthroscopic in case of a labral cyst or open in case of different site nerve compression or scapular fracture involving the nerve. When possible, arthroscopic technique is less aggressive, but it must be performed by a skilled surgeon.

Brachial plexus lesions
When they are minor by traction and compression, they are described by the players as “burning” or “pricks”, in other words, paraesthesias. Before the brachial plexopathies, the conduct is expectant with complete abstention from the sport activity of about 3 months. If after this period there is no clinical improvement it will be necessary to consider surgical repair.

Quadrilateral space syndrome
Quadrilateral space syndrome consists in compression of the axillary nerve at the level of quadrilateral space. It produces in the athlete pain and paraesthesias when performing overhead activities, so goalkeepers are the most affected players in soccer.
Rest and sports activity modifications are the most effective treatment, with surgery required in exceptional cases.

Paralysis of the long thoracic nerve
This disease causes the medial dissociation of the scapular margin from the thoracic wall due to serratus anterior disfunction. It is caused by a post-traumatic compression or traction of the long thoracic nerve (in this case usually occurring when weightlifting in the gym or after game trauma).
Treatment is usually conservative, leading to symptom resolution in up to 18 months. In exceptional cases a pectoral major surgical transfer is required to restore function in persistent chronic paralyses.

Calcifying tendinitis and stiffness of the shoulder

None of these two entities are common in the active young or elite soccer player, generally affecting older recreational players.

Calcific tendinitis

This disease consists in a highly painful deposit of calcium in the tendons of the rotator cuff, especially in the supraspinatus. It is slightly more frequent in women, and although these deposits can be asymptomatic for years, they might turn in an active phase of reabsorption, with consistency modification becoming soft. In this phase the calcification may affect also the subacromial bursa, increasing the symptoms, producing severe pain, strongly limiting the shoulder movements in all directions. Repetitive shoulder micro-traumas can be recognized in the etiology of the disease.
X-rays are able to detect the calcium deposit in the rotator cuff tendons, but only with ultrasounds it is possible to confirm the subacromial bursitis and to assess the consistency of the calcification, in order to properly address the treatment (fig. 9).
Conservative treatment is effective in most of the cases, with NSAIDs, rest, and physiotherapy while the calcium deposits are spontaneously absorbed or turn back into a silent phase, with hard consistency. When the symptoms persist, in the phase of tenderness of the calcification it is possible to perform a ultrasound guided percutaneous lavage of the deposit, with successful results. Arthroscopic or open field removal of calcifications are performed in exceptional cases.

Adhesive capsulitis

It is also known as "frozen shoulder". It is characterized by pain and stiffness of the shoulder caused by a thickened and contracted joint capsule. There are numerous factors associated with its development, such as previous trauma, prolonged immobilization, undisplaced fracture of the tuberosities or systemic medical conditions, but in most cases, it is not possible to determine the cause. The diagnosis is mainly clinical, based on patient history and physical examination. As characteristic, the shoulder is limited both in active and passive movement in all directions, with intense shoulder pain when the clinician tries to force the contracture.

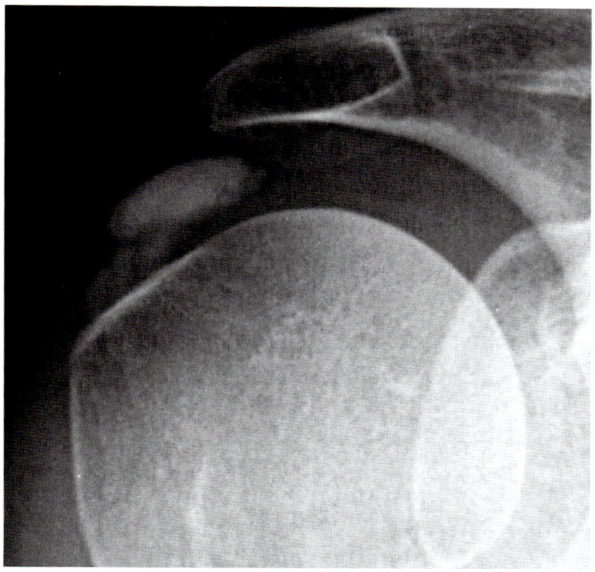

Figure 9 - X-rays of the shoulder showing calcific tendinitis

Arthrography may show a loss of axillary recess and joint capsule contracture.
Three clinical stages and four arthroscopic have been described (tab. 2).
Treatment: idiopathic frozen shoulder is generally treated with specific rehabilitation programs, sistemic NSAIDs and/or steroid infiltrations. Prolonged post-traumatic stiffness of the shoulder may take longer time to respond to conservative treatment, and some authors in literature indicate manipulation under anaesthesia and arthroscopic capsulotomy after 12-16 weeks of unsuccessful conservative treatment.

Osteochondral lesions

The osteochondral pathology of the shoulder may be found in the humeral head, glenoid cavity or both. It may be a result of direct traumas or more frequently by shoulder instability, displasya or osteonecrosis [19]. This issue is widely treated in a dedicated chapter.

Fractures

Fractures around shoulder are common occurrences in soccer players, generally occurring after direct trauma or after falls. the clavicle and proximal humerus are the most affected sites, with scapula exceptionally involved.

Stage	Name	Symptoms	Arthroscopic findings
1	Pre-freezing stage	Limited range of motion and pain with symptoms occurring at 0-3 months	Erythematous/fibrinous synovium
2	Freezing stage	Severely restricted range of motion and pain occurring 3-9 months (patients usually present during this stage)	Red, thick synovium with contracted rotator interval and thigt axillary recess with adhesions
3	Frozen stage	Severe stiffness, minimal pain, occurring at 9-15 months	Pink synovium with contracted axillary pouch and tight joint space
4	Thawing stage	Improving range of motion, minimal pain	Tight joint space but no evidence of synovitis

Table 2 - Arthroscopic stages of frozen shoulder

Clavicular fractures

Epidemiology

Clavicle fractures represent 2.4-10% of all fractures. They are especially common in the athletes, mostly affecting the central portion of the clavicle (70-80%). 25-30% affect the lateral portion, and only 2% the medial portion [20-22].

Injury mechanism

• Traumatic: they are usually produced by an indirect mechanism by a fall on the shoulder or on the hand (central or lateral third), but they can also be caused by a direct compression mechanism (more frequently in the central third) during a fall on the field.

• Stress fractures: clavicular fractures may also occurr with a fatigue mechanism.

Classification

The most used classification system was presented by Allman (groups I, II, III) (fig. 10), later expanded by Neer, Rockwood and Craig (fig. 11).

• Group I: fractures of the central third (80-85%).

• Group II: fractures of the lateral third (20%).

- Neer Type I: with coracoclavicular ligaments intact.

- Neer Type II: fracture medial to coracoclavicular ligaments.

-- Rockwood IIA: conoid and the trapezoid attached to the distal segment.

-- Rockwood IIB: conoid broken and trapezoid attached to the lateral segment.

- Neer Type III: acromioclavicular intra-articular fracture.

- Type IV Craig: typically affecting children, with undisplaced fractured lateral portion and displacement occurred at the level of the physis.

- Type V Craig: lateral fractures with a bony portion attached to the coracoclavicular ligaments.

• Group III: fractures of the medial third (5%).

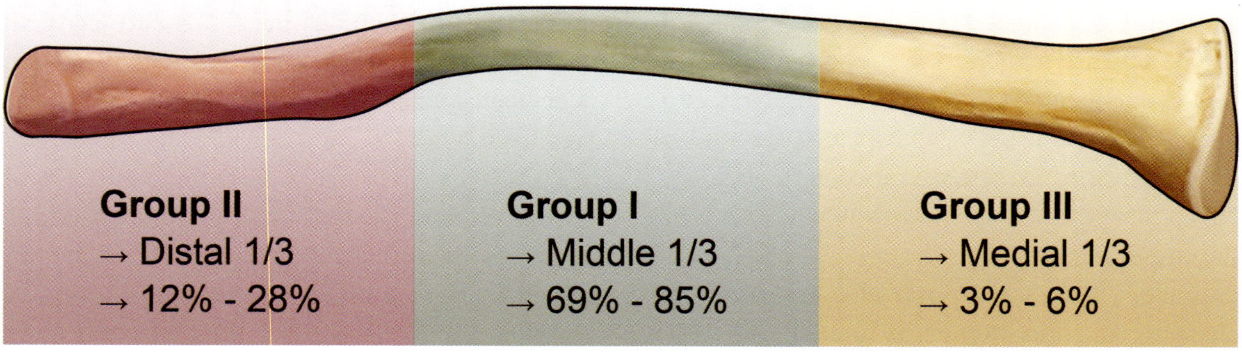

Figure 10 - Allmann classification of clavicular fractures

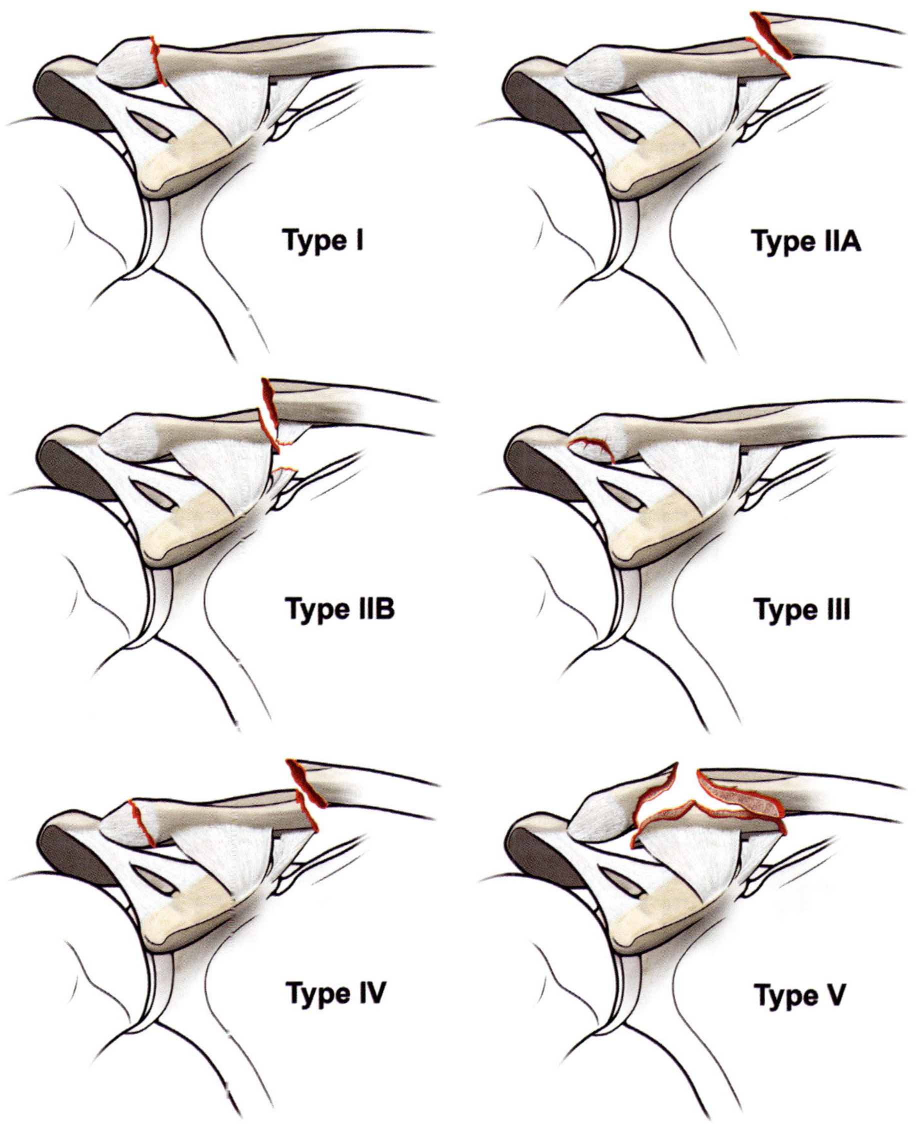

Figure 11 - Neer, Rockwood and Craig modifications of Allmann classification of clavicular fractures

Diagnosis

The athlete typically complains pain with a typical attitude of the upper limb in adduction, with the arm attached to the body held by the opposite arm. It may also present clavicular deformity and hematoma, with intense local pain at pressure.

X-ray examination must include special studies, such as oblique cephalic at 45° or the "Serendipity view" for medial fractures. CT scan is helpful in diagnosis of multifragmentary fractures or in doubtful cases, along with indicating the position and size of fragment in case of surgical treatment.

Treatment

The ideal treatment of clavicular fractures strictly depends on the location of the fracture itself.

Clavicular medial fractures usually report good outcome with conservative treatment with figure-of-8 bandage; surgery is indicated in case of vascular problems or high risk to be injured by fracture. Surgery at this level is particulary dangerous due to the big vessels in close proximity of the clavicle.

Fractures of the medial portion of the clavicle generally report good outcome with conservative treatment. The surgical indications are currently being increased, especially in athletes, due to the development of dedicated anatomical hardwares for fixation and to the possibility to early recover the sports activities. Indications for surgery are reported in table 3.

Clavicular lateral third fractures: conservative treatment with a sling is preferred for 3-6 weeks in most type I, III and IV cases. In type II and V surgical fixation is often required, due to the high

frequency of non-union (30-45%).
Recently dedicated low profile plates have been developed in order to treat the different affected sites of the clavicle: superior or anterior countured plates for medial or central third, superior with multiple lateral small size locking screws or hook plates for the lateral third. In cases of coraco-clavicular ligament lesions or avulsion (type 5) it might be useful to associate a ligament reconstruction as described for acromion-clavicular dislocations.

Proximal humerus fractures

Epidemiology

Fractures of the proximal humerus assume more than 4-5% of all adult fractures but they are unfrequent in soccer players, since they are closely related to osteoporosis being the third most frequent fractures in elderly patients. Fractures of the proximal humerus that affect athletes are usually consequence of high energy trauma, leading to displacement of the fragments, so the therapeutic approach is usually surgical in most cases [21, 22].

Mechanism of injury

The most frequent mechanism is an indirect trauma after falling with the arm in extended position, but occasionally it can be caused by direct injuries during matches or training.

Classification

The most widely accepted classification was initially proposed by Codman, who divided the proximal portion of the humerus into four main fragments, or "parts": greater tuberosity, lesser tuberosity, humeral head and shaft. Based on this interpretation, Neer established a classification taking into account the anatomy and the displacing forces affecting each fragment. By "fragment" he indicates a portion that has a displacement greater than 1cm or an angle greater than 45° with respect to the other portions.
The fracture pattern can also give clues to the risk of vascular injury to the humeral head and future risk of avascular necrosis. The longer the medial metaphyseal extension of the head, the more likely the vascularity to the humeral head is intact.

ABSOLUTE INDICATIONS

Factors dependending on the type of fracture
- Open fractures

Factors dependending on the existence of associated injuries
- Imminent cutaneous tear and irreducible fracture
- Vascular impairment
- Progressive neurological loss
- Pathological fracture displaced with associated trapeze paralysis
- Scapulothoracic dissociation

RELATIVE INDICATIONS

Factors dependending on the type of fracture
- $\geq$ 20 mm shortening
- Fracture gap of 100%
- Segmental or comminuted fractures

Factors dependending on the existence of associated lesions (bilateral fractures, polytrauma, neurological problem etc.)

Patient related factors
- Intolerance to immobilization
- Aesthetic problems
- Need for early mobilization (elite athletes, professional soccerers etc.)

Table 3: indications for surgery of the middle third clavicular fractures

The AO classification, even if not particularily used, focuses on this topic dividing fractures into three categories based on the severity of injury and likelihood of avascular necrosis of the humeral head.
- Type A fractures: no vascular isolation of articular segment.
- Type B fractures: partial vascular isolation of articular segment.
- Type C fractures: total vascular isolation of articular segment.

Each group is then subdivided numerically, with higher numbers indicating greater severity (fig. 12).

Diagnosis

The patient usually presents a swollen shoulder, often with hematoma in arm and thorax along with pain, functional impotence and a typical attitude

with the shoulder in adduction, holding the forearm with the contralateral arm.
Conventional X-rays are mandatory, often completed by a CT scan in order to better assess number and location of the fragments.

Treatment
The vast majority (80%) of the proximal humeral fractures are not displaced or have a low grade of displacement, so they are generally addressed to conservative treatment with immobilization in sling and early physiotherapy.
However, in fractures with an important displacement the risk of nonunion, malunion or avascular necrosis of the head increases significantly, leading to surgical reduction and fixation.

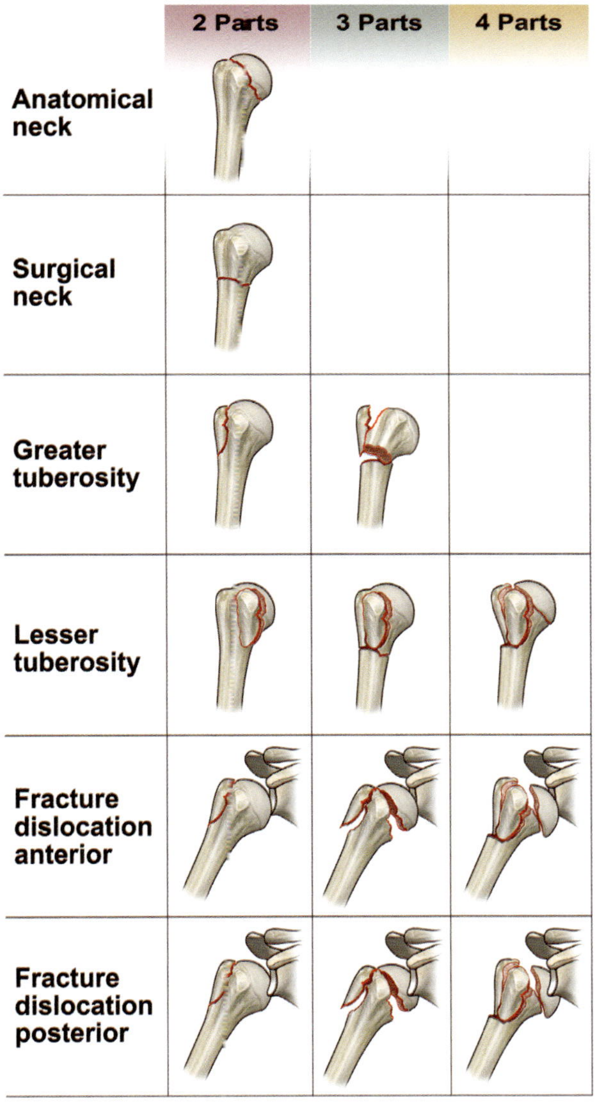

Figure 12 - Neer classification of proximal humeral fractures

- Displaced fractures of the greater tuberosity.
- Fractures of the lesser tuberosity with involvement of the articular surface.
- Displaced or unstable fractures of the surgical neck.
- Displaced fractures of the anatomical neck in young patients.
- Fractures displaced in three or four fragments with the possibility of reconstruction.
- Fractures displaced in elite athletes with high functional requirement.

Different hardwares can be used for proximal humeral fracture fixation. The most widely used are plate and screws, that allow a better reduction of the multiple fragments. Percutaneous intramedullary nailing is also used, with the advantage of less soft tissue damages thanks to the percutaneous approach, even if rotator cuff injuries are reported in literature.

Results
Results of ORIF or percutaneous nailing are strictly influenced by the fracture pattern. Good and optimal results are reported for minimally displaced and low complexity fractures, allowing a full sports recovery. With internal fixation, special attention should be paid to medial comminution, varus angulation, and restoration of the calcar.
In authors' opinion the plating technique offers a faster sports recovery, thanks to the primary intrinsic stability of plate and screw fixation. Some concerns remain with possible iatrogenic rotator cuff damages in case of anterograde humeral nailing.

Scapula fractures
Epidemiology
Fractures of the scapula in soccer are exceptional, with the incidence of less than 5% of all shoulder girdle injuries. This low incidence is due to the anatomy of the bone, its characteristic mobility and the important coverage of the muscular masses [23].
Most of the lesions occur in the body and in the spine (50%) followed by those of the neck (25%), those of the glenoid cavity (10%) and those of the coracoid process (7%).

Injury mechanism
They are usually produced by a direct high energy trauma creating fractures of the spine or the scapular body. Sometimes they can be caused by indirect trauma by means of axial compression forces with the extended arm, that produces through the humeral head an intra-articular fracture of the glenoid cavity or the scapular neck.

Classification
The fractures of scapula have been classified classically referring to the anatomy in order to facilitate the treatment. The classification of Ideberg and Goss for fractures of the glenoid cavity, that of Kuhn et al. for acromial fractures or Ogawa for fractures of the coracoid are three of the most widely used. A new classification proposed by Bartonicek based on the findings obtained with CT has recently been published.

Diagnosis
The main clinical symptoms in an athlete with scapula fracture are pain and functional impairment, with the arm in adduction and self-protected from movements. If there is an acromion fracture or fracture of the displaced neck, shoulder deformity will appear, expecially in cases of floating shoulder.
As injuries that occur after high energy trauma, the presence of other associated injuries must always be excluded, such as rib fractures, clavicle fractures, pneumothorax or, more rarely, brachial plexus or axillary vessel and nerve lesions.
Although initially radiologically examined, it may be necessary the use of TC, especially in intra-articular fractures of the glenoid cavity or the apophasis coracoid.

Treatment
Fractures of the body and spine: usually conservative with immobilization 2 to 3 weeks and, subsequently, beginning with progressive rehabilitation of scapulothoracic and glenohumeral joints.
Fractures of the coracoid process: most authors recommend conservative treatment with a sling for isolated fractures of the coracoid, although for displaced fractures with associated acromioclavicular dislocation, open reduction and internal fixation with a screw is recommended.
Acromion fractures: non-displaced fractures give good results after conservative treatment with sling for 3 weeks and early rehabilitation. The fractures displaced more than 5 mm or associated with acromion clavicular grade III dislocation are generally addressed to surgery.
Fractures of the scapular neck: undisplaced and stable fractures follow the same conservative scheme that was previously exposed. Displaced fractures (>1 cm or with 40º of angulation) or when accompanied by a fracture of the clavicle (unstable, especially in case of floating shoulder) will require surgical stabilization by the synthesis of the scapular neck or clavicle, depending on the lesion pattern.
Fractures of the glenoid: these fractures are addressed to surgery when there is the high risk of instability or long term arthritis.

Osteoarthritis

Soccer players, as well as other sports practicing people, may report symptoms due to osteoarthritis in the shoulder girdle. The most affected sites are the acromioclavicular joint and the gleno-humeral joint.

Acromioclavicular osteoarthritis
Usually soccer players are affected by post traumatic AC arthritis originated by an injury – sometimes years earlier – or by chronic mini-traumas from overuse.
The osteoarthritic process is gradual, with symptoms that may come and go and eventually worsen over time. The primary symptom of acromioclavicular osteoarthritis is pain in one or both shoulders, such as localized tenderness and intermittent pain in different positions of the shoulder. Pain is tipically increased by certain activities, such as reaching the arm across the body or lifting the ball in overhead position.
Moreover, the bone spurs caused by this type of osteoarthritis can pinch and irritate the rotator cuff tendons, resulting in even more pain.
Conventional X-rays and sometimes MRI or CT scan are the best exams to detect and quantify AC osteoarthritis, showing the typical signs of these kind of deterioration.

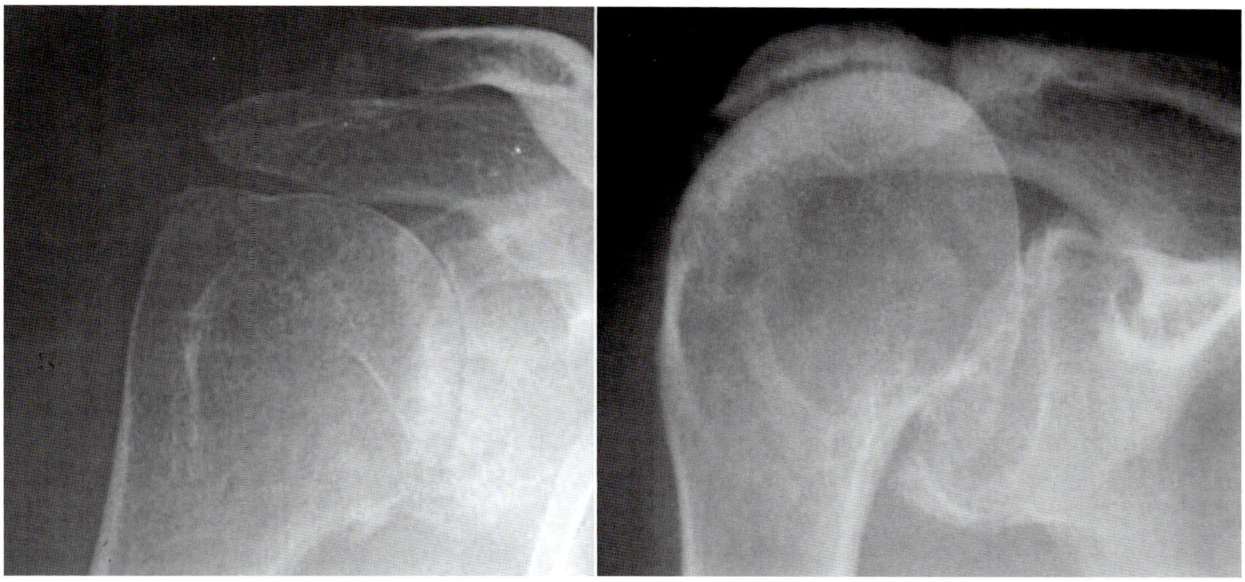

Figure 13 - X-rays showing gleno-humeral osteoarthritis. On the left a concentric arthritis is showed, while on the right an eccentric osteoarthritis with humeral superior escape

Treatments
Sistemic NSAIDs and local ice represent the first treatment line.
Certain activities and exercise will aggravate the acromioclavicular joint. Weight lifting and other exercises requiring cross-body arm movement should be avoided if they cause pain.
In contrast to other osteoarthritic joints, physical therapy has been demonstrated to be less effective for acromioclavicular patients. However, depending on the patient and concomitant specific conditions, exercises that focus on stretching and strengthening muscles and maintaining the shoulder's range of motion may be helpful.
Local aspiration and steroid injections have been proved to be an effective option, especially in the short term.
If osteoarthritis symptoms are severe and conservative treatments are not effective, surgery may be required. Surgeries to relieve osteoarthritis of the shoulder's acromioclavicular joint include:
• AC joint arthroscopy to remove loose pieces of damaged cartilage;
• resection of the distal clavicle, sometimes called distal clavicle excision, to remove a small portion of the end of the clavicle, thereby eliminating friction between the clavicle and the acromion. Eventually, scar tissue bridges the gap between the two bones. This surgery can be done with both arthroscopic or open field technique and seems to provide pain relief to most people suffering from moderate-to-severe acromioclavicular arthritis.

Glenohumeral osteoarthritis
Glenohumeral arthrosis is a degenerative disease of the articular cartilage of the humeral head and/ or the glenoid cavity (fig. 13).
In young athletes, osteoglenohumeral osteoarthritis usually is the result of recurrent shoulder instability or post-traumatic or postsurgical sequelae.
Shoulder instability has associated chondral lesions that progress towards osteoarthritis. Sometimes surgical procedures for instability treatment have been associated with osteoarthritis, like wrong anchorage placement for arthroscopic techniques or lateral positioning of the coracoid in Latarjet procedure.
Post-traumatic OA usually occurs after fractures of the proximal humerus or the glenoid cavity, especially if malunion occurs [24, 25].

Diagnosis
The athlete who starts with osteoarthritis GH will refer pain with activity, night pain, mechanical alterations such as blockages or clicks and decreased mobility, especially the external rotation. In the shoulder X-ray it is possible to observe

classic signs such as the narrowing of the joint space, subchondral sclerosis and formation of osteophytes in the humeral head and glenoid components.
CT scan is the best exam to evaluate bone changes around the joint and to assess the glenoid orientation, essential for the planning of surgical treatment.

Classification
Samilson and Prieto introduced a radiographic classification based on the size of the osteophytos that is applied in patients with GH osteoarthritis secondary to unstable shoulders.
• Minimal arthrosis: humeral osteophytes and/or glenoid < 3 mm.
• Moderate arthrosis: humeral osteophytes and/or glenoid of 3-7 mm.
• Severe osteoarthritis: humeral osteophytes and/or glenoid > 7 mm.

Treatment
The purpose of the treatment is to preserve the joint function, to prevent if possible the progression of the disease and to control the pain.
In young athletes, as we have commented, the origin of osteoarthritis tends to be secondary to an underlying pathology, so they have a worse prognosis. The treatment options are many, beginning always with a conservative treatment and subsequently surgical not prosthetics to delay the maximum possible implantation of a prosthesis.
Non-surgical treatment. The modification of life habits, whenever possible, is used in mild or moderate osteoarthritis, treatment with non-steroidal antiinflamatoros and analgesics, the infiltration of corticoids that produce a temporary relief and physiotherapy treatment. Stretching and specific muscular strenghtening are mandatory to preserve joint function, being able to slow down the degenerative process for may years and allowing the soccer player to maintain its activity level, especially in case of non goalkeepers.
Surgical treatment. In young patients with mild-moderate GH osteoarthritis, arthroscopy can be performed, often with moderate rate of success. In case of advanced arthritis the ideal treatment remains the prosthetic replacement: when the rotator cuff is not compromised it may be possible to implant stemless or short stem implants, that might be compatible with the sports activities. In case an anatomical conventional or a reverse implant is required, the sports activity is not adviced in order to avoid major complications like dislocation, components wear or peri-prosthetic fractures.

Bibliography

1. A.D. Delgado Martínez. Cirugía Ortopédica y Traumatología. Panamericana. 4ª Edición. 2018.
2. Roald Bahr, Sverre Maehlum. Clinical Guide to Sports Injuries. Human Kinetics, 2004.
3. Mark D. Miller MD, Stephen R. Thompson MD. Miller's Review of Orthopaedics. Seventh edition. 2016.
4. Snyder SJ. Diagnostic arthroscopy of the shoulder: normal anatomy and variations. In: Snyder SJ. Shoulder arthroscopy. Philadelphia, PA: Lippincott Williams &Wilkins, 2003.
5. Williams RJ 3rd, Strickland S, Cohen M, Altchek DW, Warren RF. Arthroscopic repair for traumatic posterior shoulder instability. Am J Sports Med. 2003 Mar-Apr;31(2):203-9.
6. Lafosse L, Boyle S, Gutierrez-Aramberri M, Shah A, Meller R. Arthroscopic latarjet procedure. Orthop Clin North Am. 2010 Jul;41(3):393-405.
7. Kim SH, Kim HK, Sun JI, Park JS, Oh I. Arthroscopic capsulo labro plasty for postero inferior multidirectional instability of the shoulder. Am J Sports Med. 2004.
8. Olds M, Ellis R, Donaldson K, Parmar P, Kersten P. Risk factors which predispose first-time traumatic anterior shoulder dislocations to recurrent instability in adults: a systematic review and meta-analysis. Br J Sports Med. 2015 Jul;49(14):913-22.
9. Sciascia AD, Spigelman T, Kibler WB, Uhl TL. Frequency of use of clinical shoulder examination tests by experienced shoulder surgeons. J Athl Train. 2012 Jul-Aug;47(4):457-66.
10. Kibler WB, Sciascia A. Current practice for the diagnosis of a SLAP lesion: systematic review and physician survey. Arthroscopy. 2015 Dec;31(12):2456-69.
11. Millett PJ, Horan MP, Pennock AT, Rios D. Comprehensive Arthroscopic Management (CAM) procedure: clinical results of a joint-preserving arthroscopic treatment for young, active patients with advanced shoulder osteoarthritis. Arthroscopy. 2013 Mar;29(3):440-8.
12. Elser F, Braun S, Dewing CB, Giphart JE, Millett PJ. Anatomy, function, injuries, and treatment of the long head of the biceps brachii tendon. Arthroscopy. 2011 Apr;27(4):581-92.
13. Ainsworth R, Lewis JS. Exercise therapy for the conservative management of full thickness tears of the rotator cuff: a systematic review. Br J Sports Med. 2007 Apr;41(4):200-10.
14. Tennent TD, Beach WR, Meyers JF. Clinical sports medicine update. Am J Sports Med 2003.
15. Khazzam M, George MS, Churchill RS, Kuhn JE. Disorders of the long head of biceps tendon. J Shoulder Elbow Surg. 2012 Jan;21(1):136-45.
16. Mallon WJ, Wilson RJ, Basamania CJ. The association of suprascapular neuropathy with massive rotator cuff tears: a preliminary report. J Shoulder Elbow Surg. 2006 Jul-Aug;15(4):395-8.
17. Zehetgruber H, Noske H, Lang T, Wurnig C. Suprascapular nerve entrapment. A meta-analysis. Int Orthop. 2002;26(6):339-43.
18. Safran MR. Nerve injury about the shoulder in athletes, part I: suprascapular and axillary nerve. Am J SportsMed. 2004;32:803-819.
19. Page RS. Managing chondral lesions of the glenohumeral joint. Int J Shoulder Surg. 2008 Oct;2(4):77-8.
20. Kenneth A. Egol, Kenneth J. Koval, Joseph D. Zuckerman. Handbook of fracture, 5thedition. WoltersKluwer-Health. 2015.
21. Bucholz RW, Heckman JD, Court-Brown CM,Tornetta P III, eds. Rock-wood and Green's fractures in adults, 7th ed. Philadelphia:Lippincott Williams & Wilkins 2010:1210-1244.
22. Blain TA, Bigliani LU, Levine WN. Rockwwod, Matsen, Wirth&Lippitt. The Shoulder, 3rd ed, Elsevier, 2010.
23. Molina Martínez M, Delgado Martínez AD, Pérez Caballer A. Fracturas de la clavícula y escapula.Cirugía ortopédica y traumatología. 2ª ed. Madrid: Panamericana; 2012.
24. Denard PJ, Wirth MA, Orfaly RM. Management of glenohumeral arthritis in the young adult. J Bone Joint Surg Am. 2011 May 4;93(9):885-92.
25. Casagrande D, Stains JP, Murthi AM. Identification of shoulder osteoarthritis biomarkers: comparison between shoulders with and without osteoarthritis. J Shoulder Elbow Surg. 2015 Mar;24(3):382-90.

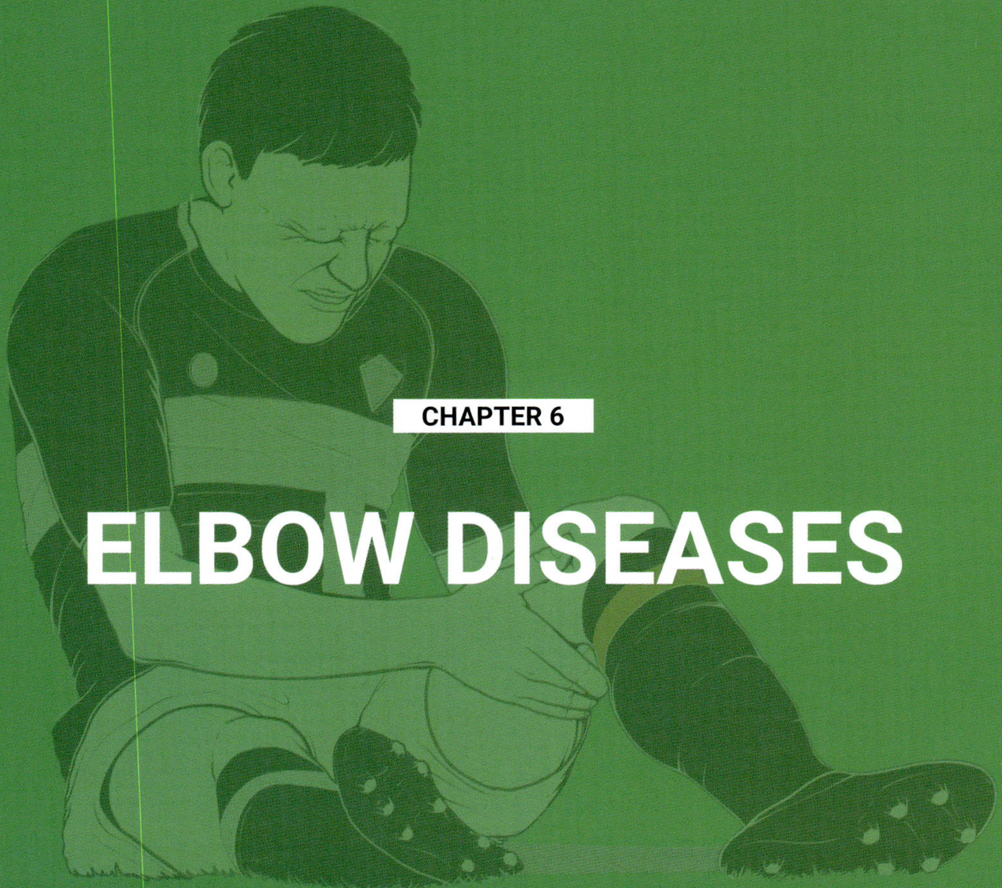

CHAPTER 6

ELBOW DISEASES

Enrico Guerra
Marco Cavallo

Shoulder and elbow Surgery (Director: R. Rotini)
IRCCS Istituto Ortopedico Rizzoli, Bologna, Italy

Introduction

Injuries and disorders of the elbow in athletes are common occurrences, especially among throwing sports. Soccer players often experience these pathologies especially in the role of goalkeeper that must throw and receive high speed balls multiple times every match and is more prone to falls on outstretched hand or directly on the elbow. Other roles are less involved, even if the contact nature of soccer always expose players to fouls play or contrasts.

Common injuries affecting soccer athletes include ulnar collateral ligament injuries, ulnar neuritis, capitellar osteochondritis dissecans, valgus extension overload with posterior olecranon impingement, olecranon stress fracture, and loose bodies, along with fractures to all the bony structures around the elbow.

For the relevance that upper limbs have in different roles, goalkeepers often experience all the “non severe” pathologies like neuritis, tendonitis or instability that are evident in a role that requires the use of upper limbs, while other players usually experience severe injuries like elbow fractures or dislocations [1].

In this chapter the main pathologies suffered by soccer players will be discussed.

Neuritis/neural impingement

Due to its anatomic conformation, the elbow is a region where in a small place three main nerves are close to bones, tendons, and ligaments: ulnar nerve, median nerve, and radial nerve. These structures can be compressed for different causes, and being stretched during elbow movements cause pain and other specific nerve compression symptoms. Systemic conditions like diabetes or hypotiroidism can increase the incidence of the nerve entrapment.

Ulnar nerve

This structure stands in the cubital tunnel in the postero-medial region of the elbow, where it can be palpated through the skin. The cubital tunnel is formed by a floor made by the medial collateral ligament and the humerus-ulnar joint, the roof is formed proximally by the Osbourn ligament (which stands between olecranon and medial epicondyle) and distally by the aponeurosis of the flexor ulnaris carpi.

The causes of ulnar nerve compression in soccer players may occur for a number of reasons and generally affect goalkeepers: traction from valgus stress, direct compression, presence of osteophyte, flexor muscle hypertrophy, or friction from a subluxing or dislocating nerve up to a snapping triceps syndrome. Athletes usually report numbness in 4th and 5th fingers during or after throwing, even if in some case only medial side discomfort is complained. The symptoms generally worsen with elbow flexion, and in the last phases it is possible to see ipotenar atrophy, lumbrical muscles, and claw hand. Tinel test is usually positive for pain.

During clinical examination elbow stability should be carefully evaluated, since valgus laxity can stress the medial structures and cause the symptoms. Diagnosis is generally clinical, to be confirmed with electromyography.

Nonsurgical treatment includes rest, NSAIDs, physycal therapy, and progressive return to sports activities. Nonoperative treatment usually allows 60% to return to sport at the previous level after 2 to 4 months.

In case of failure of conservative treatment, surgical management must be considered. This consists in ulnar nerve neurolysis that can be sufficient in case of nerve compression with preserved stability. Otherwise, the subcutaneous or submuscular anterior nerve transposition must be performed. Care must be given to perform a complete decompression proximally (intermuscular septum) and distally (flexor ulnaris carpi) in order to prevent symptoms recurrence.
The "snapping triceps" is a particular cause of ulnar nerve compression. The patient complains about a "snap" sensation during flexion from extension position. The snap is due to an hypertrophic distal medial triceps together with a congenital instability of the nerve. The recurrence of the dislocation of the nerve can induce the neuritis till the impairment of the conduction and sequent palsy. The click is easily found at palpation (many time the examiner feels two different snaps at different degree of flexion, the first is the nerve at 90°, the second is the medial triceps arond 100-110°). In these cases the simple nerve decompression is not enough, the nerve anteposition is to be performed together with a distal medial triceps plasty.

Median nerve

The entrapment of this nerve is an uncommon condition and it's related to instability or asimmetric joint load (especially in throwing athletes). A particular and slightly more frequent condition is the pronator teres syndrome (PTS), occurring at the level of proximal forearm.
In the early stages the patient reports non specific pain and numbness at the first three fingers of the hand and in the lateral region of forearm. In the later stages atrophy of the muscles innervated by the median nerve is evident: pronator teres (not involved in the pronator teres syndrome), flexor pollicis lungus, flexor digitorum lungus, and the pronator quadratus muscle.
The cause can be congenital: proximally to the joint the nerve can be entrapped below the Struthers arcade. At the joint level an hypertrophic lacertus fibrosus can be the cause of the entrapment. Distally to the joint the pronator teres can compress the nerve, leading to the interosseous nerve paralysis (motor branches that lead to only motor symptoms and slight pain).
Acquired aetiologies involve acute or chronic traumatisms that can lead to heterotopic ossifications or an hypertrophic callous that can be the cause of conflict with the nerve, usually with an association of ulnar nerve disorders. Elbow instability might induce fibrosis proximally to the pronator canal causing compression.
The diagnosis is made with the use of the electromyography that can differentiate between a nerve compression to the elbow or proximal problem like radiculopathy C5-C6 or a syringomyelia.
The treatment is generally surgical and consists in a neurolysis with the dissection of the structure causing compression, from proximal to distal following the nerve.

Radial nerve

The radial nerve crosses the antero-lateral compartment of the elbow with a direction from posterior to anterior, dividing it about 3 or 4 cm distally to the radial head, giving origin to the posterior interosseous nerve (only motor branch) that passes under the Frohse arch.
The most frequent zone of entrapment is the Frohse arc that stands between the superficial and the deep head of the supinator muscle.
Clinical presentation: the patient complains a partial or complete deficit of the extensor digitorum and the extensor pollicis longus and brevis. The beginning is typically acute with or without pain association. Wrist extension is conserved due to some collaterals from the main trunk of the radial nerve.
Aetiology is usually a congenital compression (fibrosis, vascular loop or thickened Frohse arch), with the onset of symptoms favourite by activities or sports that request repetitive elbow movements typical of goalkeepers. In rare cases the aetiology is acquired, for example post-traumatic fibrosis, post-surgery of the radial capitellum, or tumours (lipomas).
The diagnosis is clinical and it's usually (but not always) confirmed by electromyography. A specific test for this syndrome is pain during pronation-supination against resistance and the treatment is generally surgical release.

Tendinopaties

Lateral and medial epicondilitys

Lateral and medial epicondylitis, also called tennis elbow (lateral epicondylitis) and golfer's elbow (or medial epicondilytis) are pain syndromes generated in most cases by a functional overload of the epicondyloid muscles (lateral muscles that insert on the epicondyle) and of epitrochlear muscles (medial muscles that insert on the epitrochlea. Tendinosis of the elbow most frequently affects the dominant limb and patients between 35 and 50 years, although it is possible to find them in all age groups. The tennis elbow is observed in both men and women in equal measure, while epitrocleitis is more frequent in women.

Their pathogenesis remains unknown but appears to be related to a combination of local tendinopathy associated with impaired nociception and motor impairment.

During the diagnostic phase, it is mandatory to exclude the numerous pathological conditions that could simulate epicondilytis, such as the intra-articular plica, osteochondritis dissecans, radio-capellar arthritis, or posterolateral rotatory instability for example.

Most patients report pain localized to the upper half of the lateral or medial epicondyle. Pain can range from intermittent and low grade to continuous and severe, causing sleep disturbances.

The pain on the lateral epicondyle executing some movements, such as the extension of the wrist and acupressure pain are all diagnostic signs.

At the inspection, in the initial stages, there is no noticeable alteration, while in the later stages a prominence of bone on the lateral epicondyle can be detected.

The range of motion is usually not affected. The movement can be painful in later stages when it is caused by the complete extension of the elbow with the pronated forearm.

The Mills test (passive flexion of the wrist) and the Cotzen test (contrasted active extension of the wrist) are the most specific tests.

In medial epicondylitis, instead, during the objective examination there may be swelling, erythema or heat in the medial region of the elbow.

Pronation or flexion against wrist resistance causes pain and weakness of the affected arm. Range of motion is generally unaffected.

The test for medial epicondylitis is to flex the patient's wrist against resistance while the arm remains in extension and supination.

In most cases, medial and lateral apicondylitis can be diagnosed clinically. However, when clinical symptoms are not well defined imaging must be considered.

Instrumental examinations such as ultrasound, X-rays, CT scans, and MRI may be useful, evaluating case by case, to exclude other problems of the elbow and lead to a possible differential diagnosis.

Epicondylitis and epitrocleitis have a self-limiting course lasting about 12-18 months, although in some patients the symptoms may be persistent and refractory to treatment.

Most of the patients are well managed with conservative treatments and activity modifications. Rest and avoiding sports activity is the first solution to be adopted. Pain medications, NSAIDs, physiotherapy with stretching and specific muscular reinforces are often resolutive.

Laser applications or local injections with steroids, NSAIDs or PRP proved to be effective in cases that do not benefit from standard treatments, even if steroid injections have been proved to cause severe side effects along with no long lasting pain relief.

Specific braces can also help with symptom resolution.

Patients with persistent pain and disability after approximately 6 months of well-executed conservative treatment are candidates for a clinical reassessment and, possibly, surgical treatment. Open, percutaneous, and arthroscopic approaches have been used. The basic principle of surgery involves the debridement of the angio-fibrotic tissue of the extensor radialis brevis carpi (for lateral epicondylitis) or of the flexors (for medial epicondylitis) with or without repair of the affected tendon, in order to create a new well vascolarized and unpainful scar tissue. Unfortunally, the come back rate after surgery is not really high (less than 79%) [1].

Triceps tendonitis

Another common tendon disorder around the elbow in goalkeepers is triceps tendonitis. This is often caused by overuse and repetitive distraction

trauma, causing a prolonged period of pain and possibly resulting in tendon partial or complete rupture.
The assessment of these patients must be accurate: range of motion is usually reduced and the palpation of the triceps tendon insertion can show a defect: these signs indicate triceps tendon disruption. Active elbow extension can be present, but extension against gravity or resistence is painful.
Most of the triceps tendinitis and small partial ruptures in soccer athletes respond to conservative treatment, that includes rest, NSAIDs, physical therapy, and laser application.
In other cases early surgical repair is advised with tendon re-insertion at the olecranon through transosseous sutures or anchors.
Innovative therapies like PRP injections in chronic tendonitis without rupture are still ongoing to prove their efficacy.

Valgus extension overload with posterior olecranon impingement

In throwing athletes the elbow is exposed to valgus stress, lateral compression, and in the final phase of the movement to shearing stress at the posteromedial tip of the olecranon and the olecranon fossa. Repetitive throwing stresses can result in symptomatic chondral lesions, loose bodies, and marginal olecranon osteophytes. These lesion pattern injuries are known as valgus extension overload (VEO) syndrome.
Patients complain pain during the throwing process, especially after ball release and at elbow hyperextension, which might also be limited.
The extension impingement test consists in forcing the patient's elbow into full extension. Generation of pain in postero-medial area is considered positive.
Routine X-rays may detect posteromedial olecranon osteophytes and loose bodies. CT scan is mandatory, being more sensitive to visualize these conditions. MRI is useful to identify concomitant UCL injury or an olecranon stress fracture.
First line treatment consists of rest, NSAIDs, and dedicated physiotherapy.
Operative treatment is performed generally by arthroscopy that allows a better and more complete visualization of the entire articular environment and to perform posteromedial decompression removing osteophytes from olecranon and olecranon fossa. Attention must be performed to not jeopardize elbow stability with over-resection of normal bone.
When medial instability is present, the treatment should consider the medial ligament reconstruction by a tendon graft. The athlete has to be aware of the long rehabilitation required and the quite good results of these technique.

Olecranon stress fractures

Stress fractures are partial or complete fractures of a bone resulting from its inability to resist a stress applied in a repeated manner. The first olecranon stress fracture description belongs to Waris in 1946 that described the lesion of a javelin thrower. Olecranon stress fractures are an uncommon source of elbow pain in athletes, mostly occurring in throwing athletes including baseball players, gymnasts, javelin players, wrestlers, and lifters and rarely affecting soccer playing athletes. The location of the stress fracture can be the olecranon tip or the mid-articular portion; usually, these fractures show a nondisplaced pattern [2]. The possible cause of olecranon stress fracture may be the result of intrinsic forces from the muscle contraction during the terminal phase of throwing and impingement of the olecranon against the medial wall of the olecranon fossa, often according to VEO mechanism.
The treatment is generally treated conservatively avoiding sports activities. In high level goalkeepers surgical stabilization with compression screw or tension band can be performed to allow early sport resuming.

Bursitis and inflammations

Bursae are anatomical structures with a vesicular shape covered in the inner layer by a membrane similar to the joint synovium. They are generally located in the proximity of a joint or where the skin, tendons, or muscles move over a bony prominence, with the function of protecting these delicate structures from continuous friction with the bone surfaces. However, bursae can also be found between two muscular planes [3].
Inflammation of bursae is named bursitis, and can

be divided into inflammatory and hemorrhagic.

Inflammatory bursitis

This type of bursitis has triggering causes:

- repeated mechanical stress due to friction or rubbing;
- bacterial or viral infections (septic bursitis);
- systemic diseases such as gout, in which a deposit of uric acid occurs.

Hemorrhagic bursitis

In this case the triggering cause is represented by a trauma that determines the rupture of blood vessels with consequent blood extravasation inside the bursa.

Symptoms are mainly local swelling and redness of the skin, pain, functional limitation, fever (in the case of infections, hematomas; in the case of post-traumatic bursitis, bruises).

Diagnosis

The diagnosis of bursitis is, in most cases, clinical. It is however advised to investigate further in order to detect associated lesions.

- X-rays, to verify or exclude the presence of fractures or alterations of other nature at bone level like olecranon spurs.
- Ultrasound, of fundamental importance to confirm the nature and content of the bursa, as well as to evaluate the involvement of other adjacent structures affected by inflammation.
- MRI, in exceptional cases where previous examinations have not been able to clarify.
- Blood tests and possibly synovial fluid analysis, to clarify the cause of bursitis, liquid composition and the presence of any pathogens responsible for the infection.

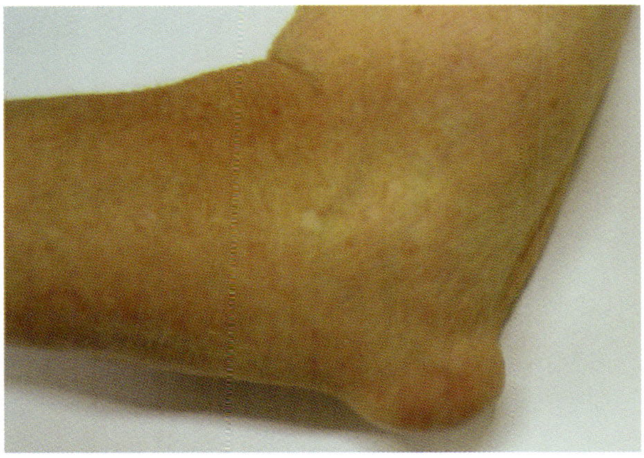

Figure 1 - Clinical presentation of bursitis of olecranon

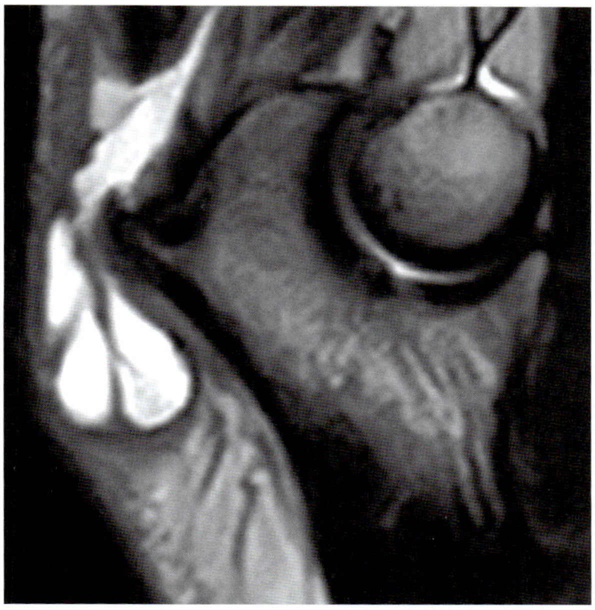

Figure 2 - MRI image of an aseptic bursitis of the olecranon: the fluid is evident between subcutaneous tissue and the deeper tissues, along with an olecranic spur that, in this case, is the cause of the recurrent bursitis

Two elbow bursitis are common: olecranon bursitis and bicipital bursitis.

The olecranon bursitis is easy to diagnose because the olecranon bursa is interposed in the thin area between the bony insertion of the triceps tendon and the skin (fig. 1). The symptomatology is mostly expressed in the presence of a round skin swelling. Usually caused by repeated micro-traumas, it is also frequent to find post-traumatic hemorrhagic bursitis, in these cases also associated with bruises. Sometimes bursitis is caused by a spur of the olecranon (fig. 2).

The acute treatment can be conservative with ice and application of compression bandage or, in the case of large swellings or bleeding, it is possible to proceed to aspirate the liquid contained inside the bag, with eventual steroid injection and subsequently applying a compression bandage.

Only in cases of recurrence and chronicity a real surgery should be carried out with bursa removal and excision.

On the other side, biceps bursitis is difficult to diagnose clinically. This bursa is located just below

the insertion of the distal biceps tendon, between it and the bone surface of the proximal radius. Therefore, the diagnosis is mostly performed by ultrasound or magnetic resonance.
In these patients the main symptom is represented by pain in the anterior cubital area which is exacerbated in the supination maneuvers and flexion against elbow resistance.
Management is mostly conservative with rest and NSAIDs. Surgical procedure of bursectomy is performed in exceptional cases.

Osteochondral lesions
Osteochondritis dissecans (OCD) of the elbow is a disabling condition affecting mostly young patients practicing sports activities. OCD usually affects the elbow at the level of capitulum humeri or, less frequently, the radial head. As all the osteochondral lesions, they mainly recognize a vascular deficiency as aetiology, made clinically relevant by traumas or microtrauma. It is well known that young gymnasts, waterpolo players or young football players often falling onto the upper limb are mainly affected.
This issue is widely treated in a dedicated chapter.

Loose bodies
Loose bodies in the elbow joint usually cause elbow pain and locking. These symptoms are caused by little pieces made of cartilage or bone, becoming trapped between the joint surfaces during the elbow movement. Most of the times the origin of these fragments is a dislocated osteochondral lesion (osteochondritis dissecans) or a broken spur in osteoarthritic environment.
The better diagnostic tool is represented by CT scan or MRI, and the treatment usually consists in arthroscopic removal of the loose body (fig. 3).
The return to sports activity is fast, unless other procedures need to be performed on the elbow during the surgery.

Instability
Elbow instability is a common disorder affecting sports people, among them soccer players. The complexity of the elbow anatomy and biomechanics and the difficulty in the diagnosis are the main causes of the unsatisfactory results in treating these problems. The new approach is to consider instability as a wide spectrum of different forms, ranging from acute forms healing in few days to extremely disabling conditions with challenging management. The aetiology is mainly post traumatic: dislocations or fracture-dislocations, with an incidence of simple elbow dislocations around 7 cases per 100,000 patients per year and that about one quarter associated with elbow fractures.

Classification
The classification of instabilities has a long history. Being a wide spectrum, it was not simple to define a classification able to take into consideration all the different forms of this problem (many attempts can be easily found in literature, with more o less success). Recently a task force of the Italian Shoulder and Elbow Society (SICSeG) developed an innovative classification system able to include all the forms of instability, in order to better address the treatment and prognosis (fig. 4).
The main parameters considered in this classification are:
- The stabilizers involved. Simple (only sof tissues damaged) or complex forms (bone and soft tissue damaged);
- Timing. Acute, chronic recurrent (i.e. elbow that

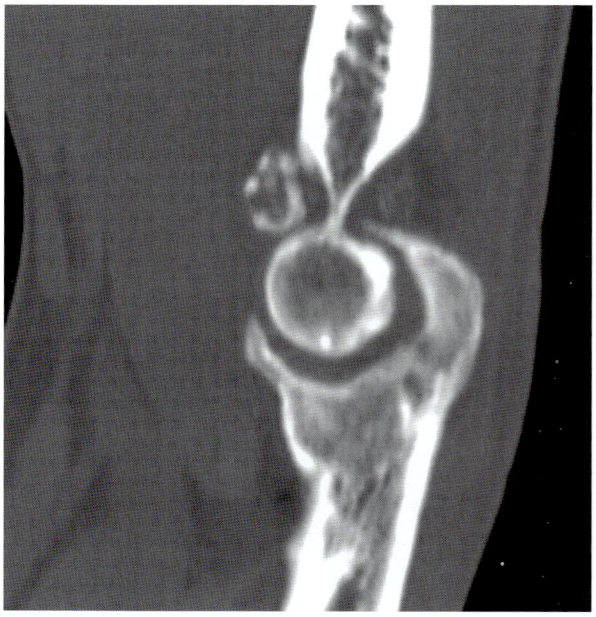

Figure 3 - CT image of a loose body in the coronoid fossa. The initial arthritic changes of the ulno-humeral joint are evident

INSTABILITY TIMING → / INVOLVED STRUCTURES ↓	ACUTE	CHRONIC RECURRENT (dynamic dislocation)	CHRONIC PERSISTENT (static dislocation)
SIMPLE SOFT TISSUE	DISLOCATION WITHOUT FRACTURES	- Post Traumatic - Over-use - Congenital Hyperlaxity - Iatrogenic *ex:* Following epicondiylitis surgery	- Post Traumatic - Neglected - Failed treatment
COMPLEX SOFT TISSUE + BONE STABILIZERS	FRACTURE OF RADIAL HEAD CORONOID OLECRANON DISTAL HUMERUS *associated with:* + LCL +\- MCL lesion	- Post Traumatic *ex:* LCL lenghtening caused by: - Cubitus varus - Coronoid bone loss - Iatrogenic *ex:* Following R.H. Excision - Congenital Dysplasia	- Post Traumatic - Neglected - Failed treatment - Congenital Dysplasia

SICSeG

Figure 4 - Omni comprehensive classification of elbow instability

passes from reduced to dislocated with movements or examination) or chronic persistent (persistent state of dislocation);

- The extent of dislocation. Subluxation or dislocation;
- Aetiology (trauma, micro-trauma, congenital, inflammatory disease, neurological disease, sequelae of infection);
- The joints involved. Humero-ulnar, humero-radial, or proximal radio-ulnar joint;
- Mechanism of dislocation/instability. Posterolateral rotatory instability (PLRI), posteromedial rotatory instability (PMRI), valgus, varus or direct axial load [4].

Considering the first two parameters, stabilizers involved and timing, it is possible to form six main groups [5]:

1. A - acute;
2. A - recurrent;
3. A - persistent;
4. B - acute;
5. B - recurrent;
6. B - persistent.

Within each group, we can divide instability according to aetiology, extent of dislocation (full dislocation or subluxation) and joints involved. For instability with traumatic or micro-traumatic origin, the lesion mechanism can be described.

Elbow acute instabilities are the most common types, all post traumatic in origin. More than 90% of elbows with chronic instability are post-traumatic and are usually the result of a lack of healing of an acute lesion, usually for a failure of the attempted treatments.

The more rare neglected forms are caused by a misdiagnosis or the decision not to treat the dislocation. Besides traumatic forms, other causes of chronic instability, recurrent and persistent, are repeated stress, typical of professional overhead throwing athletes, the sequelae of pediatric trauma (cubitus varus, deficit of coronoid), rare cases due to congenital anomalies (hyperlaxity or congenital deformity), sequelae of infection or rheumatic diseases, which lead to a progressive destruction of the joints, or neurological diseases (spasticity).

Treatment or prognosis of these conditions are extremely different and need to be focused on the broken stabilizer of the elbow.

Most of the acute simple dislocations are conservatively treated with splint and early motion, with surgery indicated in 10% of the cases (when a clear instability is present after reduction or the elbow is still dislocated in cast) with medial collateral ligament and lateral collateral ligament repair. Acute complex dislocations are often addressed

to surgery, because the main bony stabilizers are damaged. In particular the terrible triad of the elbow (association of radial head fracture, coronoid fracture and elbow dislocation) is an entyty with bad prognosis if misdiagnosed, that require proper early treatment, usually consisting in radial head fixation or replacement, collateral ligament reconstruction, and coronoid fixation.
In chronic recurrent and chronic persistent simple dislocation it is usually not possible to maintain the reduction without ligament repair or reconstruction. Especially in persistent form, the treatment involves extended arthrolysis and repair of the collateral ligaments combined or not with the use of an external fixator.
In our experience, the reconstruction of the ligaments with autologous or homologous grafts is usually required after 3 months or more of dislocation, when the local tissues are not valid enough to perform a ligament repair.

Chronic recurrent and chronic persistent complex dislocation

In this type of patients, stiffness and instability coexist and the challenge for the surgeon is to treat both situations. The treatment consists in extensive arthrolysis, radial head replacement, coronoid reconstruction usually with allograft, collateral ligaments reconstruction (generally with grafts) and if necessary an external fixator for addictional joint stabilization for the first month. In case of severe and debilitating joint damage, a total elbow replacement can be considered a surgical option, but only in old and low-demand patients.

Fractures

Although soccer is not a high demanding sport for upper limbs, it is a contact sport with the risk of falling on upper limb. Sprain or direct contact trauma (especially for goalkeeper) make the risk of elbow fracture quite elevated. Depending on the type of trauma, there can be several places that can be fractured in the elbow [6].

Diagnosis

The diagnosis of fracture involving the elbow requires a multidisciplinary approach.
The clinical presentation can move from extreme functional impairment, pain, swelling, axial deviation, loss of function and normal anatomy to tenderness and slight functional impairment, for example in cases of undisplaced radial head fractures. For this reason it is important to conduct a dedicated clinical examination, conventional X-rays and CT scan are mandatory to understand the specific fracture pattern and the bony stabilizer of the elbow involved in the lesion.
With the examination it is also important to evaluate the neurologic and vascular status, since the noble structures are extremely close to the bones at the elbow level, and it is not so difficult to observe a neuro-vascular concomitant damage, that led the injury to an emergency level.

Distal humerus

Fractures involving the distal humerus often require surgery, since the intrinsic stability of most of them is low and most of the time they are displaced fractures. Despite the improvements in the surgical treatment, it still remains a demanding procedure.

Classification

The most widely used classification was proposed by Sanchez-Sotelo, distinguishing four major patterns for distal humerus fractures: each type presents specific peculiarity for surgical approach (fixation technique).
Four major patterns for distal humerus fractures: (1) supra-intercondylar column fracture, (2) capitellar and trochlear fractures, (3) low transcondylar fracture, (4) partial articular fracture (fig. 5).
1. Supra-intercondylar/column fracture: the fracture involves the whole distal humerus, going through the columns and the articular surfaces, presenting different degrees of severity, based on the comminution at the articular and supracondylar level.
2. Capitellar and trochlear fractures: the fracture damages the articular surface of the distal humerus on the frontal plane. The fracture runs from a single big fragment to a complete destruction of the troclea.
3. Low transcondylar fractures, extra-articular fracture, exiting through or below the lateral epi-

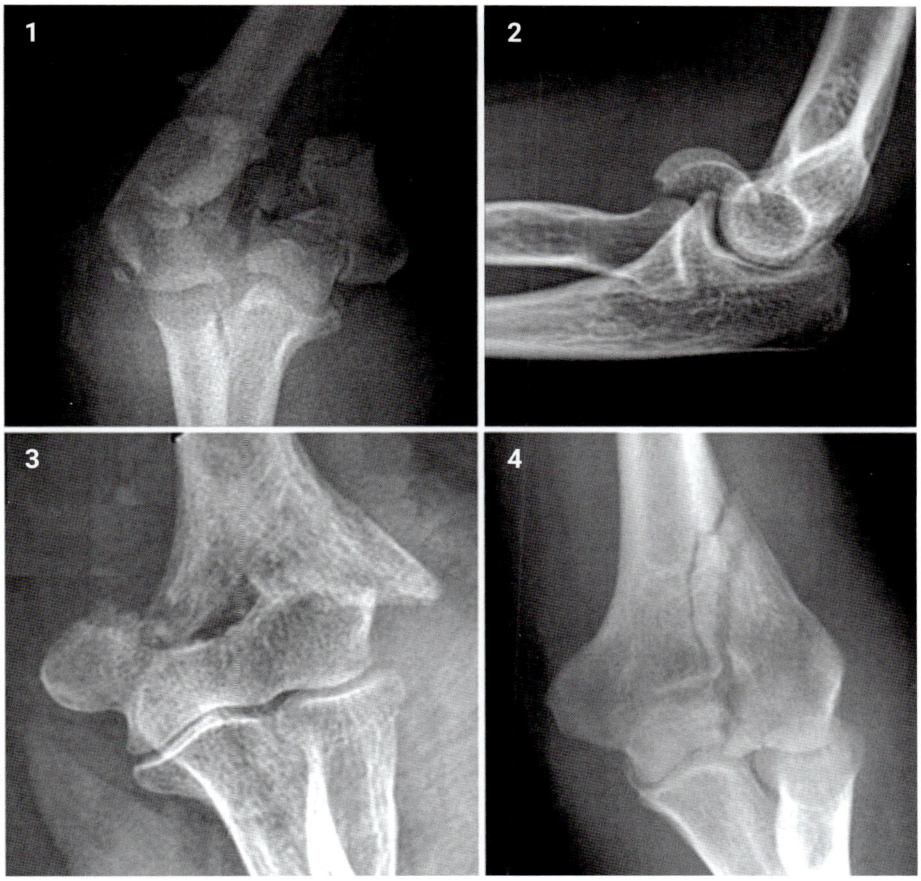

Figure 5 - Sanchez-Sotelo classification of fractures involving distal humerus:
1) Supra-intercondylar column fracture
2) Capitellar and trochlear fractures
3) Low transcondylar fracture
4) Partial articular fracture

condyle and at the level of or just above the medial epicondyle: these fractures, typical in elderly female patients, present difficulties in fixation, especially if distal or marked osteoporosis.
4. Partial articular fracture: "uni-columnar" involves a large portion of the articular surface and its adjacent column, usually in a single piece.
Routine use of a double-pre-contoured plating technique: these plates guide the anatomical reduction and allow a more stable fixation, optimizing the number and the direction of the screws in the distal fragments. The plates can be used at 90° or parallel in order to obtain the better reduction and fixation depending on the fracture pattern (fig. 6) [7, 8].

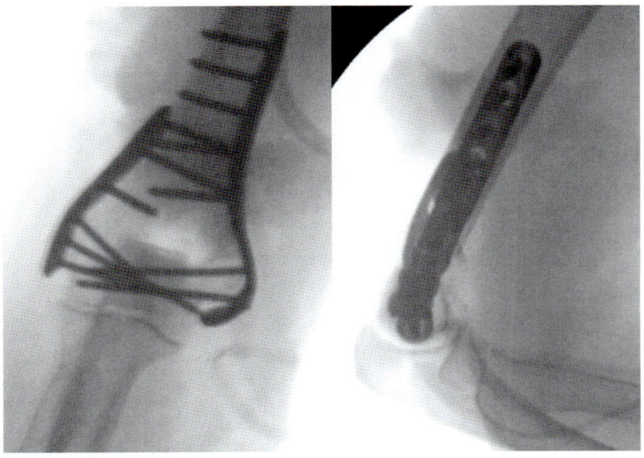

Figure 6 - Post-operative control of a distal humeral fracture treated with double plating parallel technique

Return to sports activity requires an intense rehabilitation programme, nowdays the hydrokinesis teraphy is widely associated to the normal reabilitation program hoping in a faster recovery of range of motion. Soccer is postponed until full bony healing is reached, usually at 3-5 months after surgery.

Capitellar and trochlear fractures

Capitellar and trochlear fractures are infrequent partial articular fractures of the distal humerus. The difficulties encountered in these rare types of fracture are that small and often impacted articular fragments have to be addressed through different approaches and fixed with small countersunk screws beneath the joint surface.
Several classifications have been proposed over time, and nowdays the most used is the one pro-

posed by Dubberley et al. in 2006, with the name of "capitellar and trochlea fractures". This system identifies as prognostic factors the extension of the fracture on the coronal plane and the presence of fragmentation and of posterior comminution (fig. 7).

In these cases misdiagnosis is easy on standard X-ray, so in any doubtful case CT scan is mandatory to detect these lesions and to allow a correct preoperative planning.

Several methods have been described for the treatment of capitellum and trochlea fractures, including conservative treatment, simple excision, open reduction and internal fixation, arthroscopic reduction and internal fixation (each treatment related to the fracture patter). Nowadays it is well known that conservative treatment of displaced capitellar and trochlear fracture leads invariably to poor results and it should be considered only in selected cases [9].

Complications

Stiffness, post-traumatic arthritis, malunion, nonunion, infection, and ulnar nerve neuropathy are the most common complications.

Radial head

Radial head fractures are common occurrences in contact sports players, accounting for one third of all fractures of the elbow. Usually these fractures are caused by a fall on the outstretched arm with the elbow in pronation and slight flexion. The most used classification was introduced by Mason, identifying three main patterns: a type 1 fracture is a nondisplaced fracture, a type 2 fracture is a displaced fracture, and a type 3 fracture is a comminuted fracture. A fourth type was successively added, describing a radial head fracture with associated elbow dislocation (fig. 8).

The radial head is considered a secondary stabilizer of the elbow; however, in presence of lesion

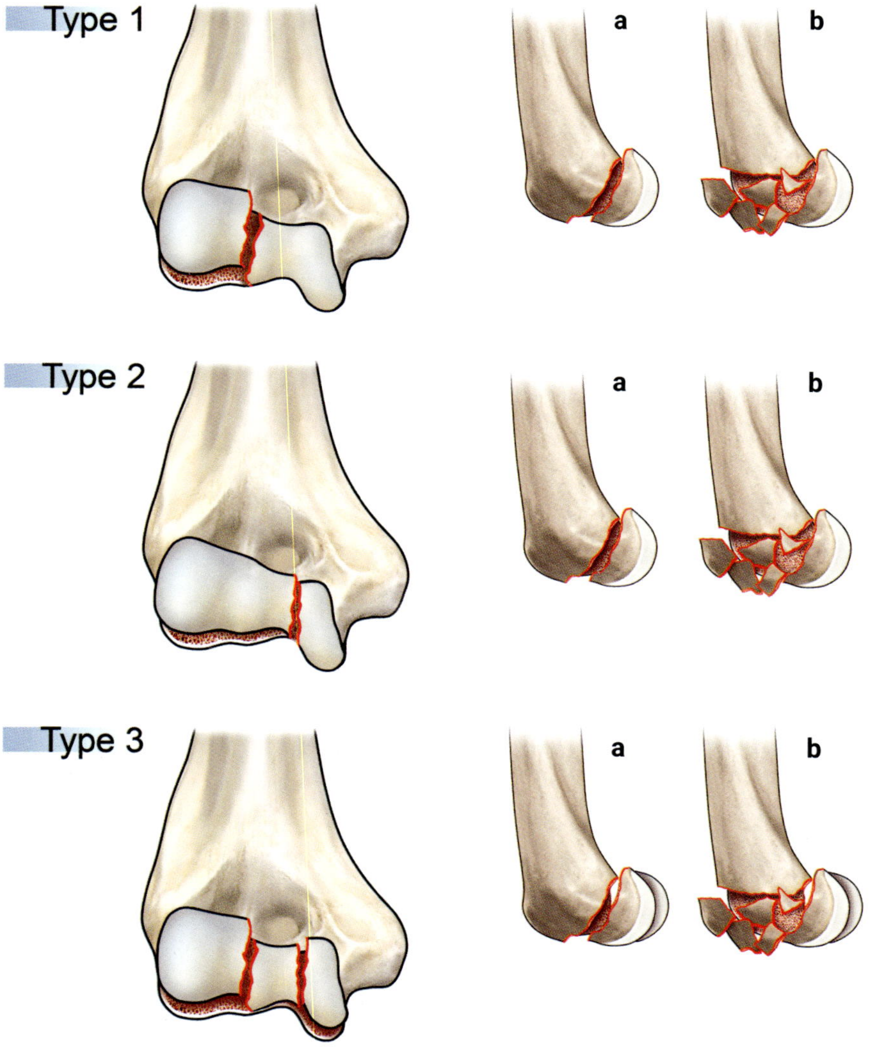

Figure 7 - Dubberley classification of shear fractures

of the primary stabilizers (coronoid, olecranon, medial collateral ligament, lateral collateral ligament) and/or impaired longitudinal forearm stability (lesion of the interosseous membrane), its role becomes primary for the stability of the elbow and forearm. In such situations and in presence of a non-fixable radial head fracture, the use of the prosthesis is indicated, due to the high risk of instability with the simple excision of the radial head, in order to prevent the onset of severe horizontal and longitudinal instability (Essex-Lopresti Syndrome), which is difficult, and sometimes impossible, to be resolved with a second surgical time.

In most of the cases the treatment of simple resection of the radial head, widely used in the past, is no longer acceptable, due to the subsequent possible instability of the elbow and wrist. Therefore, treatment options in Mason 3 and 4 fractures fall on osteosynthesis (mini-screws and pre contoured plates) or prosthetic replacement. Fixation is preferable in the presence of fracture with no more than three rhymes and with fragments of good mechanical consistency and without signs of deformation or crushing (video 1).

Radial head prosthesis is preferred when the fragments present bone loss or comminution, when there is a comminution of the neck and when there are more than three fragments (in other words when anything less is possible).

VIDEO 1

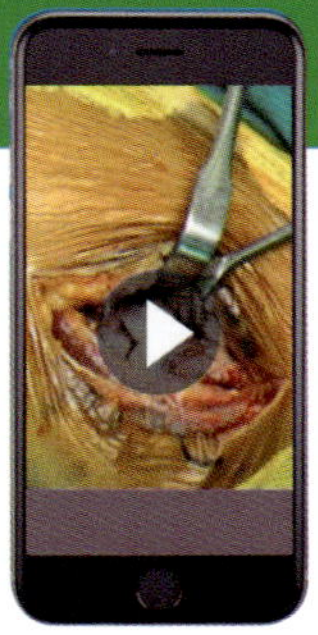

The video shows a comminuted radial head fracture in a young patient. The fragments still have the periosteum preserved, so the decision was to try a fixation with headless screws and lateral collateral ligament repair

Associated lesions are reported in 35% of the cases, involving:

- lateral collateral ligament (LCL) (80%);
- medial collateral ligament (MCL);
- a combination of MCL and LCL;
- forearm longitudinal instability (Essex-Lopresti injury with distal radioulnar joint (DRUJ) injury and interosseous membrane disruption);

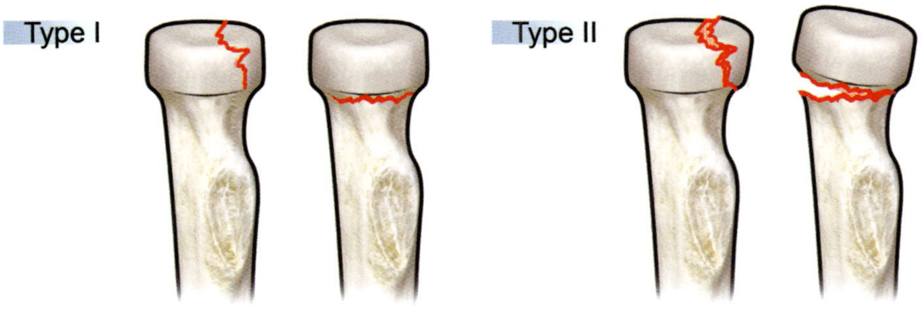

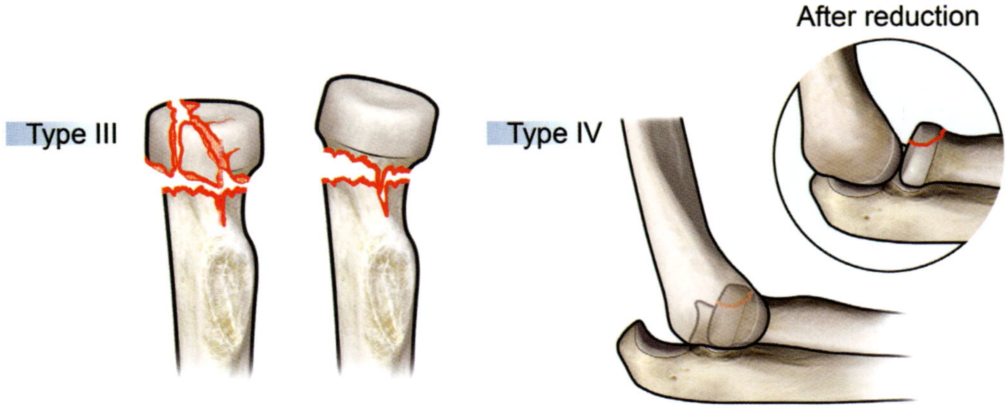

Figure 8 - Mason classification of radial head fractures (Modified by Hotchkiss and Broberg-Morrey)

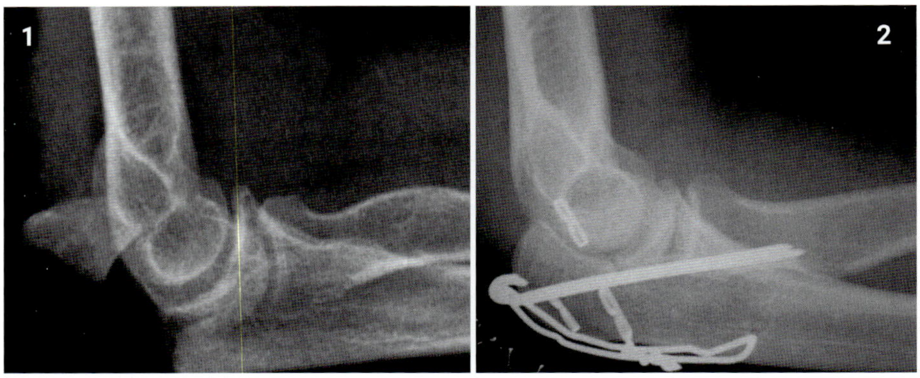

Figure 9 - Lateral X-rays showing transverse olecranon fracture (1) treated with tension band wiring (2)

• other elbow fractures (coronoid fracture or olecranon fracture) elbow dislocation such as terrible triad (elbow dislocation, radial head fracture, coronoid fracture);
• carpal fractures;
• scaphoid fracture.

Olecranon

Fractures involving the olecranon are common occurrences in sports, resulting usually after falls. These fractures can range from simple nondisplaced fractures to complex fracture-dislocations of the elbow. Displaced fractures are almost in all cases addressed to surgical treatment, exception made for old and non compliant people. Especially in soccer players, surgery must be performed early, in order to obtain a fast recovery and return to sports activity. Non displaced fractures in common population are generally treated conservatively, while sometimes in high level soccer players they are addressed to surgery in order to shorten the rehabilitation protocol and the return

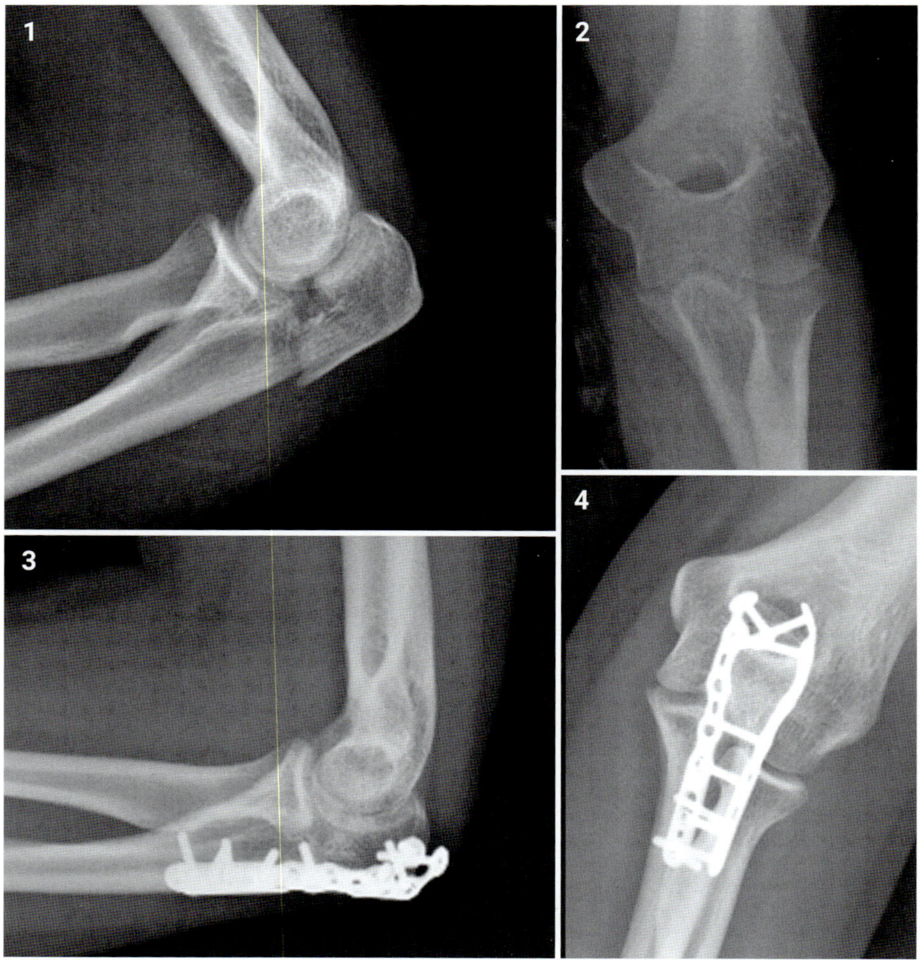

Figure 10 - Complex olecranon fracture (1, 2) treated with double plating and screws (3, 4)

to sports activities. Several treatment options for internal fixation have been reported, including metallic tension-band, plate fixation (with single plate or double plate), intramedullary screw fixation. The type of fracture usually addresses the fixation method: simple transverse fractures are generally treated with tension band wiring (fig. 9), while more complex or comminuted fractures are generally plated (fig. 10).
One of the main goals of the treatment is to obtain a fixation that is stiff enough to allow early mobilization of the elbow, in order to avoid post operative stiffness.

Coronoid

Coronoid fractures of the ulna are quite uncommon, even if often unrecognized. These fractures are often associated with elbow dislocations and constitute a major cause of elbow instability. The coronoid acts as a bony barrier to prevent posterior dislocation, especially with its medial part, named sublime tubercle, which gives the insertion to the medial ulnar collateral ligament. The anterior joint capsule and the brachialis muscle are the other major soft tissues that are inserted in this process. Injured patients often report diffuse swelling, local tenderness and limited range of motion. Conventional X-rays are important, especially to detect elbow dislocation or signs of instability. Some coronoid fractures can be undiagnosed with this exam, so it is mandatory to perform a CT scan with 2D and 3D reconstructions in order to precisely evaluate the fracture pattern and the associated lesions. In particular, the association of coronoid fracture, a radial head fracture, and posterior or posterolateral elbow dislocation is called "terrible triad of the elbow". The correct management of coronoid fractures associated with elbow dislocations is still on the edge.
O'Driscoll et al. described a new classification system involving three fracture types. Type 1 is a tip fracture, type 2 is an anteromedial facet fracture, and type 3 is a fracture through the base.
Undisplaced fractures or tip fractures non associated with dislocations are generally treated con-

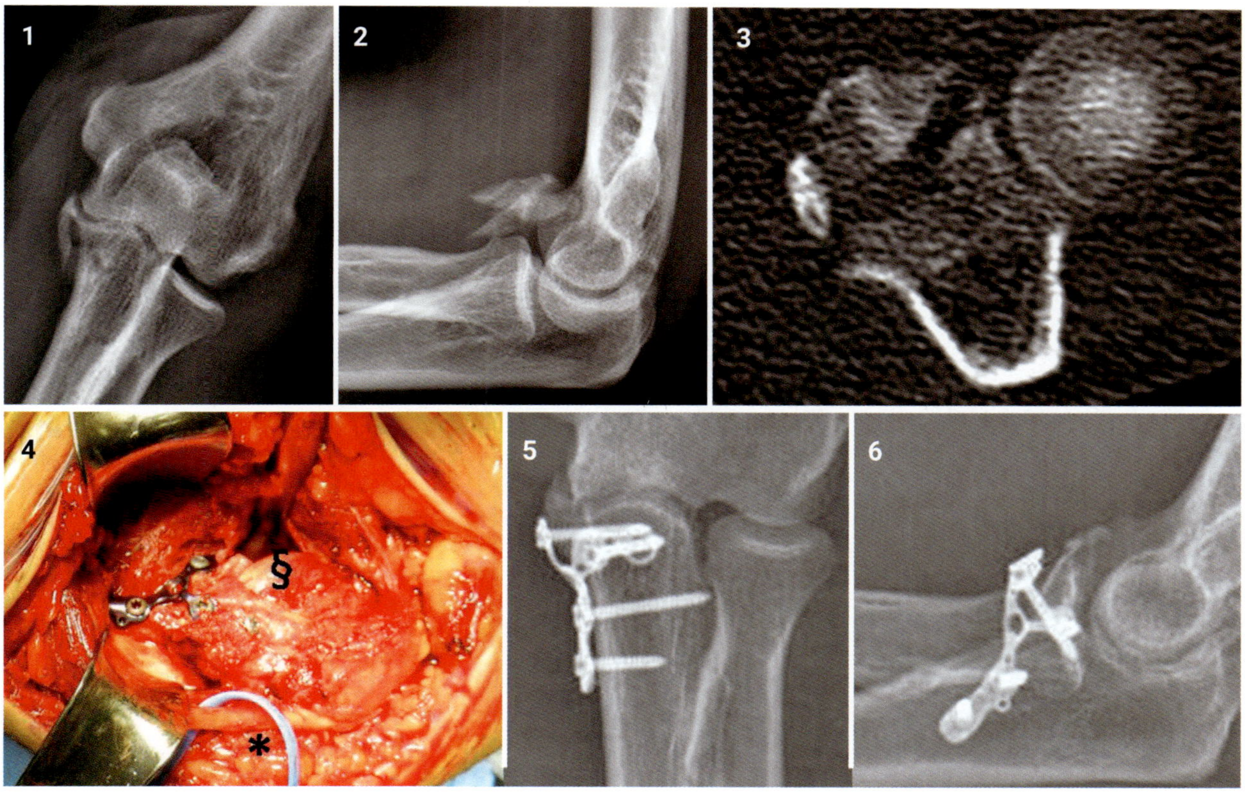

Figure 11 - X-ray (1, 2) and CT scan (3) of antero medial fracture of the coronoid (O'Driscoll type 2). This fracture was treated with plate and screws (4, 5, 6). In figure 4 the symbol § indicates the capitulum humeri and the symbol * the isolated ulnar nerve servatively with splint and early mobilization. Displaced fractures or fractures of the sublime tubercle jeopardizing the elbow stability must be surgically treated with reduction and fixation, which can also be performed by arthroscopy in some isolated single fragment fractures. In case of associated lesions or more complex fractures it must be fixed with conventional surgery with screws, K-wires, osteosutures, or pre countured plates (fig. 11). Attention must be kept to fix all the damaged ligaments, since collateral ligaments, as well as coronoid process, are primary stabilizers of the elbow.

Arthritis

As all the contact sports, soccer is a risk factor for elbow degeneration and arthritis progression. In particular, repetitive falls on outstretched hand, previous elbow fractures or instability are main causes of athritic changes over time. This problem is mainly complained by goalkeeper, since elbow are particurarly stressed in this role.

The most common symptoms of elbow arthritis are diffused pain and loss of range of motion, usually progressive over time. These symptoms can be associated with a "grating" or "locking" sensation in the elbow. The "grating" is due to loss of the normal smooth joint surface, because of cartilage damage. The "locking" can be caused by loose bodies or ostheophytes. In the later stages of osteoarthritis of the elbow nerves can be involved in the process, especially the ulnar nerve (the "funny bone").

Treatment in soccer player is generally conservative, especially in the early phase, with physiotherapy, steroid intra articular injection, or NSAIDs.

When the stiffness is stongly limiting, surgical treatment of bone and soft tissue release can be performed, preferably by the scope. The arthroscopic ostheocapsular arthrolysis is the removal of the loose bodies, osteophytes and contracted capsule in order to restore the joint volume and motion. The same surgery can also be done in open surgery obviously with an higher surgical aggressiveness and paying attention to not compromise the elbow stability. Ulnar nerve release and/or anterior transposition is to be considered every time a good recovey of motion is expected or in case of EMG positive.

Total elbow replacement is to be considered only in older people because of the strong limitation that this surgery carries on, so it is absolutely contraindicated in soccer players. In cases of advanced elbow osteoarthritis, when pain and stiffeness requires an answer, a temporary solution (before an elbow replacement) could be the interposition arthroplasty. This surgery is a really aggressive reshaping of the ulno humeral joint with a complete reléase of the collateral ligaments. A graft is left between the joint surfaces and the stability restored by an external fixator for two months. It goes without saying that these cases have to be really selective.

Bibliography

1. Cain EL, Moroski NM. Elbow Surgery in Athletes. Sports Med Arthrosc Rev. 2018 Dec;26(4):181-184.

2. Nuber GW, Diment MT. Olecranon stress fractures in throwers. A report of two cases and a review of the literature. Clin Orthop. 1992;278:58–61.

3. National Federation of State High School Associations. 2012-2013 High school athletics participation survey. 2013.

4. An K-N, Morrey BF. Biomechanics of the elbow. In: Morrey BF, editor. The elbow and its disorders. Philadelphia: WB Saunders; 1985. p. 43-61.

5. Marinelli A, Guerra E, Rotini R. Elbow instability: are we able to classify it? Review of the literature and proposal of an all-inclusive classification system. Musculoskelet Surg. 2016 Dec;100(Suppl 1):61-71.

6. Sanchez-Sotelo J. Distal humerus fractures. In: Antuna S, Barco R, editors. Chapter 4 Essentials in elbow surgery. London: Springer-Verlag; 2014. p. 47-60.

7. O'Driscoll SW. Optimizing stability in distal humeral fracture fixation. J Shoulder Elb Surg. 2005;14:186S–94S.

8. Marinelli A, Guerra E, Bettelli G, Cavaciocchi M, Rotini R. Surgical approaches based on the fracture patterns. In: Castoldi F, et al., editors. Chapter 24 Simple and complex fractures of the humerus. Italia: Springer-Verlag; 2015. p. 269-77.

9. Marinelli A, Cavallo M, Guerra E, Ritali A, Bettelli G, Rotini R. Does the presence of posterior comminution modify the treatment and prognosis in capitellar and trochlear fractures? Study performed on 45 consecutive patients. Injury. 2018 Nov;49 Suppl 3:S84-S93.

CHAPTER 7

WRIST AND HAND DISEASES

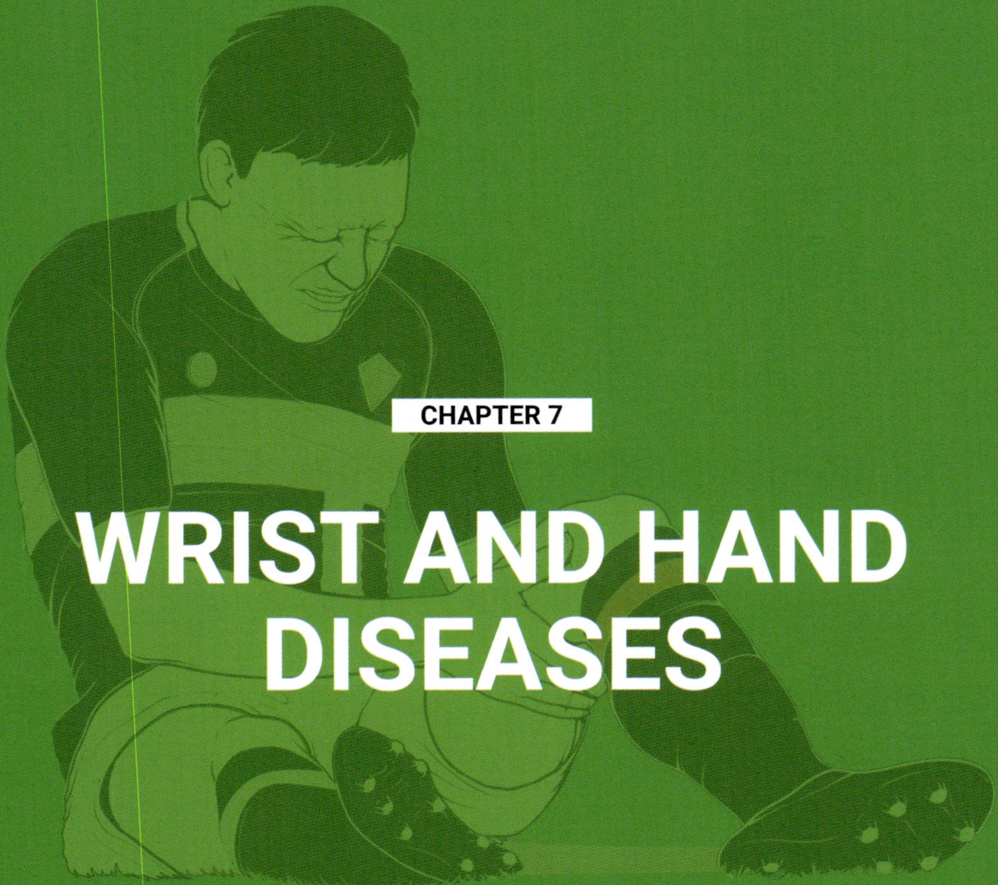

Riccardo Luchetti [1]
Loris Pegoli [2]

[1] Rimini Hand Rehabilitation and Surgery Center, Rimini, Italy

[2] Hand and Microsurgery Service
Humanitas Pio X Clinic, Milan, Italy

Introduction

Wrist and hand injuries in soccer players could seem an unusual reality since football is a sporting activity that takes place with the lower extremities. Upper-extremity injuries accounted for only 2% to 15% of all injuries in all age groups in both men's and women's leagues [1].

However, if you consider the goalkeeper, who uses his hands to parry or intercept a ball, you can understand how these injuries are specific and important in this category of players.

Finally, the soccer players themselves want to take, cling to or block the opponent, so that even occasionally, and not specifically, they can damage their hand or wrist.

In general, it is possible to do a differentiation between the specific injury due to sport and generic injury, but the treatment remains always the same. The most frequent ligament and osteocartilagineous lesions will be first taken into consideration to finish with some special injuries (tendons and nerves).

The description of the types of traumatic injuries will start from the wrist to continue towards the fingers through the hand.

Ligament injuries of the wrist

The most frequent ligament injuries of the wrist are those of the triangular fibrocartilage complex ligament (TFCC) and the scapho-lunate (SL) ligament.

TFCC Injury

The most common traumatic mechanism is the fall on the hyper-extended wrist in pronation or supination [2]. It can frequently be associated with fractures of the distal radius [3, 4] or isolated. Its rupture causes an ulnar pain around the ulna's head and sometime DRUJ instability. The classification of the traumatic lesions of the TFCC is divided into four forms (A, B, C, D), but there are also atypical ones. The various forms can also be associated. If the lesion involves its insertion site to the fovea (B1 proximal or complete in accordance with Atzei's classification) [5], an instability of the distal radio-ulnar joint (DRUJ) will be present. If the lesion is more distal (B1 distal), DRUJ instability will be minimal or absent but the ulnar pain (fig. 1) will be always present overall during prono-supination and the clinical tests.

The injury can be minimal or extensive in relation to the traumatic event. Some forms of damage of the triangular ligament can heal with immobilization, but unfortunately they are almost never recognized and surgical treatment becomes necessary for the persistence of symptoms. In painful forms, clinical evaluation by an hand surgeon and specific assessments are required.

Precise localization of the ulnar pain and the evaluation of the DRUJ stability must be evaluated. The fovea sign, the piano test, and the ballotment test have always to be checked [5].

Among the instrumental examinations, x-ray images may rarely lead to suspect of TFCC ligament damage due to an evident diastasis of the DRUJ (fig. 2). Magnetic resonance imaging (MRI) is the main exam, but it is not always able to define the lesion [6, 7]. Foveal detachment is sought, but it is not always hidden in the proximal or complete B1 forms. A certain degree of alteration of the TFCC tissue ligament signal is almost always present. Type C and D lesions are not well definable.

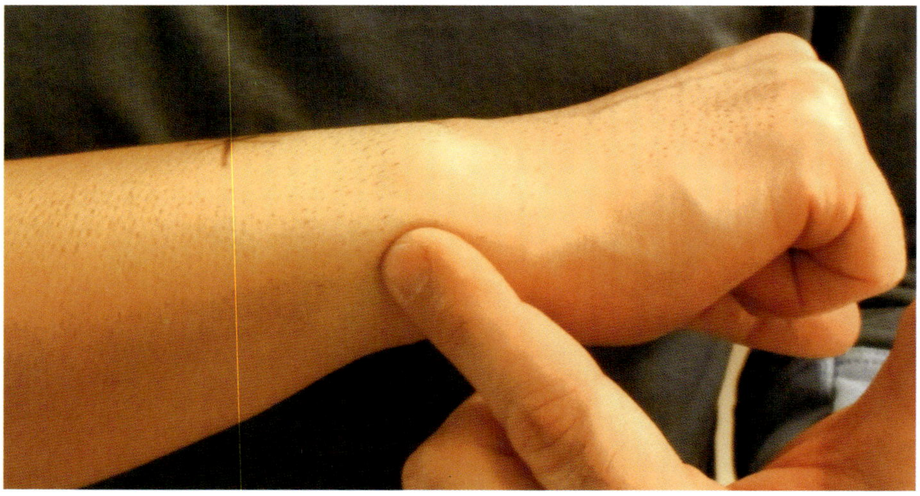

Figure 1 - Soccer player with ulna wrist pain after accidental fall during a soccer match. Index finger of the contralateral hand localizes the site of pain (Ballotment test of the DRUJ was positive)

For this reason, arthroscopy is used to identify and certify the lesions and at the same time it allows specific treatment (fig. 3). Conversion into an open surgery is always possible.
The healing time lasts one month of immobilization and two months of rehabilitation with progressive loading of the wrist (figg. 4, 5). Complete functional recovery will be possible in a period of about 3 months.
The soccer player is allowed to return to training in around two months, but the competition is granted only after the third month. For the goalkeeper the time of return to active sport is more than three months, that is after a complete healing considering an appropriate rehab.

SL ligament injury

The lesions of the SL ligament are the most frequent ligament lesions of the wrist. Hyperextension wrist traumas are the traditional traumatic mechanism [3, 8]. Rarely it occurs with a wrist flexed. The stages of SL ligament injury were classified by Geissler [9] from 1 to 4, while Messina et al. [10, 11] modified the classification by introducing subgroups to better correlate damage with clinical symptoms and choice of treatments. The 4th stage corresponds to the complete injury of the SL ligament with SL joint diastasis (dissociation) and possible rotation of both the scaphoid and the lunate (DISI deformity). This stage is often associated with other ligament injuries (secondary stabilizers), thus explaining the severity of the ligament lesion. The other stages correspond to partial or complete tears in the SL ligament without involving secondary stabilizers. Pain is located in the radial and/or dorsal-radial and/or volar-radial side of the wrist associated with limitation of motility. Frequently, radiographic findings are negative in the 1st, 2nd, and 3rd stage. In the 4th stage, a SL dissociation is appreciated and recalls the ligamentous lesion (fig. 6). Unfortunately, even this level of ligament injury is sometimes missed in the reporting of the x-ray examination.
MRI confirms the SL ligament lesion only in the major stages (4th), but high percent of failures are possible in the minor stages (2nd, 3rd) [12].
In acute cases, the treatment is conservative for the minor stages of SL injury; surgical option is recommended for stages 3 and 4. In the chronic forms, that is in the conditions in which the patient comes to visit for painful wrist after a trauma occurred months before and without improvement of symptoms despite a correct conservative treatment, the treatment is surgical but an arthroscopic investigation is needed to determine the stage of SL ligament damage and give the correct indication.
Dorsal SL ligament capsulodesis [13] is the most frequent type of surgical treatment for 2nd and 3rd stage (figg. 7, 8). Arthroscopic techniques are also available [14]. In the 4th stage the indication is the ligament reconstruction by tendon grafting by open or arthroscopic surgery [15, 16]. The results are better with capsulodesis treatment rather than with reconstruction, but this is valid to prevent a fast progression towards cartilage degeneration (SLAC wrist). The immobilization considers a

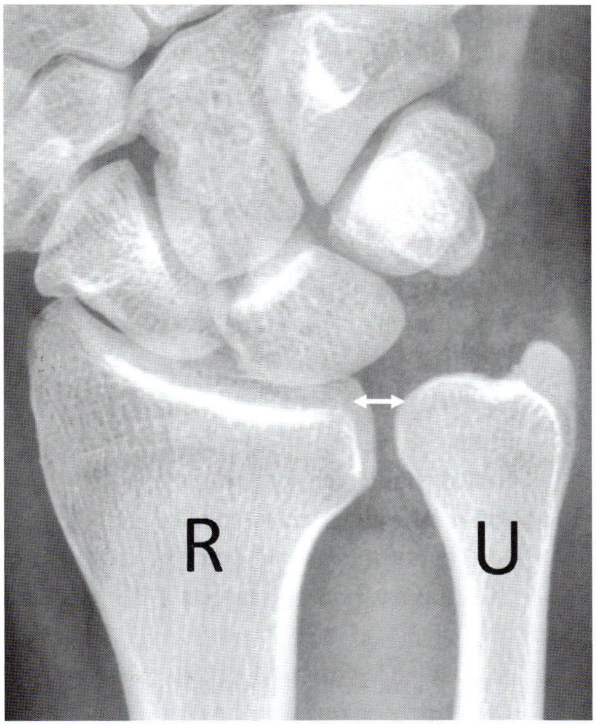

Figure 2 - X-ray image showing the diastasis between the ulna head (U) and the distal radius (R) corresponding to TFCC ligament tear

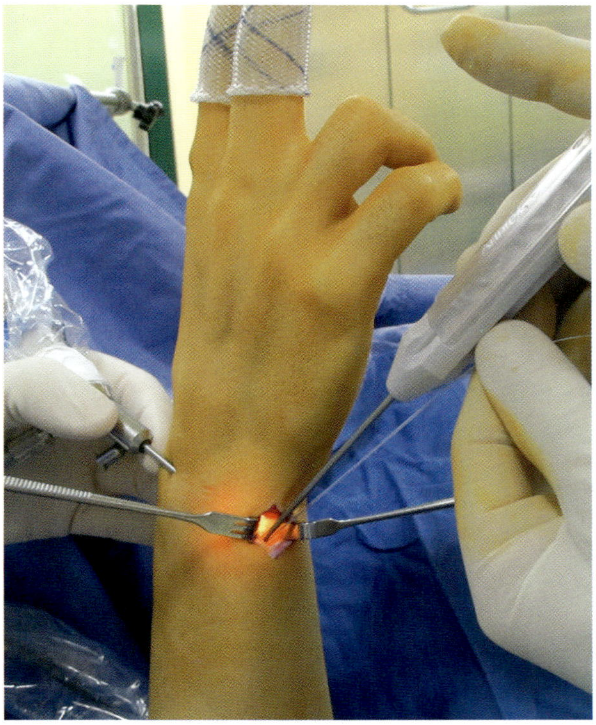

Figure 3 - Intraoperative image showing the technique of arthroscopic foveal TFCC refixation

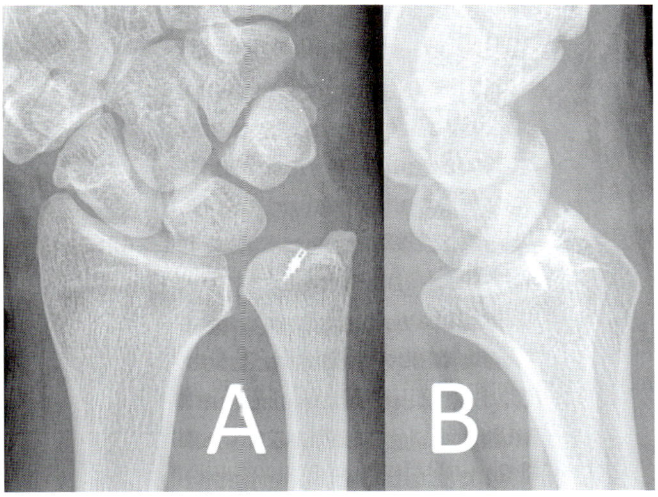

Figure 4 - Postoperative x-rays images (A, B) showing the position of the suture anchor used to refix the TFCC

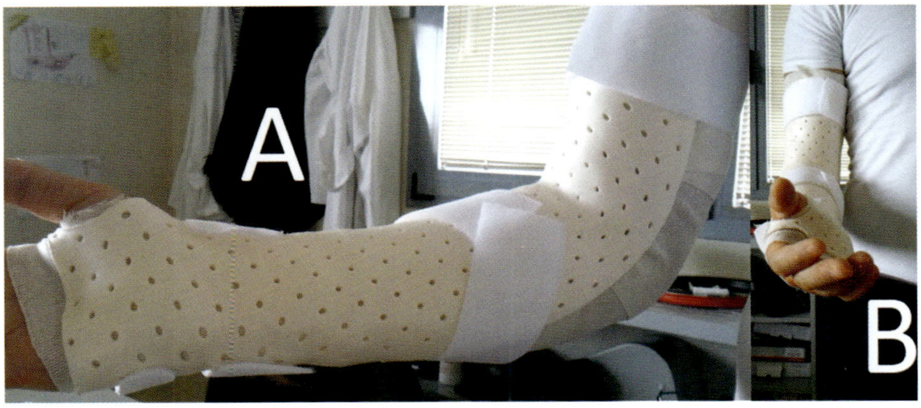

Figure 5 - Postoperative hand to above elbow thermoplastic splint used to protect the wrist from a prono-supination motion.
A) lateral view;
B) antero-posterior (AP) view

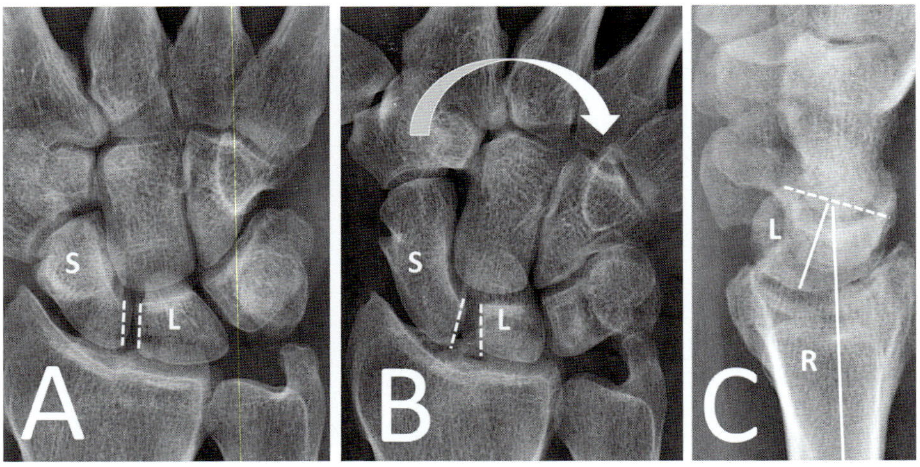

Figure 6 - Soccer player with X-rays images of a right wrist affected by scapho-lunate (SL) ligament injury. A) AP view showing a minimal increase of the space between the lunate (L) and the scaphoid (S); B) AP view of the wrist with ulnar deviation in which the SL joint space shows a clear dissociation; (C) lateral view of the wrist in which the radio-lunate angle was augmented with minimal DISI deformity

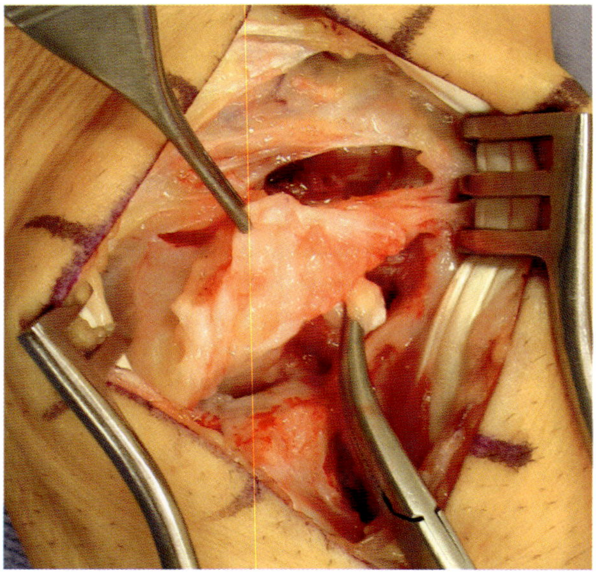

Figure 7 - Intraoperative image showing the technique of dorsal capsulodesis using a ligament flap radially based rotated from the dorsal intercarpal ligament

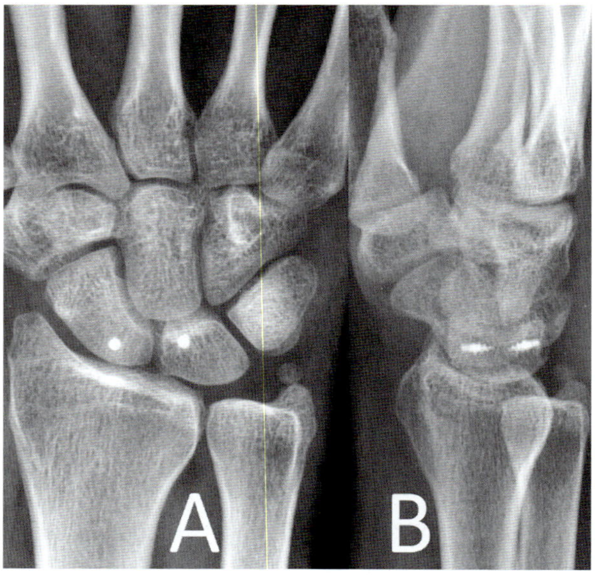

Figure 8 - Postoperative X-rays result of volar and dorsal capsulodesis for stage 3C of SL ligament tear. In the AP (A) and lateral view (B) the suture anchors are well located into the scaphoid (palmar) and lunate (dorsal)

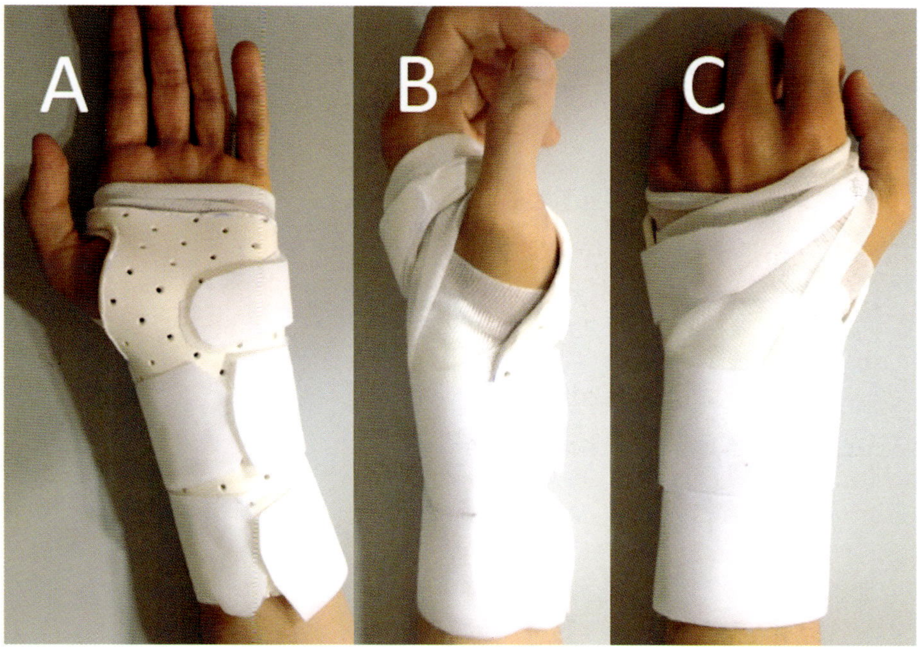

Figure 9 - Typical wrist splint for distal radius fractures (A, B, C) and/or carpal bone injury

wrist splint (fig. 9) for a month followed by specific rehabilitation for two months. The return to sport activity is fast enough for the player with a non-goalkeeper role, even before the third month. In goalkeepers, due to the obvious use of hands in sporting activities, the return to competition must await for a complete functional recovery that takes place in a period of time greater than 3 months.

Fractures

Scaphoid fractures

Scaphoid fractures are the most frequent conditions of carpal bones fractures. Scaphoid fracture is traditionally due to violent wrist hyperextension trauma with overload of the carpal bones which determines the scaphoid fracture. SL ligament injury and distal radius fracture can be associated.
The fracture of the scaphoid can be clearly visible and diagnosed at the first radiographic investigation and then it must be treated by cast or surgically if displaced or unstable. However, surgical treatment has been also proposed for undisplaced fracture. Scaphoid fixation is performed using a percutaneous Herbert screw at the level of the STT joint (fig. 10). Vice versa the proximal pole fracture of the scaphoid is fixed through a dorsal mini-approach. In the sports field the tendency to perform a surgical treatment prevails over the conservative treatment, this in favor of an early return to sport activity. The advantage of surgical treatment in athletes also lies in the lower immobilization of joint structures and early rehabilitation with return to sport. However, one must be careful to identify the associated injuries that must be treated at the same time and sometimes require longer time healing and immobilization. Not recognizing the associated injuries will result in incomplete recovery with secondary damage to the wrist. Arthroscopy of the wrist might be helpful in this situation.
In the presence of suspected scaphoid fracture, x-rays are the first imaging investigations to be performed. If the scaphoid fracture is negative at the first x-ray exam, a second radiographic examination should be requested 7-10 days later. To speed up the times a MRI should be done. CT-scan can also be helpful in identifying the fracture and its typology. In essence, the scaphoid fracture is a condition not always easy to be revealed in emergency. During the assessment period, the wrist must be protected with a simple wrist splint. When a scaphoid fracture is found, the surgical treatment is mandatory in the athletes even for undisplaced fractures. The only non-surgical scaphoid fractures are those with MRI images of "intracortical fractures", that is without interruption of the cortical bone. In these cases, a wrist splint (fig. 11) and biophysical stimulation technique, capacitive and mechanical systems [17] promote bone healing even if in a long time.

Intra-cortical scaphoid fractures should be monitored over time with x-ray and MRI to verify their healing or that they do not turn into clear fractures which will need a surgical treatment.

Distal radial fractures

Distal radius fractures are not frequent in soccer players. X-ray investigation will provide to confirm the fracture. In sport athletes, surgical treatment is preferred to shorten recovery times (fig. 12). However, undisplaced fractures can be treated with a wrist splint and monitored over time by radiography. The displaced and articular, multifragments distal radius fractures need open reduction and internal fixation (ORIF technique) using a volar and/or dorsal plate in relation to the type of fracture (figg. 13, 14) [18, 19, 20, 21, 22].

After surgery the wrist is immobilized for about a month. Specific sport activity will be excluded especially for goalkeepers. The situation becomes more complicated when associated lesions coexist, for example ulna head and ulnar styloid fractures and/or ligament injuries. Often, the associated bone or ligament injuries are underestimated and not treated [23]. Incorrect or incomplete initial treatment, incorrect immobilization, or early mobilization will lead to persistence of wrist pain and subsequent joint disorder. The ulna fractures must be surgically treated just like the distal radius and the same is for the ulna styloid, according with the level of fracture. Ligamentous injuries should be operated at the same time of surgery of the distal radius fracture, while lesser degree of ligament lesions can be treated with correct immobilization. Wrist immobilization (fig. 9) is sufficient for the carpal ligament injuries, but over elbow immobilization (fig. 5) is needed for the TFCC lesion, avoiding the pronosupination. The early mobilization in this situation should be avoided.

Therefore, it is clear that a hand surgeon, specialist in this field, should be contacted in order to treat these fractures in the best way (fig. 15).

Carpal dislocations/fracture dislocation of the carpal bones

It is a very important chapter since it concerns a very delicate and complex anatomical site. The lesser or the major arch of the wrist can be involved producing a different type of lesions [24]. Traditionally fractures of the distal radius and/or carpal bones coexit with ligament injury (fig. 16). This association configures a type of lesion that is called perilunate fracture dislocation of the carpus, because the ligaments involved are all around the lunate. When there is no fracture of any bones of the wrist and the lunate is dislocated, it is called perilunate dis-

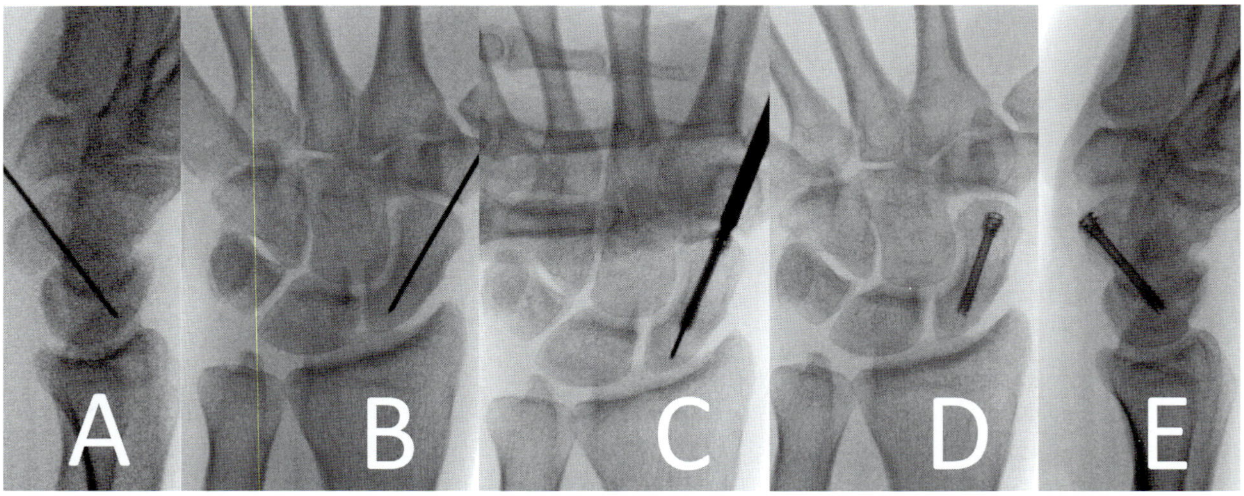

Figure 10 - Goalkeeper 21 female affected by right scaphoid fracture due to a traumatic wrist hyperextension. X-rays view of Herbert screw introduction into the scaphoid for acute fracture without displacement (A-E). A dedicated k-wire was percutaneously introduced first into the scaphoid in a distal to proximal direction under fluoroscopic control (A-B). As the perfect location of the k-wire was defined, a Herbert screw was introduced through the k-wire to fix the scaphoid fracture (C). The k-wire was removed allowing to confirm the correct position of the Herbert screw (D-E)

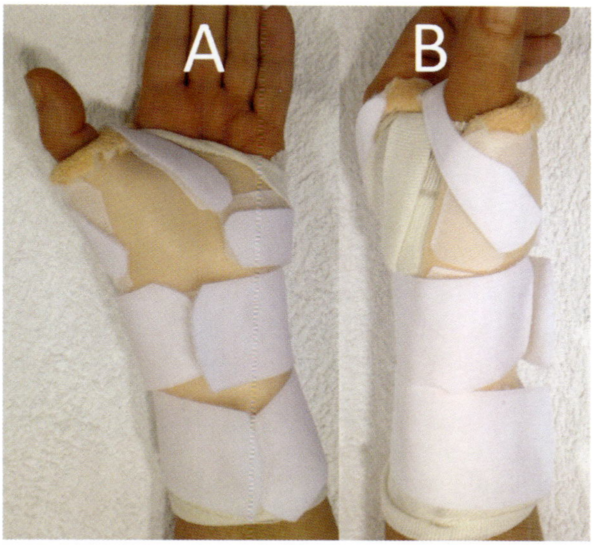

Figure 11 - Thermoplastic splint (A, B) to use after scaphoid fracture fixation: part of the thumb is included

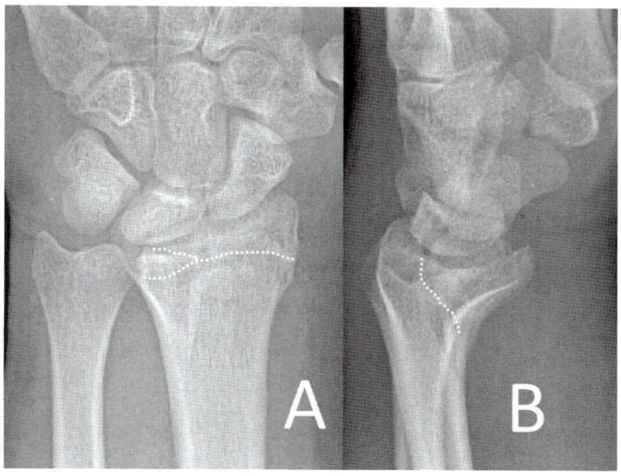

Figure 12 - X-ray images (A, B) showing an intra-articular distal radius fracture (white dotten lines) of a left wrist

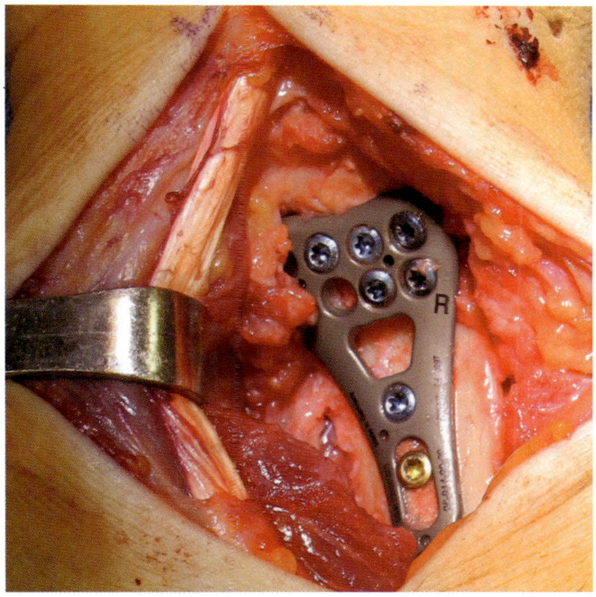

Figure 13 - Intraoperative image of distal radius fracture in which a volar plate was used to fix the fracture

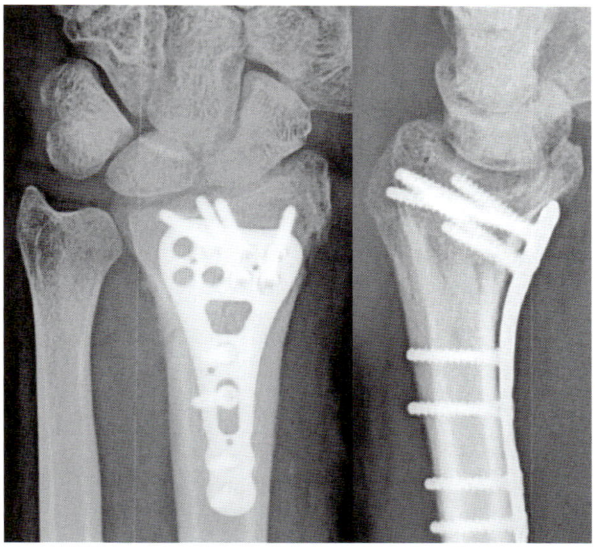

Figure 14 - Postoperative X-rays results of the distal radius fracture treated by palmar plate

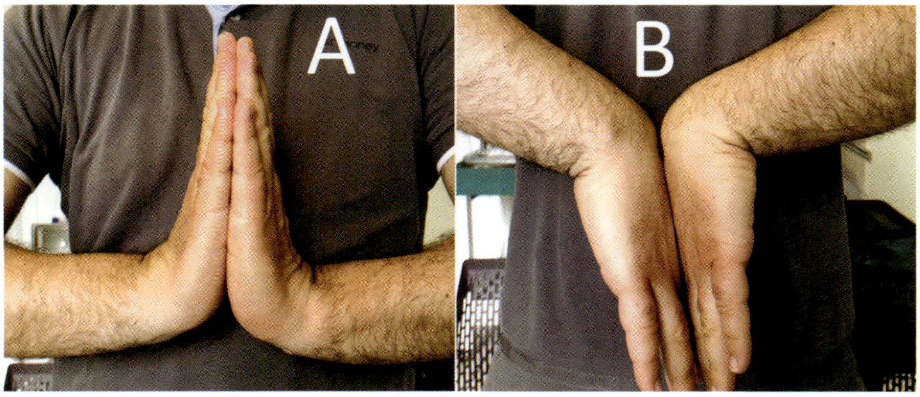

Figure 15 - Postoperative clinical result. A) complete wrist extension; B) minimal defect of the wrist flexion

location of the carpus according with the Mayfield classification [25]. However, it exists a lot of variety of mixed forms that includes bones and ligaments. Moreover, when the lunate returns to the original anatomical position after the dislocation, diagnostic recognition of the perilunate dislocation becomes difficult at the standard examination. This condition is called perilunate instability, in which different degrees of ligament injures (SL and LT) around the lunate can coexist without possibility to be detected by classical tests (x-ray, MRI). It represents a picture of carpal instability with pain persistence despite the negative imaging findings.

These clinical conditions have to be investigated by arthroscopy to verify the amount of the lesions and subsequently to address the treatment. The most serious injury involves more ligaments and skeletal parts of the wrist such as the radius, scaphoid, capitate, lunate, triquetrum, which can be fractured in various ways and association. These must be treated correctly, often surgically (figg. 17, 18), also with the help of wrist arthroscopy. All of these injuries involve a long period of treatment with clear functional limitations of the wrist at follow-up. The worst consequence of this wrist damage is the arthritis with pain and reduction of wrist motility and strength grip.

Metacarpal fractures

The 3rd, 4th, and 5th metacarpals are the most frequent metacarpals involved in the fractures [26, 27]. The metacarpal fractures, displaced or not, should be subjected to ORIF with plate (figg. 19, 20) [19] to allow early rehabilitation and return

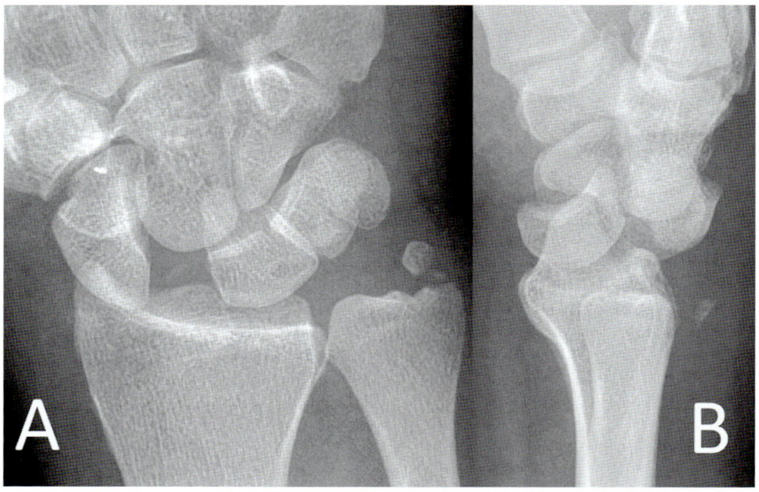

Figure 16 - X-rays images (A, B) of perilunate fracture dislocation of right wrist. The soccer player kicked the ball upside down by resting the wrist of the upper right limb on the ground. The violent wrist hyperxtension with rotation produced the fracture dislocation of the carpal bones. Note the ulnar styloid fracture and the small fragment dorsal to the SL articular space. In the X-ray lateral view this fragment is located just behind the dorsal margin of the distal radius

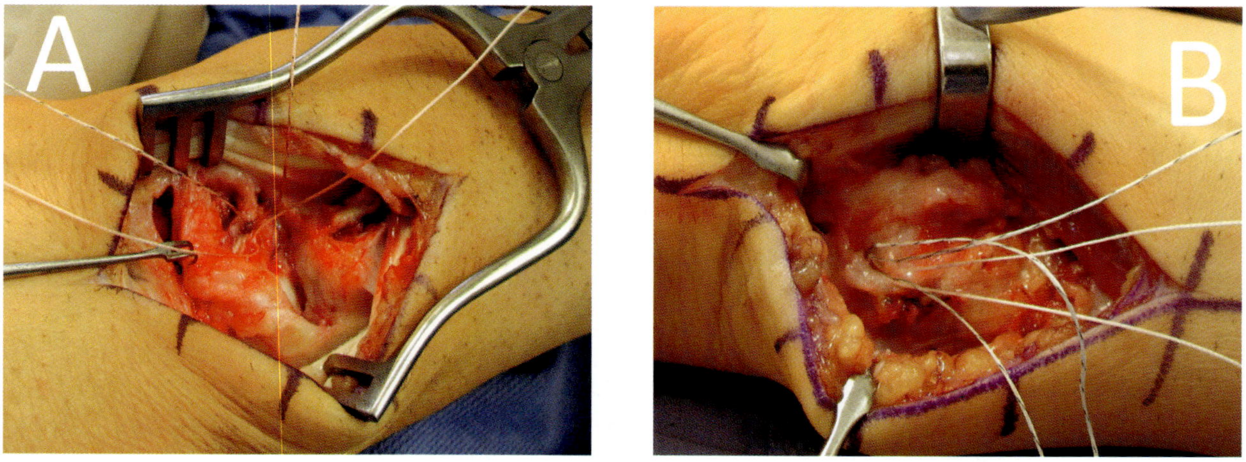

Figure 17 - Intraoperative images of the technique of reduction of the dislocation and ligaments repair using a dorsal capsulodesis for the SL ligament dissociation (A) and TFCC foveal fixation though a palmar approach (B) using a suture anchor. No temporary k-wires were used to maintain the carpal bones position reached by simple bones relocation and ligament suture. A wrist splint was used for 30 days

to activity even if protected (this concept is valid for the soccer players but not for the goalkeeper) (figg. 21, 22). The articular fracture of the 1st or 5th metacarpal bones, when involves their carpo-metacarpal joint, must be submitted to careful reduction and fixation. Special postoperative splints and taping are used to permit an earlier return to play (fig. 23). In particular cases, the first CMC joint arthroscopy might be used by skilled arthroscopists to achieve a correct reduction of intra-articular fracture (Bennett type fracture) [28]. Recovery times are around one month with the addition of specific rehabilitation. The return to activity takes place with a specific splint or taping protection (figg. 24, 25).

Time of return to play and quality of functional recovery depend on the severity of the lesion and the type of bone fixation. All these factors determine possible final functional defects.

Metacarpal fractures can also occur by crushing trauma. In this case, more tissues are damaged such as interosseous muscles and tendons (especially extensors) as well as the skin. When the skin is involved, surgical treatment by ORIF technique is contraindicated and external fixation or cast should be used. If the skin is healthy, sur-

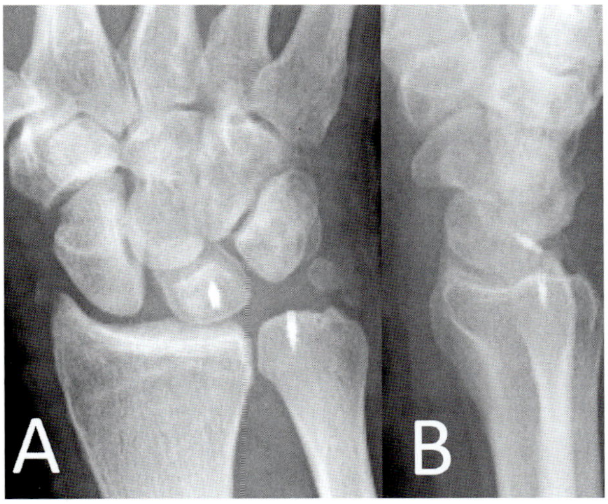

Figure 18 - Postoperative x-rays results of SL dorsal capsulodesis and TFCC foveal refixation by using two suture anchors for perilunate fracture dislocation

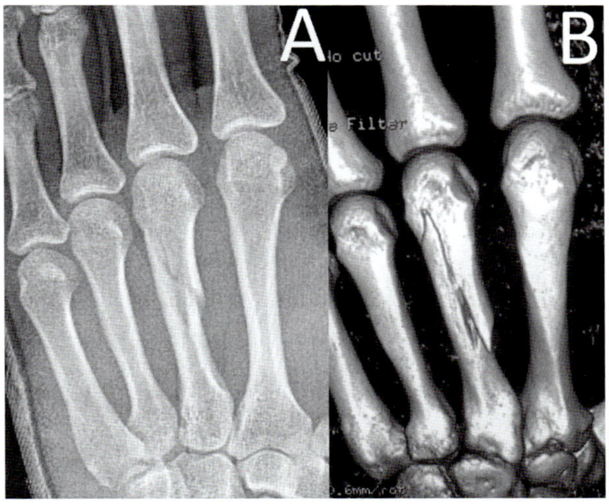

Figure 19 - Forth metacarpal fracture of the left hand of 31 male, national team player (attack), Serie A soccer player. Mechanism of injury was an accidental trauma while training, kick from another player. Treatment: open reduction, internal fixation. X-rays AP view (A) and 3D CT-scan AP view (B) in which a minimal displacement is showed

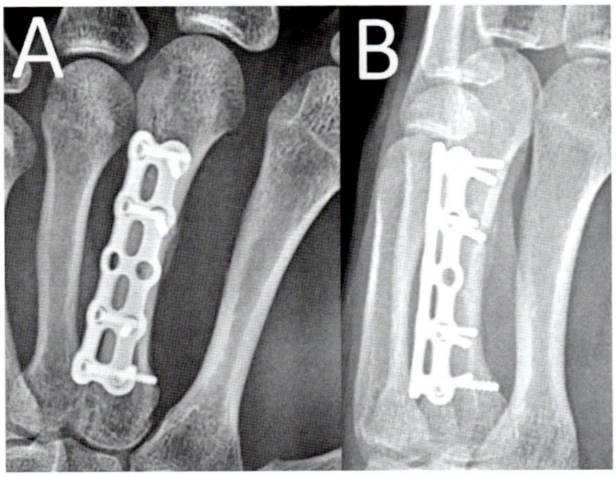

Figure 20 - Postoperative x-rays results (A: AP view; B: lateral view) of 4th metacarpal fracture treated with dorsal plate.
Patient back to play one day after. Monday: surgery. Tuesday: first training. Wednesday: training match. Friday: match.
A special thermoplastic night splint during day and night, pyrocarbon splint during the match. Follow-up at 19 months showed complete recovery of full range of motion; plate was not removed

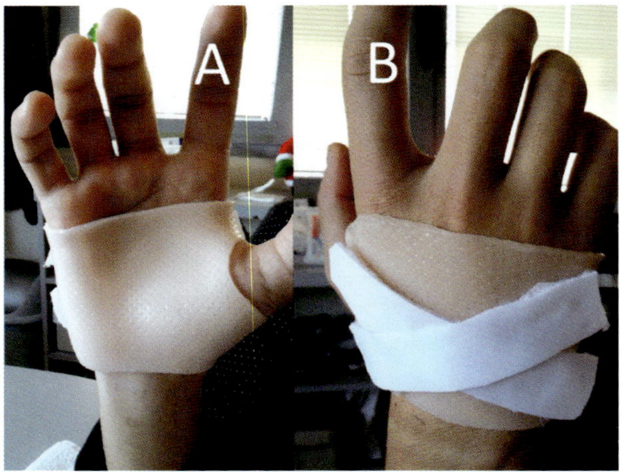

Figure 21 - Thermoplastic splint (A, B) for undisplaced metacarpal fracture

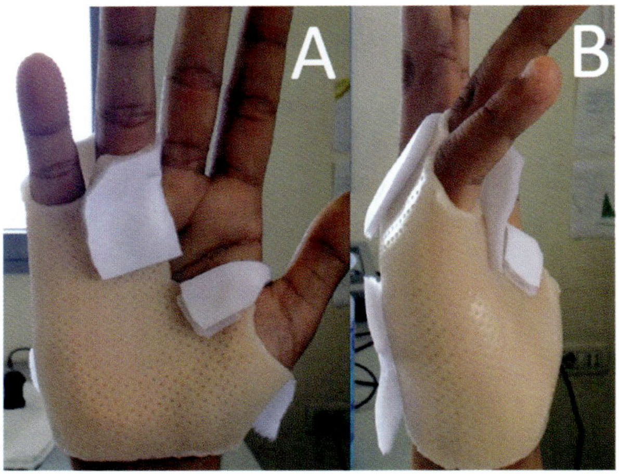

Figure 22 - Thermoplastic splint (A, B) for 5th metacarpal or base of P1 5th digit fracture

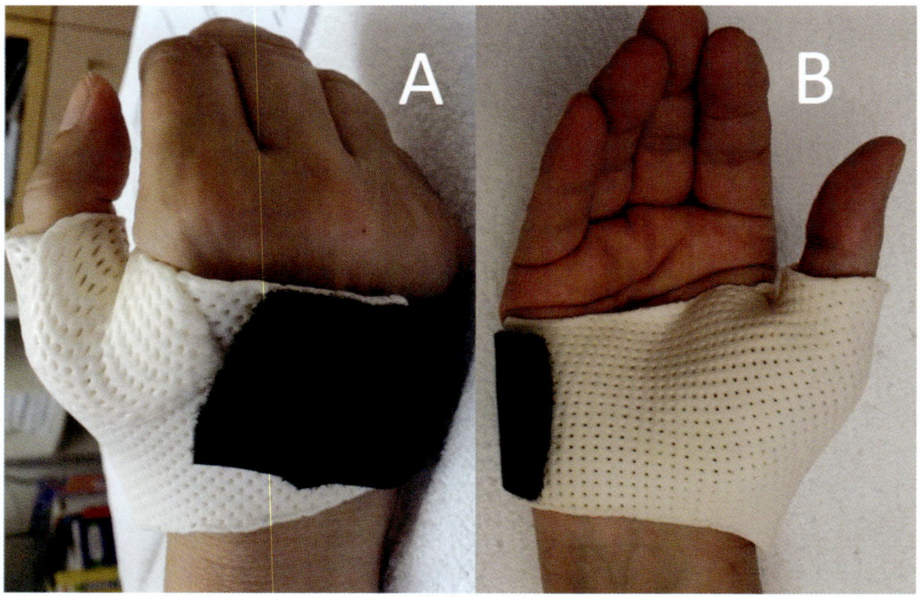

Figure 23 - Thermoplastic splint for thumb MF joint instability (A, B)

Figure 24 - Thermoplastic splint (A, B) for MP joint of the thumb. This splint is suggested one month after surgery of MP joint for protection

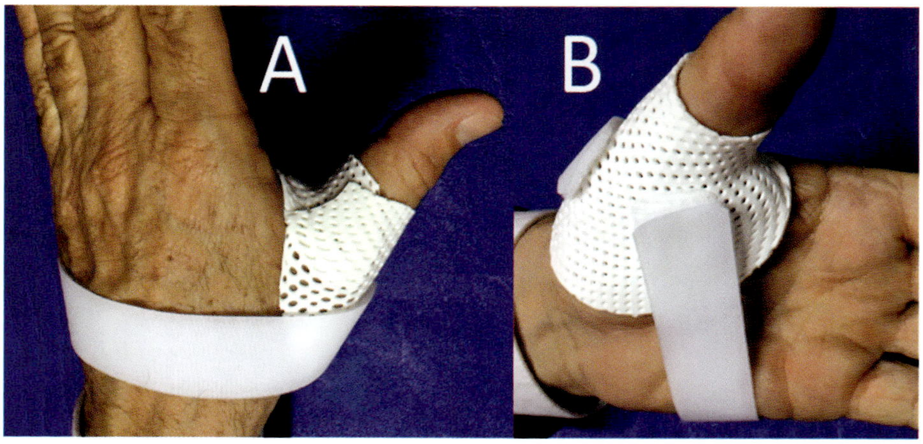

gical treatment is allowed but the damage of the other tissues will affect the complete recovery.
For the goalkeeper the procedures are the same, but the rest time is different because they have to use the hands; therefore, the risk to refracture is higher. In goalkeeper the return to the activity is postponed until healing has taken place.

Phalangeal fractures

Diaphyseal fractures should be treated by ORIF [19, 29] with plate and submitted to immediate rehabilitation.
Oblique fractures can be fixed with plate or with two or more screws. In these cases, rehabilitation must be very slow and protected. Particular attention must be paid to control the rotation and the phalangeal axis.
The fractures of the phalangeal heads must be fixed with mini-screws followed by immediate protected rehabilitation. These fractures are included into the category of articular fractures that need to be treated correctly (figg. 26, 27, 28). Ligament involvement must be recognized and treated at the same time. When the joint is involved, a reduction of the final ROM should also be expected. Hand therapist should be required to have a better rehabilitation in order to recover joint function. In soccer players, the return to ac-

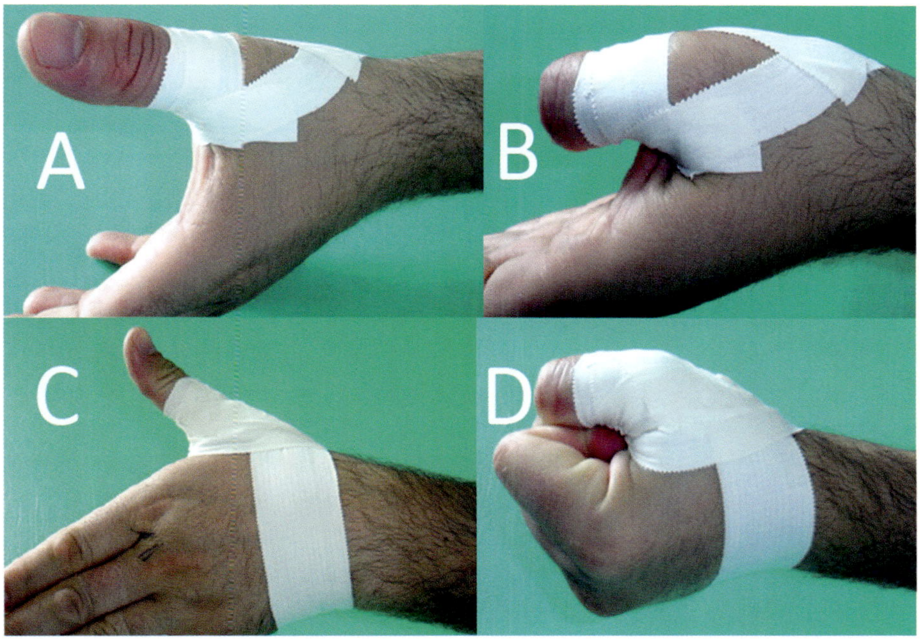

Figure 25 - Taping protecting the thumb MP joint. Pictures A and B show a crossing dorsal taping which permit an easely motion of the MP joint with external protection. Pictures C and D show a much more protective taping with the same purpose

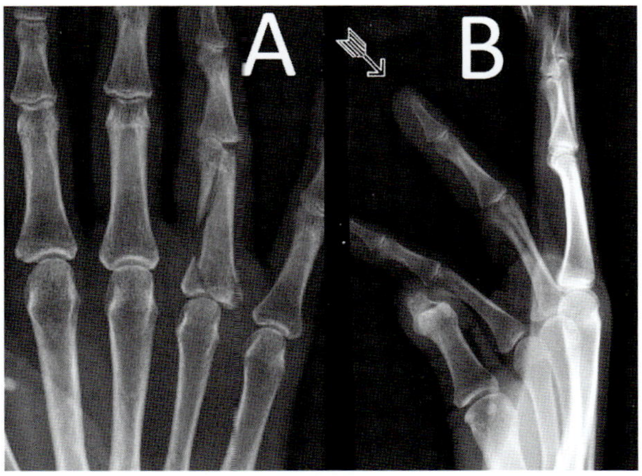

Figure 26 - Young female soccer player with bifocal dislocated articular fracture of MP and PIP joint of the 4th digit. X-rays views in AP (A) and lateral (B) position

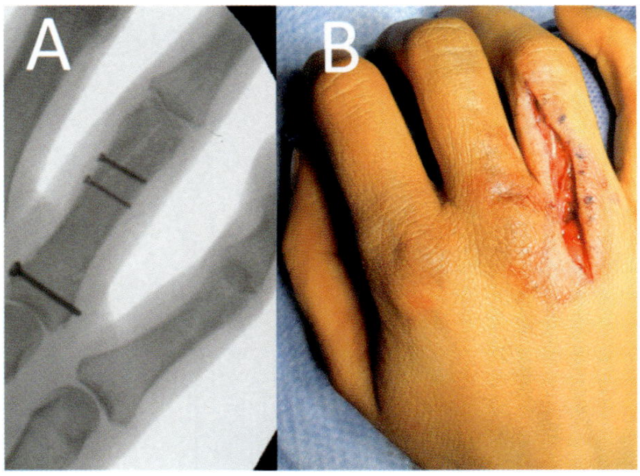

Figure 27 - Reduction and internal fixation was performed using three screws. Intraoperative fluoroscopic view (A) and intraoperative image of MP and PIP joints dorsal access (B)

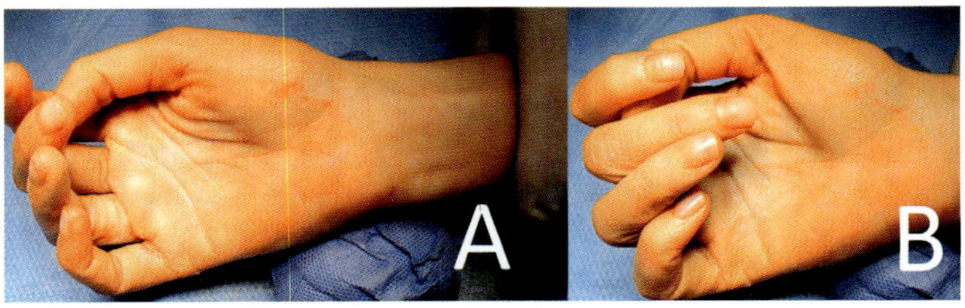

Figure 28 - Intraoperative clinical result using the Brunelli test for finger flexion squeezing the tendons proximally to the wrist crease. This method permits to evaluate the correct finger motion without rotatory or axial defect

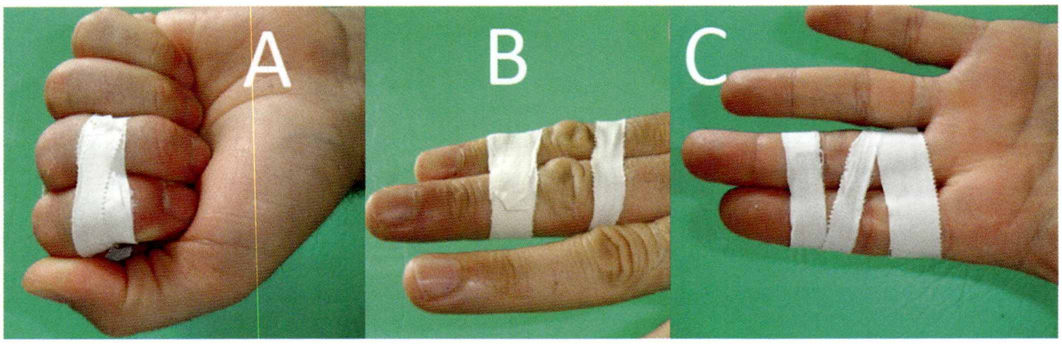

Figure 29 - Double digit taping (B, C) to protect the PIP joint of the ulnar collateral ligament of the 2nd digit or radial collateral ligament of the 3rd digit. This taping permits an easy flexion/extension of the PIP joint (A)

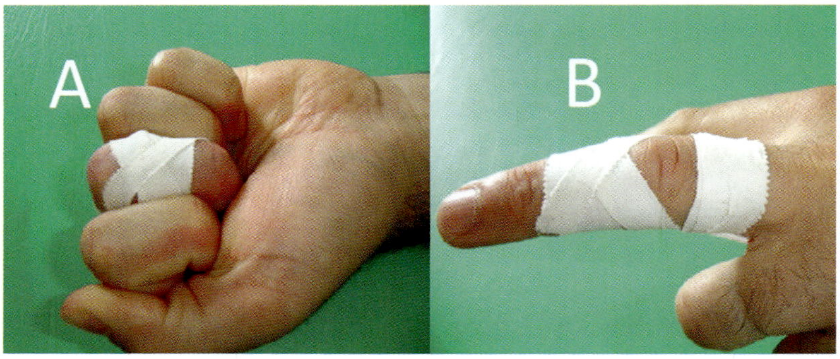

Figure 30 - Single digit taping protecting the collateral ligaments of the 3rd digit (A, B)

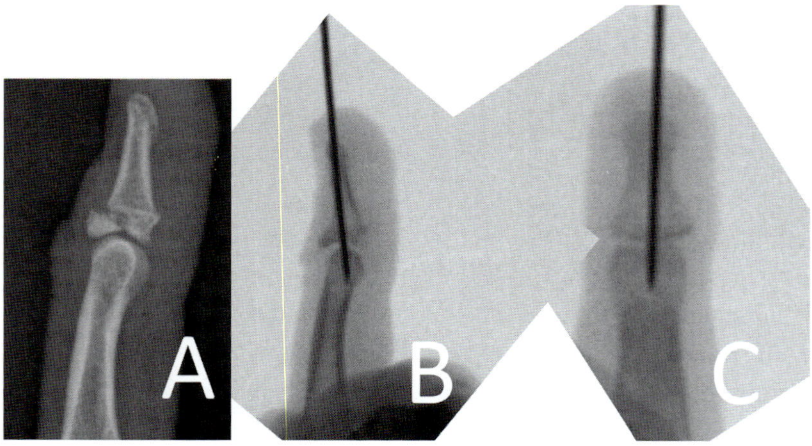

Figure 31 - Goalkeeper P3 of right 3rd finger fracture. X-rays images of mallet finger (A) with dorsal bone fragment (Segond fracture or Salter-Harris type 3 fracture of P3) treated with k-wire: B) lateral view; C) AP view

tivity is permitted by using splint and taping with parallel fingers (fig. 29), for protective purposes. In goalkeepers the return to activity will respect the times of bone consolidation and complete clinical recovery. Taping for single digit may be suggested (fig. 30).

Articular fractures from longitudinal trauma with damage to the base of the 2nd phalanx require special treatment through an immediate traction and mobilization system. This type of fracture and following treatment do not permit a return to sports activity for at least 45 days. For goalkeeper category, the rule of complete recovery is mandatory.

Distal phalangeal fractures, as for example the "mallet finger", can be operated (fig. 31) or simply immobilized with a special splint for almost 45 days (fig. 32). Surgery is also considered for displaced fractures of the distal phalanx that involve the nail. The nail plate must be reduced and if the nail has been lost it is suggested to apply a prosthesis to permit a better nail growth and contemporary healing. Even in these fractures the goalkeepers will have a prolonged protective treatment until healing is achieved.

Dislocations and ligament injury of the digits

Proximal interphalangeal joint injury

Proximal interphalangeal (PIP) joint injury is the most common ligamentous injury in the hand. The spectrum of injury ranges from a simple sprain or "jammed finger" to very challenging fracture-dislocations [30, 31].

The key to PIP joint stability is the boxlike complex well secured laterally by the collateral ligaments and volarly by the volar plate. This configuration produces a three-dimensional strength that strongly resists PIP joint displacement. To determine a displacement of the middle phalanx, the ligament-box complex must be disrupted in at least two planes. Typically, collateral ligaments fail proximally, and the volar plate avulses distally, although variable failure patterns have been reported.

Maneuvers of clinical evaluation test the stability of the joint actively and passively. Complete full or near-full range of motion despite of ligament disruption confirm that adequate joint stability remains. Re-displacement with motion indicates significant ligament lesion. Passive stability is checked helping with local anesthesia in lateral stress (at 30° of flexion and complete PIP extension) and dorsal-volar direction. Collateral ligament injuries are graduated in three levels of damage: grade I (pain and no instability); grade II (minimal instability but firm endpoint and stable arc of motion); grade III (gross instability without firm endpoint).

Radiographs (posteroanterior and true lateral view) of the digits alone are inadequate. A subtle fracture or subluxation may otherwise be missed. The joint may have spontaneously reduced, masking the pathology of a dislocation. The clinician should look for the "V" sign dorsally to identify incongruent or dorsally subluxated joints.

Ultrasonography might help in the diagnosis mostly for the collateral ligament injury with or without minimal bone detachment.

Differential diagnosis between collateral ligament sprain, volar plate avulsion, central slip disruption, dislocation, fracture dislocation, and

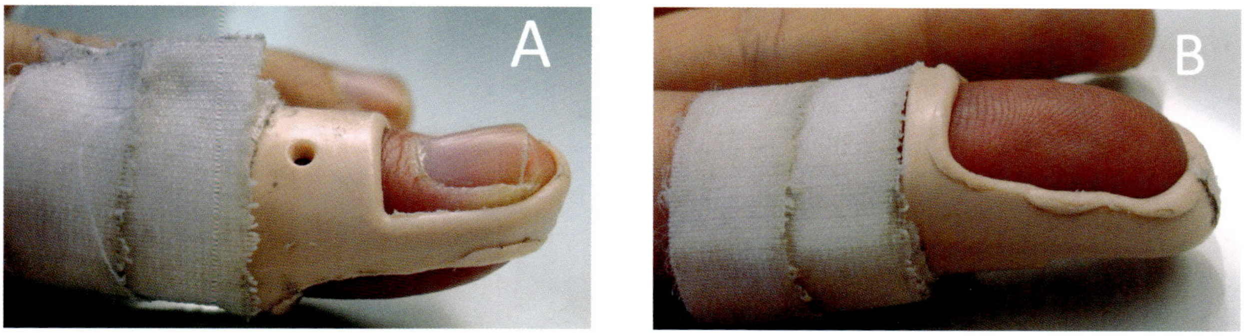

Figure 32 - Special splint for mallet finger. A) DIP joint was positioned in hyperextension; B) the volar part of the splint was opened to permit the pulp skin contact in order to preserve the sensibility

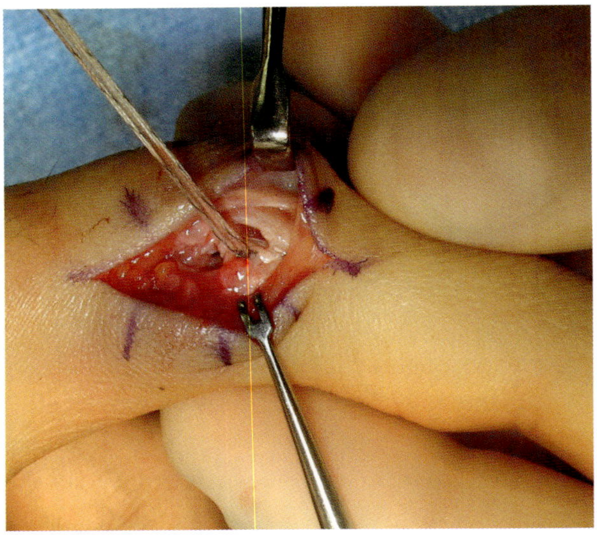

Figure 33 - Young female soccer player affected by PIP joint dislocation of right 3rd finger. Intraoperative images of radial collateral ligament refixation using a suture anchor

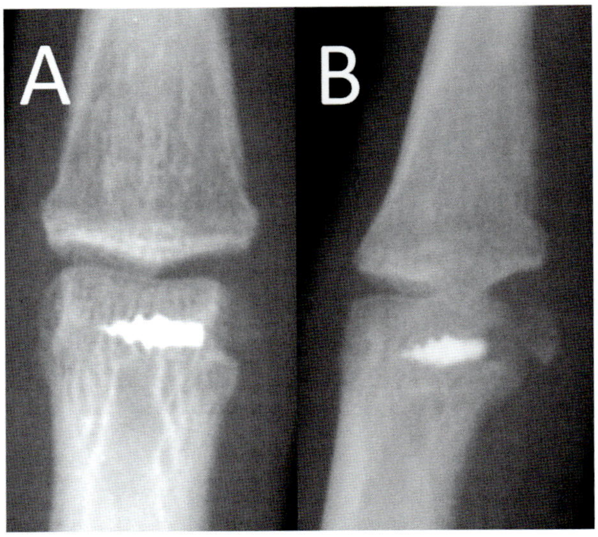

Figure 34 - Postoperative X-ray views of the correct position of the suture anchor: AP view (A) and oblique view (B) in which a small volar fragment is still evident

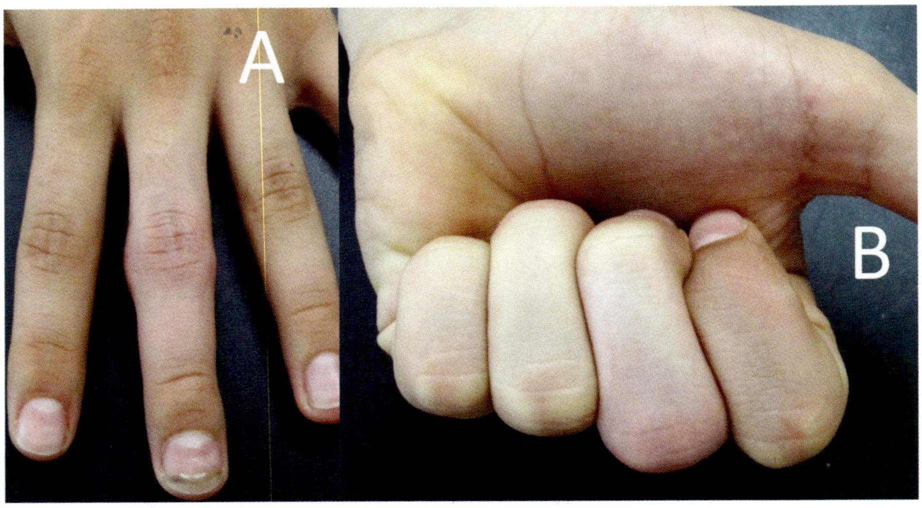

Figure 35 - Clinical result of PIP joint with complete extension (A) and flexion (B)

impacted pilon fracture-dislocation must be done before treating the damaged joint. Management of the ligament lesions depends on the grade of injury. In the minor degree of lesion with stability of the PIP joint, simple taping (fig. 30) is effective and early motion is permitted. In the middle degree of ligament injury, a splint is suggested, as for example for the volar plate injury in which the instability is appreciated but reducible; a dorsal splint is used protecting the joint at 10° more than the degree at which the joint becomes unstable. Progressive modification of splint position permits to reach the complete extension of the PIP joint with contemporary ligament healing. Patients should be counseled to expect at least 6 months of occasional pain and stiffness because recovery is typically prolonged.

Surgery will be used for irreducible dislocation: a volar approach for the volar plate injury and a lateral approach for the collateral ligaments. For the collateral ligaments suture anchors have to be used (figg. 33, 34, 35), with active motion initiated at 2 to 3 weeks, and unlimited activities allowed at 6 weeks.

In minor degree of instability early return to play is permitted for the soccer player using a taping (figg. 29, 30) [31]. In the middle degree of instability the soccer player can return to play with protection. Soccer player operated for the major instability will return to play after 45 days. The

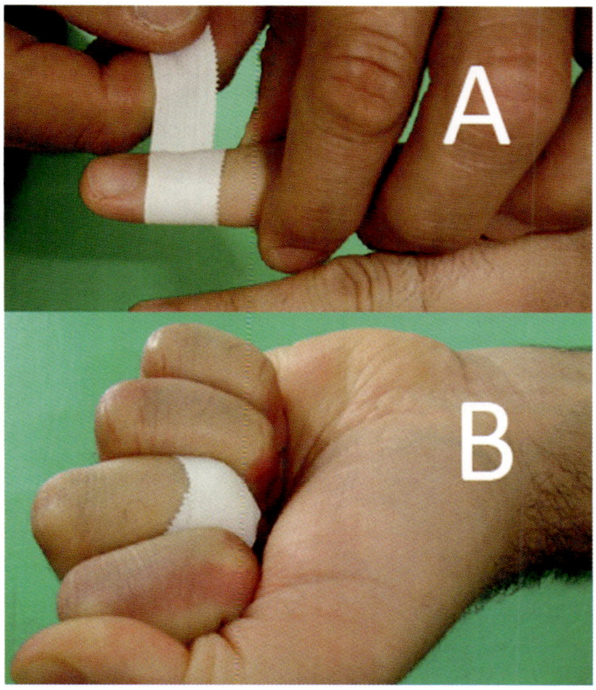

Figure 36 - Specific taping for the DIP joint. This taping permits an easy flexion/extension of the DIP joint (A, B)

goalkeeper needs to reach a complete healing of the ligament lesion before to return to play.

The most important injury of the PIP joint is the fracture-dislocation: the pilon type fracture represents the worst condition [31]. There is no particular modality of treatment of these injuries but it is the injury characteristics to guide the technical approach. Treatment is customized using several techniques, including dynamic skeletal traction, ORIF, hemihamate grafting, cerclage wiring, and volar plate arthroplasty. The minor injuries can be treated conservatively by extension block splinting. The major injuries need a more appropriate treatment. The dynamic skeletal traction method is useful in selected cases but it needs skill surgeons and hand therapists for rehabilitation. This type of treatment does not permit to return to play for almost 2 months in soccer players and 3 months for goalkeepers.

The surgical treatment is left for the fracture dislocation of the PIP joint with comminuted articular fractures joined to delayed clinical observation. All these surgical procedures stop the soccer players and goalkeepers for several months. Functional defects should be expected.

Distal interphalangeal joint injury

Dislocation of the distal interphalangeal (DIP) joints of the digits or the interphalangeal (IP) joint of the thumb are frequently dorsal or lateral [30, 31]. Treatment of these dislocations consists of closed reduction under digital or wrist block anesthesia. Post-reduction radiographs are mandatory to confirm congruous reduction. Instability after pure dislocations is rare, and the joint is immobilized in slight flexion using a dorsal splint for 2 to 3 weeks to permit a better healing of the ligaments in a correct tension. Open treatments are specific for irreducible dislocation with tendon or bone fragments interposition. Same procedure will be adopted for the proximal migration of the volar fragment attached to the flexor digitorum profundus tendon. Volar dislocation is rare and frequently is observed after spontaneous reduction. Attention should be paid to a possible extensor tendon injury or to a mallet finger as associated lesions. Splinting of the DIP (fig. 32) or thumb IP joints followed by taping (fig. 36) permit an early return to play to the soccer players but not to the goalkeepers.

Metacarpophalangeal joint injury

Finger metacarpophalangeal joint dislocations are relative frequent [30, 31]. They are most vulnerable to injury from forces directed ulnarly and dorsally. Distinction must be made between subluxation (simple) and complete (complex) dorsal dislocations. This anatomic distinction is important to plan treatment because the former is reducible by closed means, whereas the latter is not. In the dorsal dislocation, surgery is mandatory to reduce the interposed tissue. The radial collateral ligament is usually involved. Radial collateral tears should be operated in grade III. Dorsal-radial access over the ligament position is made (figg. 37, 38). The site of reattachment is cleared to bleeding bone, and a mini-suture anchor is placed directed obliquely away from the joint. The joint is immobilized for 5 to 6 weeks in 45 degrees of flexion. Range of motion of 0 to 80 degrees without pain in acute repairs can be expected. MP joint protection (figg. 21, 39) is maintained during the training and taping (fig. 40) for the match.

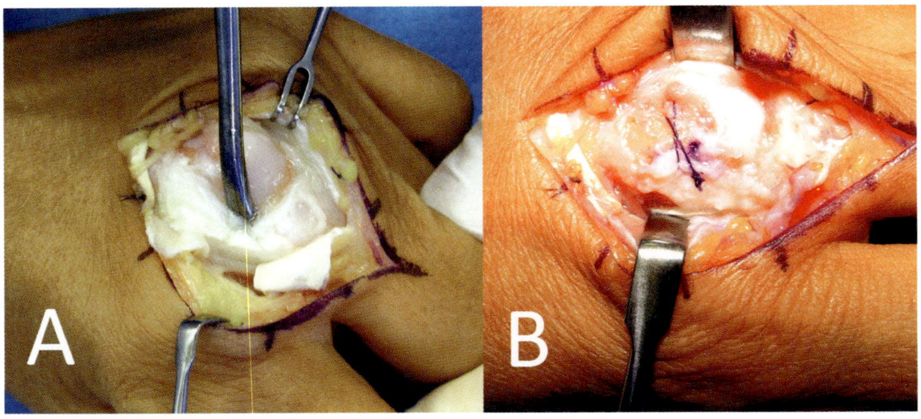

Figure 37 - Intraoperative images of radial collateral ligament tear of 3rd MP joint (A) and transosseous suture repair of the ligament (B)

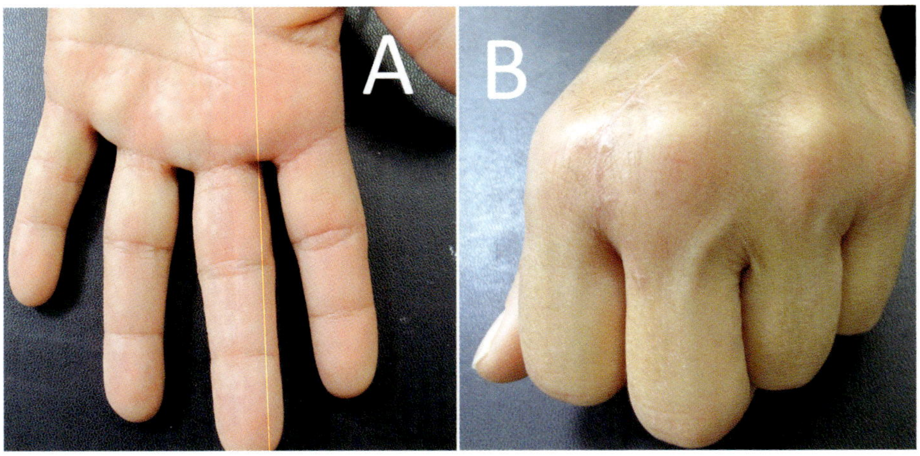

Figure 38 - Clinical result of MP joint with complete extension (A) and flexion (B)

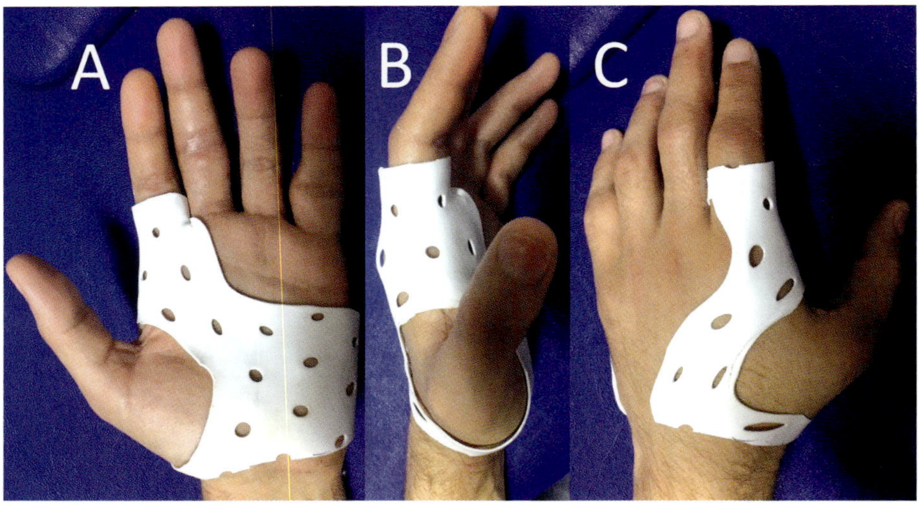

Figure 39 - Thermoplastic splint (A, B, C) for 2nd MP joint or 2nd metacarpal bone fracture

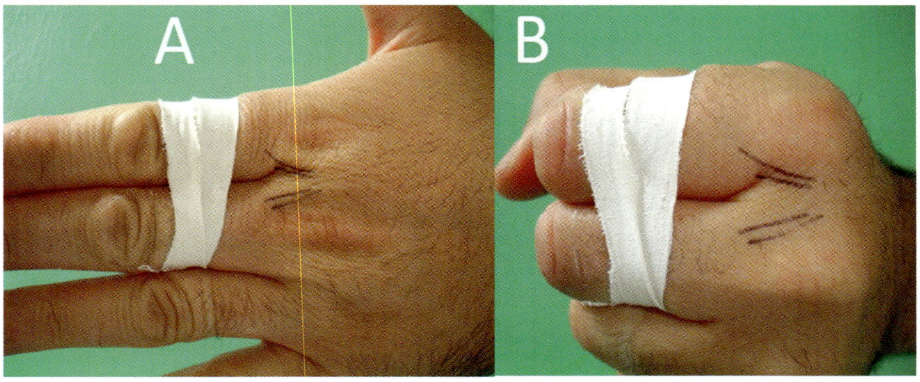

Figure 40 - Double digital taping to protect the ulnar collateral ligament of the 2nd MP joint or the radial collateral ligament of the 3rd MP joint

Post-traumatic locked MP joint is an unusual entity characterized by a moderate flexion deformity of the joint caused by several conditions such as sesamoid entrapment, spicula fracture fragment, or periarticular exostoses. The usual cause of locking is restriction of collateral or accessory collateral ligament excursion by a prominent metacarpal head radial condyle, impalement of the ligament on a marginal degenerative osteophyte, or fracture fragment. Resection of the osteophyte, fracture fragment, or sesamoid solves the problem. Goalkeeper will stop to play for almost 45 days.

Acute ulnar collateral ligament (UCL) injury of thumb MP joint is frequent [30, 31]. If clinical evaluation confirms that an acute complete rupture of the UCL is present (fig. 41), surgical repair is indicated (fig. 42). Same indication is for the radial collateral ligament (RCL) injury even if it is less frequent but with the same disabilities. In acute case simple repair is the rule followed by splinting immobilization for a month (figg. 23, 24). Rehabilitation will give almost complete recovery with minimal reduction of the flexion of the MP joint. UCL or RCL chronic ligament injury must be reconstructed by using tendon graft. Sometimes UCL and RCL injuries can coexist and both need to be repaired. Contemporary reconstruction of both ligaments should be done with box technique using a tendon graft. Taping protection for thumb MP joint is constantly used for a long period of time (2-3 months) (fig. 25).

Post-traumatic hyperextension of the MP joint is infrequent and may be the consequence of an unrecognized or undertreated tear of the volar plate injury or dislocation of the MP joint [30,31]. Simple protection with splint might be sufficient in the early phases and early stage (figg. 23, 24). More important injury of the volar plate of the thumb should be operated. The cortex of the retrocondylar fossa is decorticated, and the volar plate is advanced proximally into this area. A bone anchor is placed in the decorticated retrocondylar fossa and used to fix the proximally advanced volar plate. MP joint temporary transfixion with a Kirschner is rarely used but the thumb is splinted for 4 weeks, after which the range of motion is begun. If there has been a relatively re-

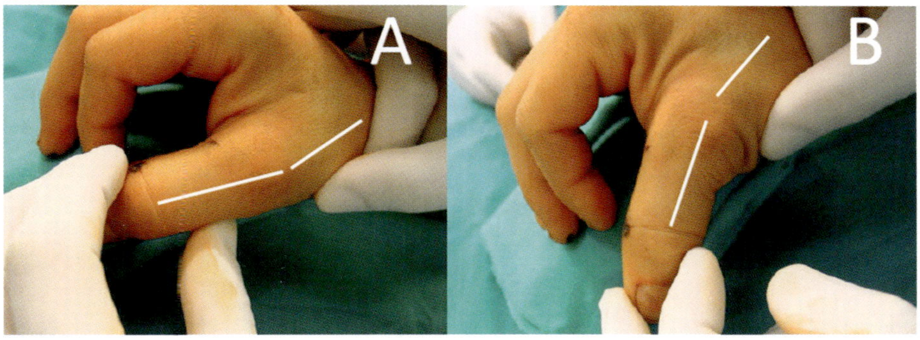

Figure 41 - Clinical test (A, B) showing the ulnar instability of the MF joint of the thumb

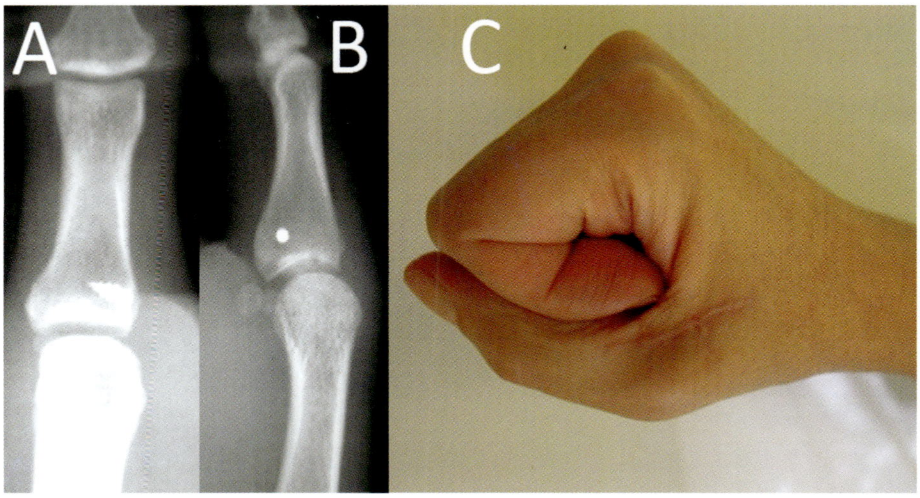

Figure 42 - X-ray images showing the right position of the suture anchor in the ulnar base of P1; C) clinical result used

cent hyperextension injury of the MP joint, it may be possible to reattach the volar plate to its metacarpal origin. A zigzag incision is used to expose the volar aspect of the MP joint. The volar plate is identified and mobilized. Its proximal end is minimally debrided and reattached to the volar aspect of the metacarpal neck with two bone anchors. The MP joint is immobilized in a cast for 1 month, after which the range of motion with a 20 degree extension block splint is encouraged for additional 2 weeks. The procedure is unlikely to be successful if the injury is chronic, and the volar plate is attenuated.
Soccer players return to play with protection after 2 weeks, goalkeepers after 45 days.

Avascular bone necrosis

Carpal bone avascular necrosis of the hand and wrist is completely unusual in the context of soccer injuries and therefore it will not be taken into consideration in detail. Lunate necrosis (Kienbock's disease) is the most frequent carpal bone avascular necrosis [32], but it can more rarely involve the scaphoid (Preiser's disease) [33, 34], as well. Surely it can occur in young players but their treatment involves first of all recognition and then staging. Based on the defined stage it will be possible to prepare a suitable treatment. Diagnosis of early stages of this pathology allows to adopt a correct treatment to promote the healing. In all other stages, treatments will lead to a partial and never complete recovery. Salvage treatments are also indicated for advanced stage, that is, bone resections and arthrodesis. Goalkeepers will have longer time of stop and sometimes the career is compromised.

Tendon injuries

The fingers are the most frequent location of tendon lesions. Flexor and extensor tendons [35] have different lesion mechanisms. The flexor profundus tendon of the 4th or 3rd finger may be involved in this type of injury due to traction mechanism during competition. The soccer players of opposing teams use to obstacle the opponent with different solutions, such as grips and pull-ups for the shirt, and an overload of traction on a single finger due to the failure of the other fingers in the grasp might cause a fracturing detachment of the P3 with the flexor tendon attacked.
The extensor tendons are also involved in the distal part of the finger, at PIP joint level [36]. It is an axial trauma that causes extensor tendon detachment from the P3 base, resulting in a hammer toe (mallet finger).
Both injuries require specific treatment. The flexor tendon must be treated surgically by fragment fixation to the P3 [36]. The extensor tendon injury with bone fragment (mallet finger) detachment may be also operated but it depends on the dimension and dislocation of the fragment itself. The Ishiguro technique [37] is the most valid procedure.
The extensor tendon injury (pure tendon lesion), on the other hand, should be treated conservatively with a splint for mallet finger for almost two months, with DIP joint in hyperextension position. In any case, these injuries cause a suspension from the specific sport for a long time (more than a month) and the role that is mostly affected is that of goalkeepers.
Other types and sites of tendon injuries involve crushing injuries of the fingers or hand often associated with fractures of the phalanges or metacarpals.
Flexor and extensor tendon lacerations need a specific suture followed by early rehabilitation [35, 36]. However, return to sport activity is forbidden for more than 45 days, mostly for the goalkeepers. Any active contraction without protection can determine detachment of the tendon sutures. Secondary surgery will not have the same chances of healing of the emergency surgery.

Peripheral nerve injuries

Nerve injuries in sports are not very frequent. Chan [38] describes that, according to the report of the Japanese Athletic Association in 1971, peripheral nerve injuries are only 0.3% of sports injuries. Among all peripheral nerve injuries treated in their center within 18 years, 5.7% were related to sports. A recent paper published in 2017 reported that sports-related nerve injuries accounted for around 0.5% of all traumatic peripheral nerve injuries (Olivo, 2017). Better understanding of sports biomechanics and preventive measures during sports could effectively reduce the number of injuries.

Nerve injury in sports could be classified into acute or chronic.

Acute injuries include:

- blunt trauma;
- sharp injury;
- fracture ends laceration;
- acute traction.

Chronic injuries are commonly caused by irritation or compression due to repetitive stress. For example:

- muscle hypertrophy, fascial edge, or increased compartment pressure causing compression;
- chronic inflammatory tissue causing compression;
- poor flexibility causing excessive traction at relative fixed point;
- subluxation with frictional injury.

The underlying pathology of chronic nerve injury is usually due to ischaemia. When the critical threshold of 40-50 mmHg compression force is reached, inflammatory response and scar tissue formation would initiate. The sequel would be neurapraxia or axonotmesis types of nerve injury. The list of common sports-related nerve injuries of upper limb do not report soccer as possible cause. The nerves of the upper limb involved in the possible damage are the brachial plexus, the suprascapular nerve, the long thoracic nerve, the musculocutaneous nerve, the ulnar nerve at the elbow and the Guyon canal, the median nerve and its anterior interosseous nerve, the radial nerve and the posterior interosseous nerve, the superficial branch of the radial nerve, and the digital nerves. All of them can be involved giving specific clinical sign at the wrist and hand. However, the digital nerves, the median nerve, the ulnar nerve and the superficial branch of the radial nerve are the specific nerves of this anatomical area. Traction, crushing, or laceration are the mechanism of nerve damage.

Clinical and instrumental investigations as nerve conduction study and ultrasonography help in the definition and staging of the nerve lesion.

Conservative treatment considers medical management and protective measures (padding, splint, gear). Surgery like nerve release or decompression or fasciotomy are rarely required. Microsurgery suture is adopted for the complete nerve lesion.

Soccer players are stopped for such a nerve lesion for almost 1 month followed by rehabilitation. Goalkeepers need more time to recover.

Simple nerve decompression allows an earlier return to play for soccer players and goalkeepers, too.

Conclusions

As it can be seen from this description on hand and wrist injuries in soccer players, it is clear that goalkeepers are the most disadvantaged athletes in terms of injury and temporary removal from the specific sport as the injury affects the most important part of their body. The hand surgeon must understand who is in front of him and must explain the type of injury and recovery time as well. This last aspect, in particular, cannot be silenced; it must be clear to the athlete and to the leaders of the company that for some of these injuries time of recovery is fundamental. There are no discounts, otherwise there will be recurrences, non-healing, or subsequent injuries.

Finally, in relation to the type of injury, the consequences of joint damage must be clear to all, such as for instance in the fractures/dislocation of the carpus because it will determine indelible marks that will sooner or later result in a degenerative pathology of the wrist.

It should also be noted that the first treatment must be as correct and complete as possible.

Bibliography

1. Emery CA. Soccer (Football). In: Caine DJ, Harmer PA, Schiff MA. Epidemiology of injury in olympic sports. International Olympic Committee, Wiley-Blackwell Publishing Ltd 2010:204-235.
2. Palmer AK, Werner FW. The triangular fibrocartilage complex of the wrist-anatomy and function. J Hand Surg Am. 1981 Mar;6(2):153-62.
3. Pechlaner S, Kathrein A, Gabl M, Lutz M, Angermann P, Zimmermann R, Peer R, Peer S, Rieger M, Freund M, Rudisch A. Distal radius fractures and concomitant lesions. Experimental studies concerning the pathomechanism. Handchir Mikrochir Plast Chir. 2002 May;34(3):150-7.
4. Hagert CG. Distal radius fracture and the distal radioulnar joint--anatomical considerations. Handchir Mikrochir Plast Chir. 1994 Jan;26(1):22-6.
5. Atzei A, Luchetti R, Garcia Elias M. Lesioni capsulo-legamentose della radio-ulnare distale e fibrocartilagine triangolare. In: Landi A, Catalano F, Luchetti R. Trattato di Chirurgia della Mano. Roma, Verduci Editore 2007, 159-187.
6. Cerofolini E, Luchetti R, Pederzini L, Soragni O, Colombini R, D'Alimonte P, Romagnoli R. MR evaluation of triangular fibrocartilage complex tears in the wrist: comparison with arthrography and arthroscopy. J Comput Assist Tomogr. 1990 Nov-Dec;14(6):963-7.
7. Luchetti R, Atzei A, Cozzolino R. Le lesioni capsulo-legamentose acute del polso e della mano. Lesioni della radio ulnare distale. GIOT 2012;38(suppl.2):79-96.
8. Luchetti R, Pegoli L, Papini Zorli I, Garcia Elias M. Le instabilità del carpo. In: Landi A, Catalano F, Luchetti R. Trattato di Chirurgia della Mano. Roma: Verduci Editore 2007;117-157.
9. Geissler WB, Haley TH. Arthroscopy management of scapholunate instability. Atlas of Hand Clinics 2001;6:253-274.
10. Messina J, Dreant N, Luchetti R, Lindau T, Mathoulin. C. Scapho-lunate tears: a new arthroscopic classification. Chir Main 2009;28:339-444.
11. Messina J, Dreant N, Van Overstraeten L, Luchetti R, Mathoulin C. Evolution of arthroscopic classification in scapholunate complex lesions. J Hand Surg 2012; 37Eu: S85-86.
12. De Santis S, Fagetti A, Cozzolino R, Luchetti R. Comparazione fra artroscopia e risonanza magnetica nelle lesioni legamentose del polso (studio retrospettivo). Riv Chir Mano 2018;55:11-17.
13. Luchetti R, Zorli IP, Atzei A, Fairplay T. Dorsal intercarpal ligament capsulodesis for predynamic and dynamic scapholunate instability. J Hand Surg Eur Vol. 2010 Jan;35(1):32-7.
14. Wahegaonkar AL, Mathoulin CL. Arthroscopic dorsal capsulo-ligamentous repairin the treatment of chronic scapholunate ligament tears. J Wrist Surg. 2013May;2(2):141-8.
15. Garcia-Elias M. Carpal instability. In: Wolf SW, Hotchkiss RN, Pederson WC, Kozin SH. Green's Operative hand surgery (sixth edition). Philadelphia, Elsevier 2011:467-524.
16. Corella F, Del Cerro M, Ocampos M, Simon de Blas C, Larrainzar-Garijo R. Arthroscopic Scapholunate Ligament Reconstruction, Volar and Dorsal Reconstruction. Hand Clin. 2017 Nov;33(4):687-707.
17. Borelli PP. The management of carpal scaphoid fractures and nonunions and the role of capacitive systems. In: Luchetti R, Pegoli L, Bain GI. Hand and wrist injuries in combat sports. Berlin, Springer Verlag 2018,193-248.
18. Fernandez DL. In: Fernandez DL, Jupiter JB. Fractures of the distal radius. Berlin, Springer-Verlag 2002:41-50.
19. Jupiter JB, Ring DC. AO Manual of fracture management hand and wrist. New York, Thieme 2005.
20. Altissimi M, Nienstedt F. Fratture del radio distale. In: Landi A, Catalano F, Luchetti R. Trattato di Chirurgia della Mano. Roma, Verduci Editore 2007;221-254.
21. Luchetti R, Atzei A, Borelli PP. Il trattamento delle fratture di polso con sintesi rigida. In: Moderni orientamenti nel trattamento delle fratture. Arto superiore e arto inferiore. Milano, Springer-Verlag 2008:519-588.
22. Wolf SW. Distal radius fractures. In: Wolf SW, Hotchkiss RN, Pederson WC, Kozin SH. Green's Operative hand surgery (sixth edition). Philadelphia, Elsevier 2011:563-640.
23. Geissler WB, Freeland AE, Savoie FH, McIntyre LW, Whipple TL. Intracarpal soft-tissue lesions associated with an intra-articular fracture of the distal end of the radius. J Bone Joint Surg Am. 1996 Mar;78(3):357-65.
24. Pilato G. Lussazioni e fratture lussazioni-perilunari del carpo. In: Landi A, Catalano F, Luchetti R. Trattato di Chirurgia della Mano. Roma, Verduci Editore 2007;209-220.
25. Mayfield JK, Johnson RP, Kilcoyne RK. Carpal dislocations: pathomechanics and progressive perilunar instability. J Hand Surg Am. 1980 May;5(3):226-41.
26. Fanfani F, Catalano F, Taccardo G. Fratture dei metacarpi. In: Landi A, Catalano F, Luchetti R. Trattato di Chirurgia della Mano. Roma: Verduci Editore, 2007;301-310
27. Day CS, Stern PJ. Fractures of the metacarpals and phalanges. In: Wolf SW, Hotchkiss RN, Pederson WC, Kozin SH. Green's Operative hand surgery (sixth edition). Philadelphia, Elsevier 2011:245-296.
28. Fontès D. A guide to diagnosis and treatment: first CMC joint articular fractures. In: Luchetti R, Pegoli L, Bain GI. Hand and wrist injuries in combat sports 2018:51-62.
29. Cugola L, Corain M. Fratture dei metacarpi. In: Landi A, Catalano F, Luchetti R. Trattato di Chirurgia della Mano. Roma, Verduci Editore 2007;311-310
30. Passaretti U, Pataia E, Fonzone A, Le lesioni legamentose delle dita. In: Landi A, Catalano F, Luchetti R. Trattato di Chirurgia della Mano. Roma, Verduci Editore 2007;195-208.
31. Merrell G, Slade JF. Dislocation and ligament injuries in the digits. In: Wolf SW, Hotchkiss RN, Pederson WC, Kozin SH. Green's Operative hand surgery (sixth edition). Philadelphia, Elsevier 2011:297-338.
32. Lichtman DM, Bain GI. Kienböck's disease advances in diagnosis and treatment. New York, Springer-Verlag 2018.
33. Vidal MA, Linscheid RL, Amadio PC, Dobyns JH. Preiser's disease. Ann Chir MainMemb Super. 1991;10(3):227-35.
34. Lenoir H, Coulet B, Lazerges C, Mares O, Croutzet P, Chammas M. Idiopathic avascular necrosis of the scaphoid: 10 new cases and a review of the literature. Indications for Preiser's disease. Orthop Traumatol Surg Res. 2012Jun;98(4):390-7.
35. Seiler JG III. Flexor tendon injury. In: Wolf SW, Hotchkiss RN, Pederson WC, Kozin SH. Green's Operative hand surgery (sixth edition). Philadelphia, Elsevier 2011:189-244.
36. Strauch RJ. Extensor tendon injury. In: Wolf SW, Hotchkiss RN, Pederson WC, Kozin SH. Green's Operative hand surgery (sixth edition). Philadelphia, Elsevier 2011:159-188.
37. Ishiguro T, Inoue K, Matsubayashi N, et al. A new method of closed reduction of mallet fractures. Cent Jpn J Orthop Traumatol1998; 131:2049–2051.
38. Chan JS, Ip JW. Upper limb nerve injuries in sport. In: Luchetti R, Pegoli L, Bain GI. Hand and wrist injuries in combat sport. New York, Springer-Verlag 2018:297-303.
39. Olivo R, Tsao B. Peripheral Nerve Injuries in Sport. Neurol Clin. 2017 Aug;35(3):559-572.

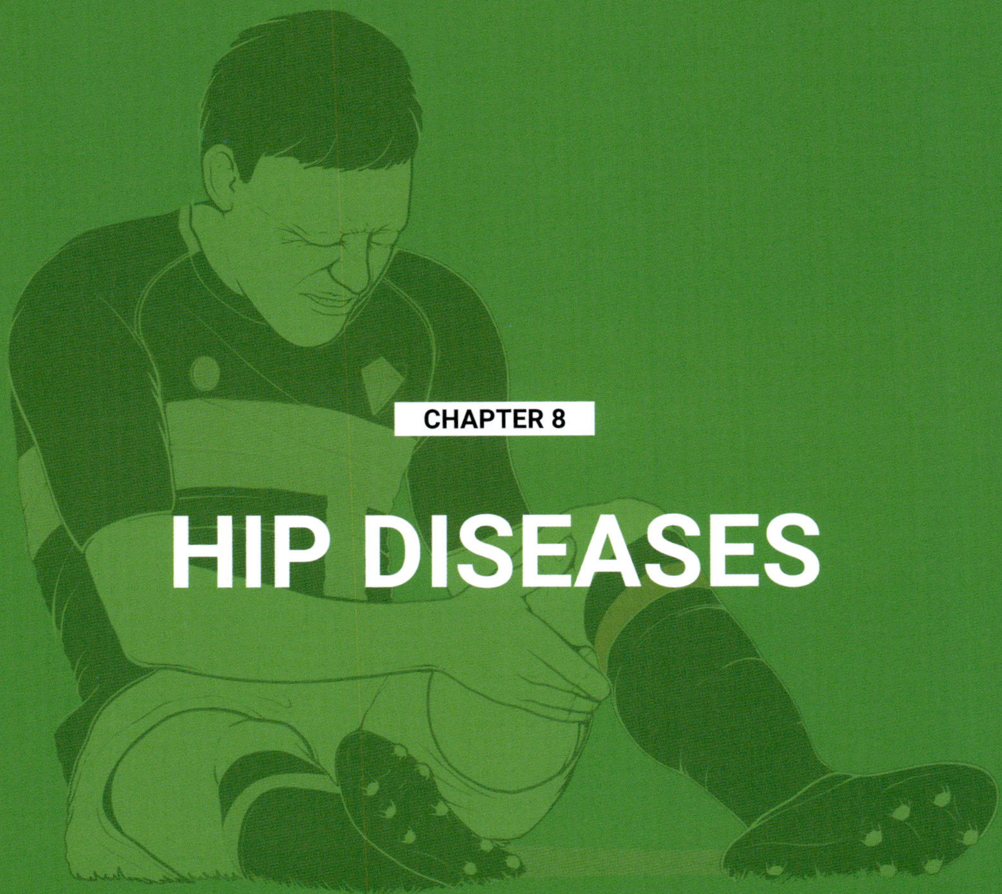

CHAPTER 8

HIP DISEASES

Francesco Traina [1, 2, 3]

Enrico Tassinari [1]

Francesco Castagnini [1]

Federico Giardina [1]

Federico Biondi [1]

[1] *Orthopaedic-Traumatology and Hip and Knee Replacement Surgery (Director: F. Traina) IRCCS Istituto Ortopedico Rizzoli, Bologna, Italy*

[2] *University of Bologna, Italy*

[3] *University of Messina, Italy*

Introduction

Hip and groin pain is more and more common in athletes at every age and at every competitive levels [1]. Groin pain accounts for 10% of all visits to sports medicine centers and groin injuries account for up to 6% of all athletic injuries. Sport activities correlated with acceleration/deceleration and cutting movements, like soccer, are more prone to hip pain. Diagnosis is challenging as hip pain recognizes multiple etiologies: some of them may coexist at the same time. Moreover, hip pain may modify the activities and movements of the athletes, leading to other important pathologies affecting knee, spine, and pelvic girdle [2, 3].

Categorization of pain and differential diagnosis are mandatory. First of all, non-musculoskeletal hip pain disorders should be ruled out. Gastrointestinal and genitourinary diseases may be considered. With regards to musculoskeletal hip pain, to date 5 clinical entities can be recognized: adductor related pain, iliopsoas related pain, abdominal wall related pain, pubic bone stress injury pain, and hip joint related pain [1, 3].

1. Adductor related (incidence in athletes: 33%): criteria for diagnosis require that palpation of adductor origin and passive stretch are painful. MRI is positive for adductor pathology.

2. Iliopsoas related (incidence in athletes: 12%): palpation, resisted hip flexion, and hip extension stretch evoke pain (modified Thomas test). Clicking is sometimes reported. Cross sectional imaging shows iliopsoas bursa or pathology.

3. Abdominal wall related (incidence in athletes: 11%): tenderness around rectus abdominis on palpation and resisted sit-up. "Sports hernia", inguinal or femoral hernia may be present (clinical diagnosis). MRI or ultrasound investigations are performed only to support unclear clinical findings.

4. Pubic bone stress injury related (incidence in athletes: 28%): tenderness over central pubic symphysis is reported, with central pain on adductor squeeze. All clinical criteria are diagnostic. MRI scan may show an increased signal at symphysis.

5. Hip joint related (intra-articular) (incidence in athletes: 56%): hip movements reproduce pain, range of motion is restricted. Diagnosis is mainly based on positive clinical criteria and radiology (radiographs or MRI), rarely on pain relief after intra-articular injections.

Intra-articular pathology and iliopsoas pain are more frequently diagnosed in female athletes, whereas males are usually more prone to other kinds of groin pain. The tendency for women to adopt greater hip adduction and knee abduction, the relative laxity of pubic symphysis, and psoas overwork in laxity may explain these findings. A common pattern observed in 22% of patients is the coexistence of hip joint pathology, pubic bone stress injury related, and adductor-related pain [2, 3].

In soccer, intra-articular pathologies are the most frequent cause of pain, followed by adductor related and pubic bone stress injury related pain. The other clinical entities are less common. When it comes to differential diagnosis, the most important issue is to differentiate intra-articular pathologies from extra-articular sources of pain [1, 3].

Intra-articular pathologies

Femoro-acetabular impingement

Femoro-acetabular impingement (FAI) is a hip pathology due to abnormal contacts between femoral head/neck and acetabular rim, resulting in labrum and cartilage damages [4]. FAI may prelude to

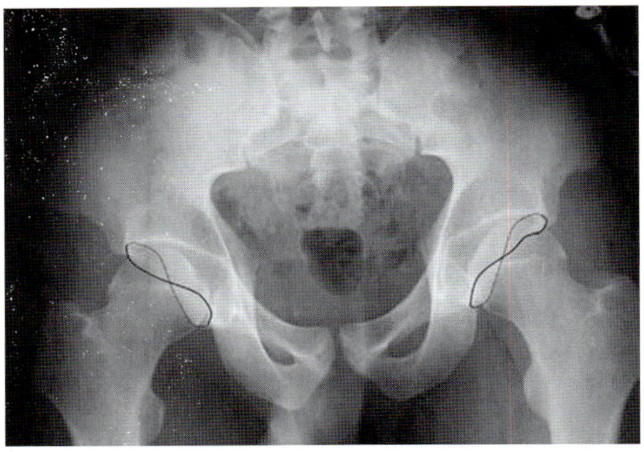

Figure 1 - Bilateral pincer deformity with a cross-over sign, showing an acetabular retroversion

osteoarthritis. FAI can be due to a prevalent acetabular deformity (pincer-deformity) or femoral deformity (cam-impingement). However, many cases are mixed, preferentially in male athletes (62%) [4, 7].

Pincer deformity is due to peripheral or global acetabular over-coverage, sustained by acetabular retroversion or protrusio acetabuli. This kind of impingement is usually associated to labral tears and countercoup chondral lesions (posteroinferior area of the hip) occurring as a consequence of subluxation (fig. 1). Articular degeneration occurs later in pincer deformities, while labrum gets torn quite precociously. By damaging the labrum, proprioceptive fibers generate precocious pain. Thus, symptomatology occurs early, before a substantial cartilage damage is evident. Females are usually more involved, between 30 and 40 years of age.

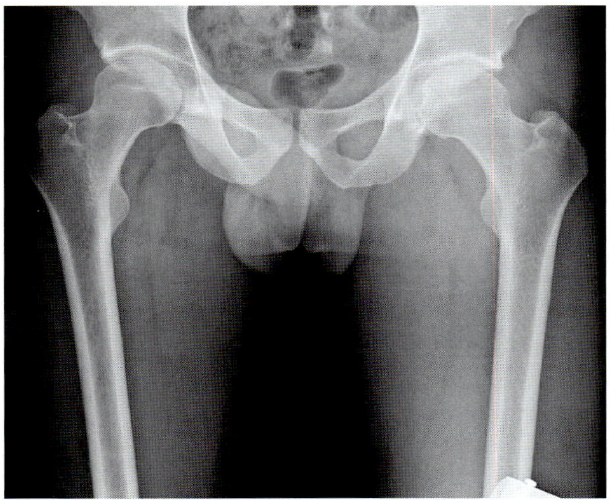

Figure 2 - Cam deformity in the right hip, with a clear femoral bump

Cam deformity is due to the loss of femoral sphericity and offset. Flexion and internal rotation cause the femoral bump to conflict with the acetabulum: an unstable chondral flap just adjacent to the labrum ensues, progressively exposing the subchondral bone (fig. 2). This is the beginning of articular degeneration in the anterosuperior portion of the hip. Cam impingement is frequent in 20-30 year old men.

FAI etiology is unknown in many cases [4, 7]. Some cases of FAI recognize specific etiologies like childhood hip disorders (developmental dysplasia of the hip, Legg-Calvè-Perthes disease, slipped capital femoral epiphysis). Overload and sport traumas are described as important causative factors. Hip injuries in soccer players were reported in 11%-16% of the cases. A prospective study showed that prevalence of FAI in elite soccer players increased from 7.1% to 22.2% of the cases in 2 years [5]. Younger players with open growth plates and high level athletes were more frequently involved (cam impingement) [5, 6]. In particular, the kicking leg was more predisposed to FAI, probably due to the femoro-acetabular impact during flexion and internal rotation [5, 6].

Diagnosis

FAI is a common origin of groin pain in young adults and athletes [4, 8]. Pain is gradual, progressive and more and more intense: it is usually elicited by prolonged sitting and cross-leg position. Some athletes report also lateral or buttock pain, but it is less frequent. C-sign is often reported: the patient's hand embraces a semicircular area around the groin. Range of motion is reduced, with internal rotation severely compromised or absent. The onset of pain, while performing passive maneuvers of flexion and rotation, can help to confirm the diagnosis, as it occurs in 99% of the FAI cases (Faber and Fadir tests). Posterior impingement is evocated with the hip hyperextended and in external rotation.

There is a wide consensus that FAI diagnosis can be made relying on a triad of symptoms, signs, and radiological features [7]. Diagnostic hip injections and cross-sectional imaging may help. Radiographic evaluation (antero-posterior and axial, possibly modified Dunn view) is mandatory [4-12]. It is important to assess the acetabular retroversion, coxa profunda, or protrusio acetabuli. These are varying degrees of overcoverage associated with pincer deformity: protrusio is the most severe and it occurs when the femoral head crossed the ilioischial line. In this case, only the cranial portion of the acetabulum is retroverted. The posterior wall should be assessed as well: crossover sign should be evaluated (two acetabular rims crossing). In case of acetabular retroversion, prominent extension of the ischial spine into the pelvis may be evident. Posterior acetabular rim lying medial to the center of rotation may highlight a lack of posterior wall coverage. Coxa profunda is not a very specific sign of global overcoverage: many athletes have signs of coxa profunda in dysplastic hips as well as non-impinging joints. Cam impingement is associated with radiographic signs of loss of offset or concavity between head and neck of the femur (pistol grip deformity).

Two angles should be measured [7, 9]. Lateral center-edge angle is subtended between a vertical axis up from the center of rotation and a line from the center of rotation and the lateral aspect of the sourcil. Lower values (<25°) indicate dysplasia, while larger angles (>39°) stand for global acetabular over-coverage. The alpha angle is important to assess the cam deformity (>60°): in the axial view, it is subtended between a line up to center of the femoral neck, from the center of rotation and the first point from which an asphericity is evident. Ct scans may improve the visualization of acetabular version and the amount of bone causing cam deformity: 2D and 3D reconstructions may be helpful [7]. MRI is another important diagnostic tool, as it allows to assess labral tear, chondral damage and subchondral bone edema [7].

Treatment

Non-operative treatments (activity restriction/modification, NSAIDs and muscular reinforcement focusing on abdominal muscles, lower back hip flexors and abductors) might be attempted, but it is unsuitable for athletes [8]. Moreover, the rate of failures is high due to mechanical symptoms and progressive chondral damages. Conservative treatments should be reserved to FAI patients with alpha angle less than 60° [8].

The Warwick agreement on FAI stated: "FAI syndrome can be treated by conservative care, rehabilitation, or surgery. Conservative care may involve education, watchful waiting, lifestyle, and activity modification. Physiotherapy-led rehabilitation aims to improve hip stability, neuromuscular control, strength, range of motion, and movement patterns. Surgery, either open or arthroscopic, aims to improve the hip morphology and repair damaged tissue. The good management of the variety of patients with FAI syndrome requires the availability of all of these approaches" [7].

Hip arthroscopy for FAI is probably the mainstay to date: it provides an adequate visualization of the joint and allows to surgically treat the mechanical symptoms, reducing the complications related to open field procedures to a minimum [9-11]. Nevertheless, the indications for arthroscopic management of FAI are not clear and guidelines are lacking. The most widespread guidelines for surgical treatment include: alpha angle higher than 60°, lateral center edge angle higher than 40°, presence of acetabular retroversion (crossover sign), MRI indicating intra-articular pathology (mostly, labral tear) and no evidence of inflammatory arthritis changes. Most of the surgeons rely on special clinical tests (70%), like Fadir, and radiology (90%) to indicate surgery. The main contraindications are related to hip arthritis and mild-to-severe dysplasia (arthroscopy may be an associate procedure more than a single surgical intervention).

After a careful pre-operative radiographic planning, surgery can be performed with the patient in lateral or supine (preferably) position [9, 11]. Traction, not prolonged for more than 2 hours, is applied and hip distraction (1 cm) is obtained thanks to a large, soft post pad. Nerve lesions (pudendal nerve) should be minimized by these precautions. The final position of the leg is 15° of flexion, 35° of internal rotation, 15° of lateral tilt, 45° of abduction. Soon after distraction, the leg is slightly adducted.

The procedure is usually performed using two portals, the standard anterolateral and the mid-anterior ones. Anterolateral portal is positioned over the greater trochanter (1-2 cm superior and 1-2 cm posterior), under fluoroscopic guidance. It is po-

sitioned in a safe zone, with the lateral cutaneous nerve far medial. It is important to avoid damages to the labrum and the chondral surfaces while inserting the instruments and setting the portal.
The mid-anterior portal is at the intersection of the tangent to the great trochanter and the tangent to the anterior-inferior iliac spine and is localized under direct visualization. The portal crosses the tensor fasciae latae and the gluteus minimum. The lateral femoral cutaneous nerve is potentially at risk: thus a careful incision and blunt dissection should be performed.
Capsular release is performed and it is necessary to easily perform the procedure. Usually, an inter-portal, T-shaped capsulotomy is enough to work, without compromising the hip stability and vascularization. The hip is visualized using a 70° arthroscopy. The central compartment should be adequately investigated: it includes labrum, articular surfaces, acetabular fossa, and a part of the femoral head. The peripheral compartment includes all the intra-capsular structures lateral to the labrum: part of the femoral head, the femoral neck, the capsule. After diagnostic visualization, the surgical procedure can be performed. The pincer impingement requires a labral repair/debridement, and the acetabuloplasty. Not infrequently, a procedure for the chondral damage is indicated (fig. 3). Cam impingement requires the femoral bump resection. Such procedure can be effectively

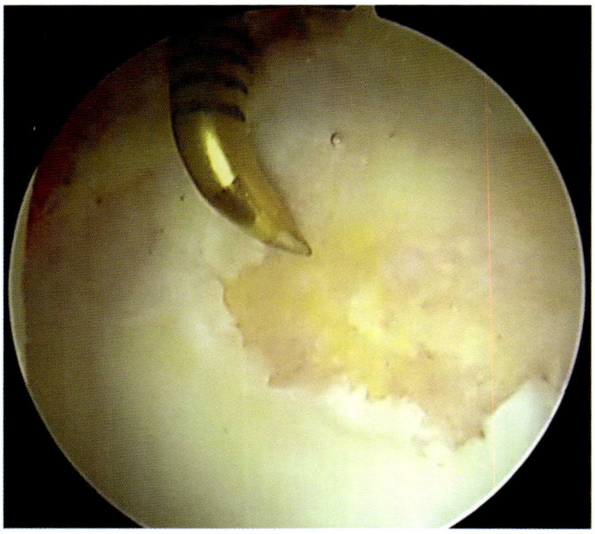

Figure 3 - Microfractures may help restore a fibrocartilage layer in acetabular chondral damages

performed using an high speed burr, in order to achieve an impingement free range of motion. The zone to be resected is defined as the convex part of the femoral head/neck passage with chondral damages and, sometimes, an herniation pit and a cyst. Lateral retinacular vessels should be addressed before starting femoral decompression. The bump is debrided with the hip in flexion, without traction, from the anterolateral working portal. Fluoroscopy and dynamic evaluation will confirm the amount of the bone to be resected: however, the exact amount of bone to be removed is not specified and it is at surgeon discretion (fig. 4). Capsular repair is recommended in order to reduce post-operative hip instability to a minimum.

Rehabilitation protocol
Evidence about rehabilitation and recovery in elite players are anecdotal and should be inferred from general patients [12]. Rehabilitation can be divided into 5 phases, according to the type of surgery and the patient's expectations. The general timetable includes:
1. Mobilization and isometric exercises (controlling pain and swelling): it takes around one month. Ice and anti-inflammatory medications play a pivotal role: a prophylaxis against periarticular ossification can be prescribed. It is important to avoid excessive weight bearing and promote exercises to improve range of motion and to prevent scars and adhesions.
2. Regain articular excursion, normalization of gait: it takes all the second month after surgery. Weight bearing is increased as tolerated, strengthening exercises and conditioning, avoiding impact activities, should be promoted. Normal gait mechanics should be achieved, with no signs of Trendelenburg limping.
3. Full strength recovery and endurance: from week 9 to week 12 after surgery. Full weight bearing, complete range of motions and strengthening exercises against resistance are usually allowed. A 90% recovery of the hip should be achieved.
4. and 5. Recovery of balance, proprioception and neuro-muscular control, functional recovery, and return to sport. Ability to complete plyometric exercises to regain the same pre-injury level without pain is the criteria for sport comeback. These two

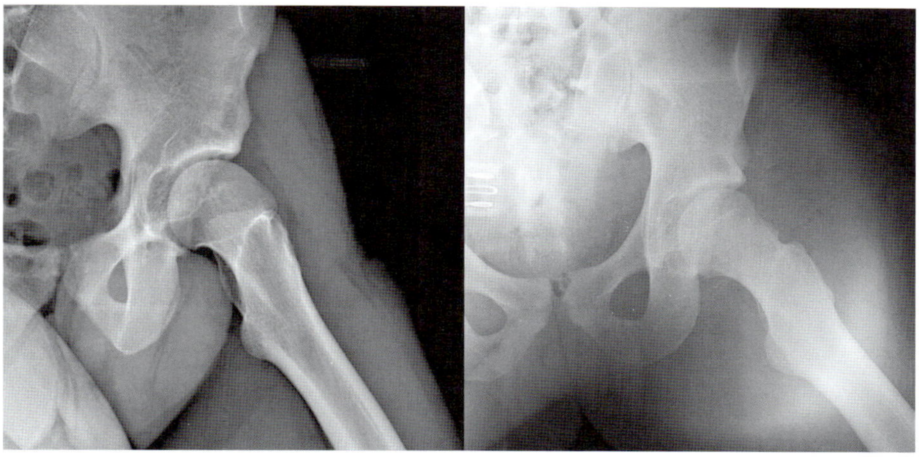

Figure 4 - Removal of femoral bump resolved the impingement symptomatology and restored the femoral sphericity (pre-operative lateral radiograph on the left, post-operative lateral radiograph after one month on the right)

phases usually take 4 months: however, athletes with a long pre-operative history of pain and limitations may need longer rehabilitation protocols. Forcing recovery is never recommended, as persistent pain, prolonged rehabilitation time, re-injury, or new injury may frequently ensue.

Outcomes of arthroscopic surgery in athletes: evidence from literature

Arthroscopic surgery was reported to be a valuable treatment for athletes: 92% of the athletes returned to sports, 88% of the players achieved the pre-injury level [11]. In a retrospective study by Locks et al. involving professional soccer players, 26 arthroscopic hip procedures in 24 athletes were evaluated [9]. All players had labral tears: focal cartilage damages (Outerbridge grade 0-2) occurred on acetabulum (69%) and femoral head (77%), with younger patients more frequently involved. Labral repair was performed in 73% of the cases, labral reconstruction in 27% of the players. Microfractures were performed in one quarter of the patients. 96% of the athletes returned to professional sport activity after a mean time of 9.2 months after arthroscopy. Professional players with national experience returned to sports after a mean of 6.2 months, earlier than younger and less experienced athletes [9, 11].

Labral tears

Labrum is a triangular tissue around the rim of the acetabulum: it is composed of fibrocartilage, a mixture of white fibrous and cartilaginous tissue [13, 14]. Together with the transverse acetabular ligament, the two structures join inferiorly to form a continuous ring. The most important role of the labrum is to seal the joint, permitting the formation of a pressurized layer of intra-articular fluid to both distribute and support compressive loads. Thus, labrum reduces stresses and strains on cartilage. The fluid provides a separation between articular surfaces. The labral seal is also crucial in maintaining hip stability through the suction effect created between the acetabulum and femoral head. Another main function is to deepen the acetabular socket and increase the contact areas. Thus, the labrum reduces cartilage contact pressure and strain. No direct involvement in mechanical loading has been described [13].

Etiologies of acetabular labral tears are traumatic, congenital (acetabular dysplasia or coxa profunda/ protrusio acetabuli), degenerative, and idiopathic [13, 14]. Many labral tears are concomitant with impingement [11]. When labral tear occur alone, most of them are caused by minor injuries from sporting (soccer and dance in particular) or even routine activities. Sudden hyperextension and external rotation (pivoting), as well as repetitive twisting movements leading to end-range hyperflexion, hyperextension, and abduction are the most common injury patterns. For a low-grade trauma without dislocation, the circumferential tearing typically occurs at the anterior region of the labrum. Circumferential tears do not compromise the stability of the joint if the lesion is shorter than 3 cm.

Diagnosis

Acetabular labral tears evoke hip pain in the inguinal region [13, 14]. Symptoms like clicking, snapping and locking, and the "dead-leg sign", are more specific. Labral tear usually occurs in the anteroposterior region, reducing the articular excursion in internal rotation and flexion. Fadir and Faber tests may recreate groin pain or mechanical symptoms by overloading the anterior-superior area of the hip. The two signs are positive in more than 95% of the labral tears. The McCarthy test is a very specific test for labral tears: the hip is flexed and then extended in external or internal rotation. The test is positive if it elicits pain or snapping during this forced movement. However, physical examination is not diriment and imaging is mandatory.

Plain radiography is useful to assess the whole joint, detecting impingement, dysplasia, or other congenital etiologies. Labral calcifications may be evident. Cross-table and frog-leg lateral radiographs are used to measure the anterior femoral head-neck morphology. 38% of the plain radiographs are normal in presence of labral tears and imaging for soft tissues is necessary.

MRI proves useful in labral tears. MRI provides detailed information regarding the soft tissues surrounding the hip, but conventional MRI is not sensitive enough for diagnosis of labral lesions. The most accurate imaging tool is MRI arthrography (fig. 5). The labral tears are classified according to Czerny et al. (0-IIIB stages) [15].

In this classification, the first stage is defined by an increased signal intensity of the labrum, not involving the surface and the triangular shape with perilabral recess. In stage 2, the contrast extends into the labrum, with no signs of detachment. In the third stage, there is a frank detachment. In all these stages, letter B stands for a thickened labrum. Only stages 2A-B and 3A-B are considered labral tears.

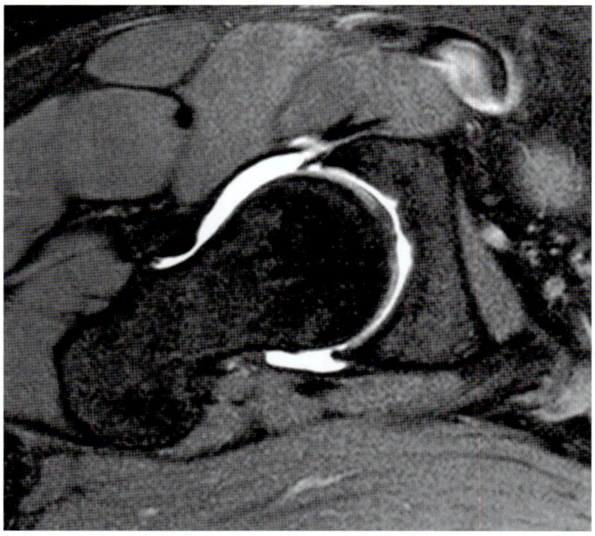

Figure 5 - MRI arthrography is the most accurate imaging tool to assess labral tear

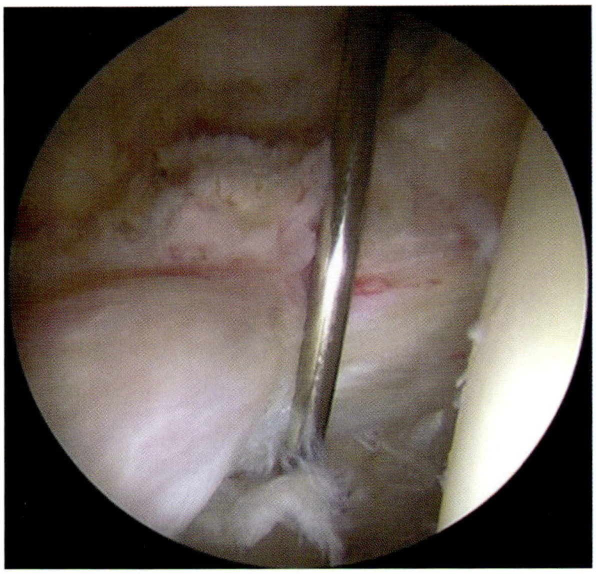

Figure 6 - A labral damage in a soccer player

Treatment

In an athlete, when a labral tear is diagnosed, the hip should be rested for 2 to 4 weeks [13, 14]. If the pain subsides, the athlete can resume activities and return to competition, following progressive rehabilitation protocols. If the conservative treatments are ineffective, surgery is warranted. Hips with a torn ligamentum teres are 16.2 times more likely to undergo surgery for failed conservative treatments [13, 14].

Labral tears may be approached with hip arthroscopy (fig. 6). Labral fraying or tears can be trimmed or shaved. Cartilage degeneration has been shown to be more prevalent post-operatively when labrum was resected. Labral re-fixation may be preferable, also because labrum heals after surgery. Thus, every attempt should be made to repair the labrum. The torn tissues are debrided, fibrocartilaginous tissue is stabilized to the rim of the acetabulum using a suture anchor positioned on the acetabular rim. Once the anchor is placed, using a suture passer, a limb of suture is positioned through a small portion of the substance of the

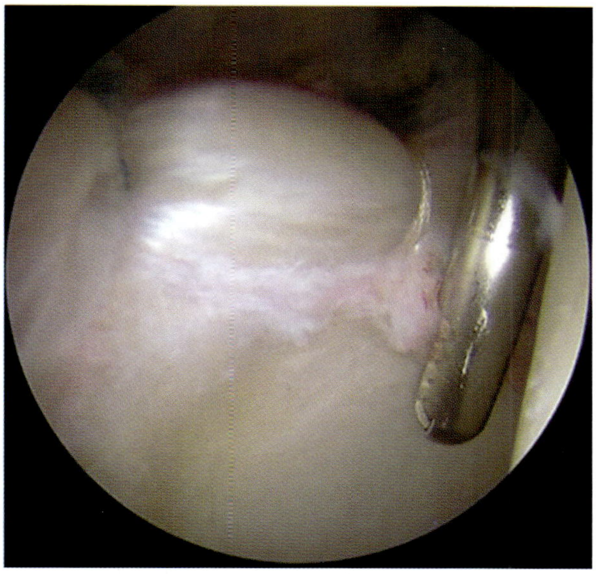

Figure 7- Labral repair in a soccer player: a concomitant chondral damage was evident

labrum. Then, the suture is retrieved and passed through the labrum a second time: a vertical mattress suture is eventually performed. The suture is tied down using standard arthroscopic knot-tying techniques (fig. 7). Recently, reconstruction has been proposed in cases where labrum cannot be repaired or is severely hypertrophic (<5 mm width) [14]. The proposed grafts are iliotibial band or gracilis tendons. When an iliotibial band is used, a small incision is performed to harvest a 20 mm wide graft. The graft is tubularized and introduced through the mid-anterior portal. The graft is sutured to the remaining stumps. Continuous passive movements are started soon after surgery. Restricted weight bearing is prescribed for 3-4 weeks similarly to labral repair.

The results in the athletes were positive: 86% of professional athletes returned to sport, 81% of the athletes returned to pre-injury level. 6 out of 7 professional soccer players resumed to sport at the same level [14]. Moreover, the histological samples after revision surgeries demonstrated histologically viable fibrovascular connective tissue with focal benign synovial type lining, showing that labral reconstruction is effective [14].

Loose bodies

Loose bodies occur in 6.3% of the athletes with intra-articular groin pain [16, 17]. Loose bodies in the hip joint can be ossified and non-ossified (cartilaginous, osteocartilaginous, fibrous, and foreign bodies). The main etiologies of osteocartilaginous loose bodies are osteophytes, osteochondritis dissecans, synovial osteochondromatosis, osteochondral fractures, and osteonecrosis [16, 17]. Foreign loose bodies may be due to broken materials during hip arthroscopy of prior hip surgery, as well as bullets.

Post-traumatic loose bodies are frequent after hip dislocations [17]. Thus, a radiograph or a CT scan is useful after reduction maneuvers to assess the presence of loose bodies. However, many loose bodies may be missed by conventional radiologic exams (even in 78% of the cases that were considered free of loose bodies after CT scan). To date, routinary hip arthroscopy after hip dislocation is not recommended [18]. However, after a traumatic dislocation, athletes may experience a constellation of intra-articular pathologies. Out of 14 athletes sustaining a simple dislocation during competition, all of these patients had labral tears and chondral defects. Half of them had chondral defects to both the acetabulum and femoral head. Most of them (11/14) had loose osteochondral fragments and the same rate of sportsmen experienced ligamentum teres tears.

Diagnosis

Clinical presentation is variable, as loose bodies may be numerous and with different sizes [16-18]. Anterior pain and locking (sometimes clicking) are frequent, usually evocated by maneuvers of flexion and internal rotation. Buttock pain could be also present and is due to loose bodies in the posterior and inferior aspect of the acetabulum.

Plain X-rays should be performed when loose bodies are suspected, looking for ossified and osteocartilaginous loose bodies. CT is useful to confirm the diagnosis. MRI may be helpful also to assess synovitis and fibrocartilaginous loose bodies. However, it should be kept in mind that MRI may fail to identify them.

Treatment

Loose bodies inside the joint deserve surgical treatment [16, 18] (fig. 8). Loose bodies are associated with joint effusion, synovitis, degradation to the intact articular cartilage, and precocious

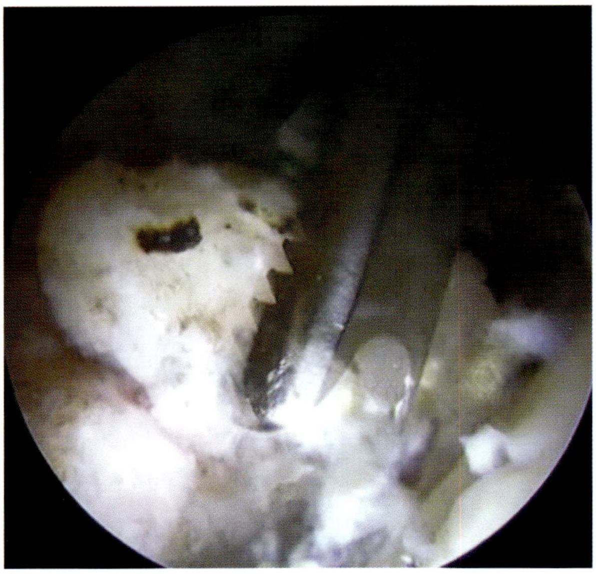

Figure 8 - Arthroscopic removal of a calcified loose body

osteoarthritis. Hip arthroscopy is useful [17, 18]. Portals should be planned according to the pre-operative imaging: for example, loose bodies next to the transverse ligament may be better approached using a posterolateral portal. Adequate distraction, mechanical morcelization of the fragment, and sequential removal of the fragments (the smallest one first, to avoid large portals and irrigation leakage) may be useful surgical pearls to ease a challenging surgery. Reparative procedures on cartilage are recommended. Prognosis is mainly related to the disease that generated loose bodies: the rate of coxarthrosis after hip dislocations is between 24 and 88% depending on the extent of acetabular damage and fracture.

Ligamentum teres injury

The ligamentum teres is a pyramidal shaped, intra-articular ligament of the hip: its course is from the acetabular notch and the transverse ligament of the acetabulum to the fovea of the femoral head [19, 20]. It is surrounded by a thin synovial lining, intimately tied to a posterior branch of the obturator artery and encompasses an undefined central sensory nerve supply. The role is unclear: it may provide additional stability in joint laxity and it is considered a secondary stabilizer. However, the ligamentum is rarely taut when distraction in hip arthroscopy is performed: thus, its role as a stabilizer is not clear. Its role in proprioception, nociception, and joint lubrication is debated as well: ligamentum teres may only be a vestigial structure. In athletes, ligamentum teres injury has been reported as one of the most common problems causing pain (and even this finding is not completely ascertained) [19]. It is a frequent finding in almost half of the arthroscopies (partial tear 43%, 4.5% degenerate tear, 3.7% complete rupture). Ligamentum teres injury can be traumatic (dislocations) but it is more commonly atraumatic associated with joint instability/microinstability. Ballet dancers are at very high risk of injury, but every athlete sustaining repetitive pivoting (external rotation and axial loading) and end-range movements may experience such a lesion.

Diagnosis

The onset of pain can be acute after a traumatic event, usually a dislocation, or subtle and persistent [19, 20]. It is located in the anterior groin or thigh, elicited during activities. Stiffness and reduce range of motion may be associated. Mechanical symptoms (catching, popping, locking, giving way) can be present but not specific. A provocative test (with the patient supine and the knee flexed to 90° the leg is moved through a full range of internal and external rotation) has been proposed. Apprehension tests for instability may be positive. MRI arthrography is the most useful imaging, despite the low sensibility and sensitivity: it is possible to distinguish between acute and chronic lesions. Arthroscopy remains the gold standard for diagnosing ligamentum teres pathology.

Treatment

Isolated tears have been associated with premature osteoarthritis, also because many ligamentum teres injuries are associated with larger sized labral tears, higher grades of acetabular cartilage injury, and femoral head cartilage defects [20]. Surgical treatment (debridement or reconstruction) has been recommended for athletes with persistent pain and instability following failed conservative management. It should be considered that in many cases restoration of hip control may compensate for a torn ligamentum teres.

Debridement is effective: the procedure is performed in slight external rotation, sometimes a more posterior portal can be used. A complete resection of the ligamentum may result in iatrogenic instability of the hip and a capsular tightening should be added to debridement. Thus, in case of partial tears, shrinkage of the ligament with a radiofrequency device, while the hip is in neutral position, may be suggested: this procedure improves haemostasis and the biomechanical strength of the remaining ligament. A limitation of external rotation of the hip may ensue. Arthroscopic reconstruction of the ligamentum teres has been performed, using artificial ligaments or semitendinosus or iliotibial autograft. Recurrence of ligamentum teres tears was reported in 17% of the patients within 12 to 48 months after the reconstruction [20]. Graft resorption or synovitis were reported as well. To date no guidelines regarding the correct surgical treatment of ligamentum teres injury exist, although debridement appears appropriate.

Extra-articular pathologies

Greater trochanteric pain syndrome

Greater trochanteric pain syndrome is a painful syndrome located at the lateral-side of the hip: it includes trochanteric bursitis, gluteus medius or minimus tears, and external coxa saltans [21]. Although greater trochanteric pain syndrome generally occurs in sedentary individuals, athletes can also be affected. Female runners, older than 40 years, are at higher risk. Gluteus medius or minimus tendinopathy and tears are the most common pathologies and are often found in patients with recalcitrant trochanteric bursitis (usually secondary to tendinopathy) [21, 22].

The pathomechanics of this syndrome is complex. Mechanical loadings drive the biological processes within a tendon, designing its structural form and load-bearing capacity through an equilibrium between catabolic and anabolic processes. Compressive (transverse) tendon load induces catabolic responses, whereas tensile (longitudinal) tendon load is responsible for catabolic and anabolic effects. A rapid increase in the intensity and/or frequency of tensile loading may start a non-equilibrated catabolic effect, in particular if compressive forces are combined. The consequence is tendon degeneration [21, 22]. The natural history of abductor tendinopathy starts with tendonitis, tendinopathy, partial thickness tears and, in the end, massive tears. Joint position (particularly excessive hip adduction) is believed to induce negative structural changes, increasing tensile force,s and shielding compressive ones. Iliotibial band tension (due to valgus knee alignment, varus neck-shaft angles, and leg length discrepancy) may exacerbate this condition.

Diagnosis

The most common clinical features of gluteal tendinopathy are pain (insidious or acute) and tenderness at the greater trochanter [21, 22]. Irradiations to buttocks, lateral hip, and groin pain are not rare due to the complex nerve supply to the peritrochanteric compartment. Patients may complain of activities that require hip abduction such as getting up from a seated position or climbing stairs. A gluteus medius avulsion involves clear limping and Trendelenburg gait (a distinct drop of the non-support pelvis indicates weakness or loss of function). Clinical examination is performed with the patient in a lateral decubitus: the examiner should palpate the anterior, lateral, and posterior aspect of the greater trochanter for tenderness. Abductor strength testing (against gravity or resistance) can be performed with knee flexed and extended. A reliable test for abductor tendinopathy was proposed by Lequesne et al.: single-leg stance should be maintained for 30 seconds, avoiding lateral trunk displacement and allowing gentle fingertip support for balance. The test is positive if pain was elicited at the lateral side. Ober's test should be performed as well. In addition, flexion, abduction, and external rotation (Faber) test may also elicit pain. Plain radiographs can be helpful to rule out intra-articular pathologies and may demonstrate calcific tendonitis. MRI and ultrasonography are more effective: cross sectional imaging for soft tissues shows bursitis, enthesopathic changes along trochanteric insertion and fatty atrophy. Thickened tendons and tears may be visualized. MRI has a sensitivity of 73 % and a specificity of 95 %.

Treatment

Conservative management is usually effective: exercise and strategies to manage tendon load, shock wave therapy, and corticosteroid injections are usually adopted [21, 22]. For athletes, controlling tendon load is fundamental: complete rest, rapid changes in training and activities involving combinations of compression, and high tensile load are not advisable. Gluteal stretching should be avoided. An appropriate rehabilitation program for athletes includes restriction of longer-distance and higher-speed running and other activities involving high eccentric abductor loads, such as hopping and bounding. Modifications of running technique (reduction of hip adduction and increase in cadence) might also be required.

When conservative treatments fail, surgical intervention is considered. Endoscopic treatment can be performed in either the lateral position on a standard table or in the supine position on the fracture table. Using the supine decubitus, the patient is positioned on a hip traction table and a 1 cm distraction is obtained. Once the tip of the greater trochanter is identified, an anterolateral portal (ALP) is established. A diagnostic arthroscopy of the central compartment is performed and intra-articular pathologies are addressed. Traction is then released and the leg is abducted 15–20°. The peritrochanteric space is entered using a 5.0 mm metal cannula through the mid-anterior portal over the vastus ridge. The cannula aimed to a point between the iliotibial band and the lateral part of the greater trochanter. The arthroscope and light source are both directed proximally: in this way, the distal peritrochanteric space is visualized. A bursectomy with shaver is performed. After bursal debridement, the gluteus medius and minimus are easily visualized. The tear is appreciated along with the quality of tissues, and the mobility of the tendons is adequately investigated. A grasper is then used to approximate the tendon to the anatomic footprint without tension. The cortical bone near the footprint is debrided to achieve bleeding. Tears are usually repaired with a single row, using one to two suture anchors. Massive tears may require a double-row suture bridge. Anchors are positioned percutaneously via a posterolateral portal. The hip is rotated to ensure anatomic reduction and fixation of the torn gluteus medius tendon. Postoperative protocol requires bracing with partial weight bearing for the first 6 weeks after surgery. Passive range of motion is suggested in order to prevent adhesions. From 6 to 8 weeks, the patient will progress to full weight bearing, protected by the harness. Repair of tears is not always effective and surgery may not provide any advantage over conservative techniques. Repair of chronic tears may be more difficult and less satisfying, in particular if fatty atrophy is abundant. Surgery for refractory lateral hip pain (including endoscopic techniques with iliotibial band release) is debated. Surgery may not address the injury mechanism, may miss the tendinopathy and may even compromise posture and muscular balance. Recently, an increasing interest in regenerative medicine has aroused: to date, there is no evidence, but some preliminary results are promising.

Internal snapping hip syndrome

Snapping hip syndrome or coxa saltans interna is a hip syndrome involving the iliopsoas tendon snapping pathologically over structures beneath it (usually iliopectineal eminence) [23, 26]. A loud audible click or clunk, associated with pain, ensues: it is due to the back-and-forth movement of the tendon over the anterior hip capsule and femoral head. Iliopsoas bursa may become inflamed or hypertrophic. Symptomatic snapping is commonly seen in activities involving large range of motion, including soccer. A symptomatic snapping has been described in 40% of the population [24].

Diagnosis

Pain, popping, clunking, and clicking may be present, often after a trauma [24, 26]. The initial pain from the injury typically never resolves, and the snap hurts: sports or activities requiring hip flexion may be painful. In supine position, the patient is able to reproduce the pain. The diagnostic test for coxa saltans interna is performed by the examiner applying pressure over the anterior hip capsule (restricting the tendon's movements): this test can eliminate the snap. External snapping hip should be excluded.

Plain radiographs are not diagnostic and may be helpful to trace out exostoses or spurs or impingement. MRI is useful to detect any thickening of the iliopsoas tendon or fluid in the bursa: intra-articular pathologies should be investigated and are a frequent concomitant finding. Pain relief by a lidocaine injection in the bursa is a valuable diagnostic test. Every other diagnosis must be excluded, in particular labral tears, synovial chondromatosis, and FAI or other predisposing intra-articular pathologies [24, 26].

Treatment

Physical therapy is frequently successful. Steroid injections may alleviate pain [24, 26]. The lengthening of the tendon performed through an open surgical approach is invasive; it may cause snapping recurrence, hip flexor weakness, and loss of sensation. Complications of the open procedure are as high as 21%. A iliopsoas tendon lengthening can be effectively performed arthroscopically. The complication rate is much lower (2.3%) and intra-articular pathologies may be adequately addressed at the same time, improving the clinical results. Iliopsoas release may be performed at three sites: at the central compartment, at the peripheral compartment, and at the lesser trochanter. Although at the three different sites the ratio tendon to muscle is different, no significant differences could be traced between the three techniques. Some sort of muscular weakness is frequently reported as a consequence of the release.

Iliopsoas impingement is another recognized pathology of the hip, occurring when an excessively thigh tendon impinges on the acetabular labrum (a repetitive traction on the anterior capsule is another possible pathogenesis) [23, 26]. This condition results in a typical labral abnormality: a direct anterior labral tears at the 3 o'clock position in the absence of bony abnormalities (differently from FAI, at 1-2 o'clock position). In some cases, the labrum appears inflamed without frank tears. Young active women involved in sports are more commonly affected. Regarding the clinical symptoms, the pattern is quite similar to coxa saltans interna, but snapping is less commonly described (17%). Positive Faber test and tenderness over the psoas are common. Surgical management of iliopsoas impingement is lengthening of the iliopsoas tendon and treatment of concurrent labral abnormality, with the same modalities and techniques described above [24, 26].

External snapping hip syndrome

External snapping hip syndrome, or coxa saltans externa, is more common than coxa saltans interna. It generally occurs in female patients with wide pelvis and prominent trochanter [27, 28]. Soccer players are at risk, similarly to all the athletes who perform repetitive extreme hip motions. It is due to the thickening of the posterior third of the iliotibial band. The band normally lies posterior to the greater trochanter in neutral position: adduction and flex-extension movements may cause the band to move over the trochanter. Pain may ensue if the trochanteric bursa becomes inflamed. However, snapping can also be asymptomatic, especially in athletes.

Diagnosis

Pain and tenderness are common over the trochanteric area [27, 28]. Flex-extension causes pain and snapping. The single leg bicycle maneuver in lateral decubitus may reproduce iliotibial band snapping. The Ober test may show a taut band, suggesting a possible surgical treatment. Gluteal muscles should be evaluated to check for weakness and tears. Coxa saltans interna must be ruled out.

Treatment

Conservative treatment is usually effective [29]. Anti-inflammatory drugs, physical therapy, cortisone injections are useful to improve many snapping hips. 66% of the affected patients returned to sports after conservative management. Surgical treatment should be reserved to those cases where a 6 to 12 month conservative management has failed. Open bursectomy and band release can be performed using an open procedure: the reported outcomes were encouraging. Also Z-plasty and open bursectomy were proposed, in order to avoid a defect in the iliotibial band, which may theoretically predispose to abductor deficiency (not proved). To date, endoscopic bursectomy and longitudinal band release are another, less invasive possible treatment in recalcitrant snapping hips. The access to the peritrochanteric space is done through the anterolateral portal (to check the central compartment), the mid-anterior portal (visualization), posterior-lateral portal (working). Through the posterior-lateral portal, an 11 blade on a scalpel is used to incise 2-3 cm of the iliotibial band, in line with the fibers. At the midpoint of the incision, two 1.5 cm perpendicular incisions are performed, anteriorly and posteriorly. Using a shaver, the flaps are debrided to achieve a final diamond configuration. The endoscopic technique was able to relieve the pain and, in many cases, managed to reduce snapping. Weakness in abduction may be a complication of the surgical treatment, in particular if the release is excessive or there is damage to the surrounding area [29].

A special condition: ischiofemoral impingement

Some cases of snapping (4-5%) do not improve with iliopsoas tendon release and subsequent revision; at the same time, they cannot be ascribed to coxa saltans interna [30, 31]. An ischiofemoral impingement may be the cause of some of these failures. This condition is defined as a narrowing of the space between the lateral aspect of the ischium and the lesser trochanter. A mechanical entrapment of soft tissues (in particular, quadratus femoris) ensues [30, 31].

Diagnosis

This condition may cause groin/buttock pain which can irradiate distally [30, 31]. A sciatica-like pain is quite common, due to nerve proximity. Popping or grating sensations may be reported. Palpation is useful to evoke tenderness around the insertion of the quadratus femoris, which easily gets entrapped in this kind of impingement. Symptoms (pain and snapping) tend to worsen during running, posing soccer female athletes at risk. Painless patients might exhibit functional leg length discrepancy due to compensatory abduction of the leg (to avoid impingement).
Radiographs may show coxa valga, or any other deformities which may predispose to the narrowing of the ischiofemoral space, and consequently to ischiofemoral impingement. Also previous osteotomies may be important predisposing factors. MRI is an useful imaging tool: it may allow to assess the entrapment of the quadratus femoris, resulting in muscular edema and fatty degeneration. Radiology allows to measure the ischiofemoral space: it has been reported that ischiofemoral impingement occurs when a narrowing of 15 mm or less is present [30].

Treatment

Conservative treatment should be attempted [30, 31]. Physiotherapy for strengthening and stretching of the quadratus femoris muscle and all the other external rotators of the hip should be performed. NSAIDs, gabapentin, added interferential current therapy, and ultrasound-guided infiltrations with corticosteroids are often effective along with physical therapy.
Surgery is rarely recommended, only in case of recalcitrant symptomatology and failure of conservative management. Open or endoscopic resection of the lesser trochanter or ischioplasty were suggested as possible surgical procedure for ischiofemoral impingement. However the literature is scarce (the condition is rare and often misdiagnosed) and evidence is currently lacking.

A special condition: subspine impingement

Subspine impingement can be defined as the presence of abnormal bony morphology between the acetabular rim and the caudad border of the anterior-inferior iliac spine, resulting in soft tissue and/or bony impingement [32, 33]. Subspine impingement can be developmental or secondary, to prior anterior-inferior ischial spine avulsion or pelvic osteotomy. Developmental impingement is commonly encountered in cases with acetabular retroversion and in some specific ischial spine morphologies (type II: bony prominence between the caudad area and the acetabular rim, or the caudad area is at the level of the acetabular rim; type III: the caudad level extends distally to the anterosuperior acetabular rim). Type II and III ischial spine morphologies may result in decreased hip flexion and internal rotation, generating subspine impingement. However, a recent study demonstrated that subspine impingement can occur in the setting of a normal ischial spine morphology, in particular when lower degrees of femoral anteversion and more limited forward flexion and internal rotation are present.
Antero-inferior ischial spine avulsion may occur after a sudden and violent contraction of the rec-

tus femoris: it is defined as "sprinter's fracture", but it is not unusual in kicking sports [32, 33]. In many cases, prodromic signs (pain and tenderness over iliac spine) can be reported. The consequences of the avulsion (exostosis, myositis ossificans, non-anatomic union) are the common reasons for subspine acquired impingement.

Diagnosis

The most common complaint is anterior hip and groin pain [32, 33]. It is usually exacerbated by straight hip flexion and sitting. Hip adduction and internal rotation may evoke pain as well. Tenderness on the ischial spine is frequent. Radiographic findings may include spine avulsion, acetabular retroversion, anterior rim sclerosis, and calcific deposits at the rectus femoris origin. A cyst at the distal femoral neck may reveal the subspine impingement and may help with differential diagnoses. CT scan better defines spine deformities, avulsion and its complications.

Treatment

Arthroscopic decompression is the preferred treatment [32, 33]. It can be achieved as an extension of the acetabuloplasty in a superior direction, above the capsule, to the insertion of the rectus femoris. This approach is particularly valuable in order to address intra-articular pathologies as well. Many case series described good outcomes after contemporary arthroscopic treatment of FAI and subspine impingements. However, the long operating time and the possible fluid leakage should be constantly monitored.

Endoscopic decompression is suggested when iliac spine deformities require a distal and inferior extension. In these cases, capsular repair may be difficult if the deformity is arthroscopically approached and instability is a significant risk. Thus, an endoscopic approach may be beneficial. The iliac spine is localized using fluoroscopy and the bony deformities may be debrided using a mechanical burr and radiofrequencies. The muscle/tendon unit (direct head of rectus femoris) should be preserved. Complications after endoscopy have not been accurately described: it is believed that preserving capsule and avoiding fluid extravasation may potentially improve post-operative results. Other major complications such as avascular necrosis, femoral neck fractures, adhesions or gluteal vessel, and sciatic nerve injuries have not been reported.

Pubalgia

Athletic pubalgia is a syndrome of the lower abdomen and groin region, affecting athletes involved in sports with repetitive twisting and turning [34, 35]. Such movements tend to increase torque and tension on the dynamic stabilizers of the anterior pelvis. Rectus abdominis-adductor complex is the most often affected compartment. Failure of the transversalis fascia and the formation of a bulge in the posterior wall of the inguinal canal are a common part of the pathomorphologic spectrum of athletic pubalgia.

A large amount of groin pathologies have been referred to athletic pubalgia, among them osteitis pubis, adductor injuries, and sports hernias. These pathologies are often the result of repetitive stresses or overuse: 44% of athletic patients with these pathologies play soccer. The vast majority of the cases related to athletic pubalgia tend to be self-limiting. However it is not uncommon that a few cases become chronic and debilitating: in these cases, conservative treatments are generally ineffective and surgical procedures should be considered.

Osteitis pubis

Osteitis pubis is a chronic, inflammatory overuse condition of the pubic symphysis and surrounding soft tissues, clinically causing pain and local tenderness over the symphysis [35, 36].

Athletes are frequently affected, in particular when sport activities involve kicking, twisting, pivoting, and sprinting. Osteitis pubis accounts for 3%-5% of injuries per year in male soccer players.

The etiology is still unclear. Repetitive stresses may cause symphysis instability and inflammation (periosteitis and osteitis). Force imbalance of abdominal and adductor muscles on the pubic symphysis may increase the stresses and implement the vicious circle of symphysitis, joint instability, and muscular imbalance. Reduced hip internal rotation has been advocated as a predisposing risk factor.

Grade	MRI findings	Prognosis: complete recovery
I	Bone marrow edema + highest mean normalized STIR SI <3 +/- periarticular edema	100%
II	Bone marrow edema + highest mean normalized STIR SI <3 + edema in the muscles around the symphyseal joint	50%
III	Bone marrow edema + highest mean normalized STIR ≥3 +/- one of the following: periarticular edema or edema in the muscles around the symphyseal joint	30%
IV	Bone marrow edema + highest mean normalized STIR >3 + periarticular edema +edema in the muscles around the symphyseal joint	20%

Table 1 - Pubalgia: MRI findings in 4 grades, with prognostic value (Gaudino et al. [36])

Diagnosis

Clinical history and the physical examination are capital [35, 36]. Anterior, unilateral groin pain, irradiated to adductors, is the most frequent clinical presentation. Pain may exacerbate and irradiate to the local areas: bilateral presentation is common in the most advanced cases.

Tenderness on palpation of the symphyseal region is common. However, other clinical examinations are not standardized: provocative tests and pain relief after anesthetic injections in the pubic symphysis have been proposed. Due to complex presentation and the subtle clinical findings, differential diagnoses should be accurately assessed.

Imaging may help complete the diagnosis, but it is not diriment. Plain radiographs may show bony sclerosis, erosion or joint degeneration, but only in advanced cases. Pelvis MRI is more informative about the symphysis and the surrounding soft tissues, tendons and bone structures: moreover, it is effective at ruling out other causes of groin pain.

MRI findings may be stratified in 4 grades, with prognostic value, as described by Gaudino et al. [36] (tab. 1). The normalized STIR parameter was calculated at the pubic zone, evaluated after normalization with the mean ipsilateral iliopsoas. Kurger et al. evaluated also the articular fluid in the symphysis, but this parameter poorly correlated with the outcome.

Treatment

Osteitis pubis is a self-limiting condition that improves with rest and physical therapy (stretching and strengthening) in 3 months [35, 36]. Local injections may alleviate pain for a short time. Management of osteitis pubis is sometimes difficult (5-10%) and athletes may not accept long periods of rest. Many different open or minimally invasive surgical procedures have been proposed, like curettage, arthrodesis, and wedge resection.

Open surgery should be discouraged. Endoscopic surgery should be evaluated with care. Saito et al. highlighted an important correlation between FAI and osteitis pubis in soccer players: after FAI treatment only, osteitis pubis strongly improved and 90% of the athletes returned to sport at the pre-injury level.

Sports hernia

Sports hernia is poorly understood and many misnomers have been attributed to this pathology [34, 37, 38]. First, sports hernia is not a true hernia. It encompass a variety of pathologic findings, with a common sign: a dilated and weak internal inguinal ring due to excessive tensions related to sport activities. This tension causes tears of inguinal structures (conjoined tendon, external oblique muscle, or inguinal ligament). Many athletes tend to experience loss of hip range of motion and FAI, as well as osteitis pubis and muscle strains.

Diagnosis

The clinical presentation is an insidious onset of unilateral, deep groin pain [34, 37, 38]. Coughing may cause pain, irradiating into the thigh or testicles. Sports hernia should meet 5 diagnostic criteria: dull or diffuse pain radiating to the medial aspect of the thigh, perineum, or contralateral side; tenderness to palpation over the pubic tubercle at the insertion of the inguinal ligament; tenderness to palpation of the deep inguinal ring; tenderness to palpation of the adductor longus tendon; tenderness or dilation of the superficial inguinal ring. Radiographs are useful to rule out other diagnoses. The only helpful imaging technique is MRI: rectus abdominis strain or tear from the pubic ramus and a partial or complete adductor longus detachment are the common findings.

Treatment

A minimum of 2 months of rest and rehabilitation (strengthening, functional movements, posture, sport-specific physical activity) before surgical approaches should be recommended [37, 38].

Treatment of sports hernia is surgical: exploration and repair of the weak posterior inguinal wall, with laparoscopic or open techniques, is generally performed. The surgical treatment is usually successful, with good outcomes ranging from 80% to 97% of the cases. The athlete can return to sport after 2 to 6 weeks after laparoscopic interventions; open procedures require longer rehabilitation (from 1 to 6 months).

Hip instability

Young athletes may experience subluxation or dislocation of the hip [39]. The first classification is in traumatic or atraumatic cases. Traumatic hip dislocation generally results from a high-energy trauma, usually accompanied by many associate lesions. The mechanism of dislocation is an axially applied force against a flexed knee with the hip in the neutral or adducted position. In children, even a low-energy mechanism may lead to hip dislocation or subluxation, but associated injuries are less likely. The most common direction of dislocations is posterior. The patient accesses to the emergency department with severe pain: the hip is held in the flexed, adducted, and internally rotated position. Plain radiographs confirm the diagnosis. Reduction is mandatory and should be performed in 6 hours: then a radiograph should be performed to check for accurate reduction. CT or MRI are indicated if an incongruent reduction and an intra-articular pathology is suspected. After reduction, restricted weight bearing is suggested for 6 weeks. Recurrent instability following closed management of a true dislocation is rare [39, 40]. In case of instability, capsular or other soft-tissue laxity may be present and should be addressed with physical therapy. If conservative management is unsuccessful, arthroscopic capsular plication effectively stabilizes the joint. If arthroscopic thermal capsulorrhaphy has been proposed, cartilage injury is a possible undesirable complication. In patients with a nonconcentric reduction, a loose body or an acetabular fracture of the posterior wall may be present and should be addressed surgically. Arthroscopy is useful to remove loose bodies, to fix fragments (Pipkin fracture) and to repair/debride labral tears.

A traumatic instability has a more subtle and chronic symptomatology: groin and/or lateral hip pain, activity-related pain relieved with rest, and limp are common [40]. The hyperlax female athlete with acetabular dysplasia is the most commonly involved patient. Radiographs are useful to detect and quantify dysplasia and joint degeneration. MRI provides information about iliocapsularis muscle and anterior hip capsule, joint degeneration, labral tears, chondromalacia, synovitis, or abnormal joint biomechanics.

A recent classification defined instability according to acetabular dysplasia, identifying three main patterns of acetabular deficiency/uncoverage.

- Anterior instability: it is suggested by pain at all the activities that put the hip near the end-range extension (anterior femoral head translation) and after prior surgeries compromising stability (arthroscopy, psoas lengthening). Clinically, apprehension test and apprehension-relocation test in an extended position may be positive. Radiographs show normal lateral center-edge angle and anterior acetabular deficiency.
- Posterior instability: it is mainly due to posterior acetabular wall insufficiency and anterior acetabular overcoverage (prevalent pincer deformity).

Pain may be exacerbated by activities that load the hip in a flexed position. Posterior pain and posterior apprehension test may be positive. Sciatica-like pain is not uncommon, as well as anterior pain. Imaging shows posterior wall deficiency (crossover sign, positive ischial sign) and normal lateral center-edge angle.

- Global instability: superolateral deficiency is typical (classic pattern of acetabular dysplasia), even if anterior or posterior wall undercoverage may be evident. Symptoms of static overload (prolonged walking) are frequent. Lateral center-edge angle is low.

Conservative treatment is the first attempt, using intra-articular injections and physical therapy [39, 40]. In case of intra-articular pathology, hip arthroscopy should be performed, even if the results in mild dysplasia and instability tend to be less satisfying and do not address the underlying pathology. In case of significant dysplasia, acetabular reorientation osteotomy should be considered. Periacetabular osteotomies in athletes were correlated with an important post-operative improvement. 85% of the athletes returned at the same level and managed to maintain the same level at a mean follow-up of 3 years. However, the subjective outcomes about athletic performances were satisfying in only 50% of the patients.

Fractures

Apophyseal avulsion

In children and adolescents, the ligaments, tendons, and muscles are much stronger than the secondary ossification centers (apophysis). Thus, avulsions are commonly encountered in young athletes due to injury mechanisms which, in adults, would preferentially lead to muscle strains [41, 42]. Participation in sports have dramatically increased the rate of apophyseal avulsion fractures of the pelvis over the last few decades. The mechanism of lesion is a sudden forceful muscle contraction, while accelerating/decelerating, or changing direction. The forceful pull against the apophysis leads to its separation from the rest of the pelvis. Sports involving such types of movements (rapid acceleration/deceleration or change in direction), like soccer, are at high risk. The ischial tuberosity (54%), the anterior inferior iliac spine (22%) and anterior superior iliac spine (19%) are more commonly involved, particularly in male athletes.

Diagnosis and treatment

The adolescent male athlete is at high risk [41,42]. The clinical presentation is a sudden pain and swelling after noncontact traumatic incident. Concomitant popping or snapping may be reported. The pain can be acute and the athlete is unable to ambulate comfortably, maintaining a position that relieves the tension in the involved muscle group. Radiographs confirm the diagnosis. The majority of these cases are treated non-operatively with an initial period of non-weight bearing, progressing to weight-bearing as tolerated. Then gentle range of motion and flexibility training can be started: gradual strengthening, proprioception, and balance are suggested. Surgical indications are generally reserved for ischial tuberosity fractures with >2 cm displacement, symptomatic nonunion, chronic pain, and impaired function.

Ischial tuberosity avulsion fractures

The ischial tuberosity is the origin of the semitendinosus, semimembranosus muscles, and the long head of biceps femoris [41, 42]. The ischial apophysis of the adolescent pelvis is quite weaker than the hamstring muscles: thus, ischial tuberosity avulsion fractures frequently involve young active population in soccer. In adults, a pathological fracture should always be ruled out. A sudden onset of disabling pain in the posterior thigh/buttock is typical, with swelling, bruising, and tenderness. Sometimes, sciatica is reported. Radiographs are confirmatory, CT and MRI should be used in more chronic or suspect cases. The treatment of nondisplaced or minimally displaced fractures is merely conservative. Open reduction and internal fixation are usually performed in case of 2 cm diastasis in order to avoid painful, fibrous nonunion: excision is an option when ORIF fails. Surgery is performed in prone decubitus. The ischial tuberosity is exposed and the proximal hamstring stump is visualized. Sciatic nerve and the posterior cutaneous nerve of the thigh are at risk and should be protected as well as the inferior gluteal nerve. ORIF can be performed. In case of proximal tendon lesions (usually occurring in adults when the bony prominence is stronger), if the stump is valid, a direct repair is performed. Otherwise, suture anchors are used.

Anterior iliac spine avulsion fractures

The ASIS is the origin of sartorius and tensor fasciae latae; AIIS is the origin of the direct head of the rectus femoris [41, 42]. Lesions to the apophysis share a similar mechanisms, after sprinting or kicking. ASIS or AIIS avulsions cause a sudden onset of pain in the anterior pelvic area and a popping. Swelling and tenderness over the spine ensue, along with reduced range of motion and antalgic position. Radiographs are confirmatory. Treatment is conservative: athletes will have a full recovery after 2-4 months. Some Authors advocated surgical treatment (ORIF), as the avulsed fragments tend to reattach more distally and abundant callus formation, malunions, and symptomatic nonunions are not so occasional. In high level athletes with more than 2 cm displacement, ORIF may be a valuable option.

Stress fractures of the femoral neck

Stress fractures may occur in young people, mainly female endurance athletes, due to overuse and repetitive microtrauma [41, 42]. When the stresses and the extent of microdamage exceed the remodeling process, fractures occur. The femur accounts for about 5% to 7% of all stress fractures. Stress fractures of the femoral neck often go unrecognized, untreated, or inappropriately managed, leading to catastrophic acute, displaced femoral neck fracture. The classic "female athlete triad", amenorrhea, eating disorders, and premature osteoporosis, is often associated. Symptoms include persistent groin discomfort, especially with activity. A recent significant increase in running sports may be reported. Stress fracture should be considered if the patient is unable to straight leg raise against resistance, a positive Trendelenberg test, the presence of a gluteus medius limp with gait testing, or pain/inability to hop on 1 foot. Radiographs may often miss the fracture. MRI scan should be performed in case of high suspect: edema extending to the cortex on either the inferior-medial and superior-lateral sides of the femoral neck is evident. Stress fractures can be classified according to the fracture pattern, distraction or compression. Distraction fracture has a transverse course starting from the superior portion of the neck (the tension side of the neck): it involves adults and may become displaced. Internal fixation with percutaneous cannulated screws is recommended before fracture displacement. The compression stress fracture involves the inferior-medial neck, usually in children. Displacement is rare. Conservative treatment is usually recommended, with protected weight bearing and activity restriction until radiographic healing.

Muscle injuries

Muscle strains are the most common muscle injury in sports, and are due to a forcible active or passive stretching of the muscle (generally through eccentric contraction) [43]. Muscles at risk of strains are involved in the range of joint motion, usually in high-speed activities with rapid acceleration/deceleration, and cutting/pivoting. Usually, the most at-risk muscles have a relatively high percentage of fast-twitch (type II) muscle fibers. Soccer players are at an elevated risk for hip and groin injuries. 20% to 37% of all time-loss injuries at men's professional levels are due to muscle injuries. The typical features of hip and groin muscle injuries among soccer players are: new injuries (87.8%), noncontact in nature (77.3%), not severe (less than 7 day loss: 67.5%), occurring during the pre-season and competition, in older players. The most common injuries are adductor strains (46.5%), hip flexor strains (27.3%), and hip contusions (10.8%). The classic classification of muscle injuries recognized: delayed-onset muscle soreness, strains (distraction injuries), and contusions (compression injuries). A more recent classification encompassed functional and structural-mechanical injuries. Functional injuries are minor fatigue-induced or neurogenic injuries causing hardening of the muscle, whereas structural mechanical injuries are muscle tears or strains of muscle fibers or bundles. From an histologic perspective, muscle fibers are torn near the myo-tendinous junction. Hemorrhage with surrounding edema ensues: the inflammatory process occurs a day or 2 after the injury. After about a week, the inflammatory phase is markedly reduced and fibrous tissue replaces the torn muscle.

Diagnosis

An acute episode of pain during an intense activity is the most typical presentation. The athlete will experience further pain after the initial injury, in particular with eccentric activation. Tenderness, swelling, and ecchymosis are common, as long as limited range of motion and muscular weakness. The diagnosis is clinical, imaging is generally not necessary. MRI may demonstrate edema, hemorrhage, and muscle fiber disruption, showing the exact localization.

Treatment

The acute treatment includes rest, ice, NSAIDs, compression, elevation for 48 hours [43, 44, 48] (tab. 2). Rehabilitation can be started as soon as pain relieves. The aims are to increase range of motion and restore muscle strength. Strength is an important predictive factor for occurrence and reoccurrences, much more than flexibility. A program including active strengthening, resistive exercises, balance training, and core strengthening of the surrounding muscles is the mainstay. An adequate pre-exercise warm-up is very important to prevent injuries, along with strengthening exercises and sport specific training. The goal is to achieve an adduction strength at least 80% of the abduction strength.

Iliac crest contusion ("hip pointer")

"Hip pointers" are contusions of the iliac crest and the overlying soft tissues (gluteal muscles, tensor fasciae latae, abdominal muscles) [41, 42]. The injury is due to a direct blow to the iliac crest. A severe and debilitating pain is common, along with tenderness, ecchymosis, swelling, and hematomas. Fluid may even dissect the interval between the iliac crest and the surrounding soft-tissues. The diagnosis is clinical: plain radiographs may rule out iliac wing fractures or apophyseal fractures

Phase I (Acute)	**Phase II (Subacute)**	**Phase III (Sport specific training)**
- RICE (rest, ice, compression, and elevation) for first 48 hours after injury - NSAIDs - Massage - TENS - Ultrasound - Submaximal isometric adduction progressing to maximal isometric adduction - Passive range of motion (PROM) in pain-free range - Non-weight-bearing hip progressive resistive exercises (PREs) without weight in anti-gravity position (all except abduction) - Upper body & trunk strengthening - Flexibility program for noninvolved muscles - Bilateral balance board	- Bicycling/Swimming - Sumo squats - Single limb stance - Concentric adduction with weight against gravity - Standing with involved foot on sliding board moving in frontal plane - Adduction in standing on cable column or Theraband - Seated adduction machine - Bilateral adduction on sliding board moving in frontal plane - Unilateral lunges (sagittal) with reciprocal arm movements - Multiplane trunk tilting - Balance board squats with throwbacks - General flexibility program	Phase II exercises with increase in load, intensity, speed and volume
Main aim: concentric adduction against gravity without pain	**Main aim:** involved adductor strength at least 75% that of the ipsilateral abductors	**Main aim:** adduction strength at least 90-100% of the abduction strength and involved muscle strength equal to that of the contralateral side

Table 2 - Adductor strain post injury program (Tyler et al. [48])

in the adolescent athlete. Conservative treatment (rest, ice, NSAIDs), followed by physical therapy (stretching and strengthening) leads to a complete recovery in 2 to 4 weeks. However, complications may be troublesome and can include myositis ossificans and muscle fibrosis.

Piriformis syndrome

Piriformis syndrome is a clinical condition due to sciatic nerve entrapment at the level of the ischial tuberosity [45]. Piriformis may get inflamed or entrap the sciatic nerve due to biomechanics causes (poor body posture), anatomic anomalies of piriformis muscle and sciatic nerve, acute injury in internal rotation, muscle hypertrophy during preseason conditioning.

Diagnosis

The clinical presentation is a sciatic-like pain in the gluteal/buttock region, with numbness in the buttocks and tingling sensations. The diagnosis is clinical and is one of exclusion. Stretching maneuvers elicited the pain, as well as manual pressure around the sciatic nerve. Forceful internal rotation of the extended thigh, resisted abduction and external rotation of the thigh, flexion, abduction, external rotation, flexion, adduction, internal rotation maneuvers may allow reproduce the symptomatology. Diagnostic modalities such as ultrasound, MRI, CT, and EMG are mostly useful in excluding other conditions (mainly lumbosacral pathologies).

Treatment

Conservative treatments like short-term rest, muscle relaxants, NSAIDs, and physical therapy should be attempted first [45]. In some patients, steroid injection around the piriformis muscle may be beneficial.

Surgery (decompression) is the last consideration in patients with piriformis syndrome. The results after surgery are unpredictable.

Athletes with piriformis syndrome may return to activities when they can demonstrate the pain-free range of motion, increased strength of the affected side, and performance without any discomfort. Stretching and warm-up before sport activity are fundamental.

Neurological conditions

Meralgia paresthetica

Meralgia paresthetica is an entrapment syndrome of the lateral femoral cutaneous nerve [46]. This sensory nerve leaves the lumbar plexus and normally appears just proximal to the iliac crest. Then the course is lateral over the iliacus where it is covered by the fascia. The nerve exits anteriorly through the fascia lata, several centimeters distal to the inguinal ligament, innervating the skin of the anterolateral aspect of the thigh. The lateral femoral cutaneous nerve is commonly entrapped where it perforates the inguinal ligament, approximately 2 cm medial to the anterior superior iliac spine. Compression of the nerve causes numbness, tingling, a burning sensation, or pain in the anterolateral thigh, limiting the daily life and the sport activities.

The pain can be elicited by palpation of the nerve. A positive pelvic compression test and Tinel's sign can be used to identify nerve entrapment. The pelvic compression test is performed applying a downward force to the pelvis while the patient's symptomatic side is facing up in lateral decubitus, in order to reduce tension on the inguinal ligament and relieve the patient's symptoms: sensibility and sensitivity are over 90%. Trial anesthetic injection may relieve symptoms and can be useful for diagnostic purposes (and even for treating the nerve entrapment). An associated injury (traumas like anterior superior iliac spine avulsion or iatrogenic causes) or a possible predisposition to this entrapment syndrome can be detected in many cases (other etiologies: spontaneous or metabolic).

If conservative treatments are ineffective (NSAIDs, rest, antiepileptic drugs), surgery may be suggested: decompression, resection, transposition were described. Surgery is not always effective, also due to the anatomical variations of the nerve. However, early outcomes after surgery showed that 90% of the athletes returned to sport with occasional pain or no pain, even after vigorous activities.

Iliacus hematoma syndrome

The iliacus hematoma syndrome is a compression neuropathy of the femoral nerve due to hemorrhage in the iliac fossa [47]. It is associated with coagulopathies or surgeries, but it has been rarely reported in athletes after a trauma. The clinical presentation is severe pain in the groin and inguinal areas: an antalgic position ensues with the hip flexed, abducted, and externally rotated to reduce tension on the iliopsoas muscle. Sensory impairments of the femoral nerve can be reported, with loss of sensations over the anterior thigh and anteromedial leg: loss of muscular force (quadriceps muscles) may be evident, too.

On physical examination, a mass or swelling in the iliac fossa and ecchymosis are frequent. Quadriceps muscle should be assessed and paralysis due to atrophy in the subacute and chronic settings may be evident. There may be decreased or absent knee jerk reflex. MRI scan is the most useful diagnostic tool. It allows for better soft tissue differentiation than CT.

Treatment is debated: delaying surgical evacuation of the hematoma can lead to permanent disability. Surgical management is more likely in younger athletes if there is progression of femoral nerve symptoms and the MRI scan shows a collection of blood impinging on the femoral nerve. The drainage of the hematoma can be performed percutaneously using ultrasound guidance if the hematoma remains unclotted. After surgical evacuation, 74% of the patients achieved complete neurological recovery of the femoral nerve with the balance resulting in incomplete or variable recovery.

Bibliography

1. Sherman B, Chahla J, Hutchinson W, Gerhardt M. Hip and Core Muscle Injuries in Soccer. Am J Orthop (Belle Mead NJ). 2018 Oct;47(10).

2. Rankin AT, Bleakley CM, Cullen M. Hip Joint Pathology as a Leading Cause of Groin Pain in the Sporting Population: A 6-Year Review of 894 Cases. Am J Sports Med. 2015 Jul;43(7):1698-703.

3. Tummala SV, Chhabra A, Makovicka JL, Patel KA, Hartigan DE. Hip and Groin Injuries Among Collegiate Male Soccer Players: The 10-Year Epidemiology, Incidence, and Prevention. Orthopedics. 2018 Nov 1;41(6):e831-e836.

4. Ganz R, Parvizi J, Beck M, Leunig M, Notzli H, Siebenrock KA. Femoroacetabular impingement: a cause for osteoarthritis of the hip. Clin Orthop Relat Res. 2003;417:112–20.

5. Lahner M, Walter PA, von Schulze Pellengahr C, Hagen M, von Engelhardt LV, Lukas C. Comparative study of the femoroacetabular impingement (FAI) prevalence in male semiprofessional and amateur soccer players. Arch Orthop Trauma Surg. 2014 Aug;134(8):1135-41.

6. de Silva V, Swain M, Broderick C, McKay D. Does high level youth sports participation increase the risk of femoroacetabular impingement? A review of the current literature. Pediatr Rheumatol Online J. 2016 Mar 11;14(1):16.

7. Griffin DR, Dickenson EJ, O'Donnell J, Agricola R, Awan T, Beck M, Clohisy JC, Dijkstra HP, Falvey E, Gimpel M, Hinman RS, Hölmich P, Kassarjian A, Martin HD, Martin R, Mather RC, Philippon MJ, Reiman MP, Takla A, Thorborg K, Walker S, Weir A, Bennell KL. The Warwick Agreement on femoroacetabular impingement syndrome (FAI syndrome): an international consensus statement. Br J Sports Med. 2016 Oct;50(19):1169-76.

8. Emara K, Samir W, el Motasem H, Ghafar KA. Conservative treatment for mild femoroacetabular impingement. J Orthop Surg (Hong Kong). 2011;19(1):41–5.

9. Locks R, Utsunomiya H, Briggs KK, McNamara S, Chahla J, Philippon MJ. Return to Play After Hip Arthroscopic Surgery for Femoroacetabular Impingement in Professional Soccer Players. Am J Sports Med. 2018 Feb;46(2):273-279.

10. Barastegui D, Seijas R, Alvarez-Diaz P, Rivera E, Alentorn-Geli E, Steinbacher G, Cuscó X, Cugat R. Assessing long-term return to play after hip arthroscopy in football players evaluating risk factors for good prognosis. Knee Surg Sports Traumatol Arthrosc. 2018 Mar;26(3):963-968.

11. Alradwan H, Philippon MJ, Farrokhyar F, Chu R, Whelan D, Bhandari M, Ayeni OR. Return to preinjury activity levels after surgical management of femoroacetabular impingement in athletes. Arthroscopy. 2012 Oct;28(10):1567-76.

12. Spencer-Gardner L, Eischen JJ, Levy BA, Sierra RJ, Engasser WM, Krych AJ. A comprehensive five-phase rehabilitation programme after hip arthroscopy for femoroacetabular impingement. Knee Surg Sports Traumatol Arthrosc. 2014 Apr;22(4):848-59.

13. Kang C, Hwang DS, Cha SM. Acetabular labral tears in patients with sports injury. Clin Orthop Surg. 2009 Dec;1(4):230-5.

14. Boykin RE, Patterson D, Briggs KK, Dee A, Philippon MJ. Results of arthroscopic labral reconstruction of the hip in elite athletes. Am J Sports Med. 2013 Oct;41(10):2296-301.

15. Czerny C, Hofmann S, Neuhold A, Tschauner C, Engel A, Recht MP, Kramer J. Lesions of the acetabular labrum: accuracy of MR imaging and MR arthrography in detection and staging. Radiology. 1996 Jul;200(1):225-30.

16. Randelli F, Randelli P, Banci L, Arrigoni P. Intra-articu-

lar loose body removal during hip arthroscopy. Orthopedics. 2010 Jul 13;33(7):476.
17. Ross JR, Larson CM, Bedi A. Indications for Hip Arthroscopy. Sports Health. 2017 Sep/Oct;9(5):402-413.
18. Newman JT, Saroki AJ, Philippon MJ. Hip arthroscopy for the management of trauma: a literature review. J Hip Preserv Surg. 2015 Jun 24;2(3):242-8.
19. Mayes S, Ferris AR, Smith P, Garnham A, Cook J. Atraumatic tears of the ligamentum teres are more frequent in professional ballet dancers than a sporting population. Skeletal Radiol. 2016 Jul;45(7):959-67.
20. de SA D, Phillips M, Philippon MJ, Letkemann S, Simunovic N, Ayeni OR. Ligamentum teres injuries of the hip: a systematic review examining surgical indications, treatment options, and outcomes. Arthroscopy. 2014 Dec;30(12):1634-41.
21. Grimaldi A, Mellor R, Hodges P, Bennell K, Wajswelner H, Vicenzino B. Gluteal Tendinopathy: A Review of Mechanisms, Assessment and Management. Sports Med. 2015 Aug;45(8):1107-19.
22. Grimaldi A, Fearon A. Gluteal Tendinopathy: Integrating Pathomechanics and Clinical Features in Its Management. J Orthop Sports Phys Ther. 2015 Nov;45(11):910-22.
23. Henning PT. The running athlete: stress fractures, osteitis pubis, and snapping hips. Sports Health. 2014 Mar;6(2):122-7.
24. Potalivo G, Bugiantella W. Snapping hip syndrome: systematic review of surgical treatment. Hip Int. 2017 Mar 31;27(2):111-121.
25. Ilizaliturri VM Jr, Camacho-Galindo J. Endoscopic treatment of snapping hips, iliotibial band, and iliopsoas tendon. Sports Med Arthrosc Rev. 2010 Jun;18(2):120-7.
26. Via AG, Basile A, Wainer M, Musa C, Padulo J, Mardones R. Endoscopic release of internal snapping hip: a review of literature. Muscles Ligaments Tendons J. 2016 Dec 21;6(3):372-377
27. Strauss EJ, Nho SJ, Kelly BT. Greater trochanteric pain syndrome. Sports Med Arthrosc Rev. 2010 Jun;18(2):113-9.
28. Flato R, Passanante GJ, Skalski MR, Patel DB, White EA, Matcuk GR Jr. The iliotibial tract: imaging, anatomy, injuries, and other pathology. Skeletal Radiol. 2017 May;46(5):605-622.
29. Pierce TP, Kurowicki J, Issa K, Festa A, Scillia AJ, McInerney VK. External snapping hip: a systematic review of outcomes following surgical intervention: External snapping hip systematic review. Hip Int. 2018 Sep;28(5):468-472.
30. Gollwitzer H, Banke IJ, Schauwecker J, Gerdesmeyer L, Suren C. How to address ischiofemoral impingement? Treatment algorithm and review of the literature. J Hip Preserv Surg. 2017 Aug 31;4(4):289-298.
31. Stafford GH, Villar RN. Ischiofemoral impingement. J Bone Joint Surg Br. 2011 Oct;93(10):1300-2.
32. Aguilera-Bohorquez B, Brugiatti M, Coaquira R, Cantor E. Frequency of Subspine Impingement in Patients With Femoroacetabular Impingement Evaluated With a 3-Dimensional Dynamic Study. Arthroscopy. 2019 Jan;35(1):91-96.
33. Carton P, Filan D. Anterior Inferior Iliac Spine (AIIS) and Subspine Hip Impingement. Muscles Ligaments Tendons J. 2016 Dec 21;6(3):324-336.
34. Tyler TF, Fukunaga T, Gellert J. Rehabilitation of soft tissue injuries of the hip and pelvis. Int J Sports Phys Ther. 2014 Nov;9(6):785-97.
35. Saito M, Utsunomiya H, Hatakeyama A, Nakashima H, Nishimura H, Matsuda DK, Sakai A, Uchida S. Hip Arthroscopic Management Can Improve Osteitis Pubis and Bone Marrow Edema in Competitive Soccer Players With Femoroacetabular Impingement. Am J Sports Med. 2019 Feb;47(2):408-419.
36. Gaudino F, Spira D, Bangert Y, Ott H, Beomonte Zobel B, Kauczor HU, Weber MA. Osteitis pubis in professional football players: MRI findings and correlation with clinical outcome. Eur J Radiol. 2017 Sep;94:46-52.
37. Hopkins JN, Brown W, Lee CA. Sports Hernia: Definition, Evaluation, and Treatment. JBJS Rev. 2017 Sep;5(9):e6.
38. Farber AJ, Wilckens JH. Sports hernia: diagnosis and therapeutic approach. J Am Acad Orthop Surg. 2007 Aug;15(8):507-14.
39. Kraeutler MJ, Garabekyan T, Pascual-Garrido C, Mei-Dan O. Hip instability: a review of hip dysplasia and other contributing factors. Muscles Ligaments Tendons J. 2016 Dec 21;6(3):343-353.
40. Wilkin GP, Ibrahim MM, Smit KM, Beaulé PE. A Contemporary Definition of Hip Dysplasia and Structural Instability: Toward a Comprehensive Classification for Acetabular Dysplasia. J Arthroplasty. 2017 Sep;32(9S):S20-S27.
41. Kovacevic D, Mariscalco M, Goodwin RC. Injuries about the hip in the adolescent athlete. Sports Med Arthrosc Rev. 2011 Mar;19(1):64-74.
42. Frank JS, Gambacorta PL, Eisner EA. Hip pathology in the adolescent athlete. J Am Acad Orthop Surg. 2013 Nov;21(11):665-74.
43. Ekstrand J, Hägglund M, Waldén M. Epidemiology of muscle injuries in professional football (soccer). Am J Sports Med. 2011 Jun;39(6):1226-32.
44. Elattar O, Choi HR, Dills VD, Busconi B. Groin Injuries (Athletic Pubalgia) and Return to Play. Sports Health. 2016 Jul;8(4):313-23.
45. Jankovic D, Peng P, van Zundert A. Brief review: piriformis syndrome: etiology, diagnosis, and management. Can J Anaesth. 2013 Oct;60(10):1003-12.
46. Ataizi ZS, Ertilav K, Ercan S. Surgical options for meralgia paresthetica: long-term outcomes in 13 cases. Br J Neurosurg. 2019 Apr;33(2):188-191.
47. Kounis NG, Macauley MB, Ghorbal MS. Iliacus hematoma syndrome. Can Med Assoc J. 1975 Apr 5;112(7):872-3.
48. Tyler TF, Campbell R, Nicholas SJ, Donellan S, McHugh MP. The effectiveness of a preseason exercise program on the prevention of groin strains in professional ice hockey players. Am J Sports Med. 2002;30(5):680-683.

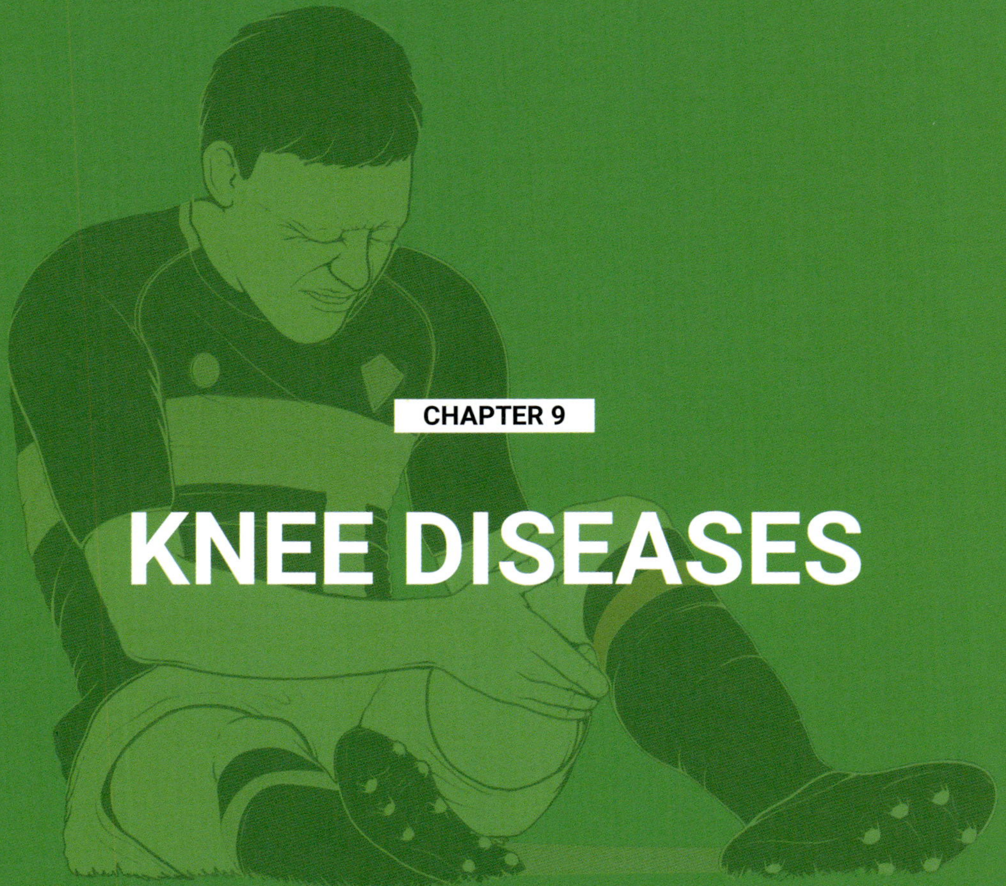

CHAPTER 9

KNEE DISEASES

Stefano Zaffagnini [1,2]

Alberto Grassi [1]

Luca Macchiarola [1]

Massimo Pirone [1]

Gian Andrea Lucidi [1]

Nicola Pizza [1]

Piero Agostinone [1]

[1] *2nd Orthopaedic and Traumatologic Clinic (Director: S. Zaffagnini) IRCCS Istituto Ortopedico Rizzoli, Bologna, Italy*

[2] *University of Bologna, Italy*

Introduction

The International Federation of Football Associations (FIFA) estimates that the number of soccer athletes worldwide is close to 270 million, of whom approximately 62 million live in Europe and 5 million live in Italy [1]. Given these huge numbers, it is extremely common to find ourselves in front of a patient suffering from soccer-related knee trauma. Virtually, the type of patient that we could deal with cannot be stereotyped: males or females, old or young, professionals or amateurs.

Meniscal injuries

Anatomy and functions

Menisci are two intra-articular fibrocartilaginous structures, triangular in section; they are positioned between the tibial plate and femoral condyles, increasing the contact area of the articular surfaces. The medial one is shaped like a "C"; it is firmly linked to the joint capsule and is the least mobile on the concave surface of the medial tibial plateau. The lateral one is shaped like an "O" and has a greater degree of freedom of movement on the convex surface of the lateral plateau (fig. 1).
In fact, the menisci are linked to the tibial plate center mainly through their roots and, although other minor ligaments have been described, meniscal bodies are forced to move back and forward on the tibial plateau when the knee flexes and extends [2]. Their blood supply comes mainly from the geniculate arteries that vascularize the capsule, thus the blood flow is significantly greater in the meniscal periphery than in the central portion.
This anatomical feature has very concrete clinical consequence since the peripheral zone (red-red) has the best potential for healing while the central zone (red-white) and a central zone (white-white) are less prone to healing when sutured [3]. If during the 80' and 90' menisci were almost considered to be needless structured and their lesions were often treated simply removing them, during the last years extensive research has been carried on and the role and function of the menisci have been somehow rediscovered. Firstly, the menisci are able to withstand different forces such as shear, tension, and compression, playing a crucial role in load-bearing, load transmission, shock absorption. The contact forces on the menisci within the human knee have been studied. It has been calculated that the intact menisci occupy approximately 60% of the contact area between the articular cartilages, while they transmit >50% of the total axial load applied in the joint. However, these percentages highly depend on the degree of knee flexion and tissue health. In fact, for every 30° of knee flexion, the contact surface between the two knee bones decreases by 4%. Of notable interest are the changes in the contact area and contact force following partial or total meniscectomy: for example in an experiment conducted on 10 cadaveric knees it was found that a total removal of the lateral meniscus causes a 50% decrease in total contact area, resulting in 235-335% increase in peak local contact load [4]. It has been demonstrated that this enormous increase in cartilage stress leads to premature osteoarthritis and chondrolysis. Besides this primary function, the menisci are secondary stabilizers of the knee joint; this factor may be of crucial importance in soccer medicine. Medial and lateral menisci contribute to knee stability acting as restraints for anterior displacement and rotations, respectively [5]. Previous in-vitro studies investigated the knee stability after medial meniscectomy [6], evaluating the residual laxity in Lachman

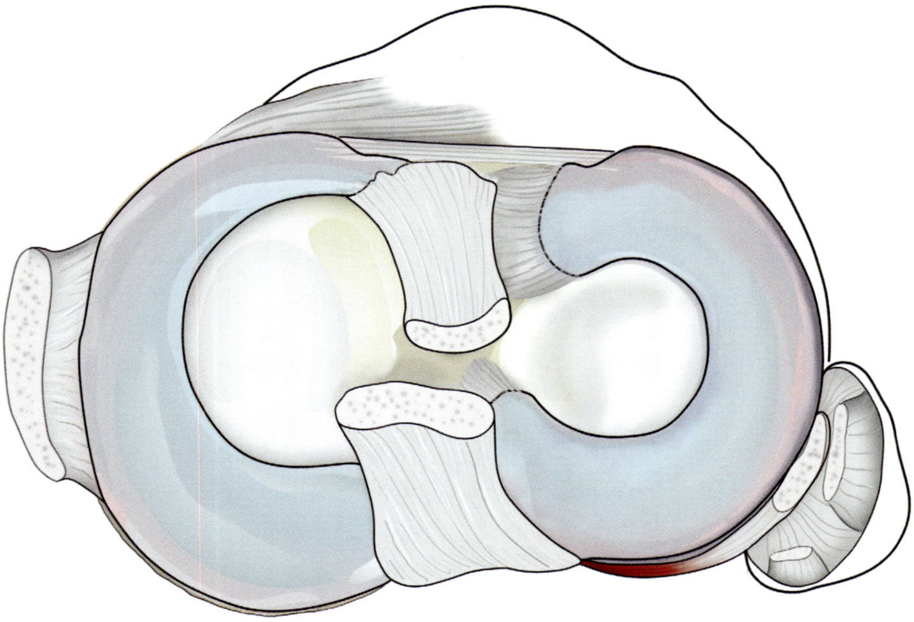

Figure 1 - Axial knee section: the anatomy of the menisci

and Pivot-shift (PS) test. A common result was an increase of AP laxity ranging from 5 to 7mm in ACL-injured knees. Few studies focused on lateral meniscectomy: Musahl et al. found an increase in knee dynamic instability during a mechanized PS maneuver. Moreover, an in-vivo navigation study on 56 patients with ACL injury showed a significant increase of pre-operative anteroposterior knee laxity at 30° and 90° in those with partial medial meniscus removal respect to those with intact menisci [7], confirming the evidence from cadaveric studies.

Injury mechanism

During the flexion and extension movements of the knee the menisci are not still and the mobility of the external meniscus is double, compared to the one of internal meniscus. Therefore, the compression and torsion forces between femoral condyles and tibial surface are responsible for the lesion of the menisci.

The injury mechanisms are listed below [8].

- Rotary traumas: flexed and valgus knee with the extra-rotated tibia, and flexed and varus knee with the intra-rotated tibia.
- The rapid and sudden passage from the flexed position to the extension of the knee.
- The functional overload, which progressively damages the cartilage of meniscuses.

There are four main kinds of meniscus tears [8].

- Longitudinal tear, that is parallel to the major axis of the meniscus, easy to be reduced and well suited for the placement of vertical mattress sutures [9].
- Radial tear, that is perpendicular to the same axis. When it extends to the periphery, it is biomechanically similar to a complete meniscectomy. This type of tear is difficult to be reduced and repaired [9].
- Complex tear, defined as a tear in two or more planes, that is generally not repairable. Therefore, it is treated with partial meniscectomy [9].
- The bucket-handle tear is a large unstable longitudinal tear and is commonly seen in ACL-deficient knees.

These types of lesions can be combined with each other, generating different types of meniscal lesions. For instance, the flap lesion is caused by a radial lesion plus a longitudinal lesion.

Clinical evaluation

The main symptoms are pain, swelling, knee instability, and the presence of mechanical disorders [10]. It is important to collect an accurate medical history, asking the athlete for the trauma modalities and symptoms. The pain can be sharp or medium, constant or occasional; it is never diffused, but point-like and localized at the internal or external articular line. The movements of rotation, hyperflexion, hyperextension can exacerbate the pain. The knee may swell after an acute meniscal injury. It could be a hemarthrosis when the lesion affects the red-zone, or more frequently joint effusion, usually after 12-24 hours from the trauma, but it is not constant [11]. Instead, the knee instability is a rare symptom, it is often an analgesic reflex due to pain. Moreover, the locked knee joint is the main symptom of the bucket-handle tear. This occurs when the knee does not fully straighten after it has bent; instead, flexion is always preserved [10]. It is important to distinguish the meniscal block from other causes of locked knee, in which both flexion and extension are abolished. The locked knee follows immediately the trauma, while an articular limitation that appears after hours indicates tightness, due to the intra-articular effusion. Moreover, the locked knee always regresses after a few hours, sometimes with a click [11].

The pain can be evoked by palpation or by semiological maneuvers. There are no specific tests to make a certain diagnosis, therefore the doctor must take advantage of the positivity of one or more tests and the anamnesis. The pain can be evoked through joint line palpation, McMurray test, and Apley grind test. Joint line palpation is the most basic maneuver to detect meniscal tears. The palpation of the medial edge of the medial meniscus is easier with internal rotation of the tibia. Alternatively, the external rotation allows improved palpation of the lateral meniscus. The range of sensitivity for joint line tenderness is 55% to 85%, with a specificity range of 29% to 67% [12].

Mc Murray test was described in 1940 by McMurray. The original description of the test, as described by McMurray, was: "In carrying out the manipulation with patient lying flat, the knee is first fully flexed until the heel approaches the buttock; the foot is then held by grasping the heel and using the forearm as a lever. The knee being now steadied by the surgeon's other hand, the leg is rotated on the thigh with the knee still in full flexion. During this movement the posterior section of the cartilage is rotated with the head of the tibia, and if the whole cartilage, or any fragment of the posterior section, is loose, this movement produces an appreciable snap in the joint. By external rotation of the leg the internal cartilage is tested, and by internal rotation any abnormality of the posterior part of the external cartilage can be appreciated. By altering the position of flexion of the joint the whole of the posterior segment of the cartilages can be examined from the middle to their posterior attachment. Probably the simplest routine is to bring the leg from its position of acute flexion to a right angle, whilst the foot is retained first in full internal, and then in full external rotation. When the click occurs with a normal but lax cartilage, the patient experiences no pain or discomfort, but when produced by a broken cartilage, which has already given trouble, the patient is able to state that the sensation is the same as he experienced when the knee gave way previously" [13].

In the literature there is a wide variation in the reported sensitivities (16%-58%) and specificities (77%-98%) of the McMurray test for detecting meniscal tears [12]. Therefore, it is useful to combine the McMurray test with other clinical examination tests. The Apley grind test was described by Apley in 1947. The patient is prone. The surgeon grasps one foot in each hand, externally rotates it as far as possible, then flexes both knees together to their limit. The feet are then rotated inward and knees extended. This test determines whether simple rotation produces pain [12]. Kurosaka et al. reported an overall sensitivity of 16% and a specificity of 80% [14].

Treatment

The treatment of meniscal injuries in soccer players must be individualized based on the pattern of the tear, the presence of associated injuries, the age and goals of the patient, and the level of the competition.

We will discuss the surgical treatment of meniscal tears. Firstly, it is important to treat a stable or stabilized knee, because isolated meniscal repair in an ACL-deficient knee has a high failure risk [15]. In most cases, it is necessary to remove (meniscectomy) or suture the pathological portion so that the greatest possible extension of the meniscuses is preserved. In soccer players it is recommended to suture when it is possible (based on the type of the tear), in order to prevent the occurrence of osteoarthritis and increase the stability of the knee [3]. The meniscal suture is the best surgical choice for the treatment of meniscal tear, even if this procedure involves longer recovery time (fig. 2). Only 20% of meniscal tears are suturable, such as complete peripheral or radial tears [16].

Some surgeons recommend partial weight bearing

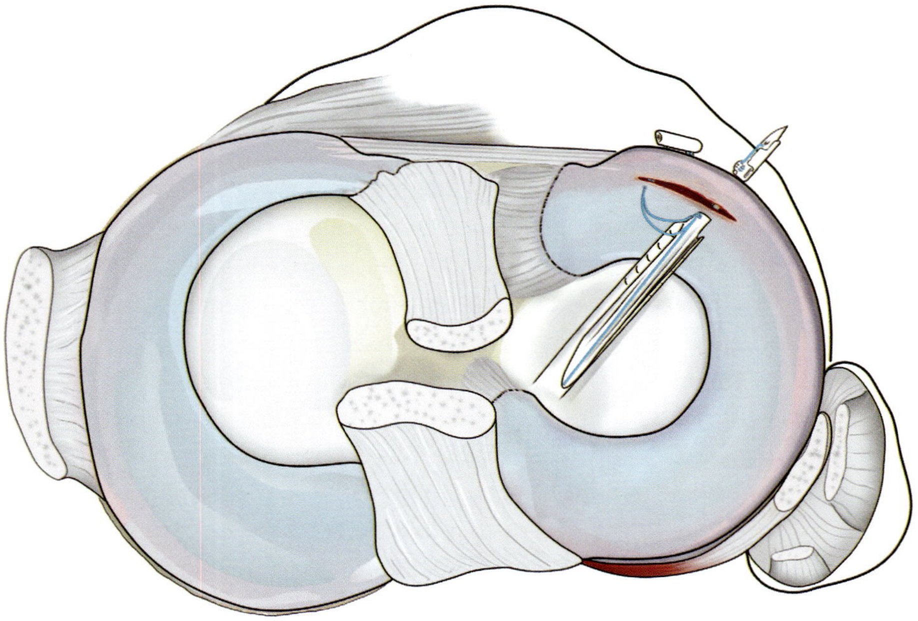

Figure 2 - Axial knee section: lateral meniscal suture

for 4 weeks [17]. It is not possible to run for the first 3 months. Usually, return to sport is permitted after 6 months, with complete knee range of motion and adequate muscle strength [17]. Instead, the partial meniscectomy is a fast and easy procedure, allowing an early return to sport without symptoms in many cases.

The main risk of partial meniscectomy is the alterations in loading patterns, that may predispose to early osteoarthritis at long-term follow-up [18]. The surgical technique is performed in arthroscopy and involves small cutaneous access to the knee, through which optical and surgical instruments are introduced to grasp and cut the pathological fragment of the meniscus.

Anterior cruciate ligament injuries

ACL injury is the most frequent ligament tear in sports practice. The anterior cruciate ligament is one of the four main ligaments of the knee, providing 85% of the restraining force to anterior tibial displacement at 30 degrees and 90 degrees of knee flexion [19]. Its function is to stabilize the joint, avoiding anterior tibial translation.

Proximal fibers fan out along the medial wall of the lateral femoral condyle; instead, the distal fibers attach in front of the intercondyloid eminence of the tibia. The ACL has two bundles, one anteromedial and one posterolateral. The first one is tense when the knee is flexed, the second one when extended [19] (fig. 3).

Injury mechanism

In literature two types of mechanisms are described: direct trauma and indirect trauma. Most ACL tears are a result of a non-contact mechanism such as a sudden change in a direction causing the knee to rotate inward. There are four main mechanisms of non-contact trauma [20].

- Knee-in and toe-out: dynamic alignment with the valgus position of the knee and the abduction position of the foot during the loading phase.
- Knee-out and toe-in: dynamic alignment with the varus position of the knee and the adduction position of the foot during the loading phase.
- Hyperextension: dynamic alignment with the hyper-extended position of the knee during the loading phase;
- Hyperflexion: dynamic alignment with the hyper-flexed position of the knee during the loading phase.

Clinical evaluation

The main symptom of ACL rupture is the knee instability and the patient feels a clear sensation, not necessarily painful, of something breaking inside the knee [21]. In acute lesions, the instability doesn't last long, because of muscular contracture and hemarthrosis. Pain and swelling resolve in about two weeks with ice, rest, and FANS. Instead, in chronic lesions, the patient reports a history of instability and pain due to the progressive rupture of the meniscal and cartilaginous structures. Other

typical symptoms include [22]:
- loss of full range of motion;
- tenderness along the joint line;
- discomfort while walking.

In clinical practice, the anterior drawer, the Lachman, and the pivot shift test are three common tests to determine ACL injuries. The anterior drawer test shows good sensitivity and specificity in chronic conditions, respectively 92% and 91%, but not in acute conditions [22]. For the anterior drawer test, the patient is supine with the hip flexed to 45°, the knee flexed to 90°, and the lower leg in neutral rotation. The examiner stabilizes the patient's foot with his thigh and places both hands behind the proximal tibia with the thumbs on the tibial plateau. An anteriorly directed force is applied to displace the tibia. Increased anterior tibial translation compared to the other side constitutes a positive test, indicating disruption of the ACL [22].

As described by the IKDC 2000 [23], the anterior drawer test is rated as normal (0 to 2 mm), nearly normal (3 to 5 mm), abnormal (6 to 10 mm), or severely abnormal (>10 mm), based on the amount of greater tibial translation on the injured side compared to the uninjured contralateral knee. Increased anterior tibial displacement in side-to-side comparison is indicative of an ACL tear.

The Lachman test has a good diagnostic accuracy to detect ACL pathology, both in acute as well as in chronic conditions. Its sensitivity is 85% and specificity is 94% [21]. It is performed with the patient lying supine and with the involved extremity on the side of the examiner. The femur is stabilized with one hand, with the patient's knee joint in 20° to 30° of flexion. The examiner's other hand is applied to the posterior aspect of the proximal tibia. The examiner applies an anteriorly-directed force to the proximal tibia and judges the amount of tibial translation [21].

According to the International Knee Documentation Committee [23], severity is graded as normal (-1 to 2 mm), nearly normal (3 to 5 mm), abnormal (6 to 10 mm), or severely abnormal (>10 mm), based on the amount of greater tibial translation

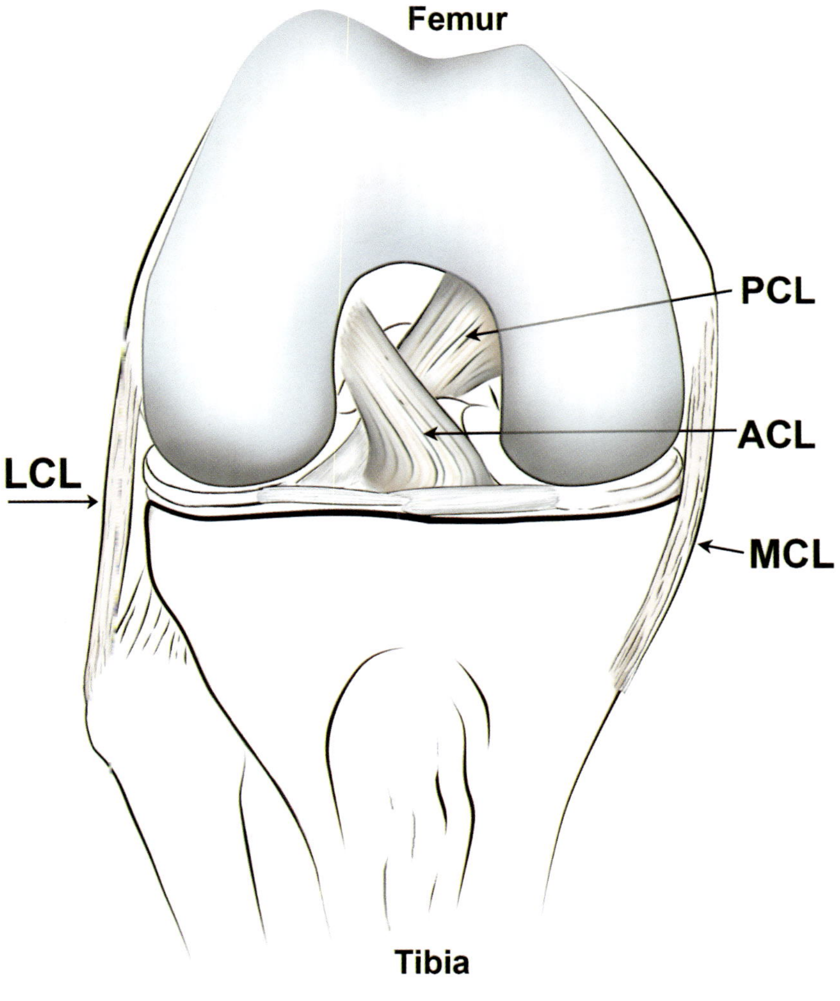

Figure 3 - The four major ligaments of the knee

on the injured side compared to the uninjured contralateral knee.

The specificity of the pivot shift test is very high, namely 98%. However, sensitivity is very poor, namely 32% and 40% in acute and chronic conditions, respectively [22]. It is performed with the patient supine. The extended leg is picked up at the ankle with the examiner's ipsilateral hand. This hand internally rotates the knee and flexes the knee from full extension, while applying valgus stress with the contralateral hand on the lateral side of the proximal tibia. A sudden reduction of the anterior subluxed lateral tibial plateau, caused by the iliotibial tract, indicates a positive pivot shift test [22]. The IKDC 2000 knee examination form [23] grades the pivot shift test as equal, glide (+), clunk (++), or gross (+++) (22).

Treatment

Surgical treatment is indicated in all subjects who practice sports even in adulthood [24]. The purpose of the treatment is to recover the stability of the knee, both static and dynamic, to restore an almost complete degree of movement, and to allow an early return to sport. Instead, in case of marked inflammation, with muscular contracture, both in flexion and in extension, the surgery must be postponed until achieving a good articulation [24]. About the reconstruction of ACL, two types of graft are commonly used:

- autografts (employing bone or tissue harvested from the patient's body);
- allografts (using bone or tissue from another body, either a cadaver or a live donor).

The choice of the type of tendon is important. It is recommended to use autologous tendons because their ability to integrate is almost certain [24]. The most used tendons are the quadriceps tendons, the central third of the patellar tendon or the hamstring tendons. The use of cadaver or synthetic allografts in the athlete is not recommended, because they are non-vascularized tissues and there is no certainty about times and transplant integration [24].

Surgery to rebuild an anterior cruciate ligament is done with an arthroscope using small incisions. There are several surgical techniques, the most used one involves the creation of two bone tunnels, in the femur and tibia, with an intra-articular emergence at the isometric points of anchorage of the native ACL (fig. 4). The graft is then secured to bones with screws or other fixation devices. After all the graft will serve as scaffolding on which new ligament tissue can grow [24].

After the reconstruction of ACL, a minimum of at least 6 months is recommended before returning to sports [25]. The risk of re-injury is higher in patients who return to sport in <7 months than those who return after 7 months [26]. Therefore, it is very important to choose the correct timing to return to sport, combining with subjective and objective criteria. Most commonly described tests are isokinetic strength tests, functional tests, clinical assessment, and subjective questionnaires [27].

The back in action (BIA) is a test battery designed for sportive users in any phase of a recovery period after an injury or in healthy conditions. BIA test battery is very easy to use, it is needed a few equipment and one room. It consists of the follow-

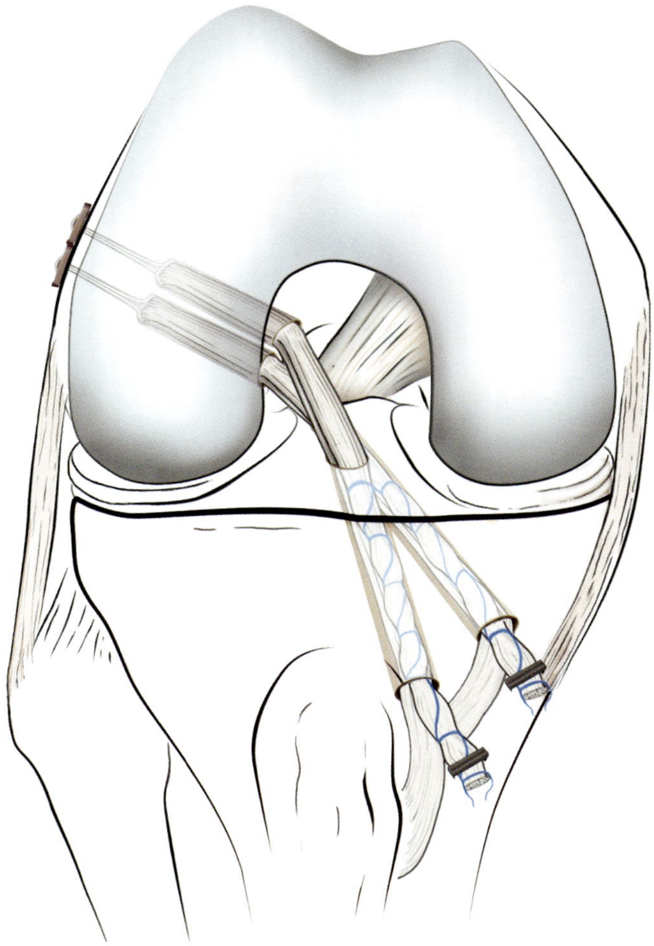

Figure 4 - ACL reconstruction with double-bundle technique

ing subtests: a two-legged and one-legged stability test, a two-legged and one-legged counter movement jump, a one-legged speedy jumps, a two-legged plyometric jumps and a two-legged quick feet test [28]. BIA test battery is used for every patient who underwent ACL reconstruction 4-5 months after surgery.
A recent systematic review reports return to play (RTP) rates of 63-65% to their preinjury level of sport after ACL reconstruction (ACLR) [29]. Returning to sport is a complex and multifactorial outcome and varies according to different physical functioning and contextual factors [29]. Many variables including patient's baseline features, surgery-related factors, and rehabilitation features affect the RTP chances for the athlete. Baseline factors, such as age, gender, pre-injury activity level are often non-modifiable. Age is the main factor that may influence the RTP rate. In fact, young age is positively associated with returning to pre-injury level of sport [30]. Other important possible predictors of functional outcome following ACLR, including RTP are the surgery factors. For example, in literature there is still no consensus about graft choice for primary ACLR; the patellar tendon autograft and hamstring autograft seem to have similar results in terms of RTP [29]. Instead, RTP rate in soccer players after revision ACLR is 43% compared to 63% for primary ACLR [31]. On the other hand, rehabilitation and psychological factors are postoperative quadriceps strength, postoperative knee effusion and pain, fewer episodes of instability, athletic confidence and motivation, and fear of reinjury. Higher postoperative quadriceps strength, less knee effusion, lower pain, fewer episodes of instability correlates with higher RTP rate [32]. About the psychological factors, higher preoperative motivation is considered a strong predictor, instead, fear of pain and especially fear of reinjury are negatively associated to RTP [33].

Medial collateral ligament injuries

Medial collateral ligament (MCL) injury is one of the most common knee injuries, especially in young athletic patients. Most MCL injuries can be managed conservatively with good results. The popularity of sports, particularly those involving valgus knee loadings such as ice hockey, skiing, and soccer, has contributed to the frequent occurrence of MCL injuries [34].

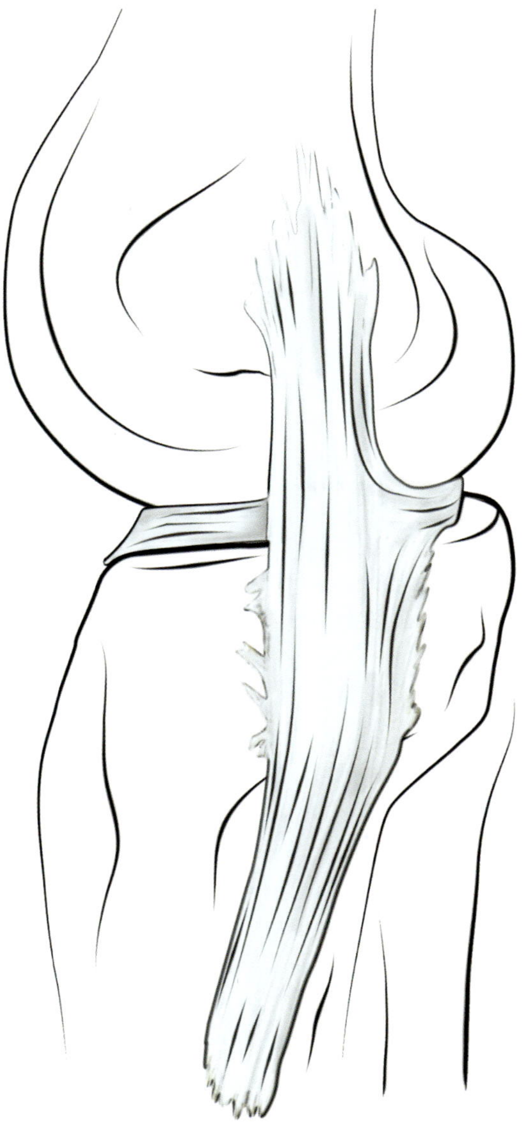

Figure 5 - Sagittal view of the knee: the anatomy of MCL

Anatomy of MCL

The anatomy of the medial side of the knee is complex, being composed of three tissue layers and multiple components with interconnections to the joint capsule, the muscle-tendon units, and the medial meniscus [35]. The medial collateral ligament (fig. 5), with its two components (superficial MCL and deep MCL), and the posterior oblique ligament are considered static stabilizers of the medial knee [36].
The superficial MCL is the primary static medial stabilizer, it is positioned between the superficial

sartorial fascia and the deep MCL. Its parallel fibers originate from the medial femoral epicondyle and insert on the medial aspect of the proximal tibia five to seven centimeters (cm) below the joint line, with an average length of 11 cm and an average width of 1.5 cm [35]. The deep MCL is extended from the femur to the mid-portion of the peripheral margin of the medial meniscus and inserted just below on the tibial articular margin, making meniscofemoral and meniscotibial portions. It is long 2 or 3 centimeters [35]. The superficial MCL, deep MCL, and posterior oblique ligament limit valgus and external rotation forces. On the other hand, the dynamic stabilizers of the medial side of the knee are the semimembranosus complex, the quadriceps, and the pes anserinus [36].

Injury mechanism

Valgus stress is the most common mechanism of injury. A minority of cases is represented by direct trauma to the lateral region of the knee with stress in valgus [37]. However, a combined flexion/valgus/external rotation injury is usually the end result. The lesion can be isolated or associated with the injured secondary restraints, such as the cruciate ligaments and the posterior capsule [37]. The degree of joint opening in millimeters contributes to the overall assessment of the severity of the instability. There are three different degrees of gravity.

- Grade 1 involves a few fibers resulting in localized tenderness but no instability.
- Grade 2 is a disruption of more fibers, with more generalized tenderness but still no instability.
- Grade 3 is a complete disruption of the ligament, with resultant instability.

Moreover, laxity system is another type of classification, according to the amount of absolute joint separation from valgus stress with the knee in 30 degrees of flexion. Therefore, there are Grade 1+, 2+, and 3+, that indicate 1-5 mm, 6-10 mm, and more than 10 mm of absolute medial separation respectively [37].

Clinical evaluation

The symptoms depend on the severity of the lesion and on the presence of associated lesions. The patient generally reports a feeling of jerking or tearing on the medial side [37]. In the absence of articular lesions, the swelling is modest and localized. In isolated lesions, the patient is usually able to complete the sporting activity. Lameness and functional limitation can arise immediately or after a few hours. The patient locates pain at the level of the internal compartment, more frequently at the femur [38]. The clinical evaluation involves performing the stress test in valgus at 0° and 30° of flexion. This test can differentiate between isolated MCL injuries and injuries involving the MCL as well as the PCL or ACL. Extensiveness laxity should lead to suspect an associated injury, whereas valgus laxity at 30° of flexion indicates that the injury involves the MCL. There are three degrees of gravity [37].

- Grade 1: 1-5 mm of joint opening.
- Grade 2: 6-10 mm of joint opening.
- Grade 3: more than 10 mm of joint opening.

Treatment

The indications for operative treatment are different for acute and chronic grade 3 medial knee injuries. In an acute injury, surgery is often indicated with multiligament injuries or knee dislocations involving the MCL. Instead, in chronic grade 3 medial knee injuries, surgery is indicated for patients who have complaints of rotatory instability and/or concurrent side-to-side instability [36]. It is also important for patients with chronic medial knee injuries to assess their weight-bearing frontal plane knee alignment. Generally, the treatment is based on the grade of lesions [36].

- Grade 1 and grade 2: the treatment is always conservative. Rehabilitation principles for acute medial knee injuries involve controlling edema, regaining range of motion, and avoiding any significant stress on the healing ligaments. For the first 7-10 days it is recommended to reduce the pain with a brace. A well-guided rehabilitation program can result in excellent functional outcomes in the majority of patients. In fact, the patient can return to sport after 4-6 weeks. Chronic instability is a very rare complication.
- Isolated grade 3: for these lesions, the treatment can be both conservative and surgical. If the lesion is at the femur, it can heal spontaneously. Instead, localized tibia lesion can heal more difficulty, so

surgical treatment is required due to residual instability.

- In case of grade 3 lesions associated with LCA tear, it is recommended the reconstruction of both ACL and MCL.
- If the conservative treatment fails and there is an important knee instability, it is recommended the reconstruction of MCL with grafts.

The surgical technique involves the use of a graft and the execution of two bone tunnels. The superficial MCL reconstruction graft is fixed into a femoral-based tunnel at the anatomic attachment site of the superficial MCL and is then fixed distally in a closed-socket tibial tunnel approximately 6 cm distal to the tibial joint line. This is the location of the native attachment site of the superficial MCL on the distal tibia [36].

Rehabilitation programs after operative treatment follow the same general protocol except for concomitant cruciate ligament reconstruction. During the phase I the knee is placed into a knee brace locked in extension for the first 4-6 weeks and passive ROM exercises are performed with a therapist [38]. It is important to progress to active assisted ROM and finally active ROM. The goal is active ROM from 0° to 120° by 6 weeks. In order to progress to phase II of the protocol, the patient should be able to fully weight bearing without any gait aids [39]. Phase II is the motor control phase, in which the patients have to strengthen dynamic knee stabilizers especially the quadriceps and hamstring and then additional lower extremity stabilizers such as gluteal musculature, gastrocnemius, and soleus [39]. The next step is to initiate straight-line jogging first in an aquatic environment and then on flat soft surfaces. Phase III is the return to sport phase during this last phase the athlete has to progress from jogging to sprinting, to incorporate soccer-specific training and at the end he has to perform performance tests to judge RTP [39].

Posterior cruciate ligament injuries

The posterior cruciate ligament (PCL) is the counterpart to the anterior cruciate ligament (ACL). The role of PCL is to restraint posterior tibial translation relative to the femur. In addition, the PCL is a secondary restraint of varus, valgus, and external

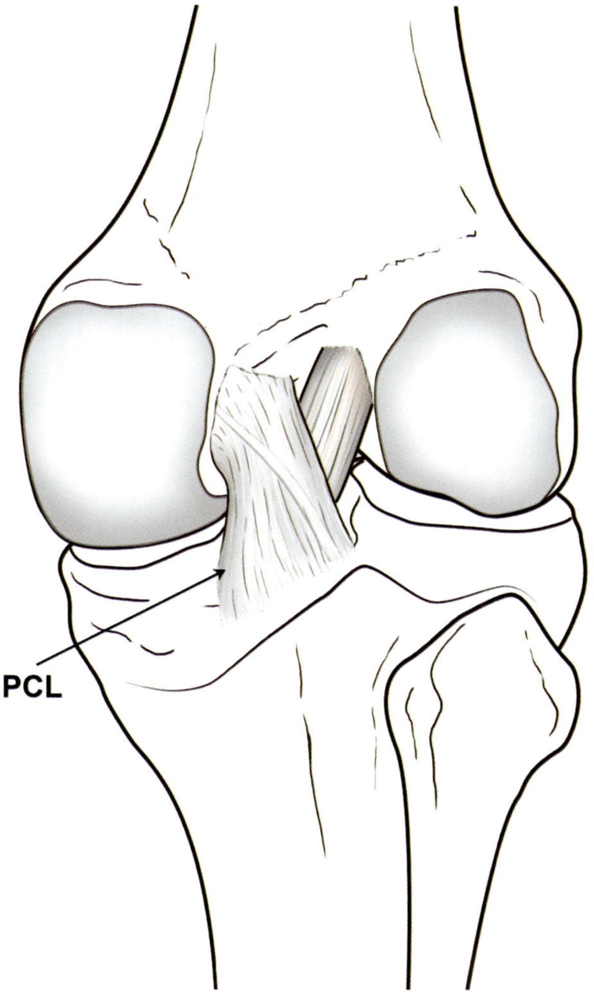

Figure 6 - Posterior view of the knee: the anatomy of PCL

rotation moments about the knee. PCL injuries are less common than ACL injuries.

Anatomy of PCL

The PCL is an intra-articular and extra-synovial structure, similar to the ACL. The length of the PCL is typically between 32 to 38 mm, and its diameter is approximately 11-13 mm. The thickness of the PCL is nearly twice that of the ACL [40]. The PCL originates from the anterolateral aspect of the medial femoral condyle and inserts along the posterior aspect of the tibial plateau, approximately 1 cm distal to the joint line [41]. The PCL is composed of two functional bundles and has important implications for knee stability (fig. 6). The larger anterolateral bundle (ALB) and smaller posteromedial bundle (PMB) have different patterns of tensioning in the entire range of motion of the knee [41]. The two bundles, therefore, contribute to stabilizing the knee joint, resisting posterior tibial translation and rotation at different angles of knee flexion (specifically between 90° and 120° of knee flexion) [40].

Injury mechanism

While less common than ACL injuries, injuries to the PCL can occur from a posterior force directed on the tibia, frequently with the knee in a flexed position [42]. This type of trauma is more common in soccer goalkeepers. Furthermore, the PCL lesions can occur after a fall with hyperflexed knee and foot in dorsal flexion, or due to a trauma with hyperextended knee. PCL lesions can be isolated, as it often happens in sports or associated with other ligament injuries [42].

Clinical evaluation

In acute injury, after the trauma, the patient feels a "clunk" sensation, the pain increases with flexion beyond 90°, and there may be a variable hemarthrosis [41]. Instead, in chronic injury the patient can complain of anterior patellofemoral pain, and only in associated lesions the patient reports instability and episodes of swelling [41].

In clinical practice, the posterior drawer test, reverse pivot shift, posterior sag test, step-off, Whipple test are important tests to determine PCL injuries.

Posterior drawer test

During a posterior drawer test, the patient lies supine. The examiner flexes the patient's hip to 45°, flexes the knee to 80° and then applies a force directed posteriorly. A positive result for PCL injury is indicated by clinically significant posterior translation movement on one side. The amount of posterior translation involved can help determine the grade of the injury. Knee ligament injuries can be graded on a scale from 0 to III, as follows [42].

- Grade 0 represents a normal ligament without injury.
- Grade I involves a few fibers resulting in localized tenderness but with no real laxity; associated with 0 to 5 mm of translation.
- Grade II is a disruption of more ligament fibers with detectable joint laxity and a good endpoint; localized pain and tenderness; between 5 and 10 mm of translation.
- Grade III is a complete tear of a single ligament, with gross laxity and instability; greater than 10 mm of translation.

Instead, Whipple test is performed while the patient lies prone. The examiner flexes the knee to 70° and then applies a force directed posteriorly [42].

Reverse pivot shift test

The reverse pivot shift test is a dynamic test and it is performed with the patient in a supine position. The examiner flexes the knee to 90° and the leg is in extra-rotation due to the posterior subluxation of the lateral tibial plate. The examiner then extends the knee, and the lateral tibial plateau shifts from a posterior subluxed position to a reduced position in full extension, resulting in a characteristic clunk [43].

Posterior sag test

It is a static test without applied active force, resulting in a posterior translation of the tibia when the knee is flexed to 90° and the foot is fixed by the examiner on the crib. The main parameter in this test is the step-off of the tibial plateau. Normally, the medial tibial plateau is 1 cm anterior to the medial femoral condyle, but is decreased (Grade I) or even absent (Grade II) or inverse (Grade III) in injuries to the posterior cruciate ligament [43].

Dial test

Dial test is used to evaluate isolated injuries of the posterolateral corner as well as injuries that affect the posterolateral corner and the PCL [43]. The patient is lying prone with the knees flexed to 90° and heels together and then with the knees flexed to 30°. The examiner has to observe the external rotation of the legs and the position of each foot. In case of posterolateral corner injury in combination with a PCL injury, an asymmetry of more than 10° is seen between the right and left foot at both 30° and 90° of flexion. Instead, a positive result for an isolated posterolateral corner injury is considered if an asymmetry of more than 10° is present with the knees at 30° of flexion but not at 90° [43].

Treatment

The extent of injury determines the management

strategy [42]. As with other ligament injuries, conservative treatment is recommended for grade I and II injuries of PCL [44]. Therefore, these types of injury are usually managed with physical therapy, rest, and exercises to strengthen the quadriceps muscle and thus provide greater stability to the knee.

In the first week after the injury, rest, ice, compression, and elevation, as well as the temporary use of crutches are recommended to reduce inflammation [44]. Once swelling and edema have decreased, strengthening the quadriceps muscle with physical therapy will help compensate for the PCL injury [44].

Instead, the complete isolated rupture with marked clinical and instrumental posterior laxity requires reconstruction surgery [43]. As for LCA reconstruction, to rebuild LCP it is preferable to use autologous tendons, such as the central third of the patellar tendon, the quadriceps tendons, or the hamstring tendons. Reconstruction surgery of LCP is done with an arthroscope using small incisions. There are several surgical techniques, the most used one involves the creation of two bone tunnels, in the femur and tibia, with an intra-articular emergence at the isometric points of anchorage of the native LCP. The graft is then secured to bones with screws or other fixation devices [43].

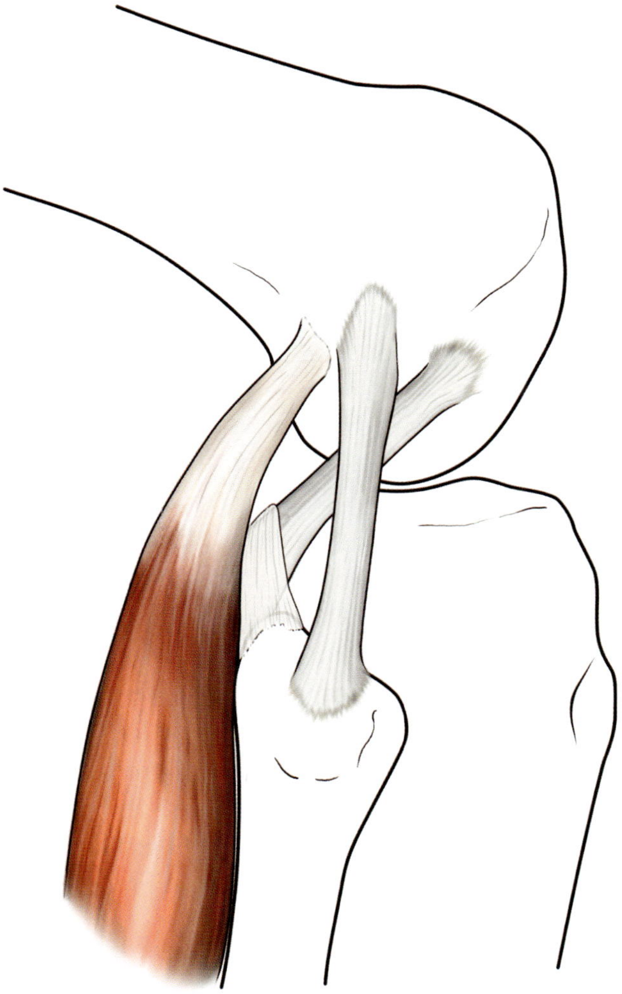

Figure 7 - Lateral view of the knee: the anatomy of the posterolateral corner

Posterolateral corner and fibular collateral ligament injuries

Posterolateral corner (PLC) injuries are infrequently seen but they can lead to chronic instability and articular cartilage degeneration if not treated [45]. PLC is a complex anatomical region of the knee and its knowledge is required to get the right and successful treatment. The most important structures of the posterolateral corner are the fibular collateral ligament (FCL), popliteus tendon (PLT), and popliteofibular ligament (PFL) [46]. These elements are responsible for the posterolateral stabilization and they help resist varus angulation, posterior tibial shift, and excessive external rotation of the knee [46].

FCL injuries are not common among soccer players. In fact, it only occurred in 1,1% of 17,379 sport injuries, as described by Majewski et al. in their study [47]. Instead, isolated PLC injuries are less than 2% of all acute knee ligament injuries [47]. Injury to the posterolateral corner of the knee is usually associated with other ligaments tears, especially with PCL tears (from 43 to 80%) [48].

Anatomy

The posterolateral corner of the knee contains a variety of structures, some of which are inconstantly present (fig. 7) [45]. These structures are fibular collateral ligament (FCL), lateral head of gastrocnemius, fabella bone in the lateral head of the gastrocnemius tendon (if present), fabellofibular ligament, popliteofibular ligament (PFL), popliteus tendon (PLT), biceps femoris tendon, iliotibial tract, and arcuate ligament [45].

The FCL originates from the posterolateral aspect of the femoral condyle, directly anterior to the origin of the lateral head of the gastrocnemius. FCL and the tendon of the biceps femoris form the con-

joint tendon and insert on the fibular head [45]. FCL helps prevent varus angulation of the knee, particularly between 5° and 25° of flexion [46].
The popliteus tendon originates at the lateral condyle of the femur, it passes under the lateral collateral ligament and the arcuate ligament. After the popliteus hiatus, it inserts on the proximal 10 to 20 cm of the posterior surface of the tibia [45]. It is the primary dynamic lateral stabilizer of the knee, and its primary function is to internally rotate the leg [46]. Moreover, the contraction of the popliteus muscle unlocks the full extension of the knee. The popliteus tendon sends attachments to the lateral meniscus (the popliteal meniscal ligament) and to the styloid process of the fibula (the popliteal fibular ligament) [45]. The arcuate ligament is a Y-shaped thickening of the capsule, found superficial to the popliteus tendon, and it helps prevent external rotation and varus angulation of the leg [49].
The fabella is a sesamoid bone, it is present in 20% of the population and it is found in the lateral head of the gastrocnemius. The fabellofibular ligament extends from the styloid process of the fibula to the fabella; if the fabella is absent, the fabellofibular ligament extends to the lateral femoral condyle [49].
The lateral head of the gastrocnemius muscle originates from the posterior aspect of the lateral epicondyle of the femur and it joins with the medial head of the gastrocnemius, soleus, and plantaris muscles to create the calcaneal (Achilles) tendon, which inserts on the calcaneal tuberosity. The lateral head of the gastrocnemius muscle helps stabilize the posterolateral aspect of the knee [46].
The tendon of the biceps femoris fuses with the FCL, forming a conjoint tendon, and inserts into the anterolateral aspect of the head of the fibula.
Another anterolateral knee stabilizer is the iliotibial tract. It is on the lateral side of the knee but anterior to the tendon of the biceps femoris and it inserts onto the anterolateral tubercle of the tibia [49]. Therefore, the primary structures responsible for the stability of the posterolateral corner are the FCL, popliteus tendon, and PFL [46] [49].

Injury mechanism

Injuries of the lateral compartment of the knee are less common than injuries of the medial compartment [47]. However, injuries of the lateral structures may be more disabling because these structures are subjected to greater force during gait. FCL injuries are caused by varus force with internal rotation of the tibia [48]. Instead, the mechanism of posterolateral injury is either direct varus force while the tibia is externally rotated or sudden hyperextension of the knee [48].

Clinical evaluation

In the case of FCL injury, the symptoms depend on the severity of the lesion and on the presence of associated lesions. The patient generally reports a feeling of jerking or tearing on the lateral side [50]. The clinical evaluation involves performing the varus stress test at 0° and 30° of flexion. This test can differentiate between isolated FCL injuries and injuries involving the FCL as well as the PCL or ACL [50]. Measurable varus laxity at 0° of flexion should lead to suspect of an associated injury, whereas a 30° laxity should lead to suspect FCL isolated injury [50].
FCL injuries can be divided into 3 different degrees of gravity.

- Grade 1: minimal tear, 1-5 mm of joint opening.
- Grade 2: partial tear, 6-10 mm of joint opening.
- Grade 3: complete tear, more than 10 mm of joint opening.

Fanelli and Larsen described another type of grading system, that classifies PLC injuries as types A, B, and C [51]. Fanelli grade A describes an isolated injury to PFL, clinically manifested with increased external rotation [51]. Fanelli grade B involves injury to PFL and partial FCL, so external rotation is increased and mild varus instability is present, too [51]. Fanelli grade C is the most severe PLC injury. It describes a complete injury to PFL, FCL, and cruciate ligaments with a significant rotational and varus instability [51].
When a posterolateral corner injury is suspected, the examination of the knee should be done with more tests, such as the posterolateral drawer test, dial test, reverse pivot shift test, external rotation recurvatum test. The examination findings are considered positive if one knee is different from the other [50].
Injuries to the posterolateral corner of the knee can be assessed with the posterolateral drawer test,

dial test, reverse pivot shift, external rotation recurvatum test, and varus stress tests.

Posterolateral drawer test

During a posterior drawer test, the patient lies supine. The examiner flexes the patient's hip to 45°, flexes the knee to 80°, externally rotates the leg 15°, then he applies a force directed posteriorly.

A positive result for PCL injury is indicated by clinically significant posterolateral translation movement on one side [50].

Dial test

Dial test is used to evaluate posterolateral corner and PCL injuries. The patient is lying prone with the knees flexed to 90° and heels together and then with the knees flexed to 30°. The examiner has to observe the external rotation of the legs and the position of each foot. In case of posterolateral corner injury in combination with a PCL injury, the extra-rotation of the affected knee is greater than the non-affected knee at both 30° and 90° of flexion.

Instead, a positive result for an isolated posterolateral corner injury is considered if the asymmetry between the right and left foot is present with the knees at 30° of flexion but not at 90° [50].

Reverse pivot shift test

The reverse pivot shift test is a dynamic test and it is performed with the patient in a supine position. The examiner flexes the knee to 90° and the leg is in extra-rotation due to the posterior subluxation of the lateral tibial plate. The examiner then extends the knee, and the lateral tibial plateau shifts from a posterior subluxed position to a reduced position in full extension, resulting in a characteristic clunk [50].

External rotation recurvatum test

In this test, the examiner determines if there is an increased amount of knee hyperextension compared to the contralateral side. The test is performed while applying a stabilizing force to the distal thigh while one lifts the great toe to assess the amount of knee recurvatum present.

A positive result is confirmed when the lower leg falls into external rotation and recurvatum, indicating a posterolateral corner injury [50].

Treatment

Non-operative management is recommended for grade I and grade II isolated PLC injuries (grade C of Fanelli classification is automatically excluded) and it may offer good outcomes [51]. The patient returned to the previous level of activity without surgical treatment after only rehabilitation. Appropriate rehabilitation and gait training may be helpful in treating grade I or grade II injuries [51].

Instead, grade III, grade II posterolateral corner injuries associated with other structural injuries and Fanelli grade C can be treated with surgical management [51].

Acute injuries, an injury that happened within 3 weeks prior to treatment, can be managed with direct repair or augmentation. If the grade of injury is severe, the primary repair is not recommended. The hamstring tendon, biceps tendon, and ITB are candidates for allograft [52].

Instead, chronic injury (more than 3 weeks following injury) can be treated with reconstruction. In chronic injury, the most important factor to consider is the lower limb alignment. In fact, diagnosis and treatment of limb malalignment should not be overlooked in the management of chronic ligamentous instability. If there is more than 3° of varus deviation, high tibial osteotomy can be considered. The most used surgical technique was described by Larson in 2005. It is an anatomic reconstruction of the PFL and LCL using the fibular-based technique and the Achilles tendon as an allograft, that can make the popliteal complex and LCL balanced appropriately [52].

The recommendations about postoperative rehabilitation in isolated PLC injuries expect unlocked hinged knee brace, passive range of motion from 0° to 90° for 2-4 weeks, and protected weight-bearing for the first 4-6 weeks [53]. A normal gait pattern should be achieved 8 weeks after surgery, then the patient can regain full of motion of the knee including quadriceps-strengthening and progressive resistance exercises [53]. Return to sport may begin 4-6 months after surgery [53]. Instead, in case of multiple-ligament injury during the first 12-16 weeks, one of the aims of rehabilitations protocol is to protect the reconstructed cruciate ligament [53]. Restricted weight-bearing of 5-10 kg is recommended for the first 4-8 weeks and physiotherapy should focus on regaining ROM, muscle activation, strength, and balance [53]. At this point, after 12 weeks the player can start greater weight-bearing activities. After 16 weeks he can initiate to recover basic motor skills and then soccer-specific skills [53]. A gradual and safe return to sport is possible after 8-12 months, but a return to play to the pre-injury level is highly unlikely [53].

Articular cartilage injuries

Articular cartilage injuries of the knee are included in high-impact sport, especially in soccer [54]. The constant loading stress in soccer players is the cause of articular cartilage modifications, such as the decrease of proteoglycan levels and the increase of degenerative enzyme levels, leading in chondrocyte apoptosis [55]. This process will result in features modifications of articular cartilage, such as volume and stiffness leading to cartilage defects [55]. Moreover, the capacity to potentially heal is limited due to poor supply of vessels and nerves [56].

The prevalence of articular cartilage lesions was calculated in a systematic review by Andrade et al. [54], which reported 217 articular cartilage defects in a total cohort of 183 soccer players. The overall prevalence was 1.19 cartilage lesions per each knee assessed. The majority of the chondral lesions in soccer players is at the femoral condyles, especially the medial femoral condyle (51%), followed by patellofemoral joint (18%) and tibial plateaus (4%) [54]. The defect size varies from 0.6 to 7.0 cm^2.

Mechanism of injury and clinical evaluation

Generally, chondral defects are caused by forceful and repetitive mechanical stresses on the knee joint during the soccer practice [57]. If the cartilage defect is very superficial, athletes may be asymptomatic. Instead, if the damage reaches the subchondral bone, the patient complains knee pain, swelling, catching, and locking [58]. In asymptomatic athletes it is important to diagnose articular cartilage defects, because, if not treated properly, they may lead to an early onset of knee osteoarthritis [59].

There are no specific tests to make a certain diagnosis; the pain can be evoked through joint line palpation. Therefore, the doctor must take advantage of the anamnesis and magnetic resonance imaging (MRI), used to estimate the size of articular cartilage defects during the preoperative time. However, the size of the lesions is underestimated compared with final post debridement size as measured during arthroscopic knee surgery [60].

Treatment

The treatment of chondral defects is complex and multifactorial. In fact, surgical technique decision depends on player's age, defect size, level of competition, career status, and time into the season [61]. The choice of treatment is also based on the type of lesion according to Outerbridge classification. It is divided into four degrees of severity [62]:

- Grade I: softening and swelling articular cartilage.
- Grade II: fragmentation and fissuring of articular cartilage affecting an area of less than 0.5 inches.
- Grade III: fragmentation and fissuring of articular cartilage affecting an area greater than 0.5 inches.
- Grade IV: cartilage erosion to the bone.

Non-operative treatment should only be considered when there is a superficial focal and small lesion (grade I and grade II of Outerbridge classification) and it includes chondroprotective pharmacotherapy, nonsteroidal anti-inflammatory medication and tramadol, physiotherapy, and hydrotherapy [63].

Instead, surgical treatment is recommended in case of high-grade articular cartilage damage (Outerbridge grade III and IV) and the most commonly used are microfracture, mosaicplasty or osteochondral autograft transplantation (OAT), autologous chondrocyte implantation (ACI), and matrix-induced autologous chondrocyte implantation (MACI) [64]. Large articular cartilage defects (>2cm^2) benefit the most from ACI/MACI procedures [65]. These two techniques have a delayed return to sports but provide a durable and higher-quality repaired tissue [64]. Instead, OAT/mosaicplasty and microfracture allow a faster return to competition; however, they have lower durability and quality [64].

The postoperative rehabilitation should be an individualized program according to surgical technique, to the athlete's specific demands, and to biologic phase of healing [61]. In phase I it is recommended to avoid excessive mechanical overload, allowing graft integration and proliferation. The goals are the progressive regain of range of motion, weight bearing and muscle control [61]. To start phase II the athlete must achieve full passive knee range of movement, muscle activation, and normal gait. Phase II provides progressive loading and functional joint restoration with the introduction of sport-specific movement patterns [66]. Finally, in phase III, while remodeling and maturation of repair cartilage, the athlete can start late stages to reestablish the preinjury level, improving muscle power and coordination, neuromuscular control, speed and endurance performance, metabolic capacity, self-efficacy, and sport-specific movement patterns [66].

Bibliography

1. FIFA Big Count 2006: 270 million people active in football. FIFA Communications Division, Information Services, 31/05/2007. Document online: http://bit.ly/37KQ31y

2. Kohn D, Moreno B. Meniscus insertion anatomy as a basis for meniscus replacement: a morphological cadaveric study. Arthroscopy. 1995 Feb;11(1):96-103.

3. Melton JT, Murray JR, Karim A, Pandit H, Wandless F, Thomas NP. Meniscal repair in anterior cruciate ligament reconstruction: a long-term outcome study. Knee Surg Sports Traumatol Arthrosc. 2011 Oct;19(10):1729-34.

4. Makris EA, Hadidi P, Athanasiou KA. The knee meniscus: structure-function, pathophysiology, current repair techniques, and prospects for regeneration. Biomaterials. 2011 Oct;32(30):7411-31.

5. Musahl V, Rahnemai-Azar AA, Costello J, Arner JW, Fu FH, Hoshino Y, Lopomo N, Samuelsson K, Irrgang JJ. The Influence of Meniscal and Anterolateral Capsular Injury on Knee Laxity in Patients With Anterior Cruciate Ligament Injuries. Am J Sports Med. 2016 Dec;44(12):3126-3131.

6. Musahl V, Citak M, O'Loughlin PF, Choi D, Bedi A, Pearle AD. The effect of medial versus lateral meniscectomy on the stability of the anterior cruciate ligament-deficient knee. Am J Sports Med. 2010 Aug;38(8):1591-7.

7. Zaffagnini S, Signorelli C, Bonanzinga T, Grassi A, Galán H, Akkawi I, Bragonzoni L, Cataldi F, Marcacci M. Does meniscus removal affect ACL-deficient knee laxity? An in vivo study. Knee Surg Sports Traumatol Arthrosc. 2016 Nov;24(11):3599-3604.

8. Lento PH, Akuthota V. Meniscal injuries: a critical review. J Back Musculoskelet Rehabil. 2000 Jan 1;15(2):55-62.

9. Beaufils P, Hulet C, Dhénain M, Nizard R, Nourissat G, Pujol N. Clinical practice guidelines for the management of meniscal lesions and isolated lesions of the anterior cruciate ligament of the knee in adults. Orthop Traumatol Surg Res. 2009 Oct;95(6):437-42.

10. Solomon DH, Simel DL, Bates DW, Katz JN, Schaffer JL. The rational clinical examination. Does this patient have a torn meniscus or ligament of the knee? Value of the physical examination. JAMA. 2001 Oct 3;286(13):1610-20.

11. Jackson JL, O'Malley PG, Kroenke K. Evaluation of acute knee pain in primary care. Ann Intern Med. 2003 Oct 7;139(7):575-88.

12. Fowler PJ, Lubliner JA. The predictive value of five clinical signs in the evaluation of meniscal pathology. Arthroscopy. 1989;5(3):184-6.

13. McMurray, TP. The semilunar cartilages. Br J Surg 1942;29:407-14.

14. Kurosaka M, Yagi M, Yoshiya S, Muratsu H, Mizuno K. Efficacy of the axially loaded pivot shift test for the diagnosis of a meniscal tear. Int Orthop. 1999;23(5):271-4.

15. Steenbrugge F, Van Nieuwenhuyse W, Verdonk R, Verstraete K. Arthroscopic meniscus repair in the ACL-deficient knee. Int Orthop. 2005 Apr;29(2):109-12.

16. Cannon WD Jr, Vittori JM. The incidence of healing in arthroscopic meniscal repairs in anterior cruciate ligament-reconstructed knees versus stable knees. Am J Sports Med. 1992 Mar-Apr;20(2):176-81.

17. Alvarez-Diaz P, Alentorn-Geli E, Llobet F, Granados N, Steinbacher G, Cugat R. Return to play after all-inside meniscal repair in competitive football players: a minimum 5-year follow-up. Knee Surg Sports Traumatol Arthrosc. 2016 Jun;24(6):1997-2001.

18. Smith MV, Nepple JJ, Wright RW, Matava MJ, Brophy RH. Knee Osteoarthritis is associated with previous menis-

cus and anterior cruciate ligament surgery among elite college american football athletes. Sports Health. 2017 May/Jun;9(3):247-251.
19. Ellison AE, Berg EE. Embryology, anatomy, and function of the anterior cruciate ligament. Orthop Clin North Am. 1985 Jan;16(1):3-14.
20. Kobayashi H, Kanamura T, Koshida S, Miyashita K, Okado T, Shimizu T, Yokoe K. Mechanisms of the anterior cruciate ligament injury in sports activities: a twenty-year clinical research of 1,700 athletes. J Sports Sci Med. 2010 Dec 1;9(4):669-75.
21. van Eck CF, van den Bekerom MP, Fu FH, Poolman RW, Kerkhoffs GM. Methods to diagnose acute anterior cruciate ligament rupture: a meta-analysis of physical examinations with and without anaesthesia. Knee Surg Sports Traumatol Arthrosc. 2013 Aug;21(8):1895-903.
22. Benjaminse A, Gokeler A, van der Schans CP. Clinical diagnosis of an anterior cruciate ligament rupture: a meta-analysis. J Orthop Sports Phys Ther. 2006 May;36(5):267-88.
23. International Knee Documentation Committee. IKDC Knee Examination Forms 2000. Document online: http://bit.ly/35I3xcx
24. Andernord D, Karlsson J, Musahl V, Bhandari M, Fu FH, Samuelsson K. Timing of surgery of the anterior cruciate ligament. Arthroscopy. 2013 Nov;29(11):1863-71.
25. Kvist J. Rehabilitation following anterior cruciate ligament injury: current recommendations for sports participation. Sports Med. 2004;34(4):269-80.
26. McCormack RG, Hutchinson MR. Time to be honest regarding outcomes of ACL reconstructions: should we be quoting 55-65% success rates for high-level athletes? Br J Sports Med. 2016 Oct;50(19):1167-8.
27. Kyritsis P, Bahr R, Landreau P, Miladi R, Witvrouw E. Likelihood of ACL graft rupture: not meeting six clinical discharge criteria before return to sport is associated with a four times greater risk of rupture. Br J Sports Med. 2016 Aug;50(15):946-51.
28. Hildebrandt C, Müller L, Zisch B, Huber R, Fink C, Raschner C. Functional assessments for decision-making regarding return to sports following ACL reconstruction. Part I: development of a new test battery. Knee Surg Sports Traumatol Arthrosc. 2015 May;23(5):1273-81.
29. Ardern CL, Taylor NF, Feller JA, Webster KE. Fifty-five per cent return to competitive sport following anterior cruciate ligament reconstruction surgery: an updated systematic review and meta-analysis including aspects of physical functioning and contextual factors. Br J Sports Med. 2014 Nov;48(21):1543-52.
30. Ardern CL, Taylor NF, Feller JA, Whitehead TS, Webster KE. Psychological responses matter in returning to preinjury level of sport after anterior cruciate ligament reconstruction surgery. Am J Sports Med. 2013 Jul;41(7):1549-58.
31. Andriolo L, Filardo G, Kon E, Ricci M, Della Villa F, Della Villa S, Zaffagnini S, Marcacci M. Revision anterior cruciate ligament reconstruction: clinical outcome and evidence for return to sport. Knee Surg Sports Traumatol Arthrosc. 2015 Oct;23(10):2825-45.
32. Czuppon S, Racette BA, Klein SE, Harris-Hayes M. Variables associated with return to sport following anterior cruciate ligament reconstruction: a systematic review. Br J Sports Med. 2014 Mar;48(5):356-64.
33. Kvist J, Ek A, Sporrstedt K, Good L. Fear of re-injury: a hindrance for returning to sports after anterior cruciate ligament reconstruction. Knee Surg Sports Traumatol Arthrosc. 2005 Jul;13(5):393-7.
34. Peterson L, Junge A, Chomiak J, Graf-Baumann T, Dvorak J. Incidence of football injuries and complaints in different age groups and skill-level groups. Am J Sports Med. 2000;28(5 Suppl):S51-7.
35. LaPrade RF, Engebretsen AH, Ly TV, Johansen S, Wentorf FA, Engebretsen L. The anatomy of the medial part of the knee. J Bone Joint Surg Am. 2007 Sep;89(9):2000-10.
36. Laprade RF, Wijdicks CA. The management of injuries to the medial side of the knee. J Orthop Sports Phys Ther. 2012 Mar;42(3):221-33.
37. Phisitkul P, James SL, Wolf BR, Amendola A. MCL injuries of the knee: current concepts review. Iowa Orthop J. 2006;26:77-90.
38. Wijdicks CA, Griffith CJ, Johansen S, Engebretsen L, LaPrade RF. Injuries to the medial collateral ligament and associated medial structures of the knee. J Bone Joint Surg Am. 2010 May;92(5):1266-80.
39. Kim C, Chasse PM, Taylor DC. Return to play after medial collateral ligament injury. Clin Sports Med. 2016 Oct;35(4):679-96.
40. Logterman SL, Wydra FB, Frank RM. Posterior cruciate ligament: anatomy and biomechanics. Curr Rev Musculoskelet Med. 2018 Sep;11(3):510-514.
41. Pache S, Aman ZS, Kennedy M, Nakama GY, Moatshe G, Ziegler C, LaPrade RF. Posterior cruciate ligament: current concepts review. Arch Bone Jt Surg. 2018 Jan;6(1):8-18.
42. Whipple TL, Ellis FD. Posterior cruciate ligament injuries. Clin Sports Med. 1991 Jul;10(3):515-27.
43. Harner CD, Höher J. Evaluation and treatment of posterior cruciate ligament injuries. Am J Sports Med. 1998 May-Jun;26(3):471-82.
44. Parolie JM, Bergfeld JA. Long-term results of nonoperative treatment of isolated posterior cruciate ligament injuries in the athlete. Am J Sports Med. 1986 Jan-Feb;14(1):35-8.
45. Cooper JM, McAndrews PT, LaPrade RF. Posterolateral corner injuries of the knee: anatomy, diagnosis, and treatment. Sports Med Arthrosc Rev. 2006 Dec;14(4):213-20.
46. Miller TT, Gladden P, Staron RB, Henry JH, Feldman F. Posterolateral stabilizers of the knee: anatomy and injuries assessed with MR imaging. AJR Am J Roentgenol. 1997 Dec;169(6):1641-7.
47. Majewski M, Susanne H, Klaus S. Epidemiology of athletic knee injuries: a 10-year study. Knee. 2006 Jun;13(3):184-8.
48. Covey DC. Injuries of the posterolateral corner of the knee. J Bone Joint Surg Am. 2001 Jan;83(1):106-18.
49. Watanabe Y, Moriya H, Takahashi K, Yamagata M, Sonoda M, Shimada Y, Tamaki T. Functional anatomy of the posterolateral structures of the knee. Arthroscopy. 1993;9(1):57-62.
50. Schweller EW, Ward PJ. Posterolateral corner knee injuries: review of anatomy and clinical evaluation. J Am Osteopath Assoc. 2015 Dec;115(12):725-31.
51. Fanelli GC, Larson RV. Practical management of posterolateral instability of the knee. Arthroscopy. 2002 Feb;18(2 Suppl 1):1-8.
52. Shon OJ, Park JW, Kim BJ. Current concepts of posterolateral corner injuries of the knee. Knee Surg Relat Res. 2017 Dec 1;29(4):256-268.
53. Irrgang JJ, Fitzgerald GK. Rehabilitation of the multiple-ligament-injured knee. Clin Sports Med. 2000 Jul;19(3):545-71.
54. Andrade R, Vasta S, Papalia R, Pereira H, Oliveira JM, Reis RL, Espregueira-Mendes J. Prevalence of articular cartilage lesions and surgical clinical outcomes in football (soc-

cer) players' knees: a systematic review. Arthroscopy. 2016 Jul;32(7):1466-77.
55. Lohmander LS, Roos H, Dahlberg L, Hoerrner LA, Lark MW. Temporal patterns of stromelysin-1, tissue inhibitor, and proteoglycan fragments in human knee joint fluid after injury to the cruciate ligament or meniscus. J Orthop Res. 1994 Jan;12(1):21-8.
56. Buckwalter JA. Articular cartilage: injuries and potential for healing. J Orthop Sports Phys Ther. 1998 Oct;28(4):192-202.
57. Gomoll AH, Filardo G, de Girolamo L, Espregueira-Mendes J, Marcacci M, Rodkey WG, Steadman JR, Zaffagnini S, Kon E. Surgical treatment for early osteoarthritis. Part I: cartilage repair procedures. Knee Surg Sports Traumatol Arthrosc. 2012 Mar;20(3):450-66.
58. Flanigan DC, Harris JD, Trinh TQ, Siston RA, Brophy RH. Prevalence of chondral defects in athletes' knees: a systematic review. Med Sci Sports Exerc. 2010 Oct;42(10):1795-801.
59. Vannini F, Spalding T, Andriolo L, Berruto M, Denti M, Espregueira-Mendes J, Menetrey J, Peretti GM, Seil R, Filardo G. Sport and early osteoarthritis: the role of sport in aetiology, progression and treatment of knee osteoarthritis. Knee Surg Sports Traumatol Arthrosc. 2016 Jun;24(6):1786-96.
60. Campbell AB, Knopp MV, Kolovich GP, Wei W, Jia G, Siston RA, Flanigan DC. Preoperative MRI underestimates articular cartilage defect size compared with findings at arthroscopic knee surgery. Am J Sports Med. 2013 Mar;41(3):590-5.
61. Hambly K, Silvers HJ, Steinwachs M. Rehabilitation after articular cartilage repair of the knee in the football (soccer) player. Cartilage. 2012 Jan;3(1 Suppl):50S-6S.
62. Rodríguez-Merchán EC, Gómez-Cardero P. The outerbridge classification predicts the need for patellar resurfacing in TKA. Clin Orthop Relat Res. 2010 May;468(5):1254-7.
63. Gorsline RT, Kaeding CC. The use of NSAIDs and nutritional supplements in athletes with osteoarthritis: prevalence, benefits, and consequences. Clin Sports Med. 2005 Jan;24(1):71-82.
64. Bekkers JE, de Windt TS, Brittberg M, Saris DB. Cartilage repair in football (soccer) athletes: what evidence leads to which treatment? A critical review of the literature. Cartilage. 2012 Jan;3(1 Suppl):43S-9S.
65. Kon E, Filardo G, Berruto M, Benazzo F, Zanon G, Della Villa S, Marcacci M. Articular cartilage treatment in high-level male soccer players: a prospective comparative study of arthroscopic second-generation autologous chondrocyte implantation versus microfracture. Am J Sports Med. 2011 Dec;39(12):2549-57.
66. Mithoefer K, Hambly K, Logerstedt D, Ricci M, Silvers H, Della Villa S. Current concepts for rehabilitation and return to sport after knee articular cartilage repair in the athlete. J Orthop Sports Phys Ther. 2012 Mar;42(3):254-73.
67. Teitz CC, Hu SS, Arendt EA. The female athlete: evaluation and treatment of sports-related problems. J Am Acad Orthop Surg. 1997 Mar;5(2):87-96.
68. Arnoczky SP, Warren RF. Microvasculature of the human meniscus. Am J Sports Med. 1982 Mar-Apr;10(2):90-5.
69. Masouros SD, McDermott ID, Amis AA, Bull AM. Biomechanics of the meniscus-meniscal ligament construct of the knee. Knee Surg Sports Traumatol Arthrosc. 2008 Dec;16(12):1121-32.
70. Hash TW 2nd. Magnetic resonance imaging of the knee. Sports Health. 2013 Jan;5(1):78-107.
71. Kosaka M, Nakase J, Toratani T, Ohashi Y, Kitaoka K, Yamada H, Komura K, Nakamura S, Tsuchiya H. Oblique coronal and oblique sagittal MRI for diagnosis of anterior cruciate ligament tears and evaluation of anterior cruciate ligament remnant tissue. Knee. 2014 Jan;21(1):54-7.
72. Ekstrand J, Hägglund M, Kristenson K, Magnusson H, Waldén M. Fewer ligament injuries but no preventive effect on muscle injuries and severe injuries: an 11-year follow-up of the UEFA Champions League injury study. Br J Sports Med. 2013 Aug;47(12):732-7.
73. Peterson L, Junge A, Chomiak J, Graf-Baumann T, Dvorak J. Incidence of football injuries and complaints in different age groups and skill-level groups. Am J Sports Med. 2000;28(5 Suppl):S51-7.
74. Arnason A, Sigurdsson SB, Gudmundsson A, Holme I, Engebretsen L, Bahr R. Risk factors for injuries in football. Am J Sports Med. 2004 Jan-Feb;32(1 Suppl):5S-16S.
75. Brophy R, Silvers HJ, Gonzales T, Mandelbaum BR. Gender influences: the role of leg dominance in ACL injury among soccer players. Br J Sports Med. 2010 Aug;44(10):694-7.
76. Ekstrand J, Hägglund M, Waldén M. Injury incidence and injury patterns in professional football: the UEFA injury study. Br J Sports Med. 2011 Jun;45(7):553-8.
77. Nielsen AB, Yde J. Epidemiology and traumatology of injuries in soccer. Am J Sports Med. 1989 Nov-Dec;17(6):803-7.
78. Lundblad M, Waldén M, Magnusson H, Karlsson J, Ekstrand J. The UEFA injury study: 11-year data concerning 346 MCL injuries and time to return to play. Br J Sports Med. 2013 Aug;47(12):759-62.

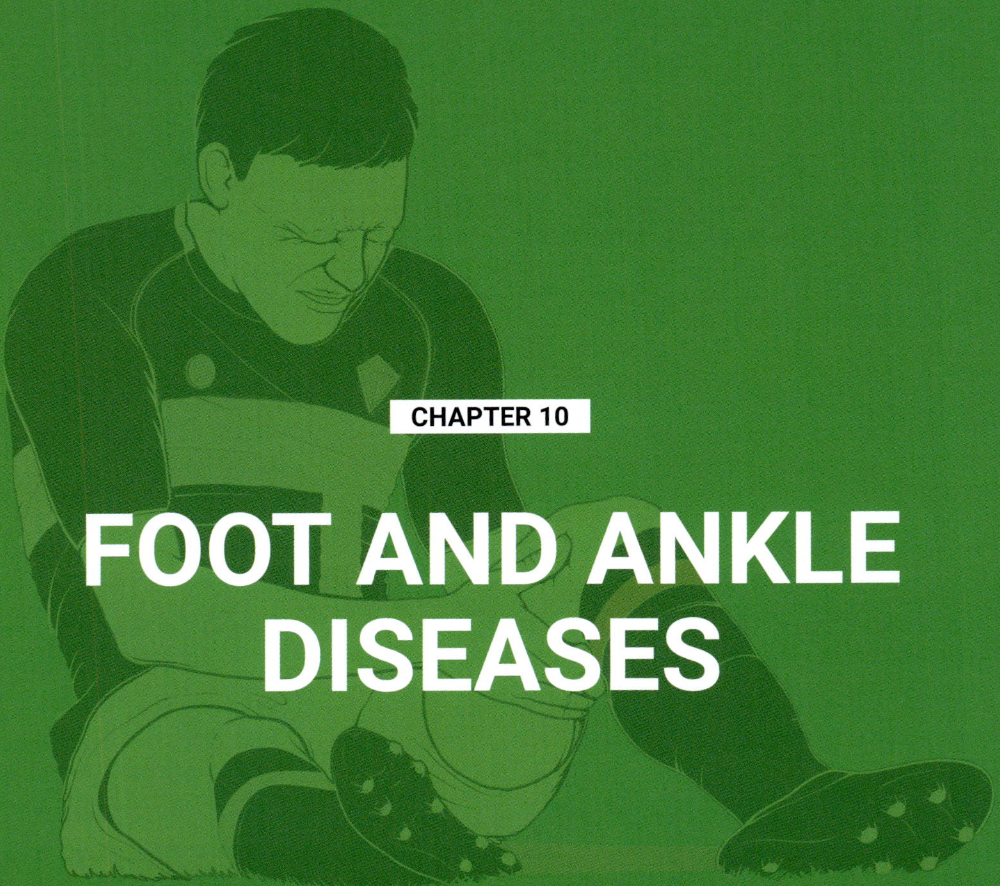

CHAPTER 10

FOOT AND ANKLE DISEASES

Sandro Giannini [1]
Antonio Mazzotti [2]

[1] IRCCS Istituto Ortopedico Rizzoli, Bologna, Italy
University of Bologna, Italy

[2] 1st Orthopaedic and Traumatologic Clinic (Director: C. Faldini)
IRCCS Istituto Ortopedico Rizzoli, Bologna, Italy

Introduction

Soccer is a popular sport, spread in over 200 countries: because of the intrinsic characteristic of this activity, foot and ankle are two of the most commonly injured anatomical sites, probably only second to those of the knee and the thigh [1-3].

Elite soccer players experience between 13 to 35 injuries per 1,000 competitive player hours [2]: above them 80% are traumatic and 20% overuse related. A study on English Premier League clubs reported that over a four season period, 20% of the injuries were at the foot and ankle level with a mean return to sport time of 54 days [2]. The incidence of injuries increases with age and is 4-6 times higher during competition than training [2, 4, 5]. The most affected sites are the ankle in 56% of cases, the hindfoot in 30% of cases and the midfoot in 4% of cases. Considering all lesions, ankle sprains are the most common [5, 12]. Other common lesions are tendon [2-23%], muscular, and osteochondral lesions: these conditions will be discussed in separate chapters [2, 3].

Fractures are rare and represent only 1% of injuries. Despite that, when a fracture occurs it impacts a much more protracted recovery. The dominant limb is affected in 79% of cases [1, 2].

The mechanism of injury is caused by direct contact from 23 to 33% of cases, followed by overuse (26%), trigging on the grass (10.5%), landing (7.5%), jumping and jumping/landing (7.5%), tackling (4.5%), being tackled (4.5%), kicking and kicking / shooting (3%), sprinting (1.5%) [3].

Several risk factors have been reported. These can be distinguished in intrinsic factors (related to the player) and extrinsic factors (related to external factors). The most common intrinsic factors are represented by ligamentous laxity, muscles tightness, previous traumas, foot morphological alterations or deformities and inadequate rehabilitation. The most important extrinsic factors include fatigue, climatic factors, playing surface type, ground conditions, equipments, training and warming defects [13]. Other foot and ankle problems in soccer are represented by deformities related pathologies such as cavus foot, flatfoot, hallux valgus, hallux rigidus, fifth toe varus, hammer toes, plantar fasciitis, nerve compression syndrome, and dermatologic problems. In this chapter all the above mentioned topics will be briefly presented.

Ankle sprains

The ankle is a highly complex anatomical structure that must provide mobility and stability, being able to absorb impacts and adapt to the irregularities of the ground. In subjects who practice sports such as soccer, it must also support important repeated efforts and stresses and guarantee excellent functionality. Three main groups of ligaments are responsible for ankle joint stability: the lateral and medial ligaments and the distal tibio-fibular syndesmosis (figg. 1, 2).

Ankle sprains are the most common traumatic injuries in soccer [1, 2, 14]. These lesions account for between 13 and 36 % of all soccer-related injuries, with an incidence varying from 1.7 to 2.0 per 1,000 hours of exposure. Moreover, of the injuries associated with the ankle, ankle sprains have been found to be the most common, accounting for between 42% and 98% [2]. Most sprains occur outside of player contact, due to the repetitive kicking motion, constant changing of direction, and frequent acceleration and deceleration [11]. The dominant leg has been reported to be the more common site of injury. Acute ankle sprains may

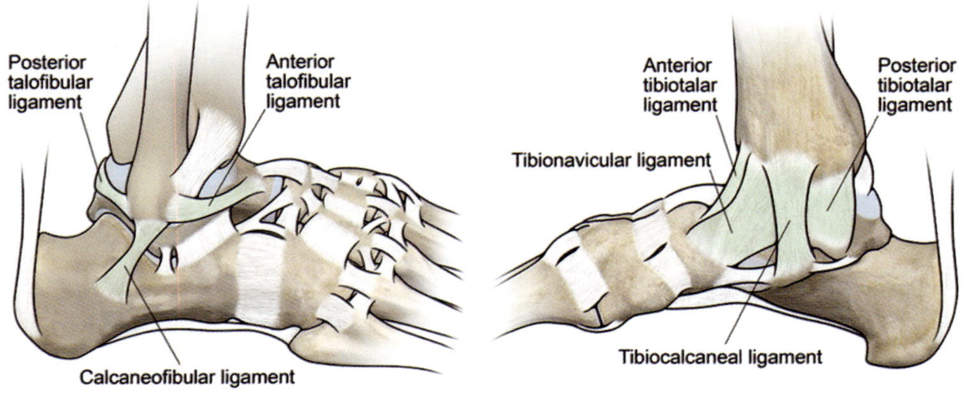

Figure 1 - On the left side, lateral ligaments: anterior talo-fibular ligament (ATFL), calcaneo-fibular ligament (CFL), and posterior talo-fibular ligament (PTFL). On the right side, medial ligaments (also known as deltoid complex): anterior tibiotalar ligament (ATTL), tibio-navicular ligament (TNL), tibio-calcaneal ligament (TCL), posterior tibiotalar ligament (PTTL)

involve both lateral and medial side [5, 15].

Like in many other sports, considering ankle anatomical characteristics, the lateral aspect is most susceptible to experience sprains (with the occurrence rate being closer to 3 lateral to 1 medial sprain) [2, 5]. Despite this evidence some authors reported that soccer players are more inclined to medial ankle injuries than other sports due to the most frequent use of the medial aspect of the foot and ankle to kick and pass the ball, and due to its common exposition to tackles.

Ankle sprain mechanisms include the prevalent actions involved in soccer, like cutting, kicking, running, tackling, being tackled, and landing.

The most common foot and ankle positions when a sprain occurs is pronation, neutral in the sagittal plane for the weightbearing limb and plantarflexion/neutral for the non-weightbearing limb. The most common rotations involved are external rotation and eversion [14]. Ankle with greater plantar flexion strength and a smaller dorsiflexion to plantarflexion ratio had a higher incidence of inversion sprains.

Ankle sprains can further be divided into contact and noncontact ankle sprains.

Contact ankle injuries are quite common and have been reported to comprise over 70% of ankle sprains. Two are the most common mechanisms specific to soccer actions that lead to contact ankle sprains: a collision contact on the medial side that leads to a laterally directed force which causes the player to land in an inverted position and a contact of an injured player and an opponent when the injured player is trying to kick the ball and this leads to forced plantar flexion [2, 16].

Another common mechanism occurs while one player comes into contact with another attempting to kick the ball.

Noncontact ankle sprains have a much wider range of reported injury mechanisms, for example when a player lands after going up for a header and, as a result, an inversion sprain occurs [2].

Many are the risk factors for ankle sprains in soccer. A history of prior sprain is a great risk factor for an ankle sprain in a soccer player. Other risk factors include player-to-player contact, condition of the pitch, weight-bearing status of the injured limb at the time of injury, and joint instability or laxity [14, 17]. Other authors also report a limitation of hip rotation and a lack of toe grip [2].

Also, there has been a reported correlation between the occurrence of ankle injuries and the age of the athlete, with older players experiencing a higher occurrence [2]. Other factors are represented by poor neuromuscular postural control [18, 22], and decreased ankle joint range of movement [23, 24]. Conversely, gender [25, 26], age [27, 28], biometry (height, weight) [29, 30], strength (ankle and hip) [23], and anatomical alignment [31, 35] still show conflicting evidence in the literature.

In addition, some extrinsic factors may play a role as a risk factor for ankle sprain, such as improper lace-up of ankle brace [36], third and fourth generation of artificial turf [37], incorrect warm-up

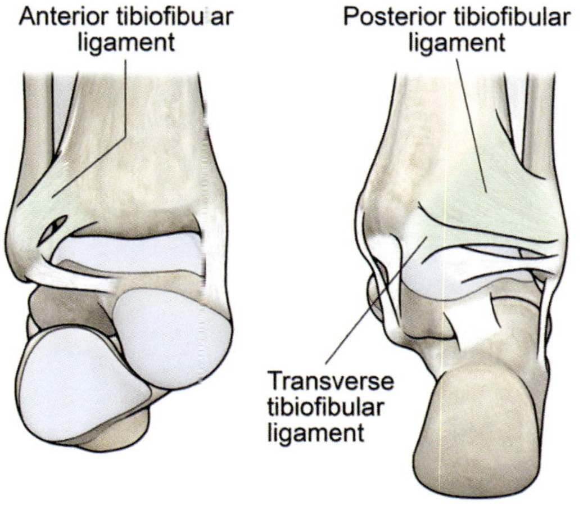

Figure 2 - On the left side, anterior view of the syndesmosis. On the right side, posterior view

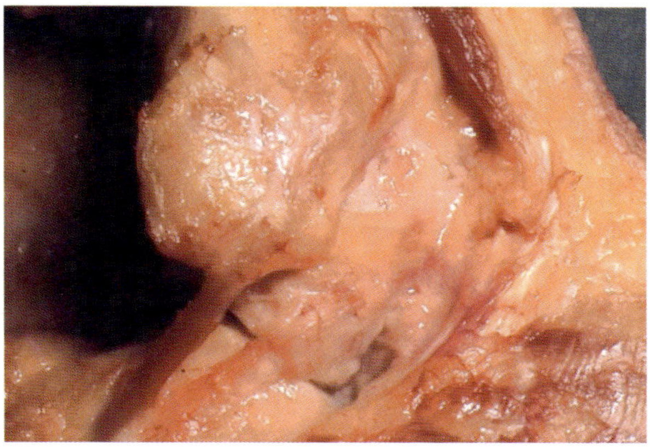

Figure 3 - Anatomical specimen showing the anterior talo-fibular ligament (ATFL), the calcaneofibular ligament (CFL), and the talo-calcaneal ligament (TCL)

[37], player position [28, 38], time into the game/season (which may be associated with accumulated fatigue), and lack of use of external support [39]. Severe or repetitive ankle injuries in soccer players may cause chronic ankle instability, which include both mechanical ligamentous laxity and functional changes.

Ankle sprain sequelae often requires a surgical procedure. Therefore, prevention, a proper initial treatment, and rehabilitation can reduce the amount of lost time from playing and avoid negative problems. Therefore, a proper diagnosis and management of ankle sprains are essential to ensure a rapid and effective recovery, to reduce the risk of relapse, as well as to prevent the development of secondary pathologies.

Lateral ankle sprains

The lateral ankle ligament complex is composed of three ligaments: the anterior talofibular ligament (ATFL), the calcaneofibular ligament (CFL), the talo-calcaneal ligament (TCL), the posterior talofibular ligament (PTFL) (fig. 3) [40]. Of these ligaments, the CFL and, medially, the intermediate layer of the deltoid ligament are isometric throughout the entire range of motion (fig. 4). Lateral ankle sprains are the most common injuries in soccer players and represent from 77% to 91% of all soccer sprains [2, 41].

Injuries to the lateral ankle ligament complex may occur in an isolated or multiligamentous fashion, with a traumatic mechanism occurring with the foot in inversion and plantar flexion.

The ATFL has been reported to be the weakest and the first to be injured when there is an ankle sprain. It ruptures in 66% of the ankle sprains as an isolated injury and, in 20% of the cases, it occurs in combination with a CFL rupture [2]. Isolated capsular lesion or partial rupture of the ATFL is only present in 1% of all the supination injuries [2, 42]. In addition, when a lateral ankle sprain occurs, the subtalar ligaments are also injured (see paragraph below), with an estimated incidence of 75-80% of individuals with chronic ankle instability [2, 43].

When lateral ankle sprains occurring with the foot in an inverted position are more severe, they can also be associated with other lesions (ligaments of the subtalar joint or fractures) [44].

The correct diagnosis is essential for a successful treatment. It is important to exclude all differential diagnosis including medial ankle sprain, high ankle sprain (involving the syndesmosis), osteochondral lesion, or fractures [45, 46]. Neural, muscular, and vascular structures should always be assessed [2]. A physical examination, performed in an acute setting, is usually not well performed, since the results may be biased or limited due to ankle mechanical pain. For this reason, a delayed physical diagnostic examination (about 4-5 days post-injury), as soon as the athlete's swelling and pain have decreased, provides better diagnostic accuracy (fig. 5) [2]. The examination must include inspection of the ankle complex, palpation of the ATFL, the talar inversion tilt test, and the anterior

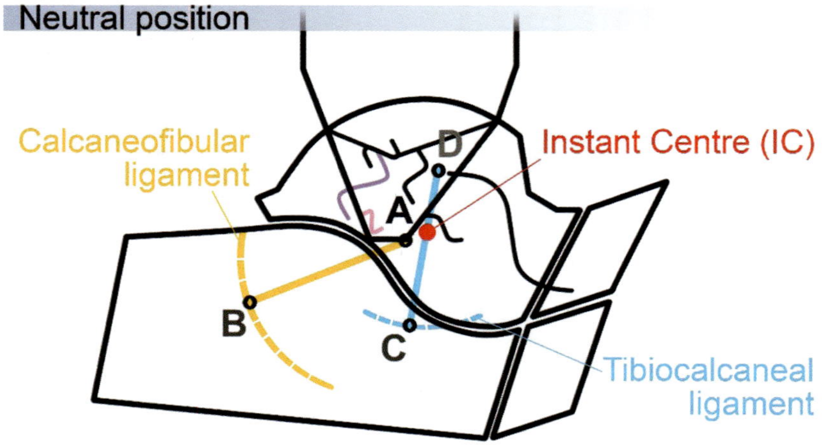

Figure 4 - The CFL and, medially, the intermediate layer of the deltoid ligament are isometric throughout the entire range of motion (Leardini A et al. [225])

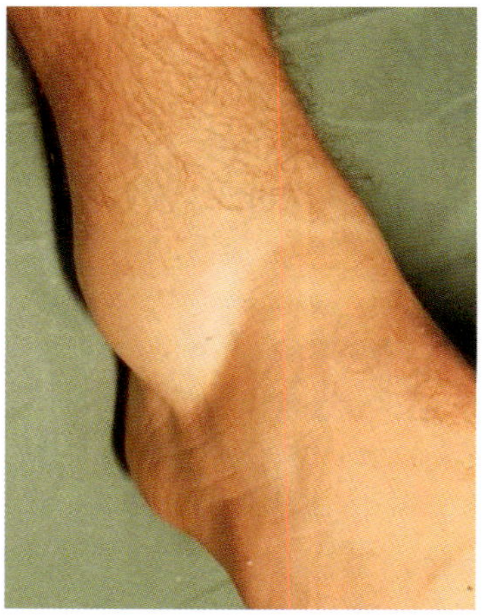

Figure 5 - Swelling in acute setting ankle sprains occurred with the foot in an inverted position

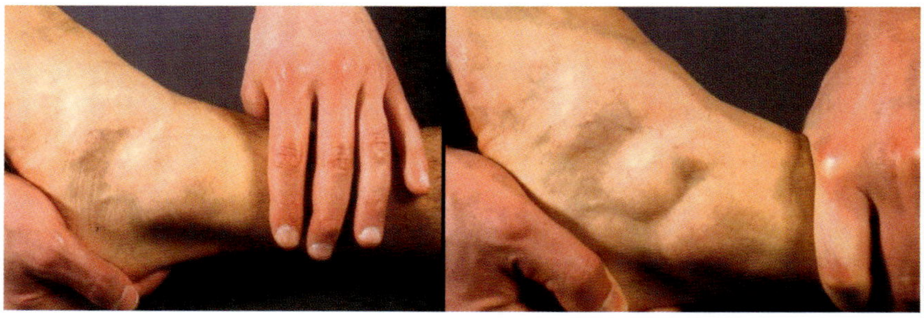

Figure 6 - The anterior drawer reveals an ATFL instability. The patient is in a supine position, the heel is resting on the palm of the examiner's hand that is resting on the table thereby stabilizing the calcaneus. The examiner pushes the tibia posteriorly observing the amount of posterior translation of the tibia and fibula at the lateral aspect of the ankle and the change in end feel

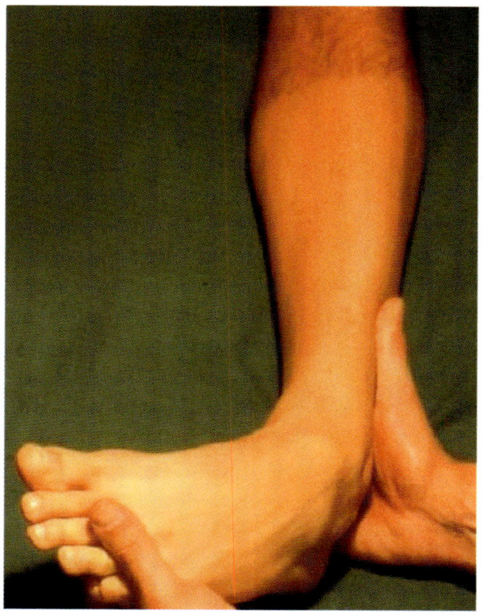

Figure 7 - Talar tilt test is performed to examine the ankle for injury of the ATFL and the CFL: patient is seated with foot and ankle unsupported. The foot is positioned in 10-20 degrees of plantarflexion. The distal lower leg is stabilized with one hand just proximal to the malleoli and the hindfoot is inverted with the other hand. The lateral aspect of the talus is palpated to determine if tilting occurs

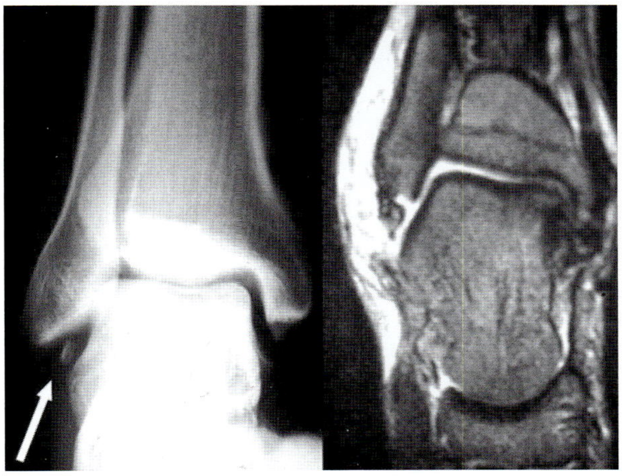

Figure 8 - Ankle X-ray showing a fibular bony fragment; MRI shows an associated ATFL rupture

drawer test (figg. 6, 7). The anterior drawer (which reveals an ATFL instability) and talar tilt (which reveals a CFL instability) tests are useful especially in evaluating ankle instability in the delayed or chronic setting; in any case, both have been shown to have limited sensitivity and significant variability amongst different examiners [2].

In addition to the previous procedures, the clinician should also assess the ankle and subtalar joint range of motion, the presence of ligamentous mechanical laxity, muscular strength, and functional performance (single-limb balance, etc.) [47, 49].

Clinical examination must always be supported by diagnostic tests including X-rays, ultrasounds (US), magnetic resonance imaging (MRI), and computed tomography (CT). When dealing with athletes with an acute lateral ankle trauma, X-rays are crucial to exclude the presence of ankle fractures (figg. 8, 9, 10) [2]. Stress radiography has no role in the routine diagnosis of acute lateral ankle ligament injuries since, during the acute setting, the evaluation may appear difficult due to edema, pain, and muscle spasms [2, 50, 51] (fig. 11). US represent a rapid and inexpensive diagnostic tool, able to provide a detailed and accurate depiction of ankle's anatomic structures and ligament integrity [52]. In detecting ankle ligament ruptures, US shows high sensitivity (92%) and moderate specificity (64%), with positive and negative predictive values of 85 and 77%, respectively (fig. 12) [2]. MRI may be useful to assess integrity and morphology of the lateral ankle ligamentous complex and its peripheral soft tissues [53] or to identify possible associated osteochondral lesions, tendon pathologies, and occult fractures [54] (figg. 13, 14, 15).

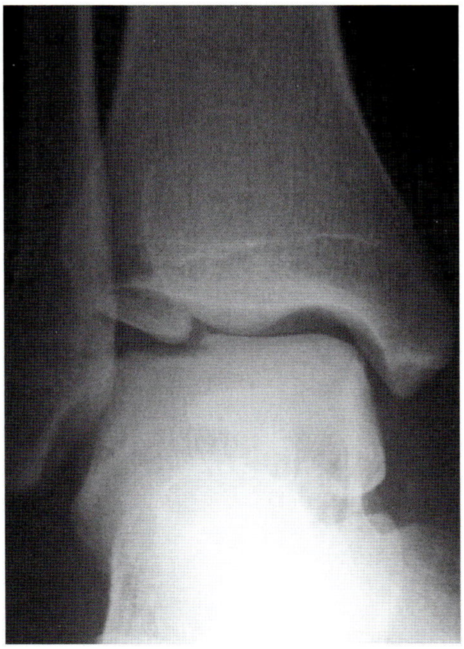

Figure 9 - Ankle X-ray showing an osteochondral fracture

When performing MRI studies the ankle should be positioned at 20 degrees of plantar flexion in order to improve the ligament visualization. CT scans may be useful to assess the articular surface, abnormal anatomy, and partial or avulsion fractures (figg. 16, 17).

Lateral ankle sprains are usually classified on a three grade classification considering joint instability.

- A grade 1 ankle sprain usually entails microscopic tearing of the ATFL. Symptoms may include minimal swelling and point tenderness directly over the ATFL; however, there is no instability. The athlete can ambulate with little or absence of pain.
- A grade 2 ankle sprain involves microscopic tearing of a larger portion of the ATFL. Symptoms may include a broader region of point tenderness over the lateral aspect of the ankle, a painful limp when the athlete is able to ambulate, and bruising and localized swelling due to tearing of the anterior joint capsule, ATFL, and surrounding soft tissues; mild instability.
- A grade 3 ankle sprain entails a complete rupture of the ATFL and may also involve microscopic or complete failure of the CFL. The PTFL is rarely injured. Symptoms may include diffuse swelling

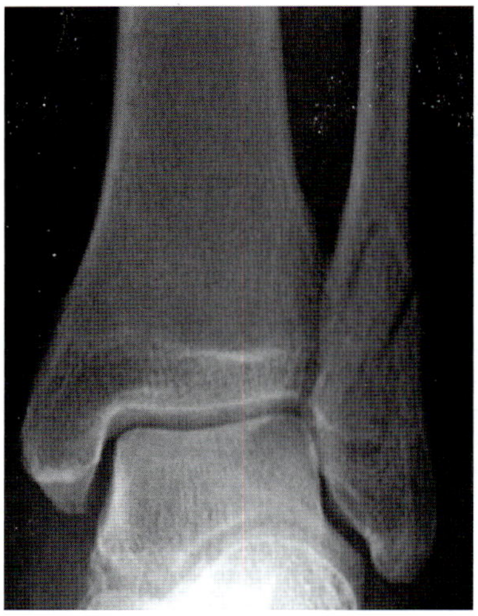

Figure 10 - Ankle X-ray showing a fibular fracture

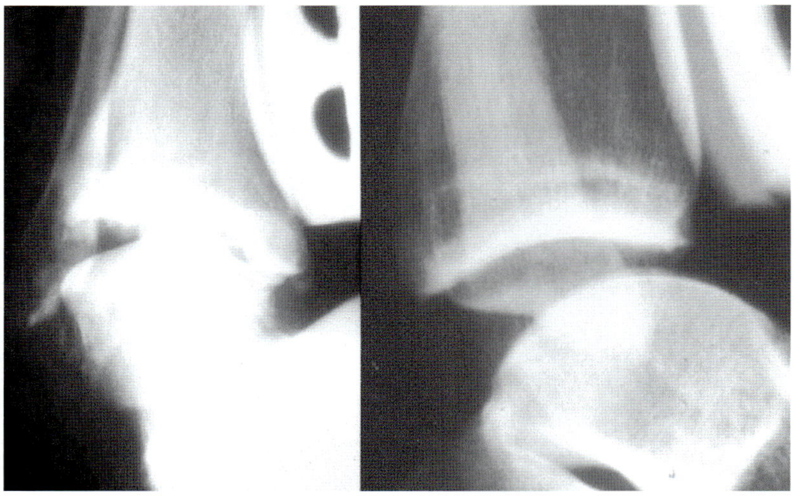

Figure 11 - Ankle stress X-rays. In the acute setting the evaluation may appear difficult

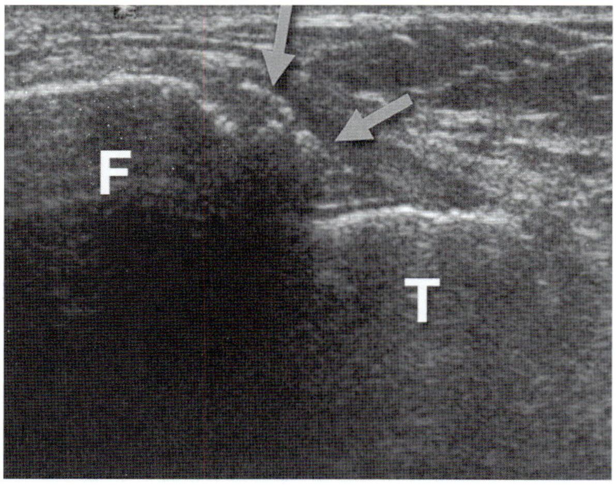

Figure 12 - US showing an ATFL rupture

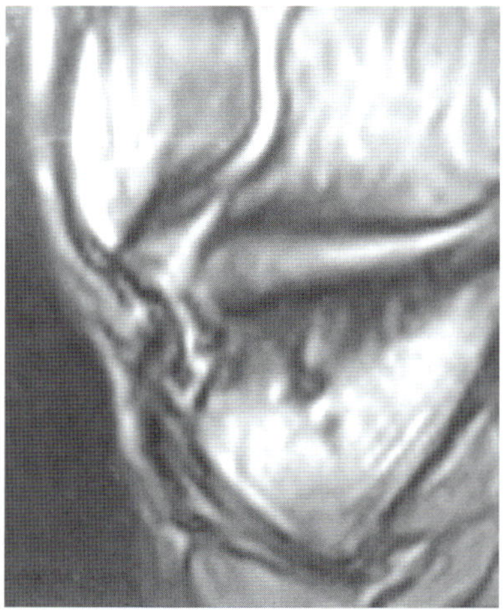

Figure 13 - MRI showing an ATFL rupture

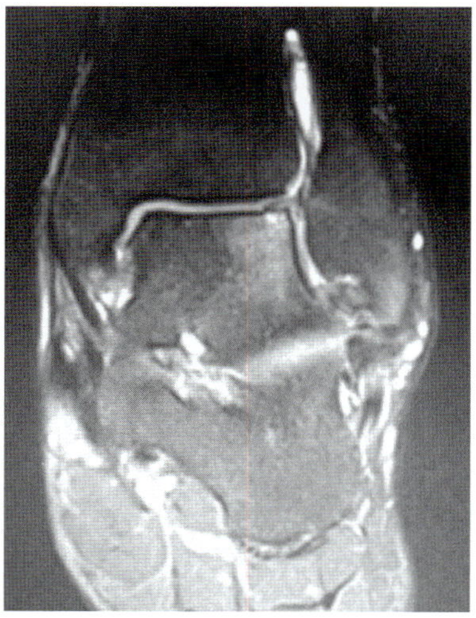

Figure 14 - MRI showing an ATFL partial lesion associated with a medial osteochondral lesion and subchondral edema

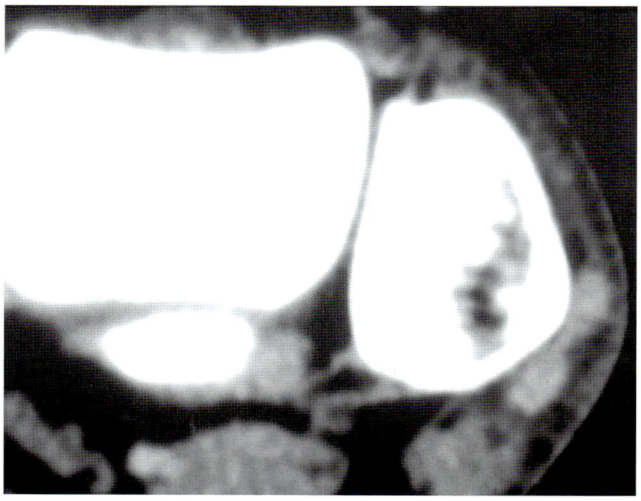

Figure 15- MRI showing anterior peroneal tendon dislocation

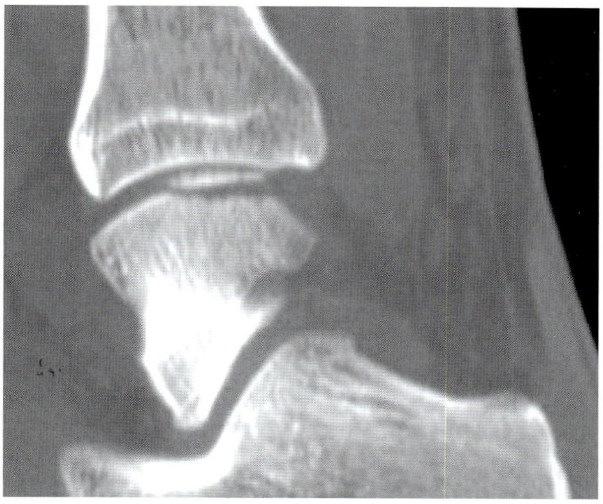

Figure 16 - Sagittal CT showing an osteochondral fracture

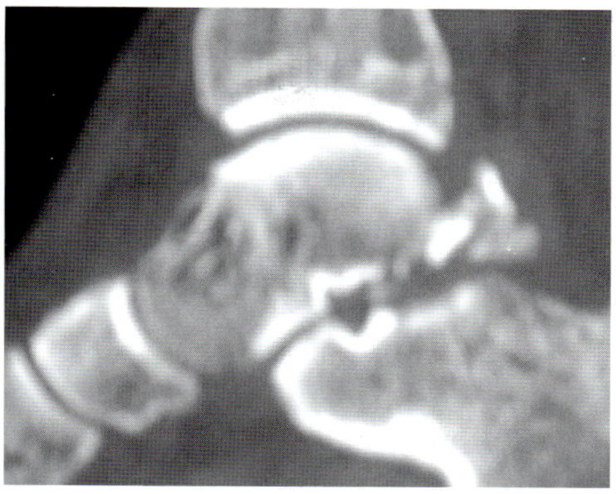

Figure 17 - Sagittal CT showing a talar posterolateral process fracture

that obliterates the margins of the Achilles tendon, inability to ambulate, and tenderness on the lateral and medial aspects of the ankle joint; instability is present.

Another classification considers only clinical features and divides lesions into mild: sprain with minimal functional loss, minimal swelling, tenderness on ATFL and CFL; moderate: moderate functional loss, pain on injured ankle, swelling; and severe: pain in weight-bearing, swelling, tenderness, complete functional loss.

Treatment may be conservative or surgical: one of the most important elements for the indication is joint stability and associated lesions which should be clinically evaluated and confirmed by instrumental exams. If the joint is stable, initial treatment will be non-operative and will consider the RICE protocol (rest, ice, compression, elevation) with the use of non-steroidal anti-inflammatory drugs (NSAIDs) during the acute phase (first 4-5 days) and a short period of immobilization (no more than 2 weeks).

Most authors agree that early mobilization followed by phased rehabilitation is warranted to minimize time away from sports [2, 55]. Prolonged immobilization (>2 weeks) has detrimental effects and may lead to a longer return to play. The rehabilitation protocol is divided into four stages. First stage: pain and edema control; second stage: range of motion (ROM), strengthening exercises; third stage: soccer specific functional training; fourth stage: prophylactic intervention with balance and proprioception exercises, Achilles and peroneal muscles stretching.

If the ankle joint is unstable and associated to a positive talar-tilt test and anterior drawer test, the treatment should be surgical. The same indication should be applied to ankle sprains associated with other lesions such as osteochondral lesions or fractures.

Although most of comparative studies between conservative and surgical treatment are in favor of surgical treatment only in professional athletes, it is important to consider the high number of complications, such as hidden osteochondral lesions, fibrous and bony impingement, chronic instability. I believe that, when instability occurs, a minimally invasive surgery is more reliable in order to explore the lateral ligament complex and to remove bony and cartilage fragments, resolve ligamentous interpositions and correctly suture and reinsert ligament stumps into the bone. It also reduces healing time and complications (figg. 18, 19, 20, 21).

After surgical repair, a Walker boot (brace) is applied for two weeks without weight-bearing; then loading is allowed in brace for another three weeks together with active mobilization, muscle strengthening and proprioceptive rehabilitation. Players will then undergo extensive physical therapy that progresses to sport-specific exercises with the ultimate goal of returning to competitive play around 4 months post-operatively [2].

Medial ankle sprains

The medial ligamentous complex is a multi-fascicular structure, originating from the medial malleolus to insert in the talus, calcaneus, and navicu-

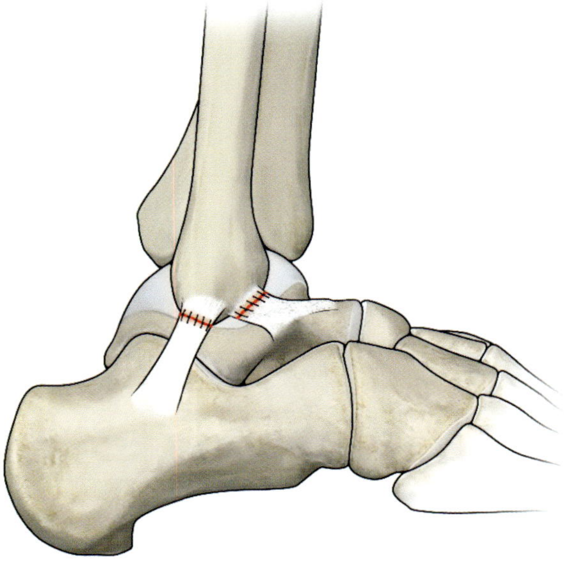

Figure 18 - ATFL and CFL repair with direct suture, according to Bostrom

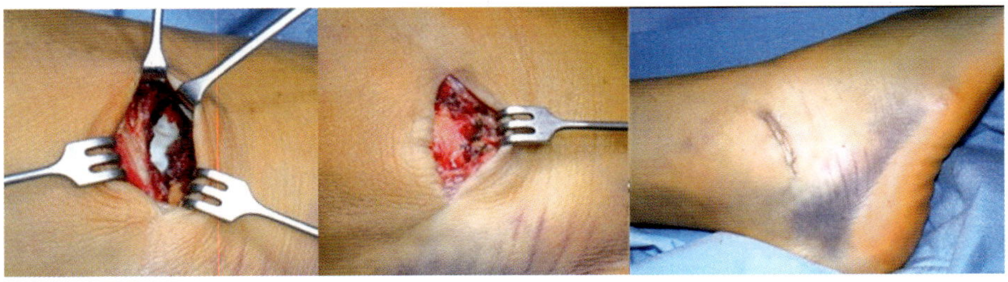

Figure 19 - ATFL repair with direct suture, according to Bostrom

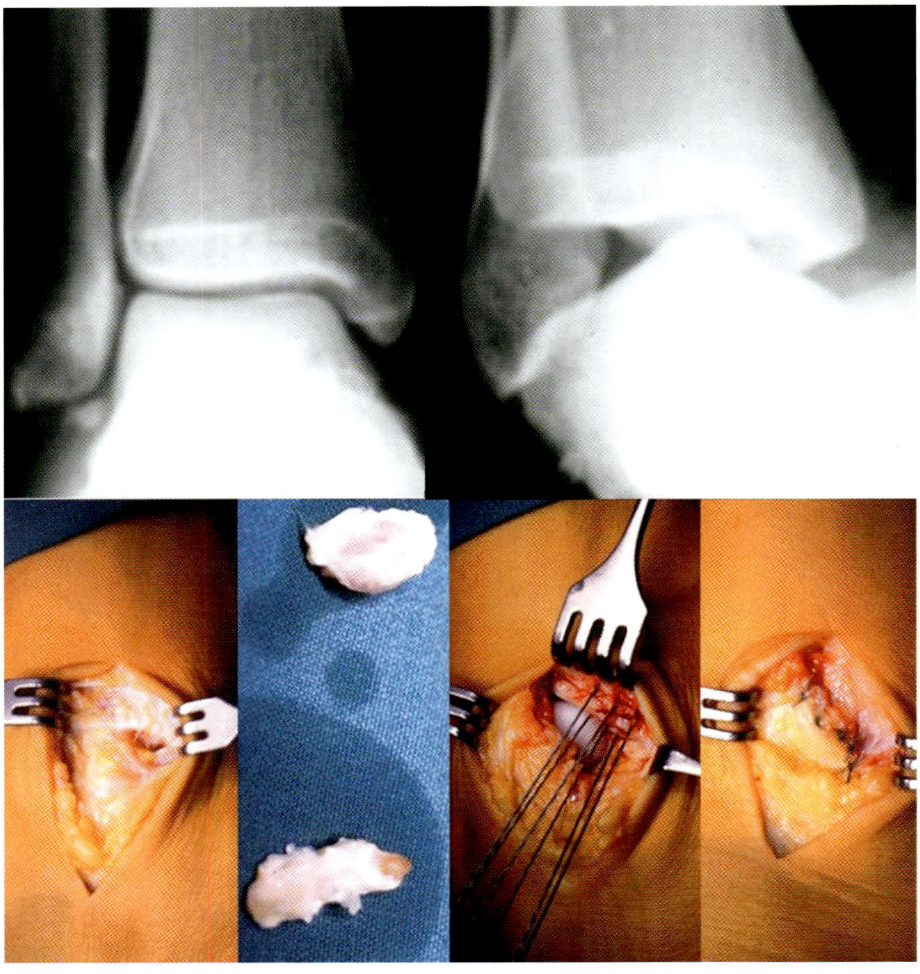

Figure 20 - ATFL repair with direct suture, according to Bostrom, associated with fibular fragment removal

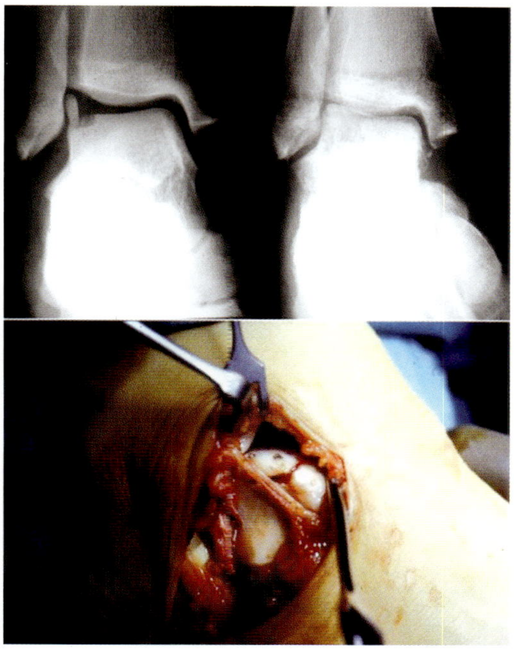

Figure 21 - ATFL repair with direct suture, according to Bostrom, associated with osteochondral fragment fixation using a bioabsorbable pin

lar bone [40]. The anatomical descriptions of this complex vary widely in the literature; however, in general, most agree that it is composed of two layers: superficial and deep [40].

The superficial components (fig. 22) are represented by the tibiocalcaneal ligament (TCL), the tibionavicular ligament (TNL), the posterior superficial tibiotalar ligament (PSTTL), and the tibiospring ligament (TSL). The deep components (fig. 23) are represented by the anterior tibiotalar ligament (ATTL) and the posterior deep tibiotalar ligament (PDTL). The medial ligamentous complex is less commonly affected compared to the lateral one, with reports of injury in soccer player of about 14% [2, 3]. Medial ankle sprains occur more often with a mechanism in eversion of the hindfoot or due to excessive external rotation movements (fig. 24).

The superficial deltoid ligament is the first to be injured in a medial ankle sprain, followed by the deep compartment and sometimes the distal tibio-peroneal syndesmosis with possible associated fibular fractures if there is an external rotation prolonged stress. When compared with other sports, soccer places an unusually high demand on both the medial foot and ankle structures. For instance, striking the ball requires the player

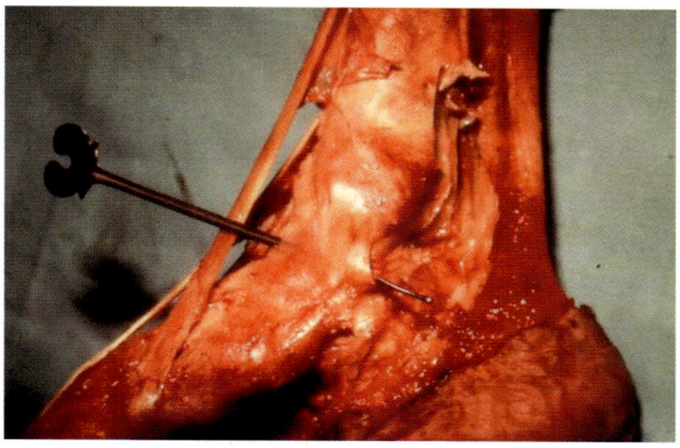

Figure 22 - Anatomical specimen showing the superficial components of the deltoid complex: the TCL, the TNL, the PSTTL, and the TSL

to abduct and externally rotate the foot, which preloads medial structures [2]. Hintermann [44], considering athletes with medial ankle instability, found that the injury commonly occurred during landing on an uneven surface, after heading the ball or jumping over a tackle. Pronation with eversion and extreme rotational injuries are well known to cause deltoid ligament injury. However, complete rupture of the deltoid ligament is rare and is more often associated with syndesmosic lesions and ankle fractures [56].

Due to its close proximity and similarly shared function in medial plantar arch stabilization with the TSL and spring ligaments, posterior tibialis tendon dysfunction is also frequently seen in medial ankle instability (fig. 25) [57]. After an acute injury, patients can present with a medial ankle hematoma and pain along the deltoid ligament. A proper diagnosis needs to exclude associated high ankle sprain, osteochondral lesion, or fractures. As for lateral sprains, neural, muscular, and vascular structures should always be assessed. The examination must include inspection of the ankle complex, palpation of the superficial components (TCL, TNL, PSTTL and TSL), and an assessment of the ankle and subtalar joint range of motion. X-rays represent the first step in order to exclude the presence of ankle fractures. Clinical examination must always be supported by X-rays (fig. 26), MRI, or CT scan [58]. US may represent a rapid diagnostic tool, but MRI offers a better picture of the lesion.

Medial ankle sprains are usually classified on a

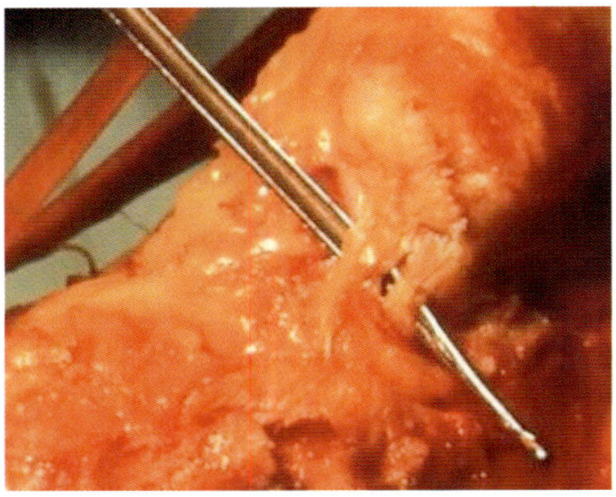

Figure 23 - Anatomical specimen showing the deep layer of the deltoid complex, represented by the ATTL

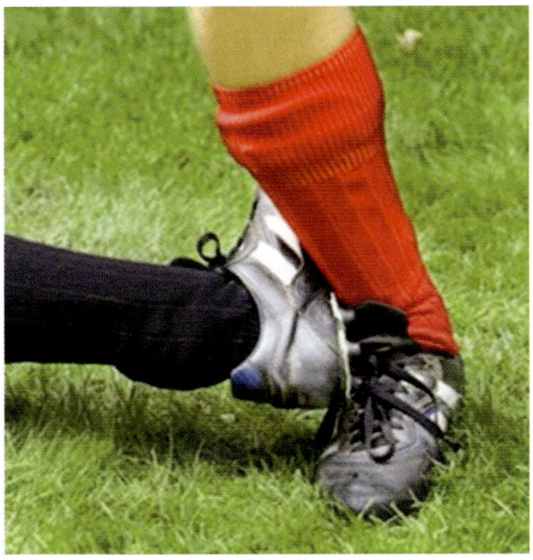

Figure 24 - Medial ankle sprains due to a direct trauma with the hindfoot in everted position

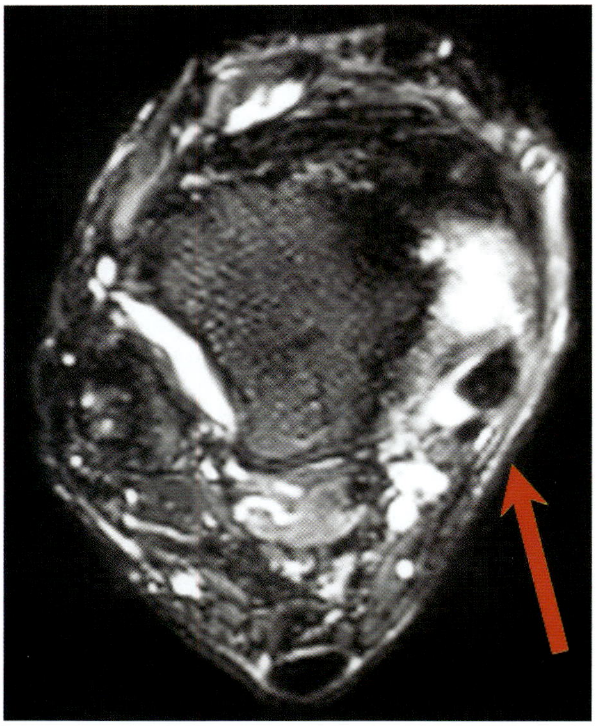

Figure 25 - Patient affected by medial ankle instability with posterior tibialis tendon dysfunction

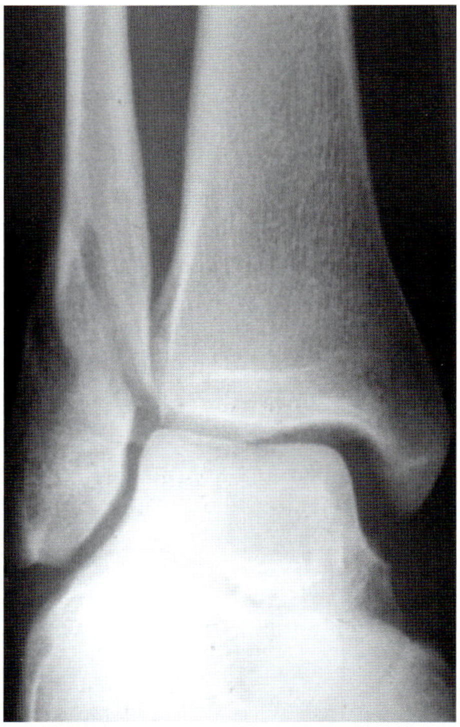

Figure 26 - Ankle X-ray showing a medial gutter widening (due to a medial ligament complex rupture) associated with a fibular fracture

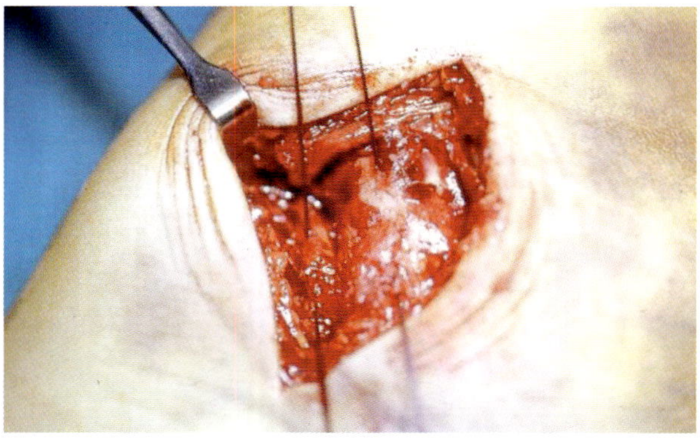

Figure 27 - Deltoid ligament repair through direct suture

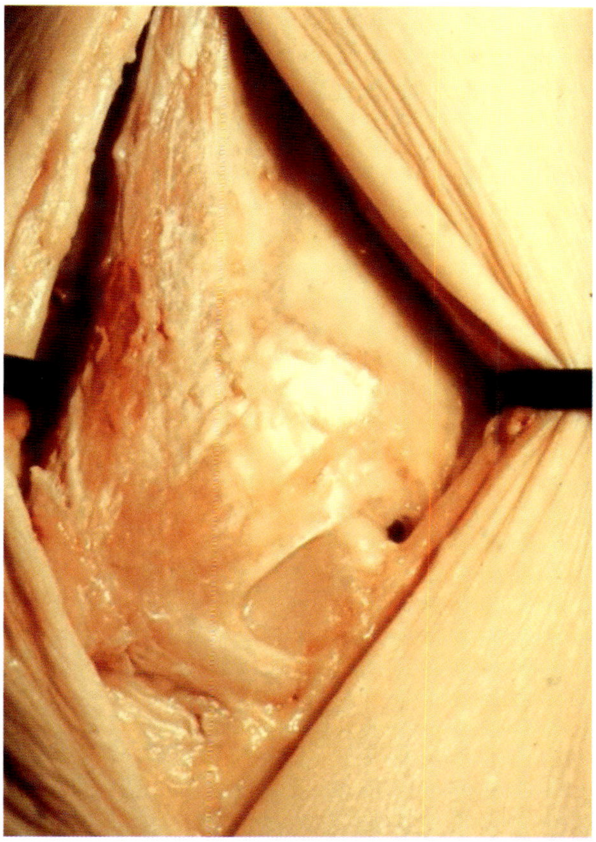

Figure 28 - Anatomical specimen of the anterior aspect of the syndesmosis showing the AITFL and the ATFL

four grade classification based on clinical features.

• A grade 1 medial ankle sprain is usually characterized by a distraction of the superficial deltoid ligament; stability maneuvers are negative.

• A grade 2 sprain is usually characterized by a rupture of the superficial deltoid ligament and a distraction of its deep portion; stability maneuvers are positive.

• In a grade 3 sprain, a superficial and deep ligament rupture occurred; stability maneuvers are totally positive.

• In a grade 4 sprain, the rupture of the superficial and deep deltoid ligament is associated to a tendon lesion (most commonly the posterior tibialis tendon); stability maneuvers are positive with associated functional impotence

If the ankle joint is stable, initial treatment will be non-operative and will involve the RICE (rest, ice, compression, elevation) protocol with the use of nonsteroidal anti-inflammatory drugs (NSAIDs) during the acute phase (first 4-5 days) with a short period (no >2 weeks) of immobilization [59]. Surgical intervention is indicated for grade 3-4 acute ankle sprains with clinical instability or if the lesion is associated to high ankle sprains, osteochondral lesions, tendon lesions, or fractures. Primary deltoid ligament tears surgical repair yields good and excellent results. In soccer players it should be considered in order to prevent problems associated with chronic tears such as instability, arthritis, and impingement syndromes [60]. When surgery is advised in an acute setting, anatomical direct repairs are made using suture threads (fig. 27). After surgical repair, a Walker boot (brace) is applied for two weeks; then loading on the brace is prescribed for another three weeks together with active mobilization, muscle strengthening, and proprioceptive rehabilitation. Players will then undergo extensive physical therapy that progresses to sport-specific exercises with the ultimate goal of returning to competitive play around 4 months post-operatively.

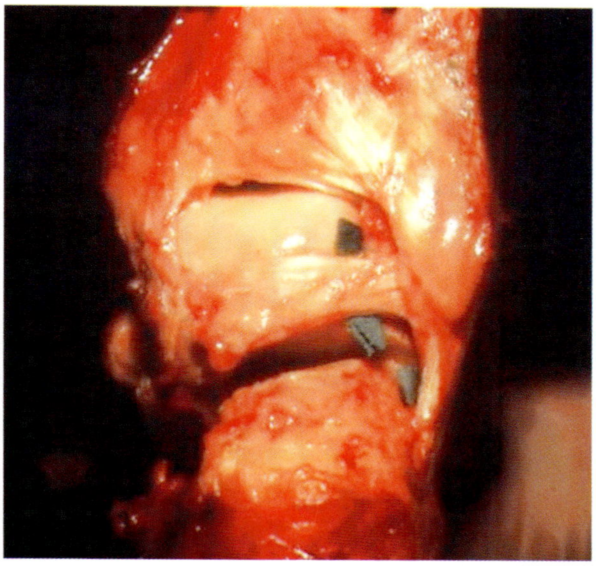

Figure 29 - Anatomical specimen of the posterior aspect of the syndesmosis showing the PITFL and the TTFL

High ankle sprains (syndesmosis)

The distal tibiofibular syndesmosis is a syndesmotic joint between the distal tibia and fibula. It is attached by the interosseous ligament (IOL), the anterior-inferior tibiofibular ligament (AITFL), the posterior-inferior tibiofibular ligament (PITFL) and the (posterior) transverse tibiofibular ligament (TTFL) (figg. 28, 29).

In soccer players high ankle sprains are much less

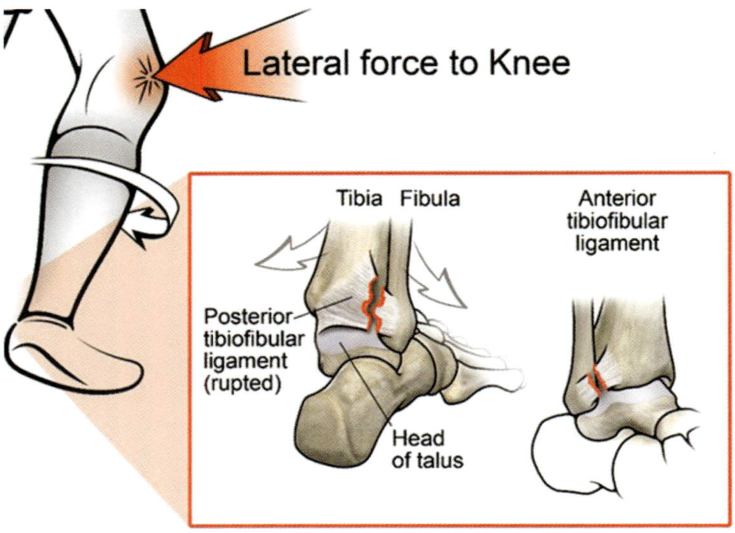

Figure 30 - Lateral impact on the leg occurring during a quick internal twist of the externally rotated foot

common than low ankle sprains; however, when they do occur they portend a lengthier rehabilitation and a poorer prognosis, especially if undiagnosed. Compared to the lateral ankle ligament injuries, tibiofibular syndesmotic injuries are rare, once they require higher loads to fail [61]. The incidence of this lesion in elite soccer player seems to be about 3-4% of all ankle lesions. This trend extends to the general athlete population, where the incidence of isolated syndesmosis sprains is low, responsible for only 10-20% of all ankle sprains [58].
Lubberts et al. [62] studied the epidemiology of isolated syndesmotic injuries in professional soccer players. They pooled data from 15 consecutive seasons of European professional soccer between 2001 and 2016. They examined a total of 3,677 players from 61 teams across 17 countries. There were 1,320 ankle ligament injuries registered during 15 seasons, of which 94 (7%) were isolated syndesmotic injuries (others associated to other ligament injuries). The incidence of these injuries increased annually between 2001 and 2016. Injuries were 74% contact-related, and isolated syndesmotic injuries were followed by a mean of a 39-day absence [42].
Incidence during match was 13 times more frequent compared to training (0.21 contra 0.02).
Moreover, soccer players may have an increased risk of syndesmotic sprains due to foot planting and cutting action [56].
Several injury mechanisms have been described; however, the most common one involves hyperdorsiflexion and external rotation of the ankle [63], which can also injure the deltoid ligament [64]. In soccer, the injury mechanism usually involves quick internal twist of the externally rotated foot with lateral impact on the leg or external lateral trauma to the lower leg (proximal to the heel), forcing the soccer player ankle to external rotation (fig. 30) [61].
Giza analyzed 76 lesions in 4 world championships by video tape: of these 52 were bruises (68.5%), 20 sprains (26.3%), and 4 fractures (5.2%). Most injuries were caused by tackles with medial and lateral forces. In 41 cases they were with one foot on the load and 35 with one foot without load. The most frequent position was pronation and plantarflexion or in external rotation [14].
Medical history may assist in determining the extent of the injury. Physical examination involves palpation of the interossal membrane, and manual test includes cotton test, dorsiflexion-compression test, external rotation stress test, fibular translation, palpation test, and squeeze test [191]. If the pain and swelling extend proximally through the interosseus membrane, an unstable ankle mortise should be suspected, since they have direct correlation [65]. Nevertheless, in the acute setting, the diagnosis may be difficult since 40% of the patients may also present pain on the anterior distal talo-fibular ligament with no rupture of the syndesmotic ligaments. The diagnosis can be made on plain X-ray when there is clear diastasis between the distal tibia and fibula. Three critical measurements on plain films are made 1 cm above the tibi-

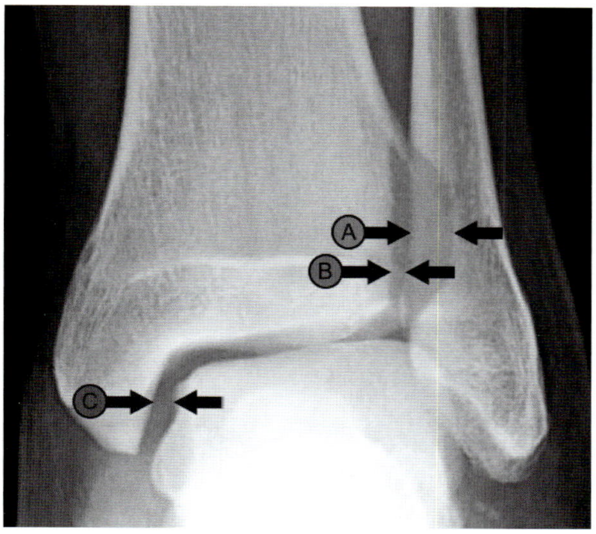

Figure 31- A: tibiofibular overlap, B: tibiofibular clear space, C: medial clear space (it's needed to be equal to the joint space)

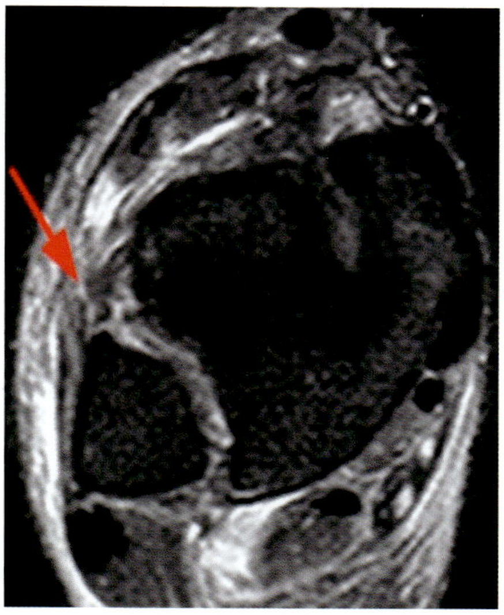

Figure 32- MRI showing the rupture of the AITFL

al plafond and are used to evaluate the integrity of the syndesmosis: tibiofibular clear space >6 mm, tibiofibular overlap <1 mm, which indicate disruption of the syndesmosis, and medial clear space (fig. 31) [66].

Stress ultrasonography may be considered as it provides a cheaper and faster examination.

More subtle injuries can be diagnosed with better sensitivity and specificity using MRI, which can also reveal secondary findings such as bone bruises, ATFL injury, osteochondral lesions, and tibiofibular incongruity [67] (fig. 32). Arthroscopy is an invaluable diagnostic tool for syndesmotic injuries with a characteristic triad finding of PITFL scarring, disrupted interosseous ligament, and posterolateral tibial plafond chondral damage [68].

Classification of the involved ligaments can aid in the selection of appropriate treatment and is divided in three grades.

- Grade 1 injuries involve AITFL tears.
- Grade 2A injuries involve AITFL and IOL tears.
- Grade 2B injuries include AITFL, PITFL, and IOL tears.
- Grade 3 injuries involve injury to all three ligaments, as well as a fibular fracture.

Another classification is based on the time from injury, as it affects the management:

acute if less than 6 weeks, subacute if between 6 weeks and 6 months and chronic if more than 6 months.

Conservative treatment is usually recommended for Grades 1 and 2A, while surgical intervention is necessary for grades 2B and 3.

The ESSKA-AFAS consensus panel [69] recommends that acute isolated syndesmotic ruptures with rupture of the anterior-inferior talofibular ligament, with or without interosseus ligament and with an intact deltoid ligament, should be treated conservatively: non-weight-bearing with initially rest, cryotherapy, and walker boot (3 weeks). Following these indications for 3 weeks, proprioceptive training, strengthening, and mobility exercises should be included into the conservative treatment [70]. Despite conservative treatment is still widely performed, syndesmotic injuries, if compared with other ankle sprains, typically require a more prolonged recovery/rehabilitation even in elite athletes. Studies in the literature suggest that these injuries require twice as long to heal. Therefore some surgeons advocate surgical intervention in professional athletes with mild sprains to expedite return to play [71].

Surgery has been well established as necessary in more severe injuries where there is clear diastasis or instability of the syndesmosis or if the acute syndesmotic lesion is associated to a deltoid ligament rupture (therefore unstable). Traditionally, screws were used for surgical fixation; however, they often required a second surgery for subsequent removal. There is no general consensus on

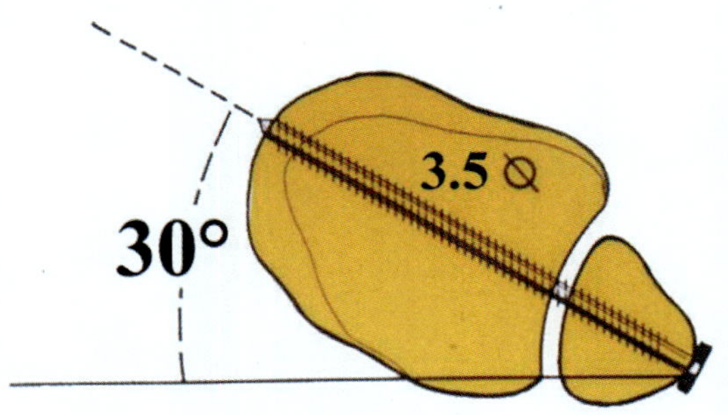

Figure 33 - The syndesmotic screw should be placed through the fibula and the lateral cortex of the tibia, just proximal to the inferior tibiofibular joint, 30 degrees from posterior to anterior, parallel to the tibial plafond, with the ankle joint in neutral position

the optimal screw size, number of screws, level of placement, or timing of removal [72] (figg. 33, 34). More recently, suture button fixation (e.g. TightRope; Arthrex) has become more popular and provides certain advantages over screw fixation, such as avoiding the need for hardware removal. TightRope (fig. 35) has been shown to provide less rigid stabilization of the syndesmosis as compared with screw fixation [73]. Another option is represented by a bioabsorbable PLLA screw (fig. 36), which at first stabilize, then it breaks and then reabsorbs. Since malreduction is the most important indicator of poor long-term functional outcome, suture button fixation should be considered in the treatment of the soccer player [74]. According to this, some authors [75] reported a lower complication rate and earlier return to sports in patients treated with knotless suture button devices compared with screw fixation.

Chronic instabilities

After an ankle sprain, if there are recurrent episodes of giving away and/or feelings of instability, the clinician should suspect for the development to chronic ankle instability [65].

In this sense, the chronic ankle instability may be subgrouped into two types of instability [76]: mechanical ankle instability and functional ankle instability.

Mechanical instability is characterized by an abnormal ankle mobility, assessed clinically using

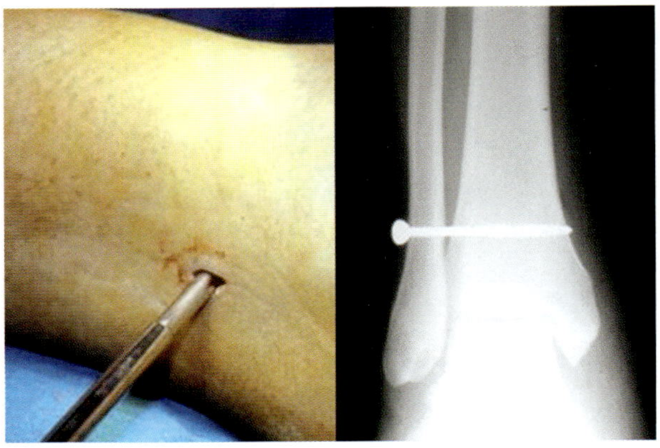

Figure 34 - Percutaneous syndesmotic screw placement

manual stress application by the anterior drawer and the talar tilt tests. Functional instability was firstly described by Freeman et al. [77] as a subjective feeling of the ankle giving way during either physical activity or during common activities of daily living. In 1985 Tropp described functional instability as a movement that is independent from voluntary control, even if the physiological range of motion is not always exceeded [78]. By subgrouping the patients into different categories, the clinician may tailor the rehabilitation protocol in accordance to the specific deficits associated with the type of instability and personalize it in order to address each player's needs and expectations. The diagnosis must exclude the presence of other pathological conditions such as sub-talar instability, nervous disorders (sural nerve or superficial peroneal nerve involvement), osteochondral lesions, tendons pathologies that can cause secondary instability, or impingement syndromes. If there is a mechanical instability of the joint, whether or not associated with functional instability, or in the case where the rehabilitation treatment has not been successful (between 3 and 6 months from the trauma) surgical treatment is indicated [79].

The literature has described several surgical techniques for the treatment of chronic ankle instability. These can be distinguished in anatomic and non-anatomic (tenodesis) reconstructions [79]. Common goals to all the techniques are: restoring the joint stability, paying attention to insertion, length, direction and tension of ligaments, allowing normal sports activities to be resumed as fast as

possible, reducing the risk of recurrence, preventing further cartilage damage and delaying or better avoiding the onset of early ankle osteoarthritis.
Anatomic techniques are simple, based on a suture and direct repair of the damaged ligament bundles. These may include the use of native injured ligament retension, reinforcements with local structures (retinacoli or periosteum), reconstructions with autograft, allograft or synthetic graft [79].
Non-anatomic procedures encompass tenodesis in order to substitute the injured ligaments, and to address the pathological ankle mobility.
These techniques, since they do not restore ligamentous isometry, often result in joint stiffness and limited range of motion, or they fail. For this reason uptoday these techniques are no longer used, especially in high-level sports patients.

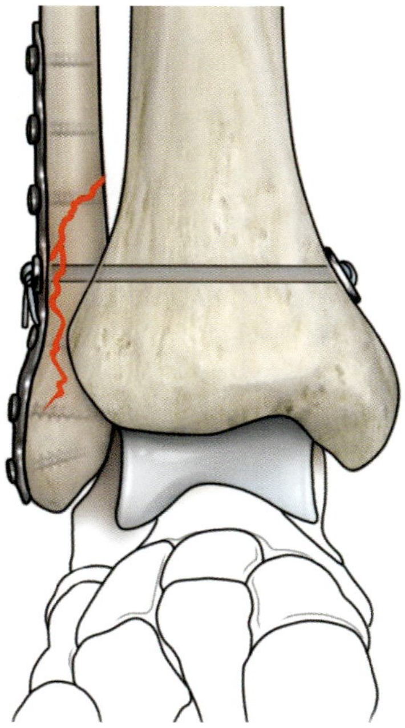

Figure 35 - TightRope system anchors the ends of the tibia and fibula together with a braided polyethylene cord, rather than with a screw

Lateral ligament repair in chronic instabilities

When facing with chronic instability, an accurate clinical and instrumental evaluation with standard and stressed X-rays and, when necessary, CT and MRI must be performed.
Surgery may include arthroscopic or open techniques, depending on the lesion type and surgeon's preferences and experience, with the common goal of being not invasive and reducing complications. Arthroscopic techniques are also very useful to perform an articular exploration before ligament repair and to treat possible associate lesions. Despite their increasing popularity, arthroscopic techniques are still more complex and require longer time for the procedure.
In open surgery, an incision of about 2.5 cm (fig. 37) parallel to the fibular bone is performed. The reinforcement choice depends on tissue consistency, laxity, and lesion type (involving one or more ligaments) [79].
One of the most common techniques is the Brostrom repair, consisting in a ligament retention. If the lesion is more complex, a regional reinforcement using the extensor retinacula, as described by Gould, may be performed. In my practice, I prefer using a periosteal flap reinforcement (fig. 38) in order to respect retinacula anatomy. In presence of poor quality local tissues, failure of previous anatomic reconstructions or when there is a general ligamentous laxity, an anatomic reconstruction using the autologous tendon of plantar gracilis or an allograft is required [79].
In presence of any associated foot deformities increasing the supination force through the lateral

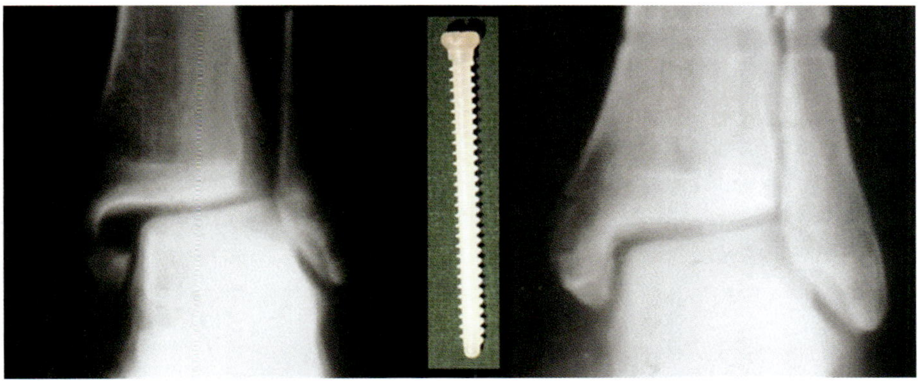

Figure 36 - Bioabsorbable syndesmotic screw. The implant is not visible on post-operative plain X-rays

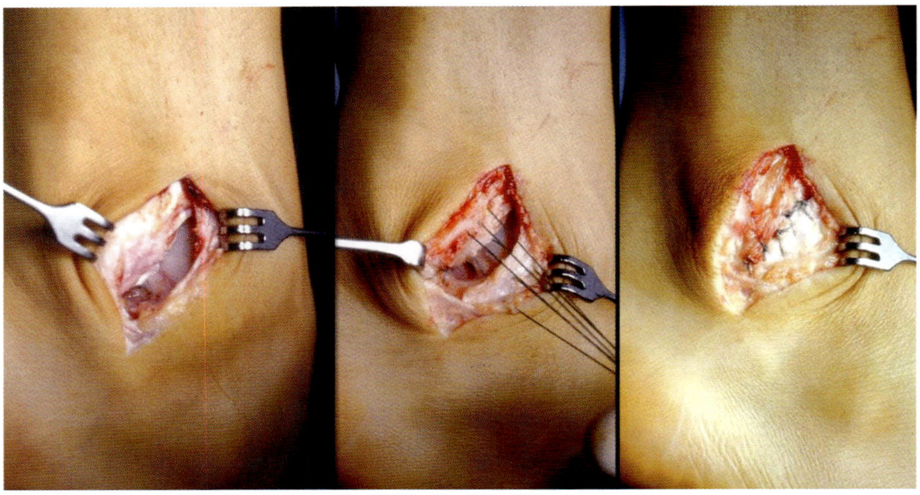

Figure 37 - 2.5 cm incision, parallel to the fibular bone. The complete rupture is sutured to the fibular bone

ankle and foot, the surgeon should address it and correct it along with the ligamentous reconstruction, using a first metatarsal osteotomy or a calcaneal osteotomy in case of cavus foot, to avoid the tripod effect.

For Brostrom-modified repair, patients' preferred position is in semilateral decubitus, under spinal anesthesia and tourniquet control.

A curved 2,5 cm incision is made from just anterior to the distal fibula and passing inferiorly to the tip of the lateral malleolus, taking care to preserve the integrity of the superficial peroneal nerve.

The inferior extensor retinaculum is retracted anteriorly to identify the joint capsule and the torn ends of the ATFL. A periosteal flap is elevated proximally from the distal lateral malleolus surface for about 2 cm long.

With the ankle at a slight everted and dorsiflexed position (about 5 degrees), repair of the ATFL is performed by pulling and reattaching the distal stump of the ATFL to the lateral malleolus using reabsorbable suture threads in transosseus fashion. The periosteal flap created on the lateral malleolus is applicated in a "vest over pant" fashion over the newly sutured ATFL (fig. 39).

In order to achieve more stability and strengthening, the inferior extensor retinaculum, previously detached for the capsule, is advanced proximally and sutured to the anterior border of the lateral malleolus. In case of reconstruction of the CFL the incision is extended distally and posteriorly while preserving the sural nerve and the lesser saphenous vein.

Then the peroneus brevis tendon is retracted in order to identify the CFL. Repair of the CFL is performed with the ankle in neutral position, by pulling proximally the distal stump of the torn CFL, and fixing it to the lateral malleolus using the same reabsorbable suture threads, as close to the anatomical origin of the CFL as possible. A regional periosteal flap may be used as a reinforcement.

In case of anatomic reconstruction using autologous plantar gracilis transfer it is important to evaluate the presence of the tendon using US because it is present in only 20-30% of the caucasian population.The plantar gracilis tendon is harvested at the ankle joint level just medial to the Achilles tendon with a 1.5 cm skin incision. Commonly, adhesions with the Achilles tendon near the calcaneal tuberosity or with the intermuscular fascia, makes the identification of the plantaris tendon challenging.

After isolation of the plantar gracilis tendon, it is harvested using an open tendon stripper and maintaining its calcaneal insertion. The graft is then tacked in its free portion with non reabsorbable suture threads. The harvested tendon is passed into the heel, throughout a drill-hole, from medial to lateral. The tendon is then passed beneath the peroneal tendons and routed into a drill-hole made into the distal fibula from posterior to anterior. The plantar gracilis tendon is inserted in the tunnel and the free tacked portion of the graft exiting on the medial side of the talus is fixed by tenodesis using non-reabsorbable stitches (figg. 40, 41). Other option is an anchor fixed to the talus at the former site of ligament insertion.

In cases of absence of the plantar gracilis tendon,

an allograft can be used. The graft is fixed on the medial border of the calcaneus using non-reabsorbable stiches or alternatively an interference screw (figg. 42, 43, 44). The subsequent surgical steps are the same described for the plantar gracilis technique. Even in this case, foot deformities must be corrected with osteotomies, as previously described [79].
Post-operative treatment includes a non-weight-bearing plaster cast for 3 weeks and then a Walker brace for another three weeks together with active mobilization. Return to competitive play usually takes about 4 months.

Medial ligament repair in chronic instabilities

Medial ankle ligament injuries are rarely isolated: the chronic symptoms may therefore depend both on a deltoid ligament insufficiency and on other associated lesions.
Chronic insufficiency is usually diagnosed based on the feeling of "giving way", pain in the medial gutter of the ankle and several degrees of valgus and pronation deformity. Arthroscopy is the most specific way to confirm clinically suspected instability of the medial ankle; however, MRI can demonstrate loss of organized medial fibers [80].
When local injured tissues are still consistent, the most practiced anatomical technique is the one described by Du Vries: the procedure requires a "cross" incision on the scar tissue and the subsequent cross-suture of the flaps in order to provide new tension at the deltoid ligament (fig. 45) [80]. Alternatively, the residual ligament may be detached from its malleolar origin and then resutured with a proper tension to the malleolus with a trans-osseous suture technique. When local tissues show a too poor condition for a direct anatomical repair, or in case of generalized ligamentous laxity or failure of previous treatments, a reconstruction using a hemitendon should be considered. The Wiltberger and Mallory technique [81] then modified by Marchetti-Giannini [80] uses a hemi-tendon of the posterior tibialis which is detached proximally by keeping its own insertion on the navicular tubercle. Once prepared, the hemitendon is then passed inside of the medial malleolus in an anterior to posterior direction and then sutured to the periosteum or using a dedicated anchor (figg. 46, 47, 48) [80].
After surgery, a plaster cast is applied for three weeks; then a loading Walker boot is prescribed for another three weeks together with active mobilization, muscle strengthening, and proprioceptive rehabilitation. Return to competitive play usually takes about 4 months.

Arthroscopic reconstruction techniques for lateral and medial side

The arthroscopic technique has been proposed in recent years both for lateral and medial chronic lesion reconstructions as an alternative to traditional open techniques. This technique however is indicated for patients with mild instability.
Several advantages are reported, such as the minimal invasivity and theoretically the more rapid functional recovery of the athlete [82].
Arthroscopic portals also allow for a more accurate assessment of the joint condition and may be useful to treat any associated lesions simultaneously.
The two most used methods are thermo-ablation, with indications limited to cases of functional instability only or slight mechanical instability, and ligament repair with anchor fixation.
In the last 20 years a vast literature has confirmed the validity of these techniques that have progressively established themselves thanks to the development of dedicated instruments and new surgical approaches [83-85].
More recent studies have used arthroscopic methods even in revision cases thanks to the use of synthetic or biological augmentations and new generation anchors.

Return to training and competition

In the majority of the soccer players that have suffered an ankle sprain, the initial inflammatory symptomatology may be resolved through conservative management in a short period of time [86,87]. Nevertheless, these athletes often present disabling symptomatology and decreased performance due to loss of strength and power and functional deficits (poor balance and neuromuscular control), which may persist even after returning to practice [88, 89]. After an acute lateral ankle sprain, there is a high likelihood of a rapid return to training and competition [90], which can be en-

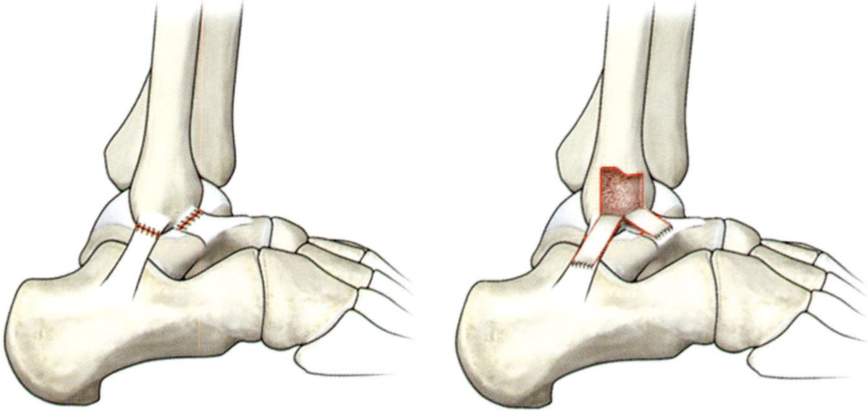

Figure 38 - After ligament suture and repair a regional periosteal flap reinforcement may be performed

Figure 39 - Lateral ligament suture associated to a regional periosteal flap reinforcement

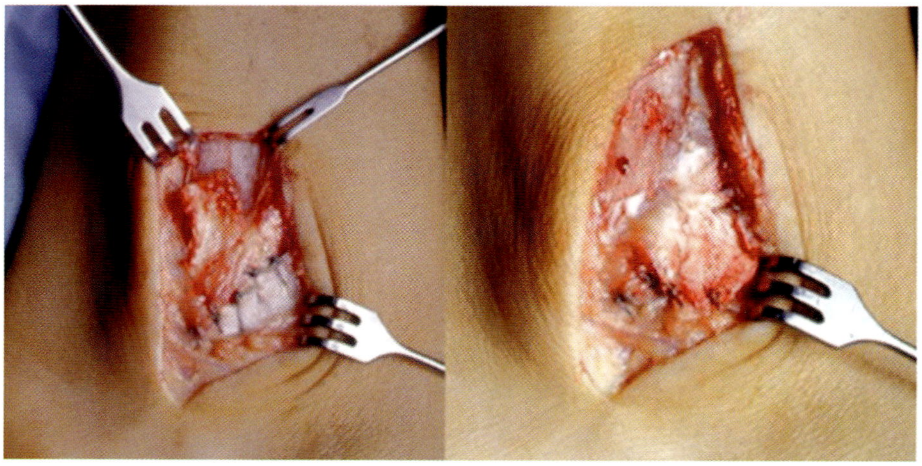

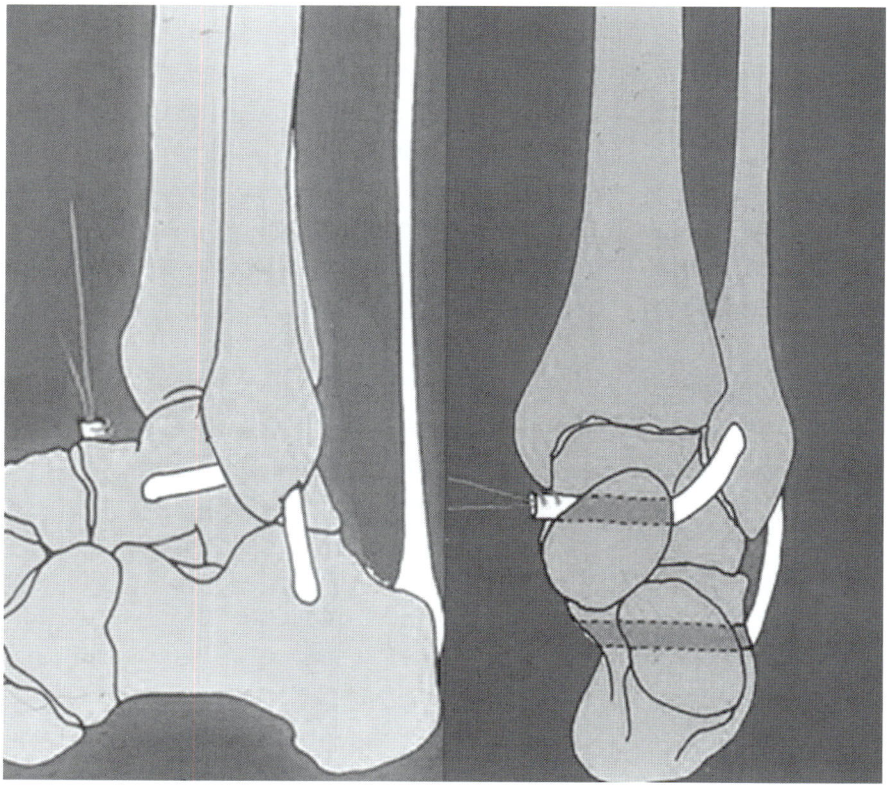

Figure 40 - Anatomic reconstruction through autologous plantar gracilis transfer

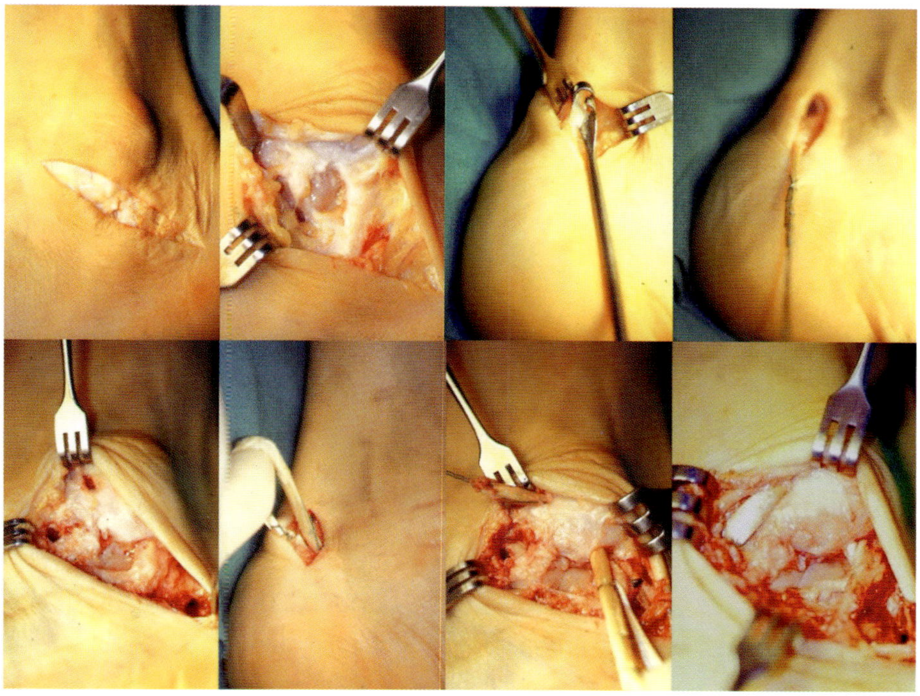

Figure 41 - The lateral lesion is detected; the plantar gracilis tendon is identified on the medial side, then harvested using a tendon stripper, maintaining its calcaneal insertion. The graft is tacked in its free portion with non reabsorbable suture thread, then passed into the heel, throughout a drill-hole, from medial to lateral. The tendon is then passed beneath the peroneal tendons and routed into a drill-hole made into the distal fibula from posterior to anterior

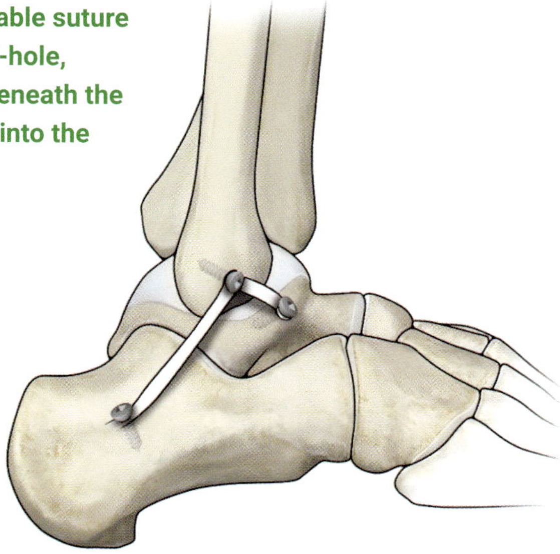

Figure 42 - Artificial allograft reconstruction. The graft is fixed on the fibula and on the medial border of the calcaneus using an interference screw or a dedicated anchor

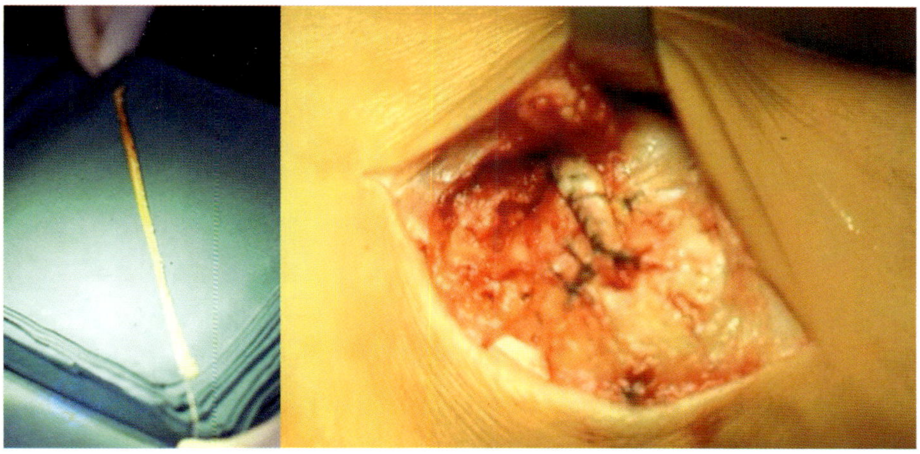

Figure 43 - Donor allograft reconstruction. The graft is fixed on the fibula and on the medial border of the calcaneus using non-reabsorbable stiches or alternatively an interference screw

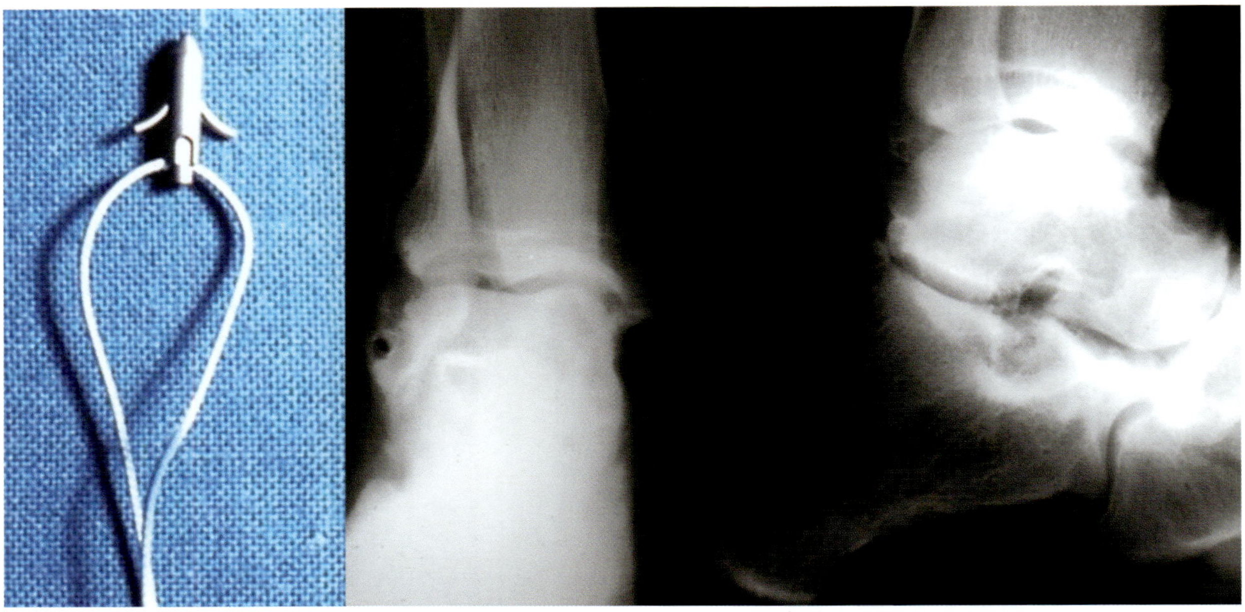

Figure 44 - Allograft reconstruction. The graft is fixed on the talar aspect using an anchor

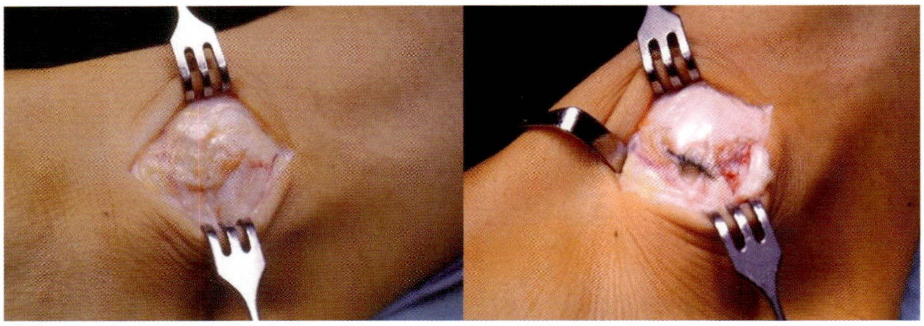

Figure 45 - The lesion is identified: a "cross" incision on the scar tissue is made, then a cross-suture on the ligament fibers is performed

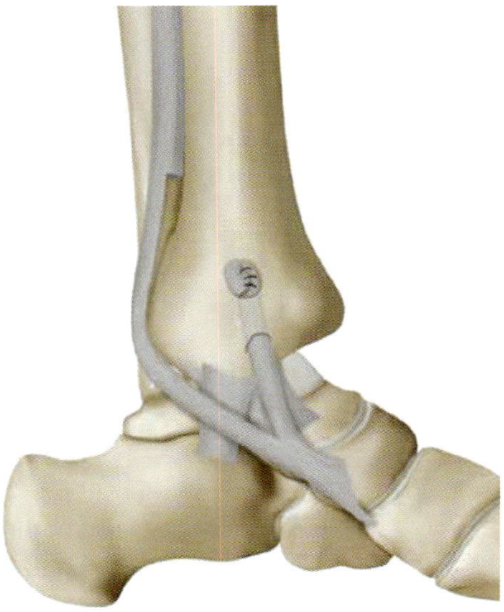

Figure 46 - Marchetti-Giannini technique uses a hemi-tendon of the posterior tibialis which is detached proximally, then passed inside of the medial and sutured to the periosteum

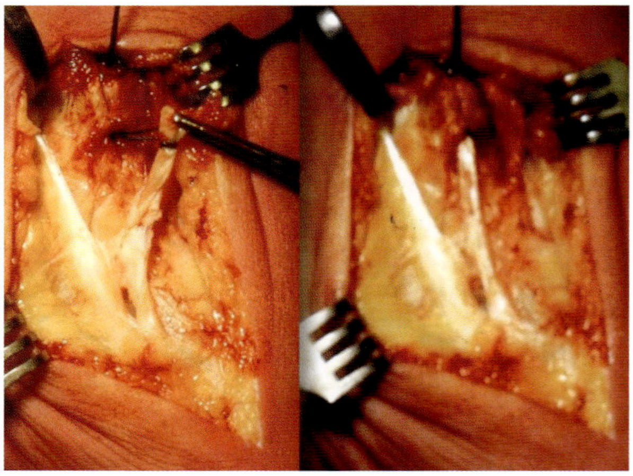

Figure 47: Marchetti-Giannini technique, surgical procedure

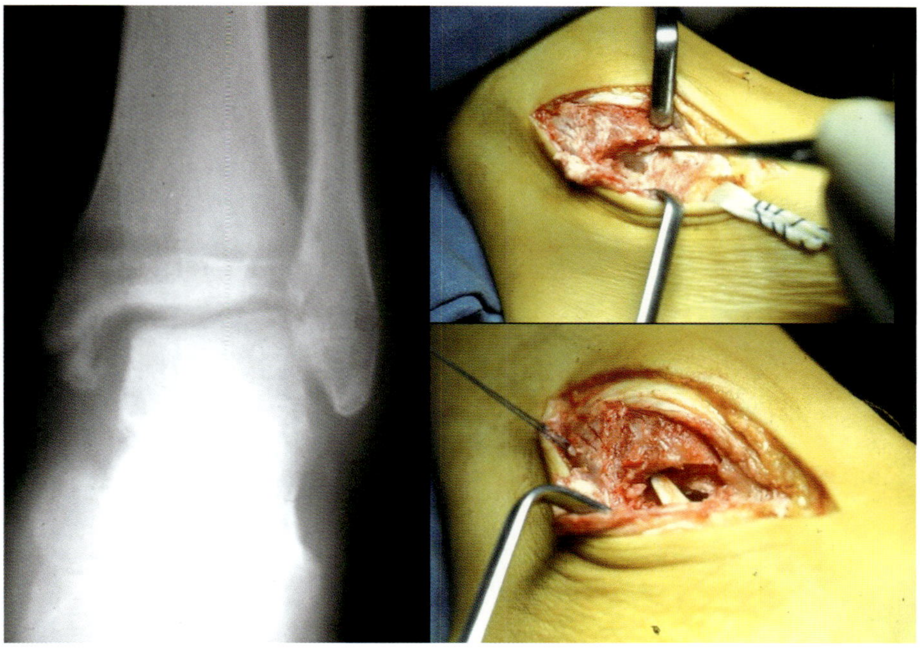

Figure 48 - X-rays showing tibial malleolus non-union associated with medial chronic instability, confirmed by the medial gutter widening. On the right side, surgical procedure: bony fragment removal and medial ligament complex reconstruction using a posterior tibialis hemi-tendon

hanced with accelerated rehabilitation protocols [91], nevertheless with a twofold increased risk of reinjury within the following year [92]. In addition, even after successful return to play residual deficits may persist leading to a higher risk of injury recurrence [93].

These include pain (30%), instability (20%), crepitus (18%), weakness (17%), stiffness (15%), and swelling (14%). It was reported that successful return to training and competition after acute lateral ligament repair (grade III injuries) was 63 days and 77 days, respectively. However, when associated injuries were present, the return was delayed to 86 days and 105 days. Still, all patients return to their pre-injury level.

In another study, with a short- to medium-term follow-up after a modified Broström repair with immediate postoperative weight-bearing, a 94% return to sports at the pre-injury levels was reported, and the remaining athletes abandoned sports due to associated injuries [94]. In a case series with a 9-year follow-up of 42 athletes after isolated ATFL ligament Broström repair, 58% of the athletes return to practice at the pre-injury levels [95].

For what concerns tibiofibular syndesmotic injuries, Calder et al. [96] found that patients with anterior inferior tibio-fibular ligament and deltoid ligament tenderness and that presented positive squeeze and external rotation tests had unstable syndesmosis at arthroscopy. They reported a mean time to return to sports of 45 days for patients treated conservatively (grade II injuries) compared to 65 days for those treated with surgical fixation (grade II injuries). Patients that had injured both the anterior inferior tibio-fibular ligament and deltoid ligament took longer to return to sports, as well as the ones that required concomitant chondral surgical procedure. The authors suggested that the cornerstone for a successful treatment relies on preserving the anatomic restoration of the syndesmosis throughout the duration of treatment until full healing is achieved. Athletes with lateral ligament surgical repair should expect a successful return to competition, within 2-3 months post-surgery. Regarding tibiofibular syndesmotic injuries, it should be expected that the return to competition is within 1-2 months and 1-3 months for patients treated conservatively or with surgical fixation, respectively.

Prevention

Acute sprains are generally treated conservatively in case of ankle stability and surgically in case of instability. Emphasis is usually placed on secondary prevention in order to reduce the risk of future sprains and progression to chronic ankle stability. In athletes, prevention of recurrent sprains is the key. Braces may help prevent ankle sprains and bracing has been shown to be superior to taping, as tape loses its restrictive properties within 20 to 30 minutes of initiating activity [97, 98].

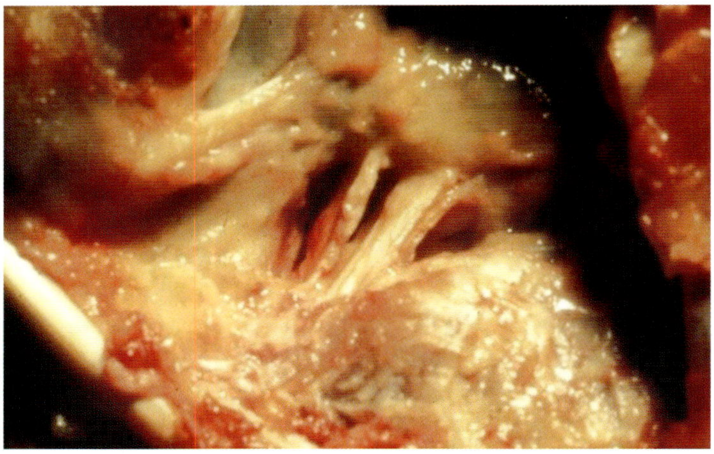

Figure 49 - Anatomical specimen showing the subtalar interosseous ligament

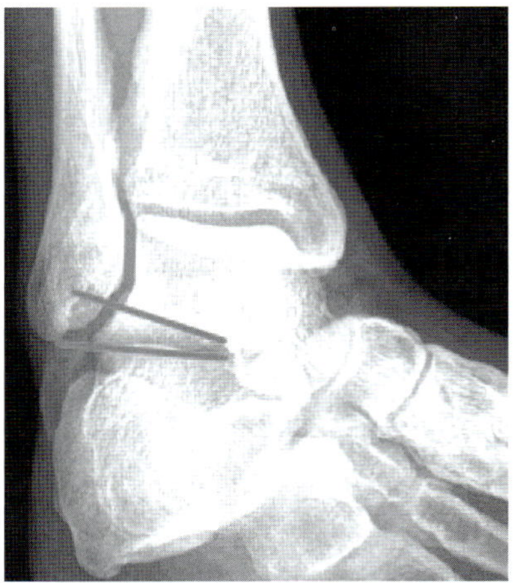

Figure 50 - Stress Broden view at 20° showing loss of parallelism at the subtalar joint

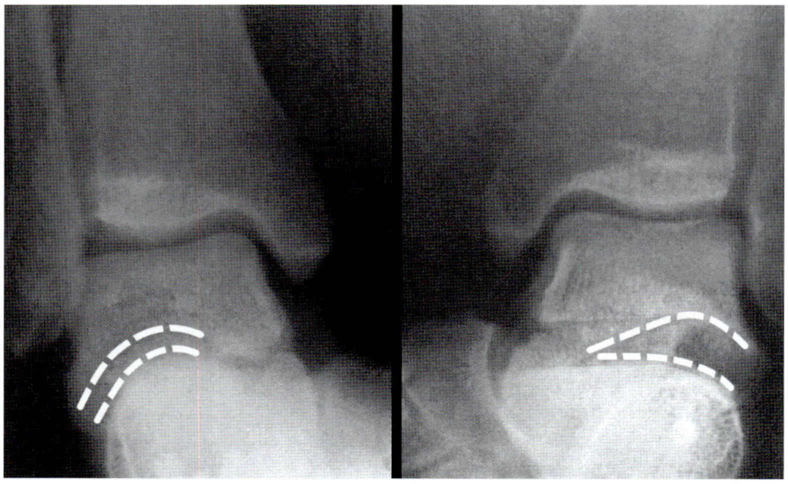

Figure 51 - On the left side, stress X-rays showing a normal sub-talar joint with parallelism of the posterior facets. On the right side, a separation between posterior facets is evident, indicating subtalar instability

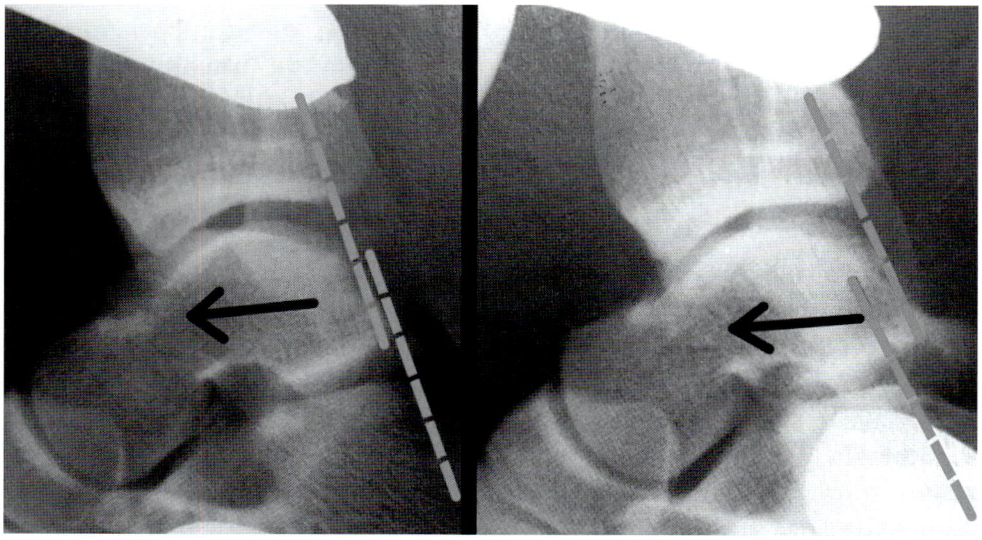

Figure 52 - On the left side, lateral X-ray showing a normal subtalar joint during the anterior drawer stress test. On the right side, abnormal subtalar joint

Application of orthosis (lace-up ankle orthosis) has been shown to reduce the incidence of ankle reinjury in soccer players with previous ankle sprains. Several studies have found minimal, if any, effect of orthoses on athletic performance [39, 99].

Low-profile braces for soccer have been developed, which allow for minimal disruption of the player's boot and space proximally to insert the shin guard. Another essential component of prevention is prophylactic intervention with balance and proprioceptive exercises. A study looking at first division men's league soccer players in Iran showed a significant decrease in reinjury rates with proprioceptive training [100].

In 2003, FIFA introduced a comprehensive warm-up program which has been shown in several studies to decrease the risk of injury in amateur soccer players [101-102]

Subtalar sprains

Most subtalar ligament injuries are associated with lateral ankle sprains. Subtalar instability occurs in about 10% of ankle lateral sprain sequelae [103]. The two subtalar joint ligaments (cervical and interosseous ligaments) control the reciprocal movements between talus and calcaneus in flexion-supination, adduction and extension, pronation-abduction (fig. 49). In addition to subtalar ligaments, the CFL, the lateral talo-calcaneal ligament (LTCL), and the inferior extensor retinacula also contributes to subtalar joint stability.

Diagnosis is not easy. The traumatic mechanism does not help in distinguishing between ankle and sub-talar sprain. A "turning heel" is usually referred especially in the presence of an irregular ground; a pain in the sinus tarsi area and tenderness involving even the peroneal tendons may be present. An increased subtalar joint internal rotation movement can be found and a slight hindfoot varus compared to the contralateral side can be detected. Standard radiographs are usually negative. Stress radiographs are useful (figg. 50, 51, 52) [103]. US, MRI and arthroscopy are useful tools for assessing and confirming instability.

Treatment varies depending on whether instability is acute or chronic. Acute lesions rarely require a surgical treatment unless associated with lateral ankle ligament lesions (common in chronic lesions). Non-operative treatment includes peroneal strengthening, triceps strenghtening, taping, braces or insoles. If conservative treatment is not successful, surgical treatment is needed. The plantar gracilis tendon, a hemi-peroneal tendon, or a tendinous allograft may be used in order to reconstruct the cervical ligament, the ATFL, and CFL (fig. 53). Post-operative treatment includes a non-weight-bearing plaster cast for three weeks, then a loading brace for another three weeks and active mobilization. Return to competitive play usually takes about 4 months.

Sinus tarsi syndrome

Sinus tarsi syndrome is characterized by pain at the level of the tarsus sinus, mostly caused by ligament injuries, instability, osteofibrosis, ganglion cysts, subtalar osteochondral lesions, or osteophytes [104]. Pain is usually reported at the level of the sinus tarsus arising following an inversion trauma. Instability is not evident but a localized swelling is common above the sinus tarsus. X-rays are usually negative. MRI can highlight the presence of fibrosis, synovitis, and fluids (fig. 54) [104]. A local injection of anesthetic may be useful for the diagnosis and sometimes can lead to a pain resolution [104]. In doubtful cases a diagnostic arthroscopy can be performed.

Initial treatment is conservative. A hindfoot re-alignement with the use of dedicated orthosis is advisable in case of flat-foot or cavus-foot deformity. When symptoms persist, surgical treatment is indicated [104]. An incision of about 2 cm is made oblique above the sinus tarsi. The fibers of the IFR are removed and the capsules are opened: the posterior subtalar joint is highlighted. Any lateral osteophyte secondary to an impingement should be removed. The undamaged ligaments are respected and the fatty-fibrous tissue, rich in nerve terminations, is removed (fig. 55).

Arthroscopy may be a valid alternative to open surgery with high percentage of good results (about 94% of cases) [104].

Midfoot sprains

A midfoot sprain involves the central region of the foot, which is composed by the 3 cuneiforms, the cuboid and by a highly complex system of ligaments attaching each of these bones to one another

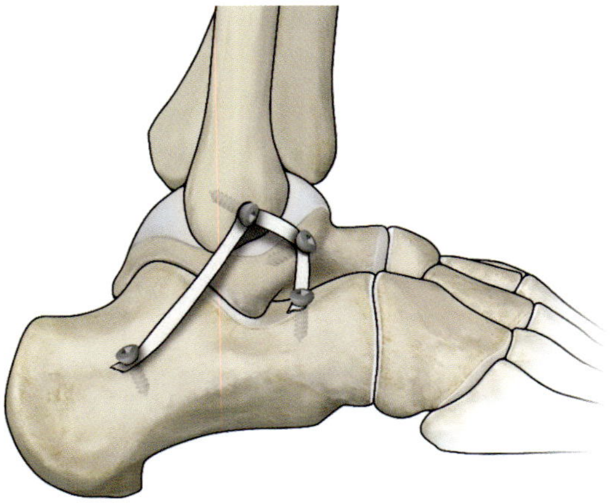

Figure 53 - Artificial allograft for CFL and ATFL reconstruction

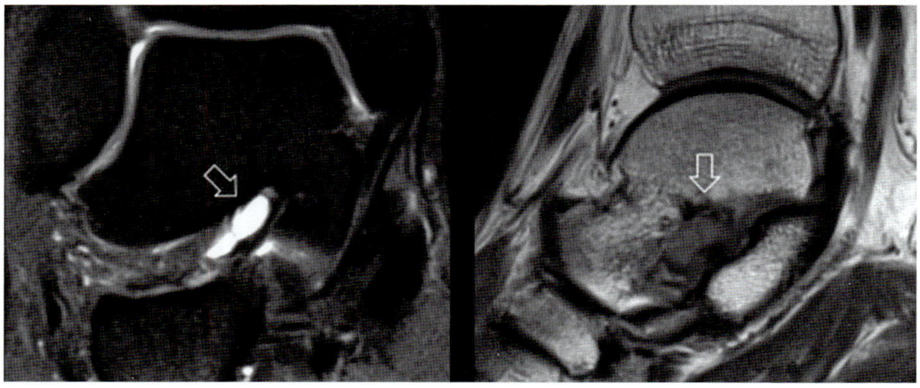

Figure 54 - MRI showing fibrosis and fluids at the subtalar level

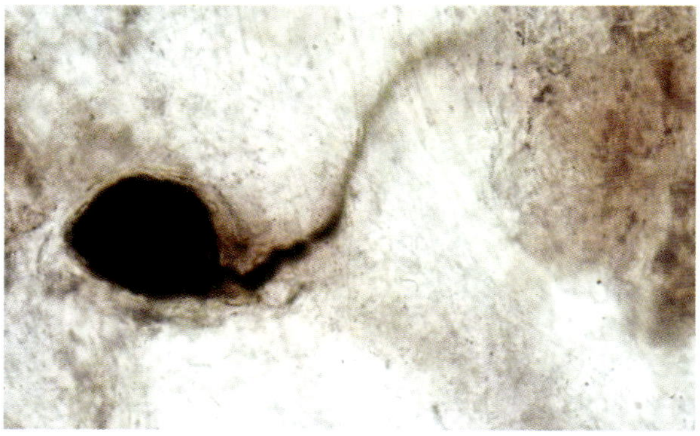

Figure 55 - Pacinian corpuscles from sinus tarsi tissue in a microscope slide

Figure 56 - The force application point is crucial in the direction of tarso-metatarsal displacement. Most direct injuries result in plantar displacement of metatarsal bases. Dorsal displacement may occur if the impact point is proximal to the joint (from Myerson MS et al. [224])

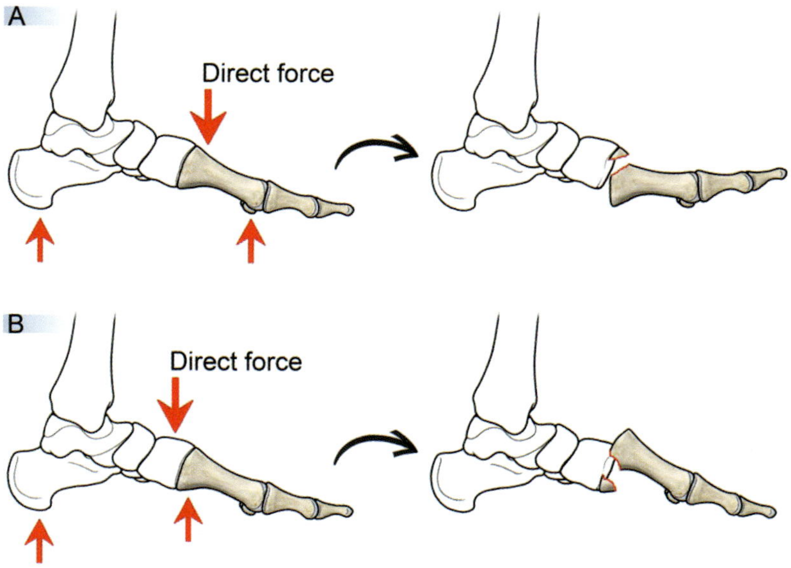

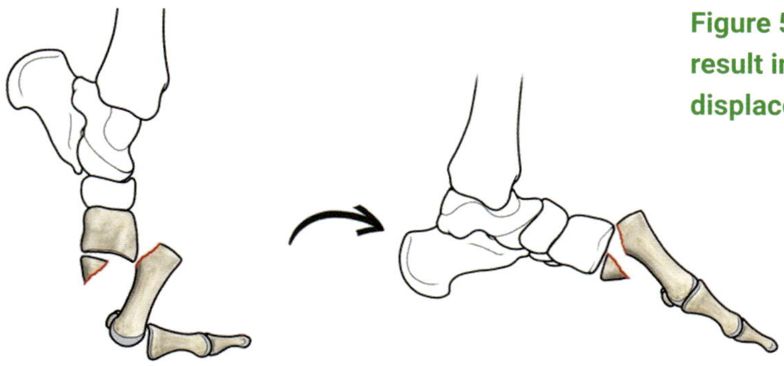

Figure 57 - The majority of indirect injuries result in the metatarsal base dorsal displacement (from Myerson MS et al. [224])

and also to the metatarsal in the forefoot [105]. Severe midfoot sprains are usually associated with fractures, but they are uncommon in soccer players. On the other hand, minor injuries are more common and if not correctly evaluated and treated, they can cause persistent pain and lack of activity for long periods [106].

Midfoot sprains are second in frequency only to MPJ sprains.

The mechanism of injury can be direct or indirect. The direct mechanism (fig. 56), depending on the force application point, more often causes a plantar displacement. The indirect mechanism (fig. 57) is mainly caused by a twisting injury due to a force with a forefoot adduction or secondary to an axial loading while the foot is in a plantarflexed position [106].

From the clinical point of view pain is referred to the foot medial side; walking is allowed but running and jumping are limited. The palpation between the first and second metatarsus bases usually causes pain even in lesions with a small joint displacement. Side to side compression of the midfoot and a dorso-plantar deviation of the first metatarsal head is positive evoking pain, as well as passive pronation and abduction of the midfoot. Radiographic evaluation requires special attention (figg. 58, 59, 60). Midfoot sprains related lesions, if not suspected and adequately investigated, are unrecognized at X-rays in about 20% of cases [107]. An under-weightbearing X-ray of the two feet in the antero-posterior view may be useful to detect the diastasis between the bases of the first and second metatarsus. A CT allows to better highlight any associated fractures (figg. 61, 62). A MRI may identify lesions of the soft tissues (fig. 63) [107].

Midfoot sprains related lesions are usually classified in three stages (fig. 64).

In stage 1 the ligament is stretched but there is no diastase, with increased bone scan captation only. In stage 2 a diastasis between the first and second metatarsus is evident due to a breaking of the Lisfranc ligament; the plantar arch is preserved. In stage 3 diastase and a medial arch reduction are present; in lateral X-rays views a reduction of the distance between the fifth metatarsal and the medial cuneiform is evident.

In stage 1 the treatment is conservative with a non-weight-bearing plaster cast for four weeks, then a walking Walker boot and progressive mobilization for another three weeks. In stage 2 a reduction and stabilization of the diastase is necessary. When closed reduction is achievable, percutaneous fixation is performed (fig. 65), otherwise an open reduction is needed.

In stage 3 lesion open reduction is advisable in order to remove any bone fragments and better visualize the reduction (fig. 66).

A non-weight-bearing plaster cast or Walker boot is prescribed for six weeks, then partial load is allowed. Full load is granted after 12 weeks. Semi-rigid insoles may be useful.

Forefoot sprains and turf toe

Forefoot sprains more frequently involve first MTP joint, usually with a hallux hyperextension trauma; less commonly, they occur due to a hallux hyperflexion movement ("sand toe") or involve lesser toes [108]. A hallux trauma due to a hyperextension sprain is known as turf-toe [109].

These injuries can lead to an important disability due to pain, usually emphasized during the push-off-phase. The most common mechanism of injury involves an axial load on the first MTP joint with the foot placed in a fixed equinus position. This causes a forced hyperextension of the joint,

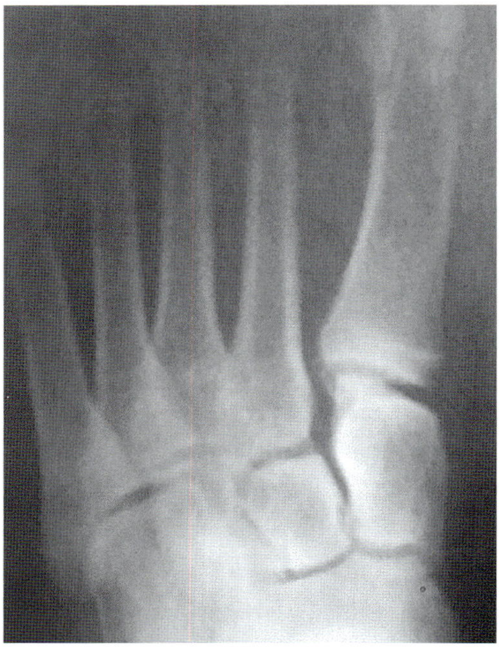

Figure 58 - Dorso-plantar X-ray showing a widening of the medial cuneifom-second metatarsal space indicating Lisfranc complex instability

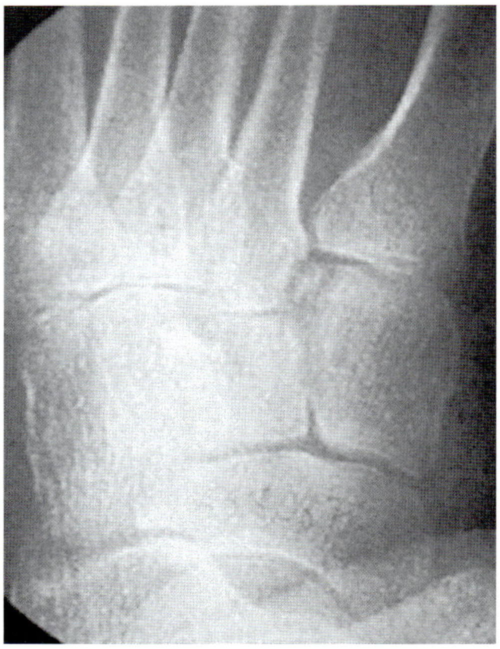

Figure 59 - Dorso-plantar X-ray showing a widening of the medial cuneifom-second metatarsal space associated with a bony fragment from the medial cuneiform

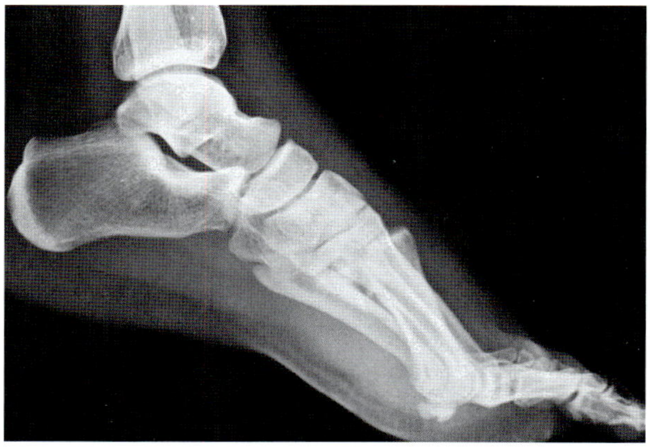

Figure 60 - Lateral X-ray showing a dorsal dislocation of the second metatarsal base

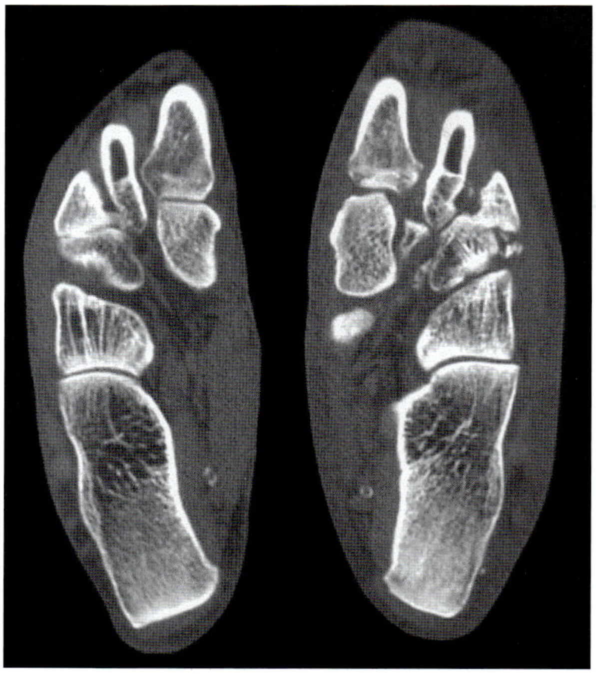

Figure 61- Comparative CT scan of both feet showing the Lisfranc injury on the right side

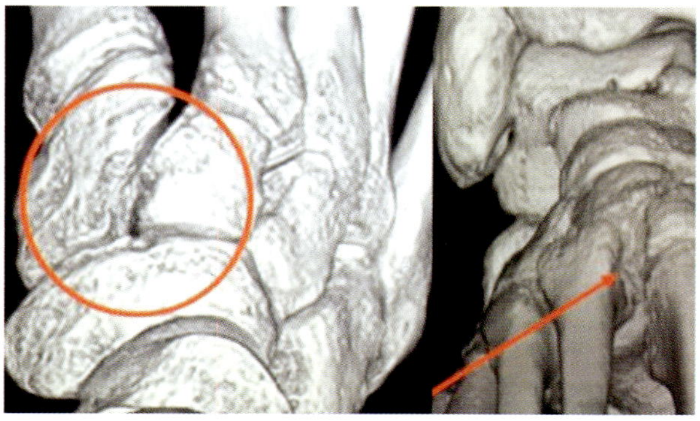

Figure 62 - 3D CT scan reconstruction showing the Lisfranc injury (red arrow)

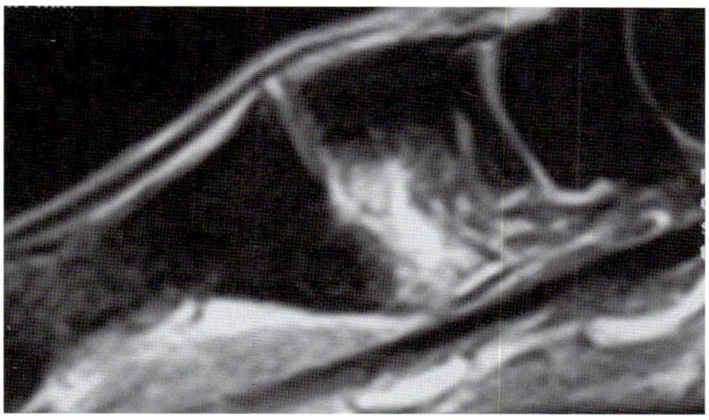

Figure 63 - MRI showing the Lisfranc complex involvement associated with bone edema

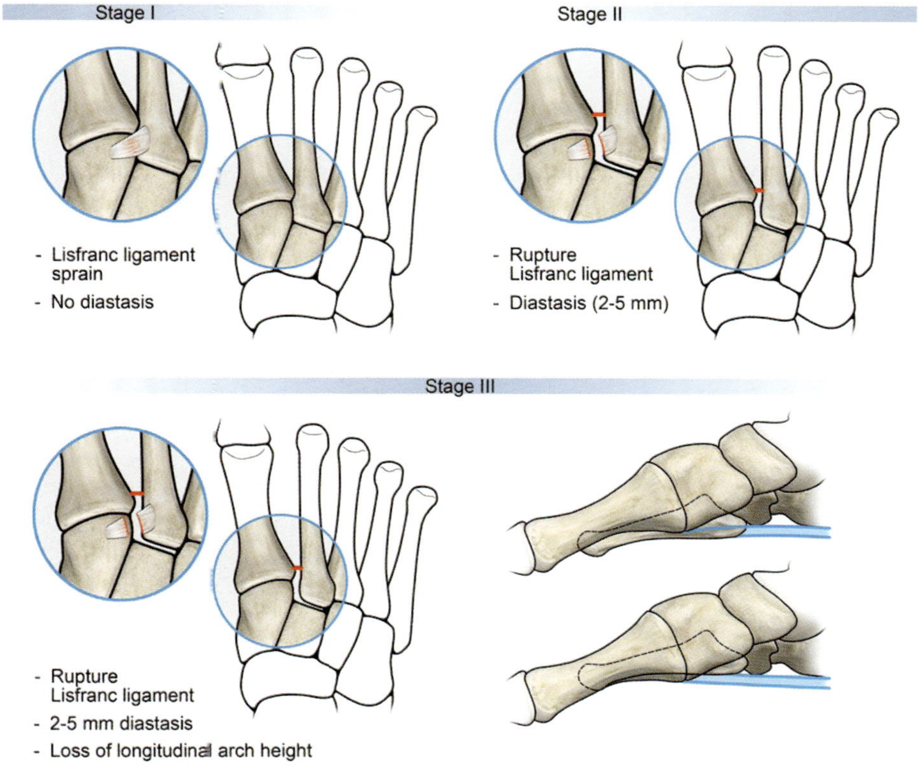

Figure 64 - Midfoot sprains lesions, III-grades classification

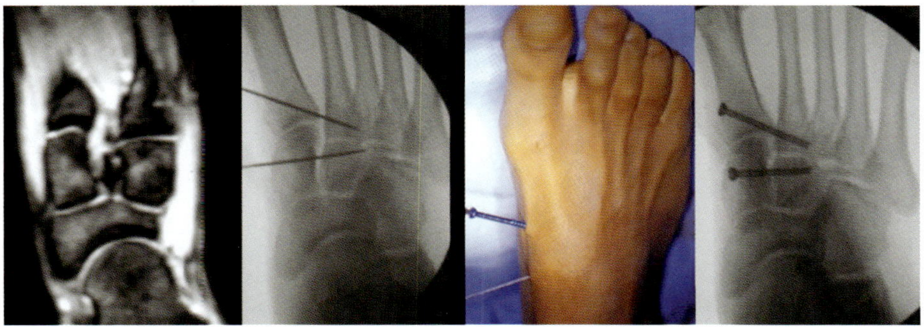

Figure 65 - On the left side, MRI showing the Lisfranc injury. The reduction is obtained with two percutaneous screws

Figure 66 - Stage 3 lesions treated with open reduction and Lisfranc complex arthrodesis with screws

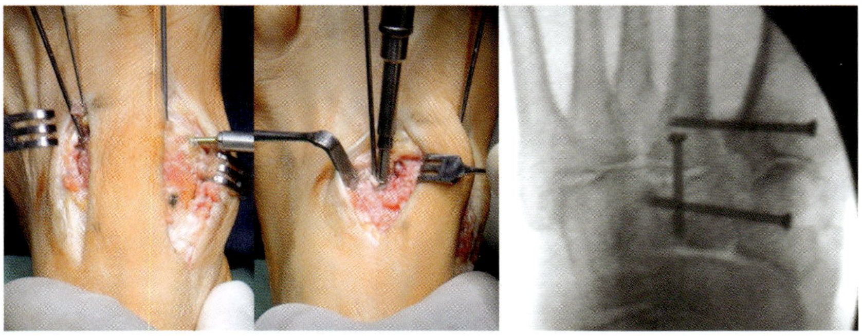

therefore producing a sprain injury of the plantar structure (fig. 67). In severe cases, it can produce a complete dislocation of the toe and osteochondral lesions of the articular surface [109].

A variation of the turf toe, known as sand toe and due to a forced hyperflexion of the first MTP joint, has been described. This type of injury involves the dorsal structures and is most common in beach soccer players due to a botched jump landing. Another variation described in literature involves a valgus directed force causing injury to the medial ligamentous, capsular and sesamoid complex; this usually causes a relative contracture of the lateral structures that appears as a traumatic hallux valgus deformity [110].

The rupture of the glenoid rim can occur distally to sesamoids, at their level, or proximally to them. Turf toe development and high incidence have been correlated to the use of shoes with flexible soles on artificial turf, and its incidence has seen significant growth since the introduction of modern artificial playing surfaces. The diagnosis of turf toe injury can be challenging. A high degree of suspicion must be kept in an athlete that suffered trauma to the first MTP joint. As with all lesions, the severity of a turf toe injury can be a spectrum ranging from a mild sprain to complete disruption of the normal articular anatomy. An acute injury usually presents itself with swelling, plantar ecchymoses, and load limitation.

During the examination is crucial to palpate the plantar sesamoid complex, the dorsal capsule, and the collateral ligaments, searching for pain and tenderness. Specifically, a tenderness proximal to the sesamoids is correlated to an often low-grade injury, whereas a distal tenderness is correlated to a more severe type of injury. Once the palpation phase of the examination is over, a careful evaluation of the range of motion and articular stability of the first MTP joint should be performed. Turf toe injuries tend to present with a restricted range of motion with a concomitant articular instability found during varus-valgus stress or a dorso-plantar drawer test [111]. In the chronic conditions a deformity known as swan neck deformity, caused by an avulsion of the flexor hallucis brevis, may be present (fig. 68).

Routinely, the initial assessment is performed using standard radiographs. Specifically, weight-bearing dorsoplantar, lateral, and axial sesamoid views should be performed. Radiographs can help identify bony abnormalities, sesamoids proximal migration, bipartite sesamoid, or sesamoid diastasis.

However, due to their nature, turf toe injuries can be often overlooked, causing long term problems especially in professional athletes. Since the radiographic diagnosis can be difficult to be performed, it is common practice to perform CT-scans and MRI-scans to better define the extent of the injury. Specifically, MRI can be helpful to evaluate the presence of bone marrow edema, loose bodies, and osteochondral lesions of the first MTP joint (figg. 69, 70).

Lesions are classified in three grades [112, 113].

- Grade 1 lesions are represented by sprain of the capsule without continuity loss, normal range of motion, no ecchymosis or instability, weight-bearing allowed.
- Grade 2 lesions are defined as a partial tear of the plantar plate and capsule, swelling, ecchymosis, pain during motion of the MTP joint.
- Grade 3 lesions are represented by a complete lesion of the plantar plate and capsule. Severe instability, weight-bearing is not allowed due to pain. It is possible to find concomitant lesions such as sesamoid fractures and osteochondral lesions.

There is a lack of trials in specialized literature for comparing treatment options regarding turf toe injuries. Nevertheless, treatment can be divided into conservative and surgical [114, 116].

Grade 1 or 2 lesions are usually treated conservatively, while in grade 3 lesions surgical treatment is often required.

Conservative treatment should always be the initial choice, whatever stage of injury, except in cases of irreducible dislocations. The RICE (Rest, Ice, Compression and Elevation) protocol is often used in combination with pain medications for the first 48 to 72 hours after the trauma. Furthermore, the use of a brace, a short leg cast or talus shoes can reduce symptoms.

In the case of grade I injuries, following the initial supportive measures, the patient benefits greatly from a taping in a slight plantar-flexed position in a rigid shoe. Care must be taken around the taping

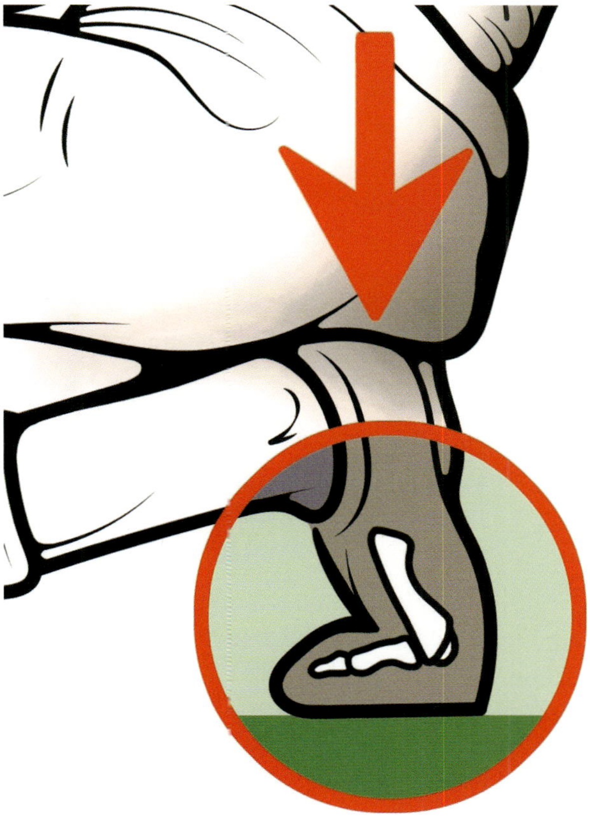

Figure 67 - Forced hyperextension mechanism

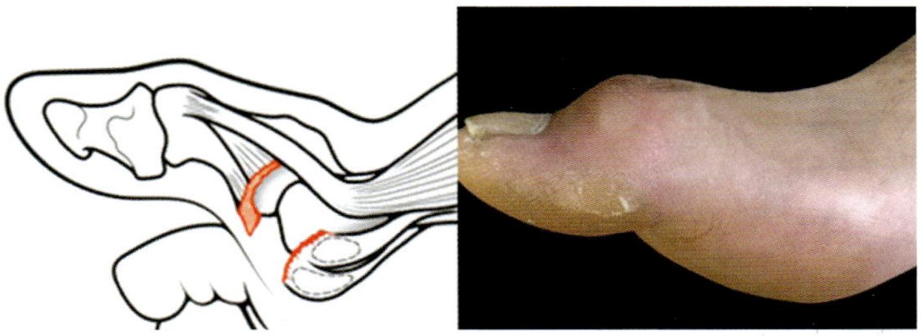

Figure 68 - The avulsion of the flexor hallucis brevis causes a swan neck deformity of the first toe

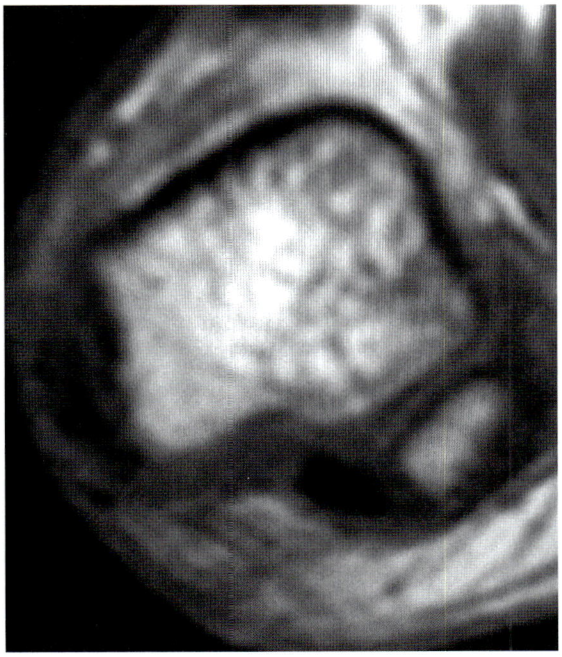

Figure 69 - MRI turf toe injuries showing capsular and chondral lesion in the dorsal aspect of the metatarsal head, bone marrow edema

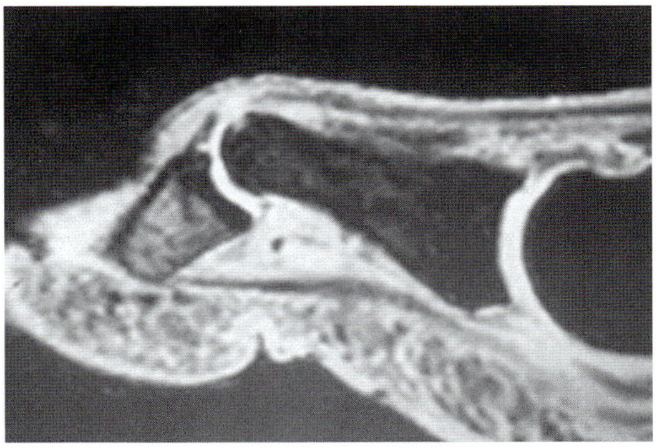

Figure 70 - MRI showing bone marrow edema at the first metatarsal head

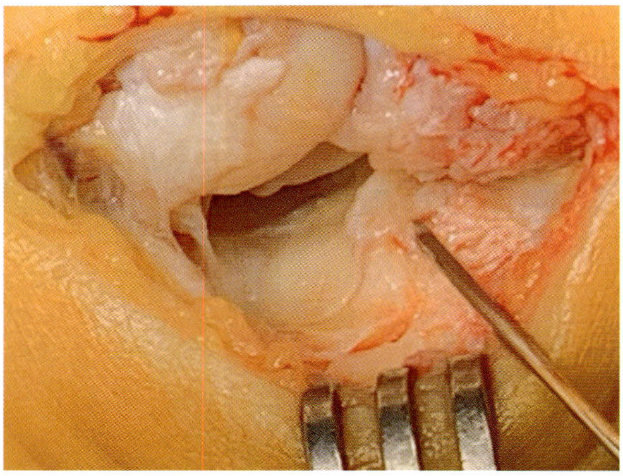

Figure71 - Isolated capsular disruption, proximal to the sesamoid complex

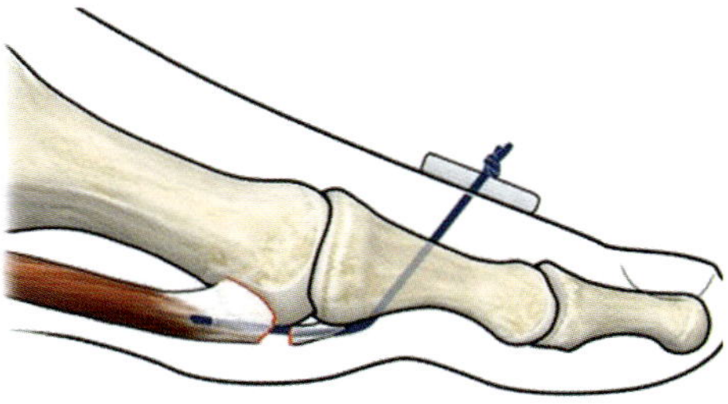

Figure 72 - Tendon re-insertion at the base of the phalanx using a dorsal pull-out technique

since it can cause vascular supply deficits due to the swelling during the first phases after the trauma. Active range of motion exercises should be initiated after 3-5 days after trauma, as well as low impact activities. Steroid injections are not recommended in these conditions. Athletes must be advised not to underestimate their injury since it can lead to a significant worsening of both the sprain and the symptomatology [114]. The recovery will be progressively faster depending on the degree of injury. A few days in type 1, two weeks in type 2, up to six months in type 3.

Grade 2 injuries see a similar conservative treatment to grade I lesions. These lesions also benefit from a plantarflexing taping of the first toe. Gentle passive motion is started after the resolution of pain and swelling. High impact activities should be progressively introduced. Athletes are preferably not allowed high impact activities for at least 2 weeks.

Grade 3 injuries need a more aggressive treatment protocol if compared with grade I and grade II lesions. Normally, conservative treatment of grade III injuries requires 8 weeks of immobilization and it may take up to 4-5 months to achieve a complete symptomatology resolution. Return to sports activities should be postponed until 50°-60° forced dorsiflexion of the first MTP joint can be achieved without pain [112].

Surgical treatment for turf toe injuries is indicated for instabilities with massive capsular lesions, sesamoids fractures, sesamoid position retraction, traumatic bunions, or osteochondral lesions [116]. Surgical technique varies depending on lesion type. In isolated capsular disruption, surgical treatment is based on an end-to-end suture of the capsule (fig. 71). Usually, the capsular suture is performed with a single medial incision. If the lesion is distal to the sesamoid complex, the tendon can be sutured or reinserted at the base of the phalanx (fig. 72).

If a fracture with sesamoid diastase is present, a cerclage is applied or the smaller fragment is removed and a suture is performed. In case of tibial sesamoidectomy it is better to perform a transposition of the abductor hallucis into the residual plantar defect (the abductor hallucis longus should be interposed to provide an active restraint to dorsiflexion) (fig. 73). In case of chronic lesions with cock deformity, a transposition of the flexor hallucis longus into the base of the phalanx associated with an arthrodesis of the interphalangeal joint of

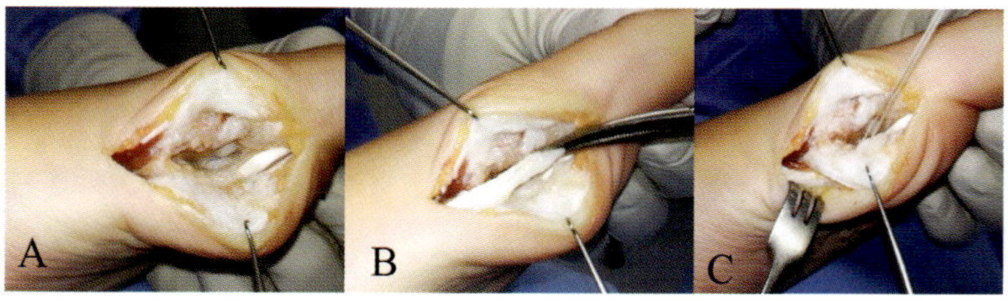

Figure 73 - In case of tibial sesamoidectomy (A) a transposition of the abductor hallucis (B) into the plantar defect is performed (C)

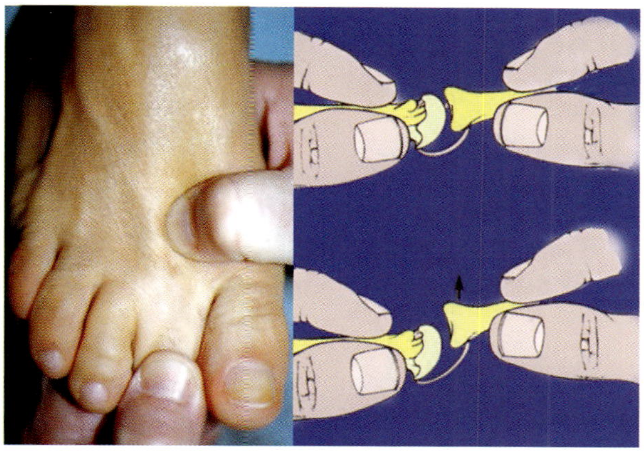

Figure 74 - The MPJ drawer test may confirm a clinical instability

the big toe can be performed.

Post-operative protocol consists in early passive mobilization in plantar-flexion started 1 week post-operatively, trying avoiding dorsiflexion movements and using talus shoes for one month. At 6 weeks post-operatively patient should start walking with a rigid sole shoe. After three months sport activity is resumed [117].

Metatarsophalangeal instability

Metatarsophalangeal Joint (MPJ) instability clinically appears as an isolated pain located under the head of the corresponding metatarsal.

More frequently it affects the second and the third metatarsal at the metatarsophalangeal joint level. The pain is due to the dorsal subluxation of the proximal phalanx above the metatarsal head which is thus pushed downwards [3]. The instability is clinically evident with the drawer test (fig. 74).

If no structured joint luxation is present, X-rays are negative. MRI may shows osteochondral lesion caused by the instability (fig. 75).

Conservative treatment consists in metatarsal head plantar discharge using dedicated orthotics insoles. A taping involving two contiguous fingers and aligning the finger thus favoring its plantar flexion can be useful.

When instability is chronic surgical treatment is indicated.

The less invasive solution is represented by the plantar release followed by the stabilization of the metatarsophalangeal joint with a Kirshner-Wire for 4 weeks in order to promote the formation of a plantar scar able to stabilize the joint

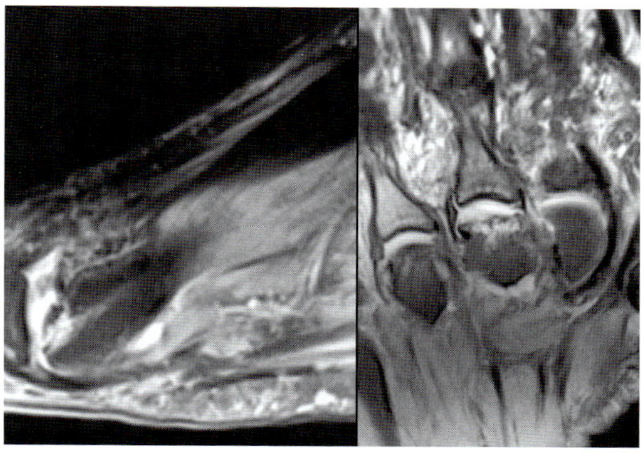

Figure 75 - MRI in a third MPJ instability showing metatarsal head chondral lesion

(fig. 76). In other cases a flexor-to-extensor tendon transposition may be performed (fig. 77).

In case of significant overload of the metatarsal head a condylectomy may be associated. When a metatarsal head chondral lesion is associated (fig. 78), microfractures may be associated (fig. 79).

Impingement

Ankle impingement syndrome is the result of a conflict between bony structures or soft tissues and is a very common condition among soccer players. According to pathoanatomy, impingement may be subgrouped in anterior and posterior [2, 118].

Anterior ankle impingement

Anterior impingement syndrome of the ankle can involve either osseous or fibrous tissue and is one of the most common causes of chronic ankle pain in athletes. Because of its incidence this condition is also known as “footballer’s ankle” [2]. The anterior bony impingement is related to the presence of tibial or talar osteophytes.

When a bony etiology is excluded, impingement is classified as fibrous or soft tissue.

Since the 1950s, a growing body of research has investigated various pathologic conditions that can be classified as anterior ankle soft tissue impingement [6]. Based on the etiology and location of the anterior ankle impingement, four anterior soft tissue impingement groups can be described: anterolateral, anteromedial, syndesmotic, and diffuse anterior soft tissue impingement [2].

Anterior osseous ankle impingement (fig. 80) is caused by anterior osteophytes on both the distal

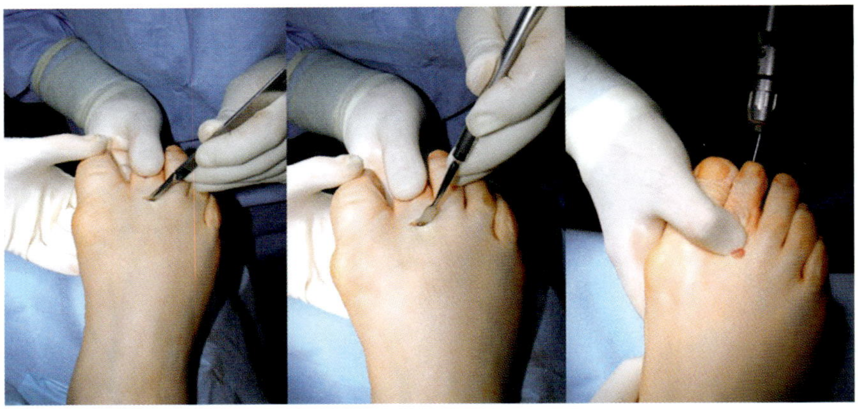

Figure 76 - Percutaneous plantar release and metatarsophalangeal joint stabilization using a Kirshner-Wire

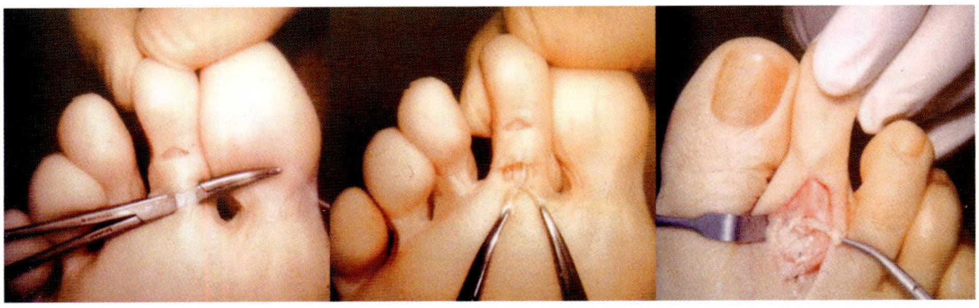

Figure 77 - Flexor-to-extensor tendon transfer. The procedure consists in splitting the FDL tendon in half after detaching it from the plantar base of the distal phalanx. A second incision is made plantarly at the MPJ, through which the detached flexor tendon is harvested. A dorsal incision over the proximal phalanx is then performed; each half of the splitted tendon is pulled and sutured dorsally

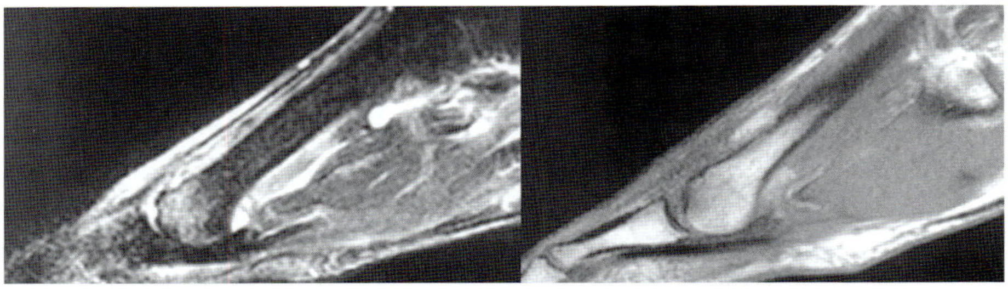

Figure 78 - MRI in a second MPJ instability showing metatarsal head chondral lesion

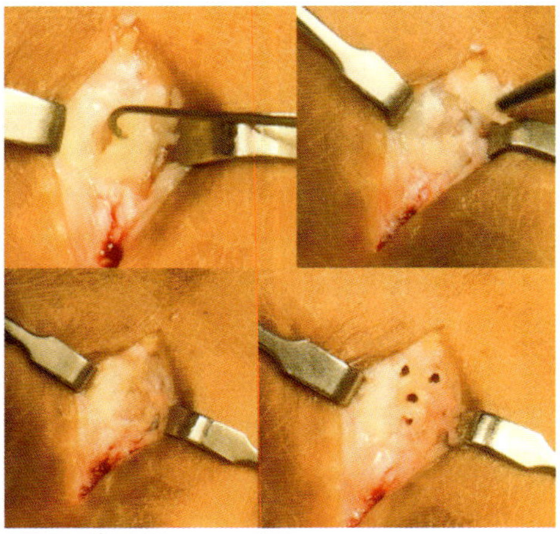

Figure 79 - The metatarsal head chondral lesion is treated with microfractures through a dorsal incision

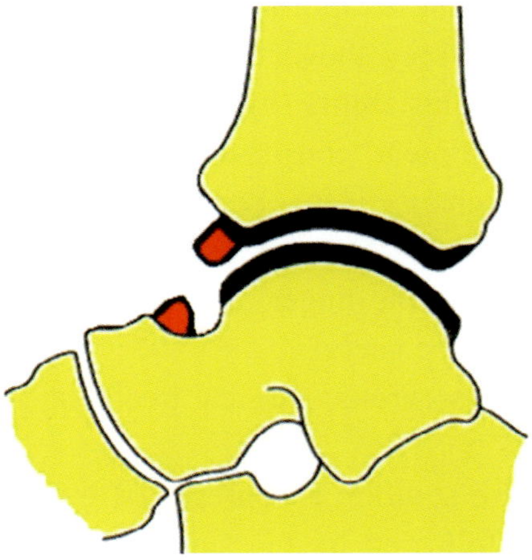

Figure 80 - Anterior osseous ankle impingement: osteophytes represented both on the distal tibia and talar neck

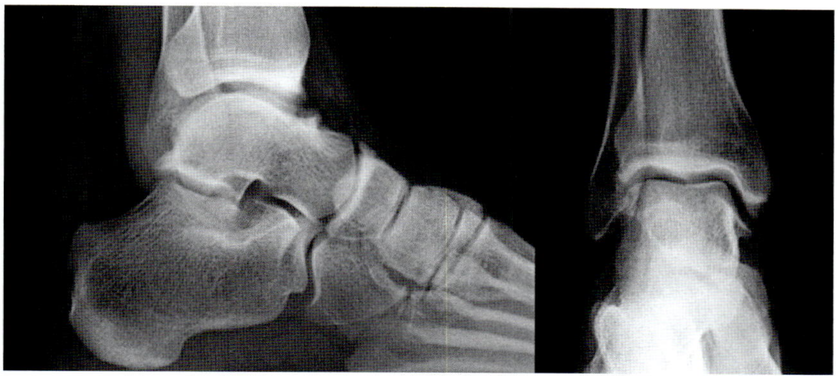

Figure 81 - Lateral ankle X-ray shows tibiotalar osteophytes. In the anterior view (on the right) osteophytes are not detected

tibia and talar neck. It is thought to be related to repetitive microtraumas to the anteromedial aspect of the ankle from recurrent ball impact [119].

It is very common among soccer players: some studies suggest that 60% of soccer players have this syndrome. It is primarily diagnosed with lateral ankle X-rays (fig. 81), which will show the osteophytes. An oblique antero-medial X-ray may increase detection of osteophytes. The early stages of anterior impingement can be treated successfully with injections and heel lifts. Treatment of lesions that fail to respond to conservative management involves arthroscopic or open excision of osteophytes (video 1).

Most patients with no pre-existing osteoarthritis treated arthroscopically will experience pain relief and return to full activity, though recurrent osteophyte formation has been noted at long-term follow-up [120].

Anterior ankle impingement is most often caused by acute ankle sprains with an inversion type of mechanism. The subsequent reactive inflammation can cause fibrosis leading to distal fascicle

VIDEO 1

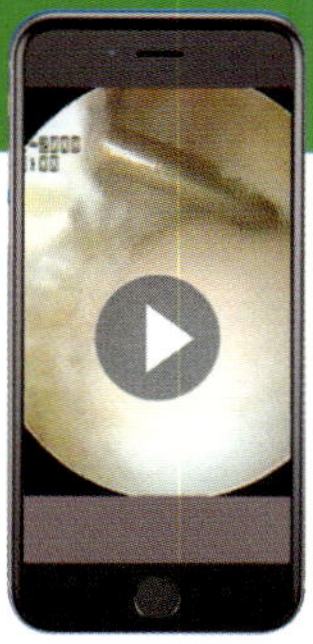

Arthroscopic osteophyte excision

enlargement of the AITFL. Impingement in the anterolateral gutter of this enlarged fascicle can also cause both chronic reactive synovitis and chondromalacia of the lateral talar dome [121].

MRI can identify abnormal areas of pathology; however, 50% of cases are diagnosed on clinical examination alone.

Patients generally present with a history of anterolateral ankle pain and swelling with an occasional popping or snapping sensation. Soccer players commonly develop anterior bony impingement due to repetitive loading of the anterior ankle from striking the ball. This repetition can lead to osteophyte formation of the anterior distal tibia and talar neck. After the osteophytes form, decreased dorsiflexion can occur due to a mechanical stop and inflammation of the interposed capsule. The patient will exhibit tenderness to palpation along the anterolateral aspect of the ankle, with pain elicited at extreme passive dorsiflexion. Initially, an injection with local anesthetic and corticosteroid can serve both a diagnostic and therapeutic purpose; however, patients who fail conservative treatment can be treated with arthroscopy or open surgery with resection of the involved scar tissue and osteophytes (figg. 82, 83).

The best results are seen in those patients with no concurrent intra-articular lesions or ankle osteoarthritis. When treated non-operatively, a player may return to play when pain resolves; however, if treated surgically with arthroscopic debridement/resection, a player must wait until his surgical scars have healed prior to attempting return to play [2].

Anterior ankle soft tissue impingement is less common. The anteromedial side is the most affected and it is associated with eversion injuries, following medial malleolar, or talar fractures [122].

Previous injury to the anterior tibiotalar fascicle of

the deltoid complex leads to ligament thickening and subsequent impingement in the anteromedial corner of the talus (fig. 84).
Adjacent fibrosis and synovitis are common consequences of impingement; however, osteophyte formation and chondral stripping along the anteromedial talus can also be seen. Patients typically complain of pain along the anteromedial joint line that gets worse with activity, clicking or popping sensations, and painful, limited dorsiflexion.
On examination, impingement can be detected through palpation over the anterior tibiotalar fascicle of the deltoid ligament and eversion or extreme passive dorsiflexion of the foot and all of which will elicit medial ankle tenderness [120].
Initial treatment consists of rest, physical therapy, and NSAIDs. Refractory cases may be amenable to arthroscopic or open resection of the anterior tibiotalar fascicle with débridement of any adjacent synovitis and scar tissue (fig. 85) [2].

Posterior ankle impingement

Posterior ankle impingement is a common cause of chronic ankle pain. It is the result of compression between bony or soft tissue structures during terminal plantar flexion. The cause and pathological anatomic features are heterogeneous, and several pathological conditions can result in posterior impingement [2, 123].
The bony structures responsible for posterior ankle impingement lie in the tibiocalcaneal interval. These include the posterior malleolus, the posterolateral talar process (trigonal or Stieda's process), an os trigonum, the posterior subtalar joint, and the posterior calcaneal tuberosity (figg. 86, 87).
In early anatomic studies, Cloquet and Shepherd independently described the presence of an os trigonum. Both authors attributed this bony variation to a fracture. Although it is sometimes still referred to as a Shepherd's fracture, Shepherd later realized that this structure was actually a separate ossification center [123-124].
An os trigonum is an accessory bone that represents a developmental analogue of the secondary ossification center of the posterolateral talus. The latter mineralizes between 7 and 13 years of age and fuses within 1 year. In 7% to 14% of adults it remains as a separate accessory bone, which is bilateral in 1.4% of cases. This structure is usually asymptomatic, but it may become painful in individuals participating in sports involving repeated plantar flexion [123].
The plantar flexion movement may play a role in generating compression of the os trigonum or posterolateral process. The posterolateral process may be acutely fractured by a single plantar flexion event. In the setting of an os trigonum, such an injury results in disruption of the synchondrosis that connects the accessory bone to the native talus. Alternatively, chronic fracture of these structures may result from repetitive stress. In some cases, forced dorsiflexion may increase tension on the posterior talofibular ligament, which can result in avulsion of the os trigonum or posterolateral tubercle. Finally, posterior impingement may result from previous fractures or degenerative arthritis that can lead to the formation of ankle and subtalar osteophytes. Impinging calcifications in the posterior aspect of the ankle may also result from chronic soft tissue inflammation [123].
The diagnosis of posterior ankle impingement is based primarily on the clinical history. The patient usually reports chronic or recurrent posterior pain caused or exacerbated by forced plantar flexion or push-off activities, such as kicking or running. The pain is usually deep and may have a mechanical component. There may be a recent or remote history of acute ankle trauma, but overuse must also be considered. On physical examination there is typically posteromedial or posterolateral tenderness. Passive terminal plantar flexion may reproduce the patient's symptoms. If passive hallux motion causes pain, flexor hallucis longus abnormality may also be present. Plain radiographs may detect an acute or chronic fracture of the trigonal process as well as the presence of an intact or fractured os trigonum. Nevertheless, the presence of an os trigonum on conventional radiographs is not necessarily clinically relevant. Calcifications may be detected about the posterior ankle and result from previous trauma, arthritis, or chronic soft tissue inflammation. With regard to advanced imaging, MRI may reveal bone marrow edema in the os trigonum or the trigonal process as well as adjacent soft issue inflammation. Other findings that may be demonstrated on MRI include chondral injury and flexor hallucis longus tenosynovitis. CT can detect or confirm the pres-

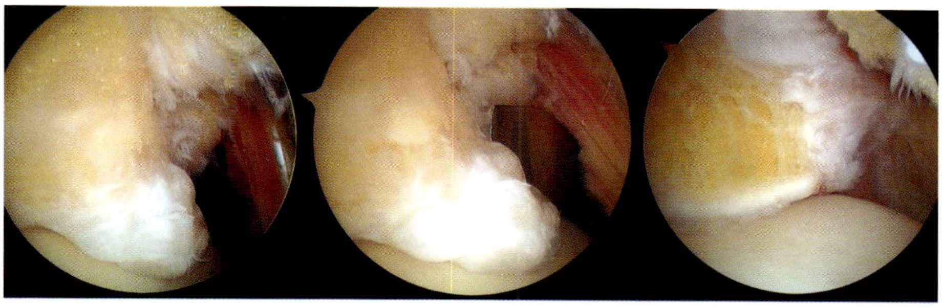

Figure 82 - Arthroscopic anterior osteophytes excision

Figure 83 - Open osteophytes excision through an antero-medial incision

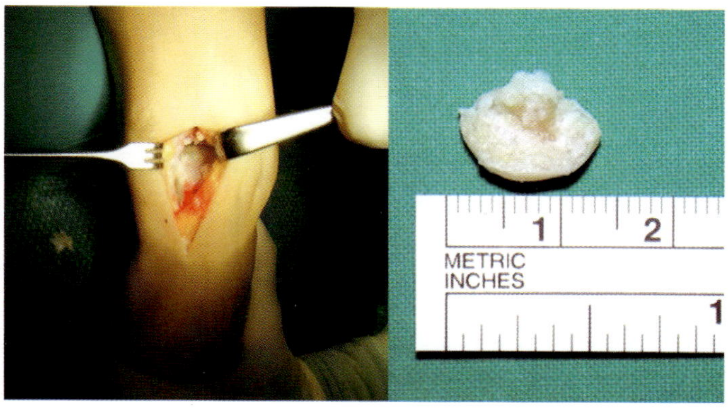

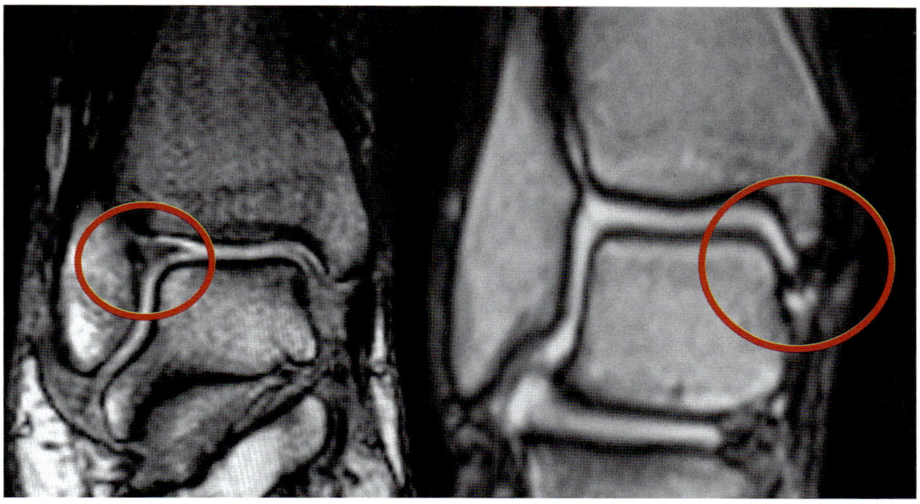

Figure 84 - MRI showing thickening and impingement in the anteromedial side of the talus

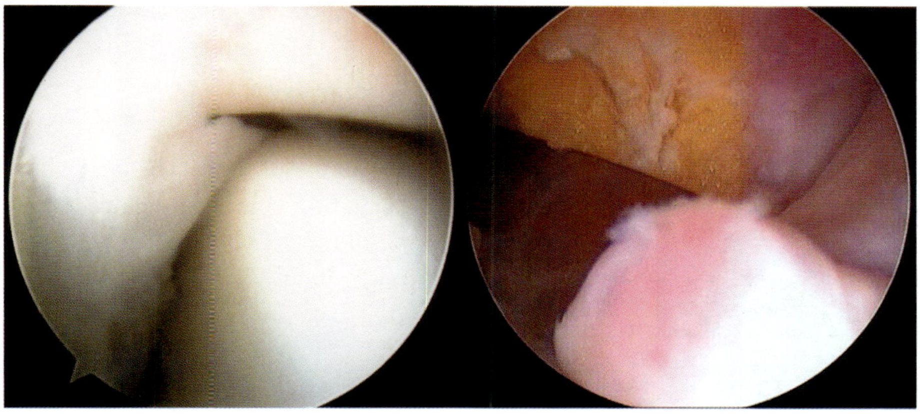

Figure 85 - On the left the arthroscopic image shows the antero-medial impingement; the procedure allows for the resection of the anterior tibiotalar fascicle with local debridement

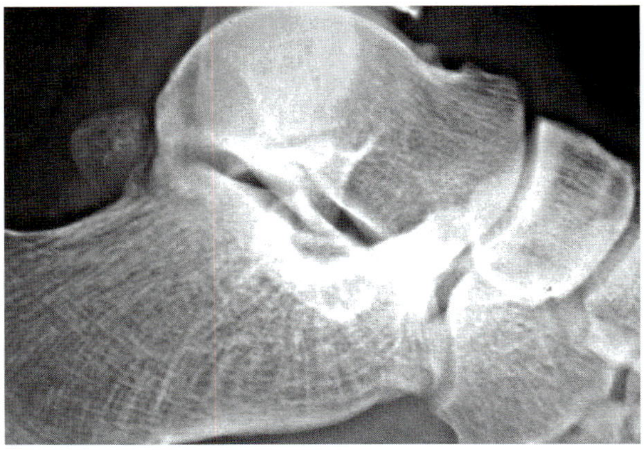

Figure 86 - Lateral X-ray showing a talar os trigonum

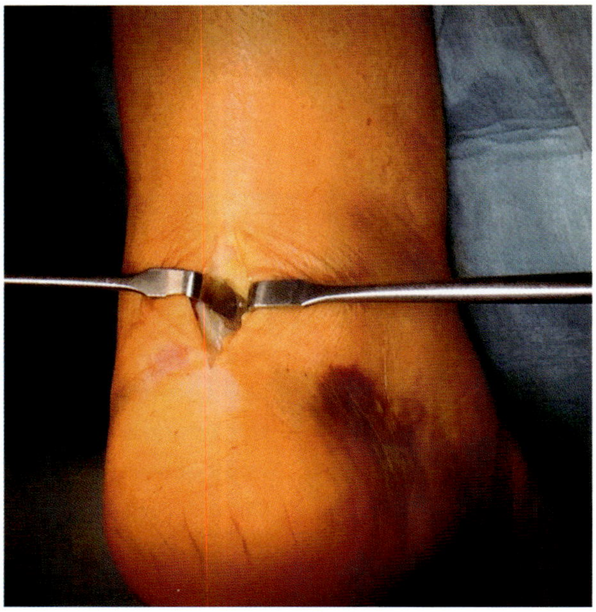

Figure 88 - Open posteromedial approach for the bony impingement removal

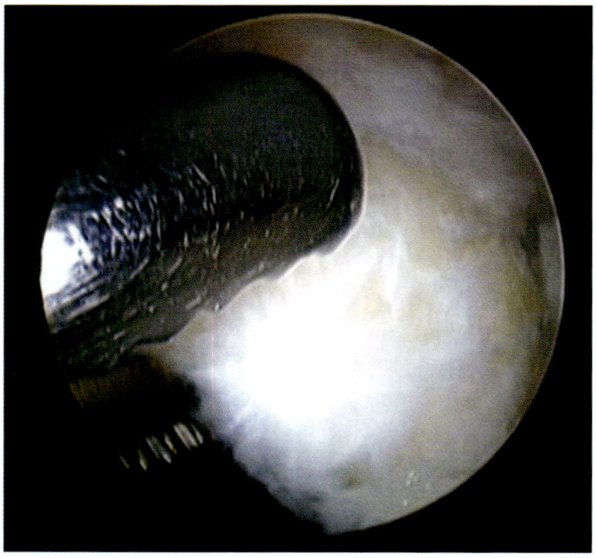

Figure 89 - Arthroscopic decompression for the posterior ankle impingement

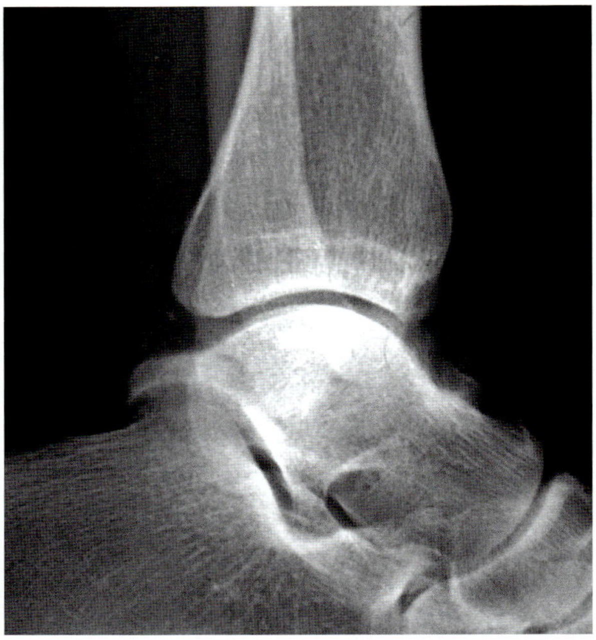

Figure 87 - Lateral X-ray showing a huge posterolateral talar process (trigonal or Stieda's process)

ence of a non-displaced or minimally displaced fracture. Finally, local anesthetic injections may also be of diagnostic value.

The initial treatment of bony impingement includes rest, ice, nonsteroidal anti-inflammatory medication, and the avoidance of extreme ankle plantar flexion. Immobilization is indicated if there is evidence of an acute fracture. Subsequent physical therapy and protective dorsiflexion taping may be helpful. Operative intervention is indicated if symptoms persist despite 3 to 6 months of non-operative care. Typically, surgery entails excision of the os trigonum. The approach may be either posterolateral or medial. The posterolateral approach between the peroneal and flexor hallucis longus (FHL) muscle is more direct and avoids the neurovascular bundle. However, the medial approach allows direct visualization of the FHL tendon. This is useful if the latter needs to be released, as in the setting of tenosynovitis. The medial approach also reduces the risk of peroneal tendinitis and adhesions, which have been reported to be a complication of the posterolateral approach (fig. 88) [124]. Arthroscopic/endoscopic decompression has been described for the treatment of posterior ankle impingement (fig. 89), demonstrating good results with low complication rates and early return to sports [123].

Fractures

In soccer players, severe ankle and foot fractures are quite rare and treatment usually does not differ from the fracture treatment applied in the normal population [2].

However, the reduction, especially when facing articular fractures, must be as anatomical as possible in order to avoid an abnormal pressure distribution during loading and therefore arthritis. Moreover, the technique should be minimally-invasive and effective so as to reduce complications and promote recovery and healing times [12, 125]. The treatment is conservative in case of non-displaced and stable fractures, while surgical in case of displacement or instability. If surgical treatment is performed, stability is needed in order to start active and passive mobilization as early as possible.

The choice whether to perform a percutaneous, a minimally-invasive or a more extended approach depends on the fracture characteristic and on the possibility of reducing it stably. This is the only way to reduce myostatic contracture, muscle atrofy, decreased joint motion, artrofibrosis, cartilagineus degeneration, bone athrophy, and decreased range of motion.

Ankle fractures

In order to assess the mechanism of the lesion, its severity and therefore the type of treatment, a X-rays evaluation with standard views (antero-posterior, lateral, and mortise view with an internal rotation of 15-20°) is necessary [2, 126]. In the mortise view the joint space should appear symmetrical and the medial and lateral joint space should be equal. The circle that forms between the lateral wall of the talus and the apex of the distal fibular malleolus should be in contact with the tibial subchondral bone (fig. 90) [127]. Another useful measurement is represented by the angle formed by the line that joins the apex of the two malleoli and the line parallel to the talus (talo-crural angle) which is usually 83° ± 4°. A too shallow angle suggests a fibular shortening (fig. 91). CT Scan is indicated for complex fractures and to evaluate fracture union.

To assess which fracture is stable or unstable it is useful to consider what proposed by Neer: the ankle with ligaments and stabilizers act as an intact ring, with a single break it is always stable, with two breaks the ring is unstable. Surgical treatment should preferably be carried out as soon as possible, within 12-24 hours, before blisters are formed and important edema occurs. In case of severe edema and soft tissue suffering it is better to wait until a clinical improvement before proceeding with surgical treatment. In addition to the timing assessment, the surgical approach and the fixation devices must be chosen. Regarding ankle fractures, posterolateral approach allows treating the fracture of the fibula and posterior malleolus [128, 129]. Medial approach is useful for treating tibial malleolar fractures [130].

In case of multiple malleolar fractures it is advisable to start from the lateral aspect in order to perform a proper peroneal length reconstruction.

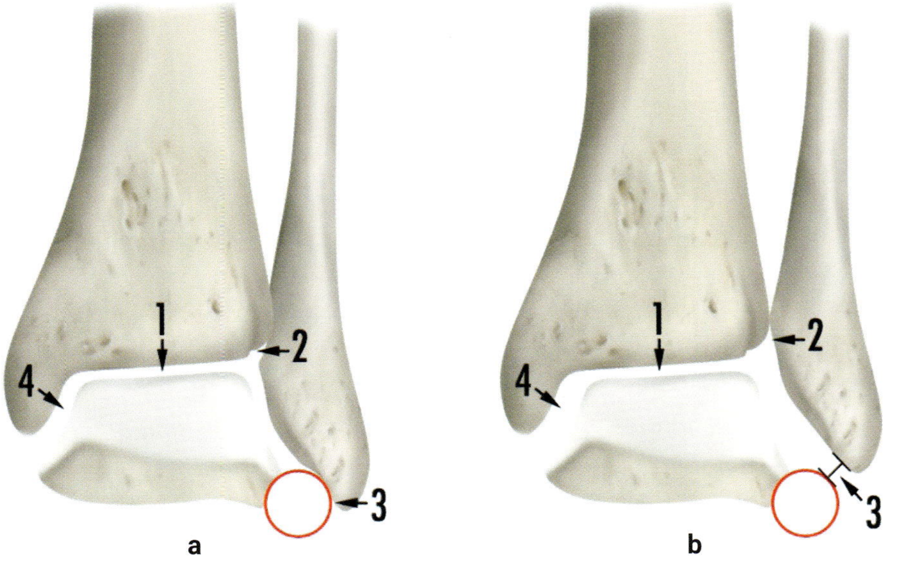

Figure 90 - The circle between the lateral wall of the talus and the apex of the distal fibular malleolus should be in contact with the tibial subchondral bone (as shown on the left). On the right, a malalignment is shown

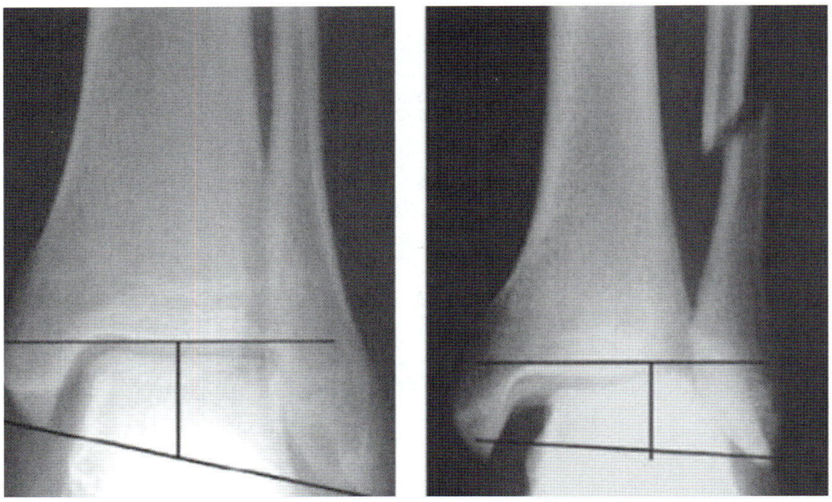

Figure 91 - On the left, a normal talo-crural angle. On the right, decreased talo-crural angle due to fibular shortening

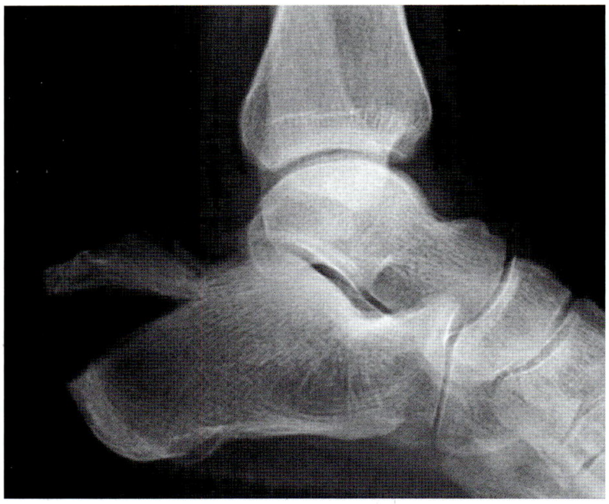

Figure 92 - Avulsion fracture of the posterior tuberosity

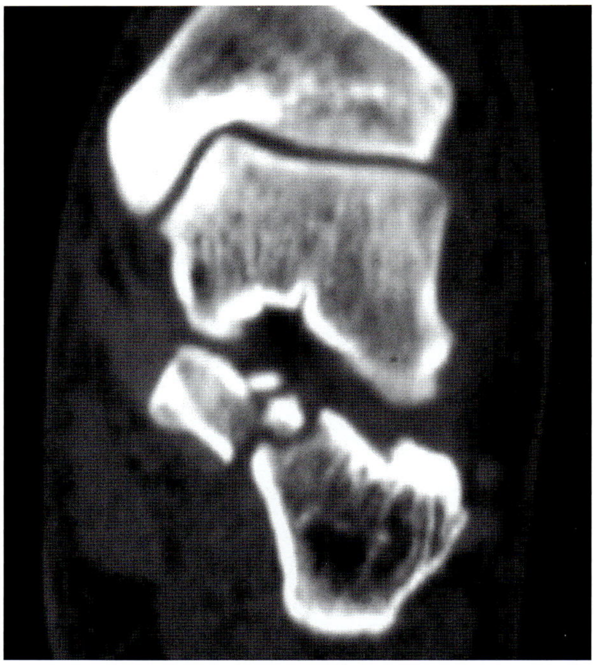

Figure 93 - CT scan showing a sustentaculum tali fracture

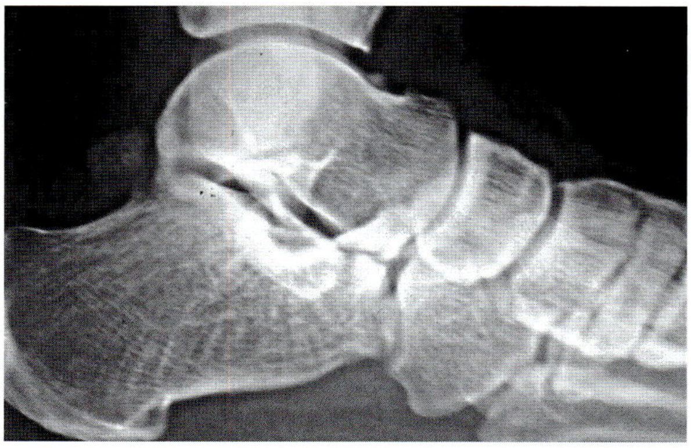

Figure 94 - Lateral X-ray showing a calcaneal anterior process fracture

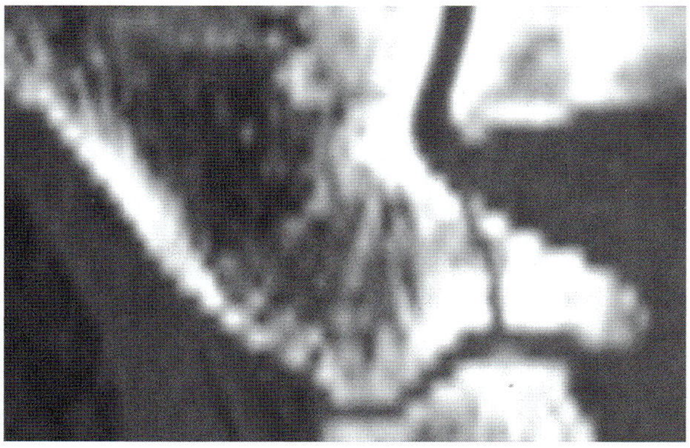

Figure 95 - CT scan showing a calcaneal anterior process fracture

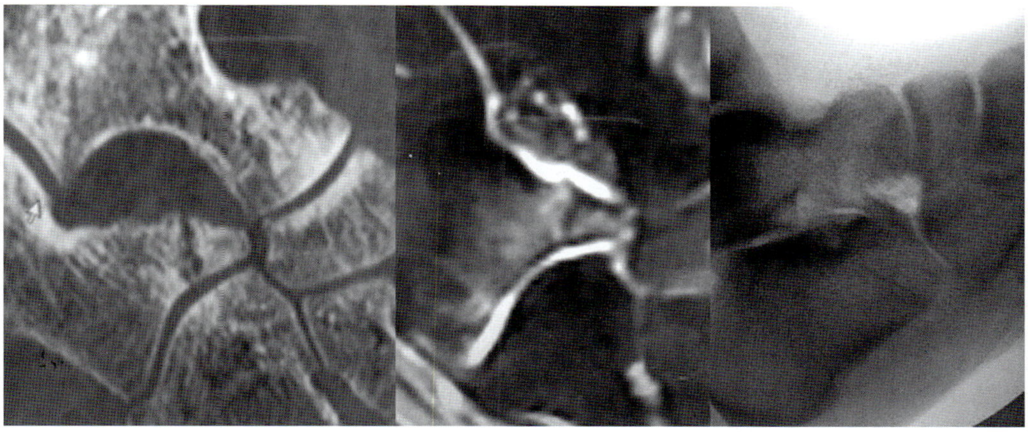

Figure 96 - On the left, lateral X-ray showing a calcaneal anterior process fracture; the fragment is detected on the MRI (in the middle). On the right, lateral X-ray after the fragment removal

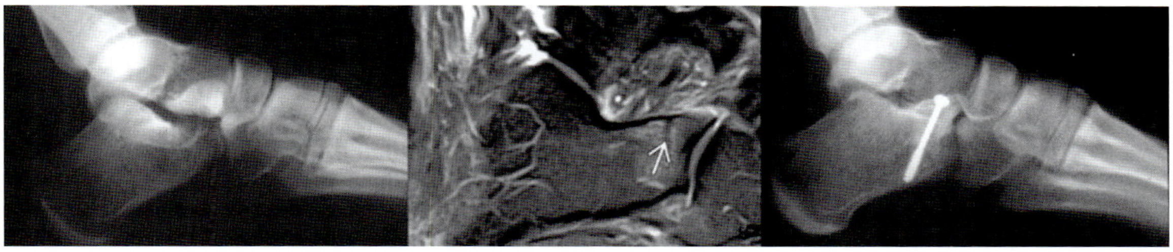

Figure 97 - On the left, lateral X-ray showing a calcaneal anterior process fracture; the fragment is detected on the MRI (in the middle). On the right lateral X-ray after the fragment reduction and fixation using a screw

It is advisable to visualize the medial aspect in order to remove possible bone fragments or ligament flaps interposition. After having performed the malleolar synthesis, it is necessary to evaluate if there is a syndesmosis instability using a small spreader.
In case of instability a screw or a TightRope should be inserted [131].
Arthroscopy may be performed in case of isolated medial or anterior malleolar fractures (video 2).

Hindfoot fractures
Most hindfoot fractures in soccer are extra-articular, caused by torsional trauma or by traction forces applied by ligaments or tendons [2, 132]. Calcaneus or talus may be involved. The most common calcaneal fractures are those caused by an avulsion of the posterior tuberosity due to a violent traction of the soleo-gastrocnemius complex (fig. 92). Another extra articular fracture is the one involving the sustentaculum, evident in a coronal CT view (fig. 93). Finally, the fracture of the anterior process, caused by a forced inversion and plantar-flexion of the foot with avulsion by the bifurcated ligament is also frequent (figg. 94, 95) [133, 134]. If the fragment is broken and small, it should be removed (fig. 96); if the fragment is bigger than 5 mm, a synthesis with a small fragment screw is indicated (fig. 97).
The most frequent talar fractures are represented by osteochondral fractures, then by the fractures of posterior and lateral processes [135, 136].
For osteochondral fractures please see the dedicated chapter.
Fractures of the lateral tubercle can be caused by a forced plantar flexion with direct contact between the posterolateral process and the tibial plafonds. Another mechanism is a forced dorsiflexion with avulsion of the posterolateral process by the talofibular ligaments [137].
The medial tubercle fractures, caused by dorsiflexion and pronation movements, are uncommon, with an avulsion occurring on the posterior part of the tibiotalar ligament [138].
Fractures of the lateral process are more common (fig. 98) and represent 24% of talar body fractures. The lateral process plays an important role since it contributes to the stability of the ankle mortise [139].

The main mechanism of fracture is due to a forced dorsiflexion and inversion of the foot.
Treatment choice depends on size and displacement of the fragment.
Non-displaced fractures are treated with a walker boot for six weeks without weight-bearing followed by weight-bearing walker boot for other four weeks. In displaced fractures, a small fragment should be removed. If the fragment is bigger, it should be fixed with screws or pins through open reduction and internal fixation [137] (fig. 99).
Articular calcaneal fractures are uncommon and after X-rays and CT diagnosis are mostly treated by osteosynthesis with screws, as well as fractures of the talar neck and body (figg. 100, 101) [140].

Midfoot and forefoot fractures
Midfoot and forefoot fractures can affect the navicular, the cuboid, the cuneiforms, the metatarsals, the phalanges and the sesamoids bones [141, 142]. Acute fractures of the navicular body are uncommon, while avulsion fractures are frequent and produced by the capsule and the dorsal ligaments traction during a sprain (figg. 102, 103, 104) [143]. Other fractures are represented by the tuberosity avulsion (fig. 105) that can occur during an eversion movement for the posterior tibialis tendon and deltoid ligament traction. Navicular stress fractures will be discussed in the next section.
If the fragment is small and not displaced the treatment is conservative with immobilization for 6 weeks; if the fragment is small and comminuted, but not big enough to be synthesized, it is removed and immobilization for 6 weeks is prescribed [143]. If synthesis can be performed, open reduction and internal fixation is the treatment of choice. A navicular tuberosity fracture, due to its capsular and tendon insertions, is usually undisplaced and its treatment is more often conservative. If a diastase greater than 3 mm is present and the fragment is not too large, the fragment should be removed and the tibialis posterior tendon sutured to the navicular. If the fragment is bigger, a reduction and internal fixation with a compression screw should be performed [143].
Cuboid fractures are generally represented by avulsion and compression fractures (fig. 106) [144].
Avulsion fractures occur in the lateral side of the foot. The treatment is generally represented by an immobilization in a Walker boot for 4/6 weeks. Only articular fractures require open reduction and internal fixation, sometimes associated with bone graft.
Isolated cuneiform fractures are rare and usually occur without displacement [145].
In case of displacement, a dislocation of the midtarsal joint has to be suspected (fig. 107). Surgical treatment is necessary only in displaced fractures, otherwise a Walker boot is prescribed for 4-6 weeks. Metatarsal fractures are common and usually caused by a direct trauma during a body contact or after a sprain [146].
Thanks to the several ligaments inserted on the metatarsals and to the insertions of the interosseous and lombricalis muscles the displacement is usually limited with the exception of fractures at the neck level in which a plantar shift occurs due to the displacing action of the flexor tendons (fig. 108) [146]. Fractures of the metatarsal base are often associated to Lisfranc involvement so it must always be carefully evaluated. Isolated fractures of the second, third and fourth metatarsals are usually treated conservatively with a talus shoe.
Displaced fractures of the base of the first metatarsal must be treated with a reduction and synthesis. Metatarsal shaft fractures, if not associated with displacement, are treated with a Walker boot [146]. On the other hand, displaced fractures must be reduced in a closed or open manner and stabilized with a Kirschner wire or more rarely with screws or plates [146]. It is important to look for an anatomical reduction to avoid metatarsalgia, impingement and bony prominences which may cause conflict with the shoe.

VIDEO 2

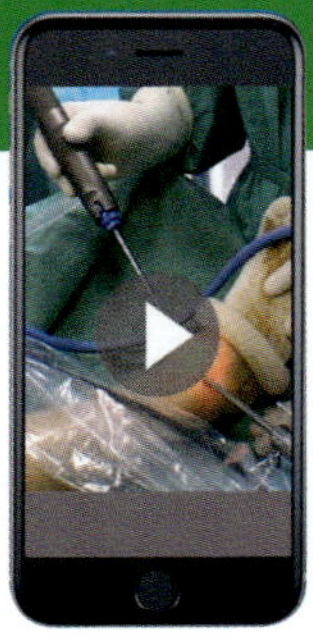

Arthroscopic assisted reduction and fixation

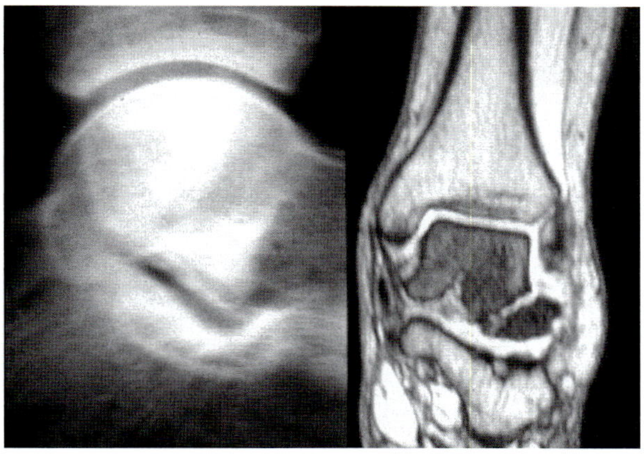

Figure 98 - On the left, lateral X-ray showing a talar lateral process fracture; the fragment is better detected on the MRI (on the right)

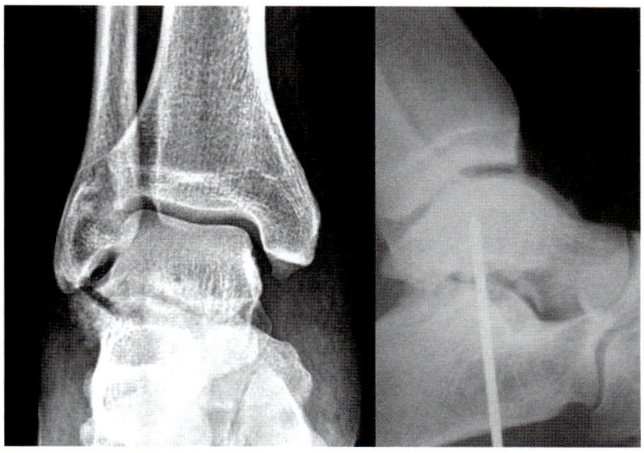

Figure 99 - Displaced lateral process fracture: the fragment is reduced and fixed with a Kirschner wire

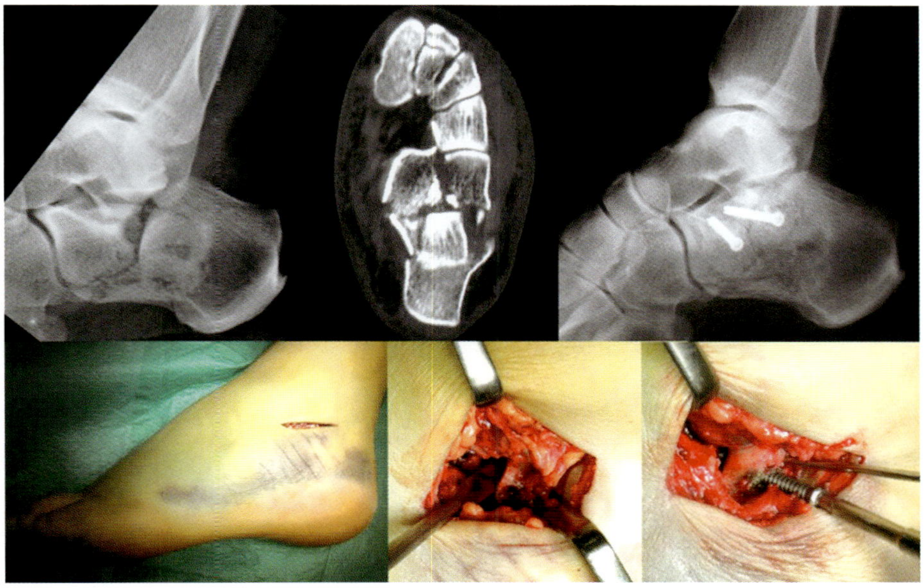

Figure 100 - Above, on the left, lateral X-ray showing complex articular calcaneal fracture; the fracture is better detected on the CT scan (in the middle). The fracture is reduced and fixed with screws (on the right). Below, surgical procedure: on the left, the incision, in the middle the subtalar and fracture reduction, on the right screws insertion

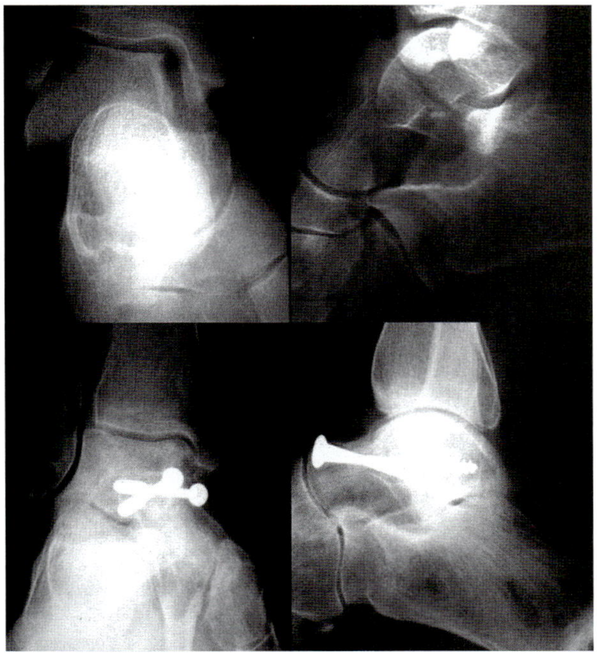

Figure 101 - Above, lateral and anterior X-rays showing a body talar fracture. The fracture is reduced and fixed with screws

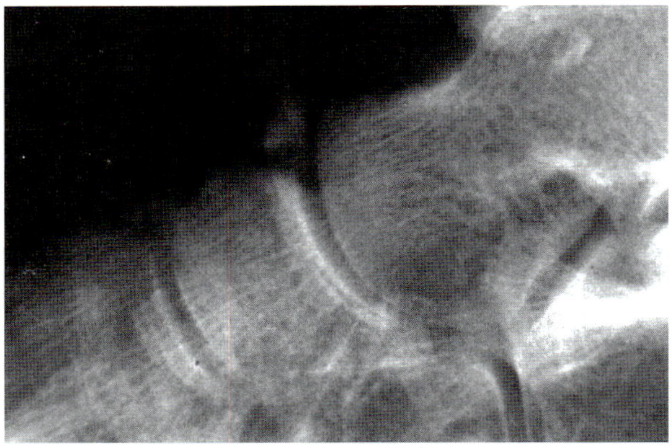

Figure 102 - Lateral X-rays showing a small dorsal navicular avulsion fracture produced by the capsule traction during a sprain

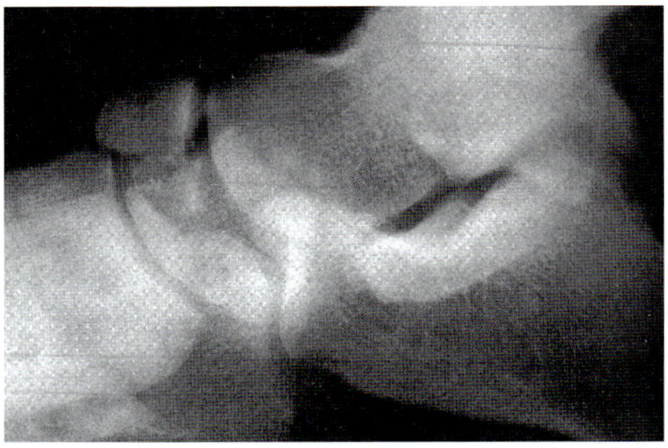

Figure 103 - Lateral X-rays showing a dorsal navicular avulsion fracture

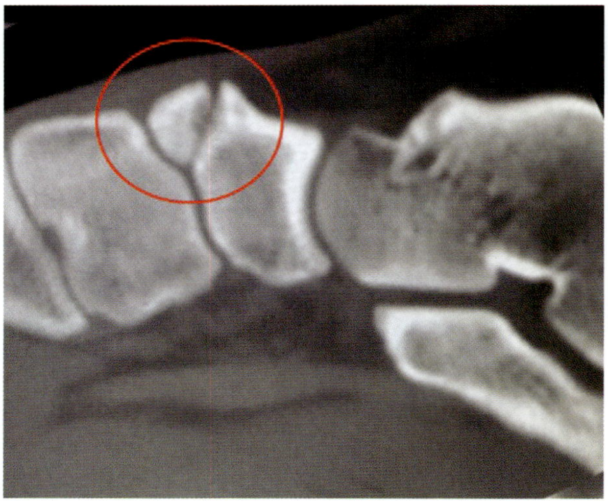

Figure 104 - CT scan showing a dorsal navicular avulsion fracture

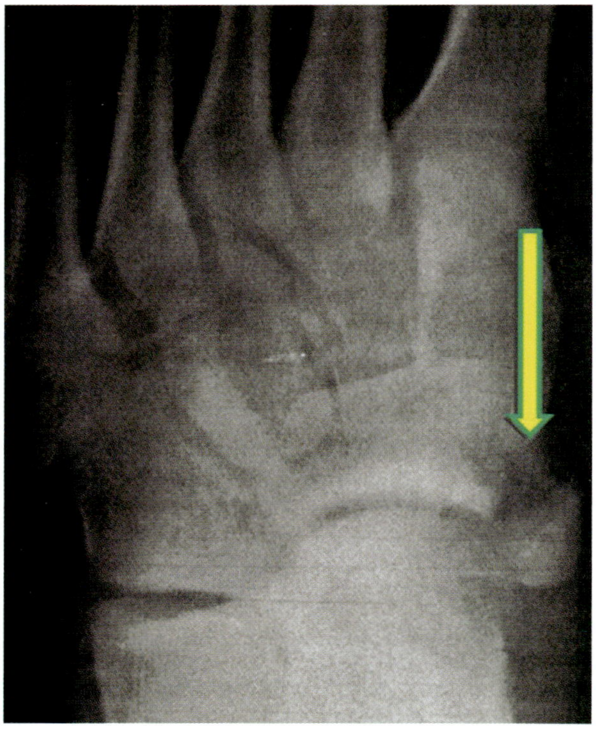

Figure 105 - Dorso-plantar X-ray showing a navicular tuberosity avulsion fracture (indicated by the arrow)

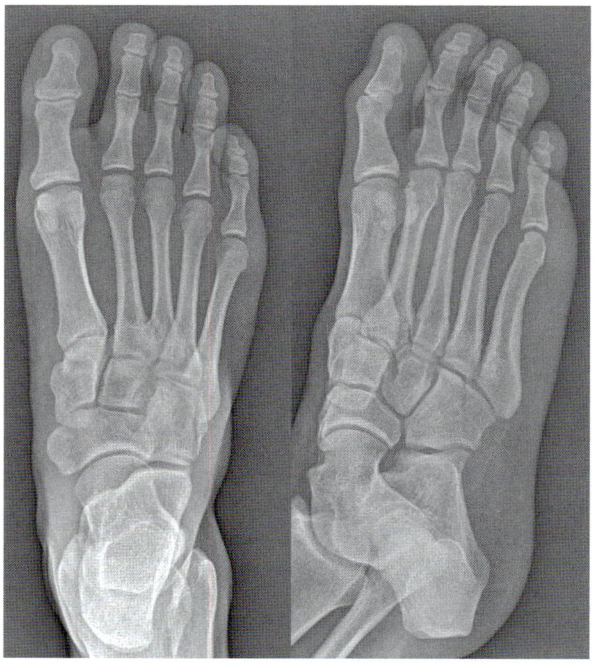

Figure 106 - Dorso-plantar and oblique X-rays showing a cuboid fracture

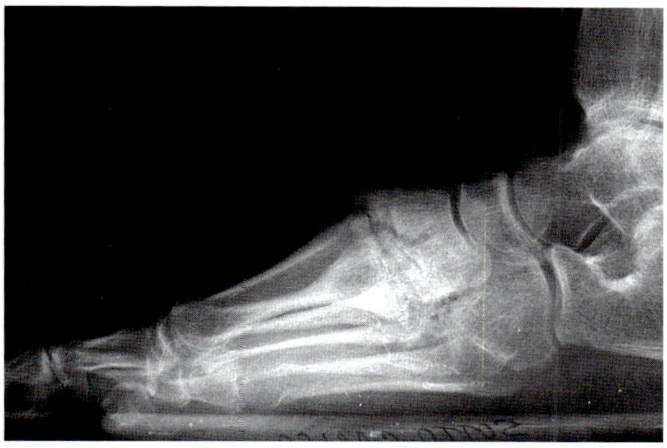

Figure 107 - Lateral X-rays showing a dorsal cuneiform avulsion fracture

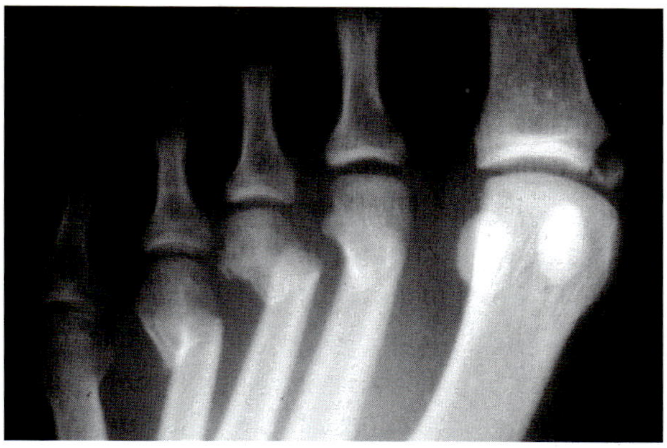

Figure 108 - Dorso-plantar X-ray showing displaced third and fourth metatarsal fractures associated with a hallux proximal phalanx base fracture. The displacement occurs due to the flexor tendons action

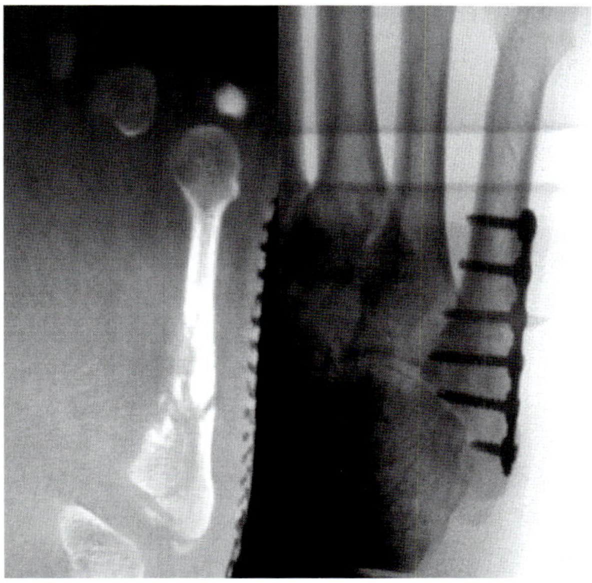

Figure 109 - On the left, TC scan showing a displaced, multi-fragments, fifth metatarsal fracture. The fracture was treated with an open reduction and internal fixation with plates and screws (X-ray in the middle)

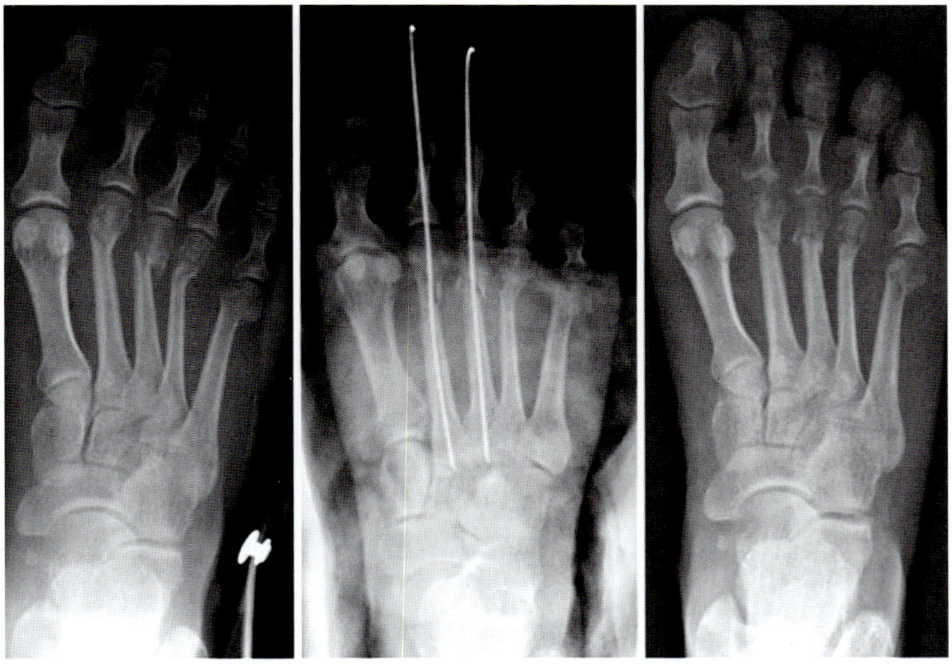

Figure 110 - On the left, dorso-plantar X-ray showing displaced second and third metatarsal neck fractures; in the middle, dorso-plantar X-ray after closed reduction and stabilization with Kischner wires; on the right, dorso-plantar X-ray after 4 months

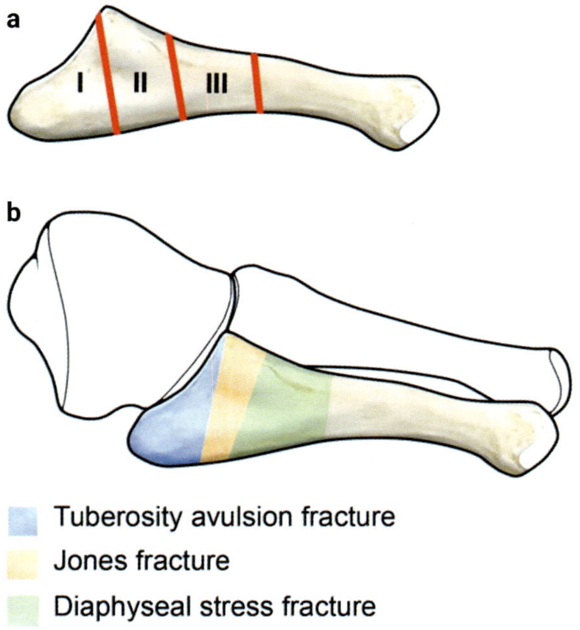

Figure 111 - Different fractures occurring at the fifth metatarsal base

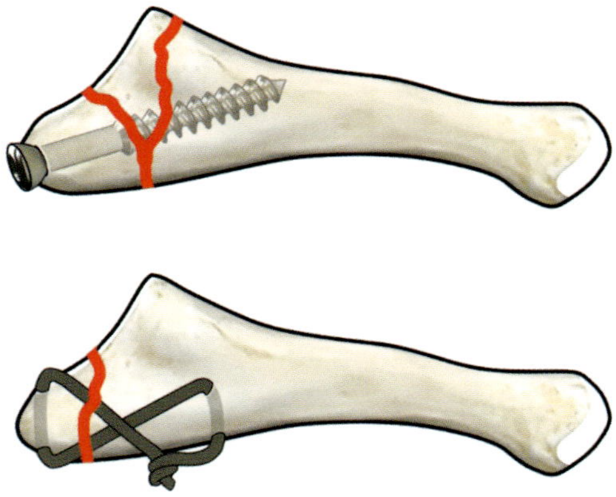

Figure 112 - Surgical option in the treatment of fifth metatarsal base fractures. Above: screw fixation. Below: tension band wiring technique

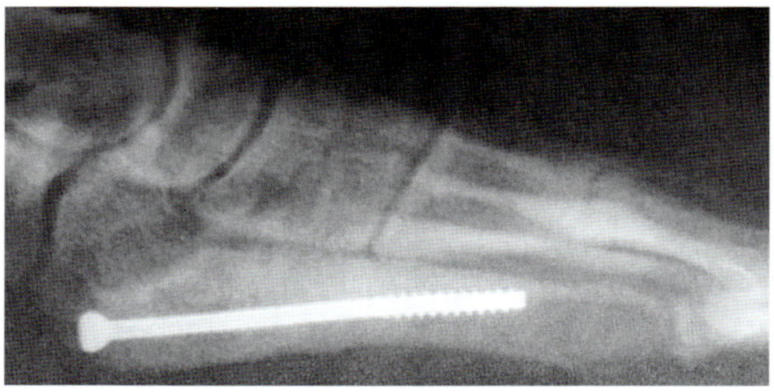

Figure 113 - Lateral X-ray showing a Jones fracture treated with osteosynthesis by means of a large diameter intramedullary screw

Diaphyseal fractures of the fifth metatarsal are usually treated nonoperatively. When displaced, with avulsion and several fragments, it is better treated with an open reduction and internal fixation with plates and screws (fig. 109). Postoperative protocol requires a walker boot without weight-bearing for 6 weeks and active and passive mobilization since the first day [147].

Metatarsal neck fractures are rarely isolated: if a satisfactory result is not obtained after a closed reduction attempt, it is better to perform an open reduction (fig. 110) [146].

Metatarsal head fractures are mostly caused by direct trauma and shear forces and are usually intra-articular fractures. They must be reduced by pulling on the corresponding finger and fixed with a percutaneous Kirschner wire. An open reduction is rarely necessary [146].

Fractures of the fifth metatarsal base are classified into tuberosity fractures, Jones fractures, and diaphyseal stress fractures (see next paragraph) (fig. 111) [147]. If no displacement occurred, tuberosity fracture treatment is conservative with a Walker boot without weight-bearing for 4 to 6 weeks. If the fracture fragment exceeds 30% of the articular surface and an articular step greater than 2 mm is present, it is better to perform an internal fixation [147].

Fractures occuring between the diaphysis and the metaphysis (Jones fracture), given the high risk of healing failure, are more often treated with osteosynthesis by means of a large diameter intramedullary screw or a tension band wiring (figg, 112, 113) [147].

Phalanx fractures are the most common forefoot fractures [142]. Fractures of first phalanx of the first toe are the most common and are generally associated with dislocation, while fractures of the distal phalanx are more often comminuted.

Lesser toe fractures occur more frequently in the first phalanx and are associated with a posterior displacement. They are caused by a trauma that most often occurs in beach soccer or secondarily to a step from the opponent. Usually the treatment of these fractures is conservative with manual reduction and stabilization by adhesive taping to the adjacent finger [148, 149]. Surgical treatment is rarely indicated and limited to exostectomies in case of dorsal prominences.

Sesamoid fractures occur during a relapse or a jump due to the compression of a sesamoid (especially the medial one) that crushes against the metatarsal head. Another cause is represented by a forced dorsiflexion of the first toe at the metatarsophalangeal level [150, 151].

The differential diagnosis is important and is carried out through an X-rays evaluation to distinguish between fracture, osteochondritis dissecans and bipartite sesamoid. When conservative treatment does not relieve pain after six weeks, surgical treatment may be needed with excision of the smaller fragment and a glenoid rim repair [150, 151].

Stress fractures

Stress fractures are common clinical features and are represented by a group of lesions ranging from subcortical edema to complete cortical interruption. They are the consequence of repeated forces that exceed the reparative capacities of the bone. Usually, these sub-maximal forces do not cause a fracture, but if the loads are not adequately dispersed and the recovery times are not respected, the rate of resorption of the osteoclasts exceeds bone formation and the bone weakens until the fracture by stress [153].

The lower third of the leg and the foot represent the most affected sites in elite soccer players and the incidence is 0.004 lesions over 1,000 hours of activity and with a clear prevalence at the level of the 5th metatarsal (78%).

Metatarsal fractures are the most frequent, while those at the navicular, calcaneus, cuboid, and cuneiform levels have a lower incidence [154]. These fractures are mostly correlated with biomechanical factors such as a difference in limb length, an incorrect way of running, a malalignment of the limb and foot abnormalities or deformities that lead to alterations of the load during weight-bearing (fig. 114). Women who have problems with oligomenorrhea or amenorrhea have shown a higher percentage of fractures than women with normal menstrual period [155].

The two metatarsal fractures that create more diagnostic and treatment problems are the fractures of the fifth metatarsal (Jones fracture), due to frequent delayed union or nonunion, and the fractures of the base of the second metatarsal [2, 155]. Both these fractures are often mistakenly diagnosed as sprains. Even tarsal fractures, especially those involving the navicular, often show diagnostic delays and inadequate treatments due to the lack of confirmation on initial radiographs [156].

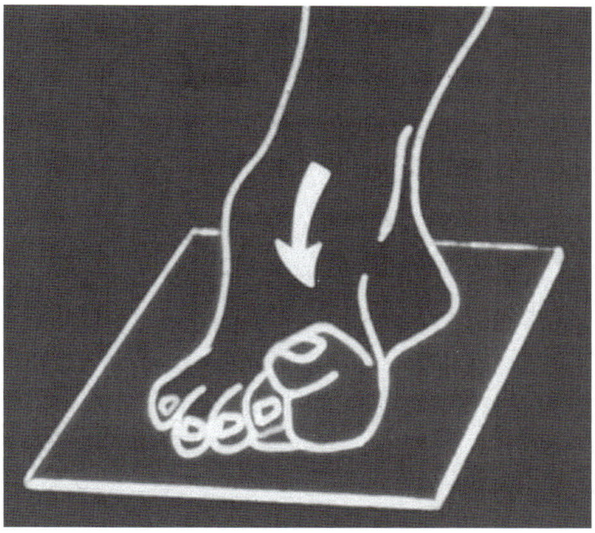

Figure 114 - Cavus foot represents a deformity that lead to gait alterations; due to the fixed deformity at the level of the first ray, which appears plantarflexed, a so called tripod effect is produced, characterized by an internal rotation of the foot, with a heel varus deviation

Another stress fracture typical of the soccer player is the fracture of the hallux proximal phalanx base, favored by a forced and repeated dorsiflexion of the metatarsal phalangeal [157], more frequent in case of hallux valgus which produces an excessive traction of the extensor hallucis longus and abductor hallucis (fig. 115).

Pain is one of the first symptoms with an insidious onset [81]. The pain appears during training or just after the activity, and it is exacerbated by impacts or stresses during prono-supination of the foot. Edema and local tenderness are common features, exacerbated by pressure and by the one-legged hop test; usually, there is no hematoma formation.

A stress fracture diagnosis must be confirmed by instrumental examinations such as X-rays in standard views and, if necessary, with oblique views. It is important to look for the presence of periosteal bone alterations, cortical sclerosis, or radiolucent lines. These are signs that usually appear two weeks after the onset of symptoms when

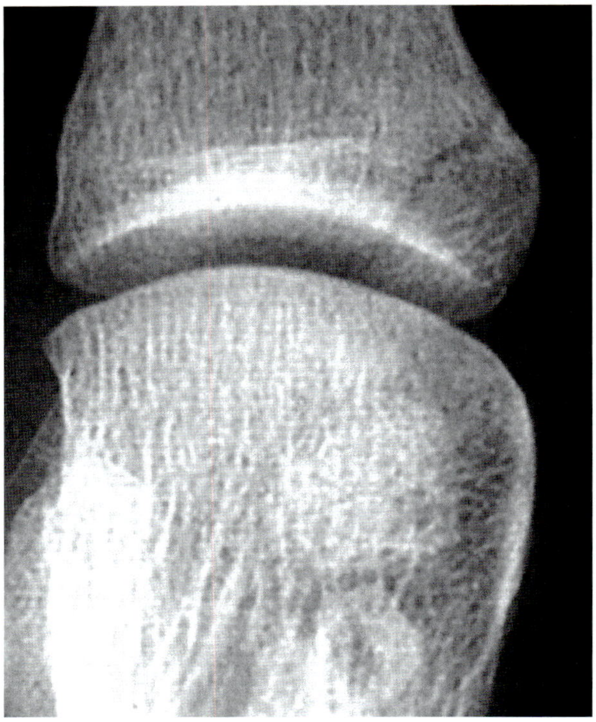

Figure 115 - X-rays showing a fracture of the hallux proximal phalanx base

the signs of osteoclastic activity appear [155, 156]. Other diagnostic exams are represented by MRI, TC, and bone scan. MRI is sensitive and specific for localization but does not allow to easily highlight the extent of the fracture gap. The CT allows to fully highlight the fracture line and the extension of the fracture as well as to be able to assess the need for bone grafting [155].

The possible causes of stress fractures are a decrease in shock-absorbing capacity due to muscle fatigue or repeated trauma to the bone that overcomes the elastic capacities of the bone with consequent microfractures. Certain factors can increase the risk of stress fractures such as anatomical deformities, cavus foot, flat foot, metatarsus adductus, long metatarsus, hormonal imbalances such as amenorrhea or hyperthyroidism. Finally, training errors and improper athletic technique can lead to stress fractures [155].

Two types of stress fractures are described: diaphyseal fractures, characterized by an interruption of the cortex that then gives rise to a dense callus in metatarsals, and subchondral fractures that appear as lines perpendicular to the directions of stress: these are more common in the calcaneus, in the navicular, and the first metatarsal [155].

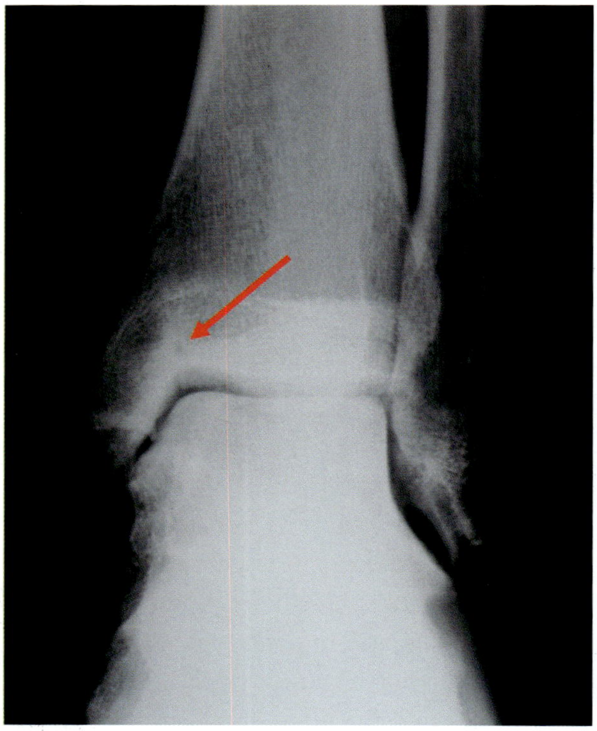

Figure 116 - Anterior X-rays showing a medial malleolar stress fracture (red harrow)

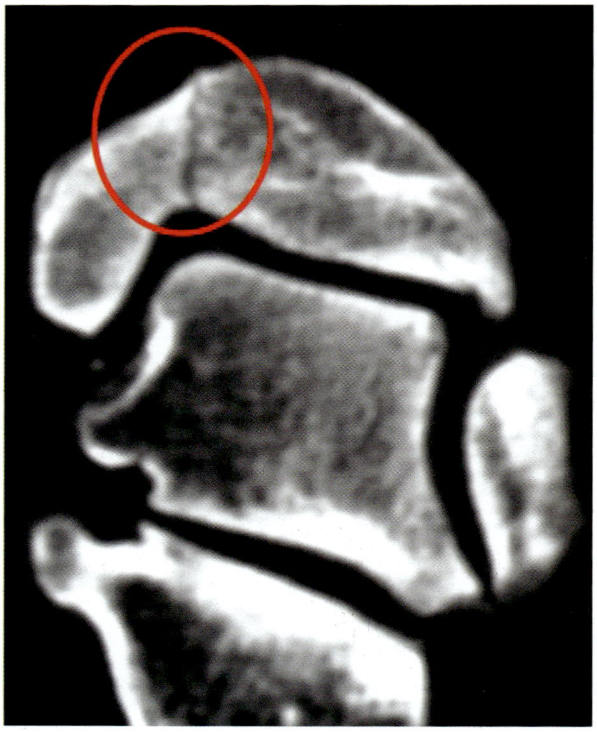

Figure 117 - CT scan showing a medial malleolar stress fracture

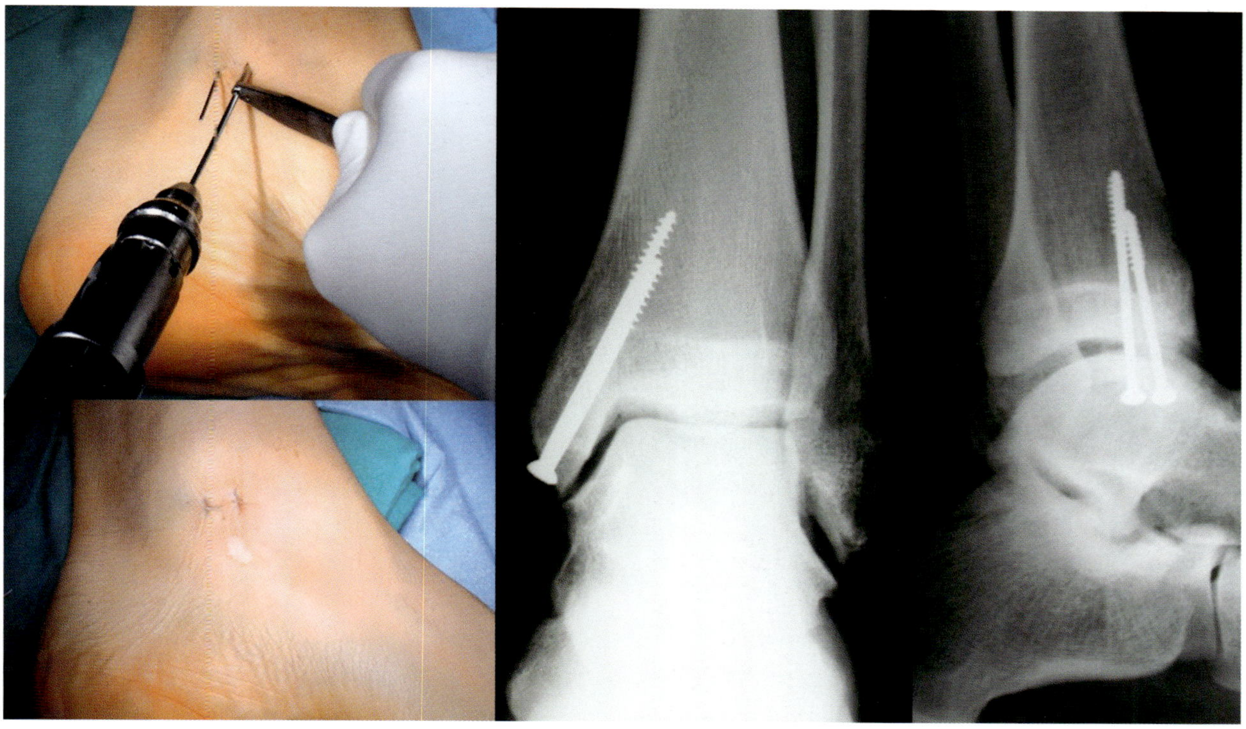

Figure 118 - A medial malleolar stress fracture surgically treated with percutaneous fixation with screws, placed parallel to the medial joint side

Tibial diaphyseal stress fractures

The most frequent localizations are at the level of the posterolateral cortex for the repeated tractions of the soleo-gastrocnemius complex which would cause subperiosteal bleeding, then responsible for the cortical fracture [158]. The first symptom is the pain that appears mainly towards the end of the sports activity. This progressively increases even after limited activity and tends to last a long time. Tenderness is present at the midshaft tibial region associated with swelling, redness, and heat. Pressure on the medial edge of the tibia is particularly painful. In the early stages, a non-high-impact activity such as cycling or swimming is mandatory, until symptoms disappear and clinical negativity is reached. A gradual recovery follows with custom-molded orthotics and insoles to compensate for load defects on the foot. Healing usually takes about 4 months [158].

A less frequent site is along the anterior cortex called block-line, a possible site for a pseudo-arthrosis.

Given the high risk of non-union, surgical treatment is often necessary. The most used techniques are excision and bone grafting, drilling of the defect, intramedullary reaming and fixation with associated electromagnetic therapy. Cancellous bone grafting or the use of demineralized bone and concentrated mesenchymal cells can be used for the treatment of non-union in order to promote bone healing [158, 159].

Medial malleolar stress fractures

These fractures account for 9% of all ankle and foot stress fractures. Usually, the fracture has a vertical course at the junction between the tibial plafond and the medial malleolus [156, 160].

They are fractures caused by repeated microtraumas in dorsiflexion and rotation or in case of excessive pronation associated with an increased internal rotation of the tibia.

Differential diagnosis can be difficult, especially with sequelae of deltoid ligament sprains, talar dome osteochondral lesions, tibialis posterior lesions, anteromedial bone impingement [160].

When fracture lines are not clear on X-rays (fig. 116), treatment is based on immobilization with a Walker boot and weight-bearing as tolerated.

If there is evidence of fracture detected by MRI, and if necessary by CT (fig. 117), surgical treatment with percutaneous synthesis with screws is required (fig. 118) [159, 160].

If displacement or pseudoarthrosis are present, the treatment consists of an open reduction and internal fixation with plate and bone graft [159, 160].

Fibular stress fractures

These fractures are localized in the distal fibula 3 to 7 cm from the apex of the malleolus [161, 162]. Radiographically they appear at 3-4 weeks from the onset of symptoms. They are usually transverse and present a minor displacement. Rarely more tests are needed. Fractures are favored by an eversion of the hindfoot that causes a repeated concentration of stress on the fibula. According to Davis [163], repeated trauma to plantar flexors that are inserted on the fibula would lead to the fracture.

Usually, the treatment is conservative with embers to be worn for 4 weeks. The recovery of the activity takes place on average after 6-8 weeks [161].

Rarely, a synthesis with screws and plaque is necessary. It is important to compensate for possible defects in pronation with orthotics or a calcaneal osteotomy [158].

Sesamoid stress fractures

Of the two sesamoids the medial, thicker, longer, and distal is more frequently involved. The medial sesamoid has a terminal vascularization and presents a congenital partition in about 20% of cases. The sesamoids have the function of distributing the load forces and, lowering the metatarsal head, to favor the pushing force of the big toe [164].

The pain is located in the plantar site at the level of the MTP joint and is aggravated during weight-bearing. Marked tenderness and signs of inflammation may be present. Over time, movement can become limited. Compression maneuvers on the sesamoid and dorsiflexion of the big toe increase pain [152].

The radiographic analysis includes AP and lateral views. Sometimes other tangential and oblique axial projections are necessary to evaluate signs of arthrosis and fracture lines. It is difficult to recognize a bipartite sesamoid from a fracture. The fracture has irregular edges at the level of the line while in the bipartite sesamoid they are smooth. Furthermore, the bipartite sesamoid is often bilateral [152]. A MRI is useful to differentiate alterations of the surrounding soft parts, of the flexor tendon and the glenoid rim, and to evaluate vascular bone disorders [164]. CT is also useful for better highlighting the fracture and to evaluate metatarsal-sesamoid arthrosis or fracture healing [164].

The conservative treatment can be decisive and consists of the discharge of the sesamoid through taping that limits movement and orthotics relieving pressure on the sesamoid [152].

If the pain remains after 3-4 months, if a functional limitation is associated or if signs of necrosis are present a surgical approach is necessary. It may consist of repair with bone graft in case of diastasis not exceeding 2 mm and no gross motion of the two fragments or partial sesamoidectomy in case of avascular necrosis, disproportionately sizes fragments or condyle lesion. Bone grafting repair is an open surgery with a medial incision. Partial resection can be performed with open or arthroscopic surgery [152].

It is better to avoid sesamoidectomy due to the consequent reduction of the toe pushing phase and the tendency to valgus deformity. If necessary, as in the case of severe comminution or arthrosis, it is useful to associate the sesamoidectomy with abductor hallucis tendon transfer into the plantar defect [150, 152, 158, 165].

Metatarsal stress fractures

They represent 14-20% of stress fractures in the lower limb [2, 166, 167]. The most frequently affected metatarsals are the second in 52% of cases and the third in 35% of cases. The first is affected in 8% of cases, the fourth and fifth in 5% [2, 166, 167]. Fractures of the central metatarsals are typically diaphyseal, those of the first metatarsal are metaphyseal with medial localization, those of the fifth metatarsal are metadiaphyseal with lateral localization [167]. The mechanical stress due to an altered relationship between the lengths of the first and second metatarsal bone may favor the fracture of the second. Flat foot can cause an increased stress on the metatarsals as it increases the tension of the plantar fascia. Muscle fatigue also reduces stress resistance by about four times. Clinically there is a dorsal swelling with diaphyseal tenderness for the central metatarsals and

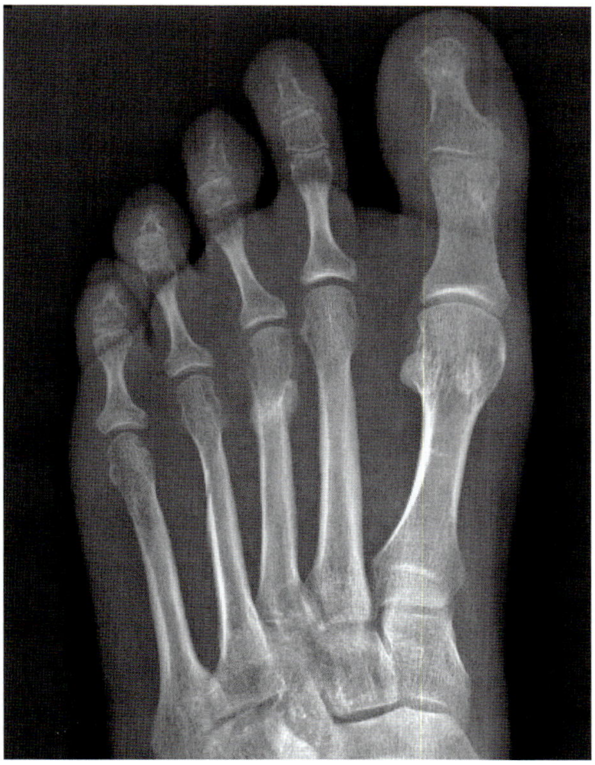

Figure 119 - Dorso-plantar X-rays show the healing process at the third metatarsal neck level

more proximal for the first and fifth metatarsal. The second metatarsal is painful mainly in the pushing phase [166, 167].
Treatment consists of restricting activities by immobilization depending on symptoms resolution. X-rays allow to establish the healing process (fig. 119) [168].
It is necessary to prevent recurrences with adequate training techniques, proper footwear, and orthotics that compensate for foot defomities such as cavus foot, flat foot, or metatarsus adductus.
In women, to avoid relapses, it is important to resolve endocrine changes such as amenorrhea or alteration of estrogen levels. Physical therapy such as magnetotherapy can be useful. The use of calcifying drugs is still not well defined.
Less frequently the fracture of the second metatarsal may occur at the level of the proximal part where the anatomical rigidity and the muscular actions of the long peroneal and the posterior tibial are particularly accentuated [169].
With conservative treatment, the average recovery time is 6-8 weeks. When the pain persists and there are no signs of consolidation, surgery with screws, plates, and bone grafting is required [166, 167].

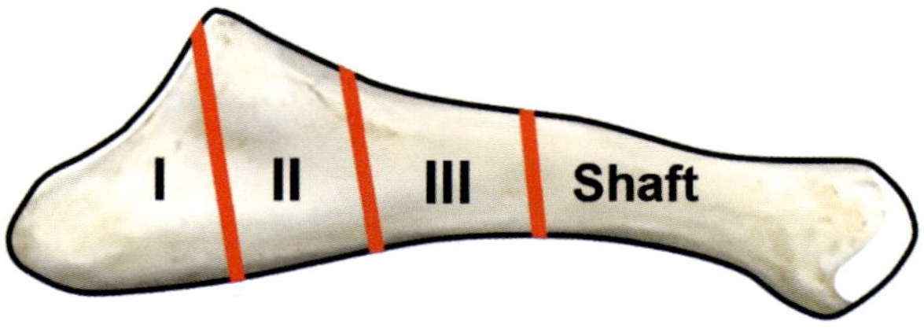

Figure 120 - 3 different fracture zones at the fifth metatarsal base level

Fifth metatarsal stress fractures
They are called Jones fractures and occur at the metaphyseal junction [170]. These fractures have a high percentage of delayed union, non-union (from 15% to 30%) and recurrence, are more frequent in men than women under the age of 30 and more frequent in women over 30 years [2, 170, 171].
There are several classifications among which the most used are the Torg one [172] based on marrow sclerosis and the one which distinguishes 3 different fracture zones (fig. 120).
Localization is in 93% of cases at the level of zone 1, 4% in zone 2 and 3% in zone 3. They are favored by a deformity as pes planus, cavus-varus, metatarsus adductus with plantarflexion of the first ray, or by a weakness of the peroneus, all factors that determine a lateral overload. Matsuda [173] reports a greater incidence in the everted hindfoot and inverted forefoot. Saita reported that a limitation of hip rotation seems to increase the risk of fracture [174]. According to Fuitaka [175] a weak toe grip strength may lead to an increased lateral load and therefore stress fracture. Other possible risk factors may be training defects or inadequate footwear.
An instrumental evaluation with gait analysis can highlight functional overload even in the absence of other clinical signs. Radiographs in AP, lateral and oblique planes represent the first diagnostic investigation. In addition to the fracture line, intramedullary sclerosis and a periosteal reaction can be observed in chronic forms. A CT scan is useful to evaluate the extension of the fracture gap and the degree of consolidation. MRI can confirm the fracture in case of normal X-ray with suspicion of injury [2, 170, 171].
Even if a conservative treatment in zones 2 and 3 with bracing for two months without load and one in charge leads to recovery up to 75% of cases

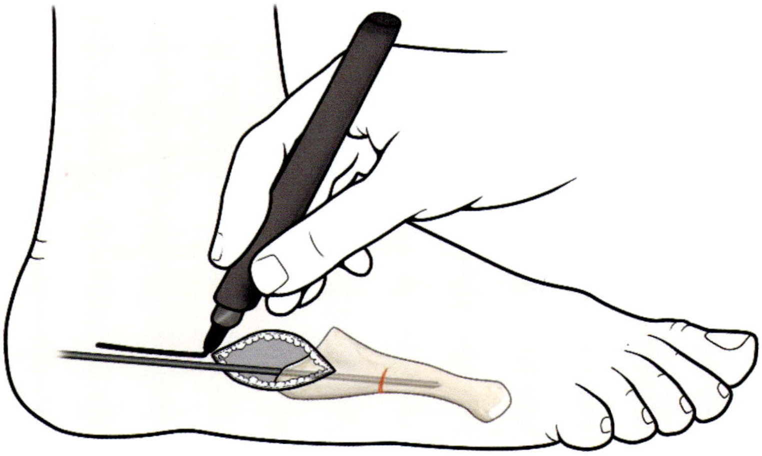

Figure 121 - An incision of 5 mm is made proximally to the tuberosity prominence; then a 1.6 mm guide wire is inserted under fluoroscopic control from the tuberosity of the base of the metatarsal

within 5 months, it must be considered that the time needed is too long. Furthermore, there is a high risk of refracture (33%) and in 50% of cases, the fracture does not heal [2, 172, 176].

For this reason, in the elite athlete, the treatment should be surgical [170]. Surgery will be percutaneous or with mini-incision at the level of the fracture if the bone reduction or grafting is required [177]. An incision of 5 mm is made proximally to the prominence of the tuberosity, a 1.6 mm guide wire is inserted under fluoroscopic control from the tuberosity of the base of the metatarsal in a supero-medial direction up inside the medullary canal to allow proceeding with the screw distally without contrast with the medial cortex due to the curvature of the metatarsal.

Marking the direction of the wire on the skin, as advised by Delee [178], helps with the introduction of drill reducing the risk of breaking the wire (fig. 121). The wire is removed and a 4.5 mm screw partially threated is introduced if the channel is narrow, and a 6.5mm screw if the channel is wide. The threaded part must exceed the fracture gap by 1.5 cm. It is important to check the final position of the screw with the fluoroscope and make sure there is no diastasis between the ends of the fracture (fig. 122).

In case of important intramedullary sclerosis, diastasis at the level of the fracture, bone resorption or in case of refracture a lateral incision of 1.5/2 cm is made at the level of the fracture and after protecting the sural nerve the fracture is freshened, perforations performed and a 6.5 mm wide and 50 to 65 mm long screw is applied: autologous cancellous bone graft taken from the proximal tibia is applied. Alternatively, DBM and bone marrow concentrate can be used.

The post-operative treatment involves the use of a brace for 6 weeks with load granted after 2 weeks. In case of revisions, the load is granted after 4 weeks. The execution of magnetotherapy at home for 4 hours a day for 4-6 weeks is useful. After a 12-week CT assessment, if consolidation is highlighted, a resumption of activity can be scheduled with the use of custom-made orthotics that compensate for any foot posture defects. If not symptomatic it is better not to remove the screw in order not to increase the possibility of refracture after removal [2, 170, 171].

The choice between conservative and surgical treatment remains debated. Eixshand and Van Dijk [179] on 13754 fractures reported that despite a surgical treatment the recovery was similar (80 days vs 74 days).

Navicular stress fractures

The incidence of these fractures varies from 14% to 30% of all stress fractures of the foot. Due to the scarcity of symptoms and the difficulty in highlighting the fracture with a standard radiographic examination, the diagnosis is often delayed, so it is necessary to suspect and search for this type of fracture when there is a persistent pain that is aggravated by activity [180, 181].

The navicular mainly articulates with the talus and anteriorly with the three cuneiforms; it suffers from high compressive forces especially in the pushing phase and in the landing phase after a jump.

The navicular has a vascularization that derives

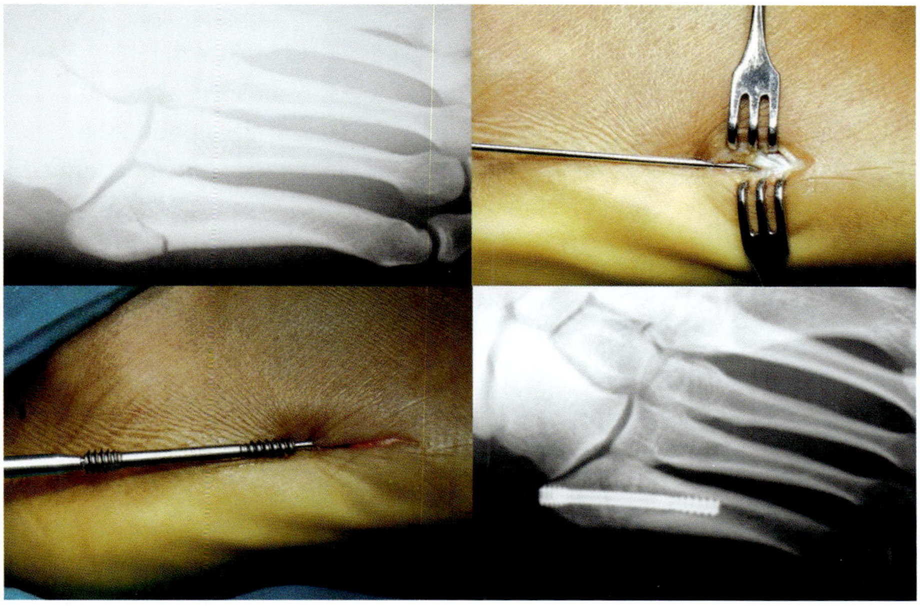

Figure122 - Fifth metatarsal base fracture treated by percutaneous screw fixation

from small branches of the posterior tibial artery and the dorsal artery of the foot [182]. Blood supply is relatively higher in the medial and lateral areas, while it is less in the central part where stress fractures occur.

Anatomical factors such as a longer first metatarsal, a metatarsus adductus, a pronated foot, a cavus foot, and limited dorsiflexion favor an increase in stress on the navicular. Other factors that can affect are a rapid increase in the intensity and duration of sports activity [156, 180].

The onset of symptoms is often insidious, referred more like a discomfort at the end of the training. Then the symptoms tend to increase over time. Frequently, the diagnosis is misleading towards midtarsal sprain, tendinitis, and plantar fasciitis [156]. Usually, tenderness and pain are present in the dorsal area over the navicular which increases with percussion and during jumps on the affected foot. This scarcity of symptoms makes the navicular stress fractures difficult to diagnose if not suspected and researched with instrumental examinations. In standard radiographs, it was found [183] that only 24% of incomplete fractures and 81% of complete fractures are diagnosed due to the difficulty in obtaining precise anteroposterior projections and to the characteristic obliquity of the fracture line (usually from dorsal to plantar and from proximal to distal). The CT exam allows us to highlight the fracture in its location, extension, direction, and displacement (fig. 123).

Usually, the fracture is localized in the central third and slightly shifted laterally. Through CT three types of fractures are identified by Saxena [184]: type I, dorsal cortical head, type II with the propagation of the line inside the navicular, type III also involving the second cortex.

MRI makes it possible to make an early diagnosis for its high sensitivity with the possibility of identifying the bone edema (fig. 124).

Conservative treatment with a plaster cast for 6-8 weeks may be indicated in type I fractures [87]. In type II and III fractures, considering the long recovery times (up to 6-8 months) it is better to perform an early surgical treatment which in 83% of cases has shown recovery times of 3.8 months. [185, 186]. The surgery is often performed percutaneously: under fluoroscopic control, 1 or 2 parallel guide wires are introduced into the navicular with dorso-lateral towards plantar-medial direction and is synthesized with two partially threaded cannulated screws perpendicular to the fracture line. The particular direction and the introduction technique of the screws are due to the oblique fracture line and also because the lateral fragment is smaller and therefore it is preferable to insert the threaded part in the larger medial fragment (figg. 125, 126). In fractures with sclerotic edges, dorsal fragments, or displacement it is best to perform a freshening of the fracture bed and use cancellous bone grafts [185, 187].

Open surgery is performed through a mini-incision

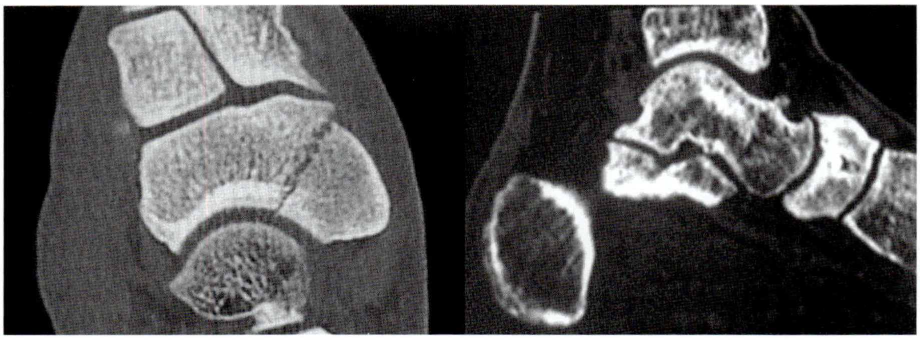

Figure 123 - CT scan allows better highlighting the fracture location

approximately 2-3 cm above the navicular. It passes between the extensors laterally and the vascular bundle medially. Present fragments are removed and after having freshened the fracture spongious graft is applied and then synthesized with 2 cannulated screws [187].

Post-operative treatment in patients with incomplete fractures involves a walker boot for 6 weeks. In the case of complete fractures, a plaster cast will be applied for 6 weeks without weightbearing. [184, 187].

The increase in activity will be based on clinical evaluation and the absence of pain. However, the resumption of activity, which usually occurs after 12-16 weeks, must be endorsed by a CT demonstrating dorsal cortical bridging.

The main complications are represented by delayed unions, pseudoarthrosis, and talonavicular arthritis (fig. 127).

Any deformity of the foot such as the cavus foot or flat foot must be compensated with orthotics

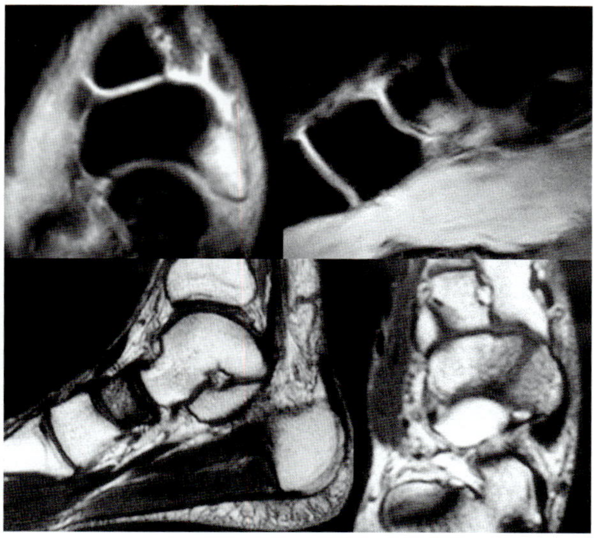

Figure 124 - Different MRI views identifying the bone edema at the navicular level

or treated with calcaneal osteotomy or metatarsal osteotomies to reduce stress at the navicular level [184, 187].

Calcaneal stress fractures

They are the most frequent stress fractures of the hindfoot and are more frequent in women [155].

Among the main causes gait alterations and flatfoot are reported. They are characterized by pain accompanied by swelling. The most frequent cause of the diagnostic error is with plantar fasciitis or with the insertional tendinopathy of the Achilles tendon. Percussion tenderness in the calcaneal tuberosity, both medial and lateral, are diagnostic [155].

The radiographic examination can be positive about 2 weeks after the onset of symptoms and is increasingly visible up to 6 weeks with a fracture line starting from the postero-superior region. The MRI allows early diagnosis (fig. 128) [155].

The treatment is conservative with bracing and load with Walker boot. Return to sport is usually possible after 8 weeks, again based on the presence or absence of symptoms. Recurrences are rare therefore surgical treatment is usually not necessary.

Nerve compression

Nerve compressions in the ankle and foot are caused by an acute trauma or repeated microtraumas. The nerves which are most subjected to trauma are the superficial branches of the intermediate dorsal cutaneous nerve and the medial dorsal cutaneous nerve, as well as the branches of the sural nerve (fig. 129).

The causes of acute compression include trauma and lacerations with scarring; among the most frequent causes of chronic compressions, there is the

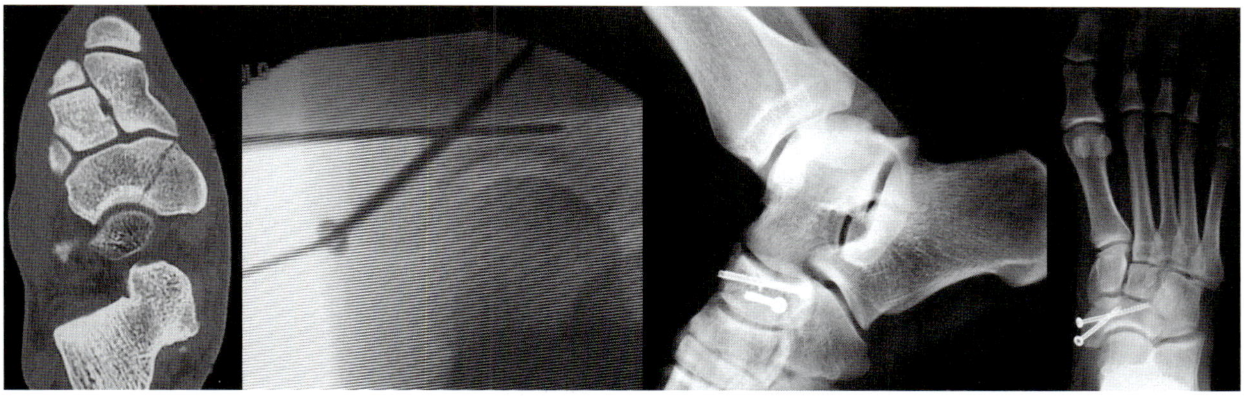

Figure 125 - CT scan shows the navicular fracture. The fracture was treated percutaneously, under fluoroscopic control: two guide wires were introduced into the navicular with dorso-lateral towards plantar-medial direction and the fracture synthesized with two partially threaded cannulated screws perpendicular to the fracture line

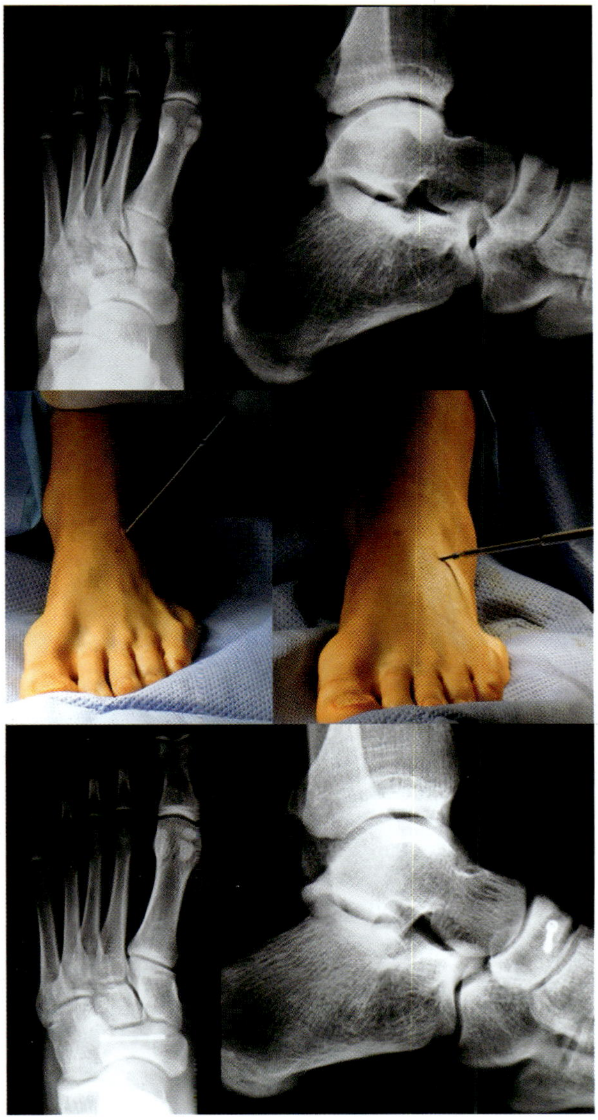

Figure 126 - Above, X-rays show the navicular fracture. The fracture was treated percutaneously, under fluoroscopic control: one guide wire was introduced into the navicular with dorso-lateral towards plantar-medial direction and the fracture was synthesized with a partially threaded cannulated screw

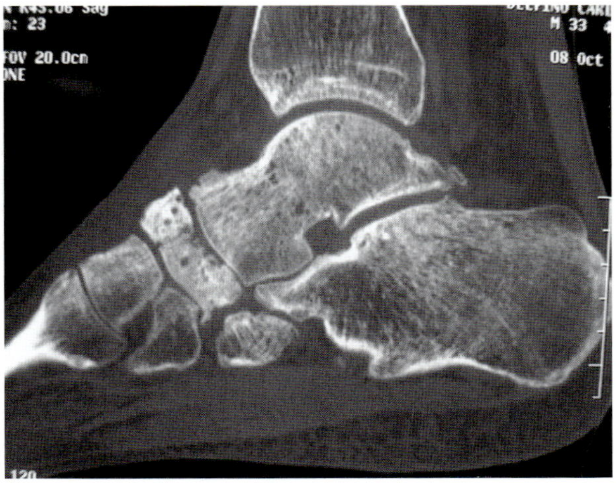

Figure 127 - CT scan, showing in the sagittal plane a navicular pseudoarthrosis

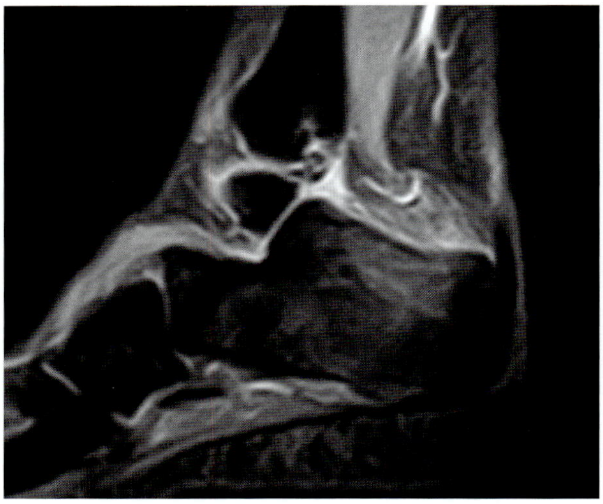

Figure 128 - MRI allows identifying calcaneal bone edema and therefore helps in early diagnosis

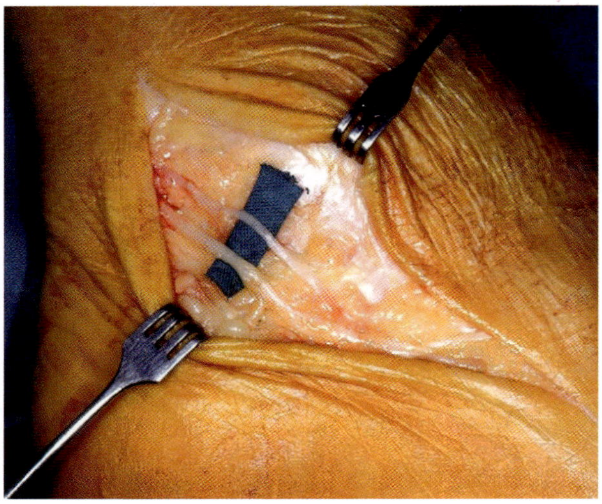

Figure 129 - Intermediate dorsal cutaneous nerve and medial dorsal cutaneous nerve

use of narrow shoes often associated with a cavus foot with dorsal osteophytes or a flatfoot deformity [188, 189].

The diagnosis is confirmed by the characteristics of pain: burning, distally and proximally irradiated, located on the back of the foot along with the distribution of the nerve. It also presents as local pain and sometimes loss or reduction of skin sensitivity distally in respect of the compression [189, 190]. A local injection of anesthetic leading to the disappearance of pain further confirms the diagnosis and may resolve the problem.

Ultrasound and an X-ray allow us to evaluate the soft parts and the presence of bony irregularities.

When conservative treatment fails, surgical treatment is necessary. Surgery is usually performed through a longitudinal incision, isolation of the nerve proximally and distally to the compression zone. In case of compression only, the nerve is freed from the scar and any osteophytes will be removed. If a neuroma is present this must be removed and the nerve separated and positioned with thin, resorbable points in a deep area not subject to trauma.

Morton's neuroma

The interdigital neuroma or better of Civinini-Morton, since Civinini first [191] described this type of syndrome, is characterized by the compression of the interdigital nerves. The etiology, although not precisely known, seems to be due to anatomical factors and micro traumatic factors [192]. The interdigital nerves are the continuation of the medial and lateral branches of the posterior tibial nerve (fig. 130): from the medial plantar nerve derive the first, the second, and third common digital nerve and from the lateral plantar nerve the digital nerve for the fourth space and the digital nerve for the fifth finger.

An anastomotic branch between the third and fourth common digital nerve makes the nerve of the third space less mobile and therefore more subject to microtraumas: this is why the third space is the most frequent site of neuroma formation. Other causes are altered metatarsal stresses such as in a pronated foot, in a supinated foot or a hallux rigidus. These repeated microtraumas lead to edema, interstitial degeneration, fibrosis, and neuroma formation. The symptoms are more frequent in women. The most affected space is the third and in about 15% of cases, it can be bilateral [192, 193].

The pain is referred to be in the plantar site at the level of the metatarsal head as burning, irradiated to the fingers corresponding to the space concerned and is accentuated by removing the shoes. The diagnosis is mainly clinical and based on the characteristics of the pain and on he physical examination with pain on palpation at the level of the space concerned and on the positive Murphy maneuver. The diagnosis can be confirmed by an ultrasound scan. MRI is rarely necessary except to exclude other types of pathology. If necessary, an

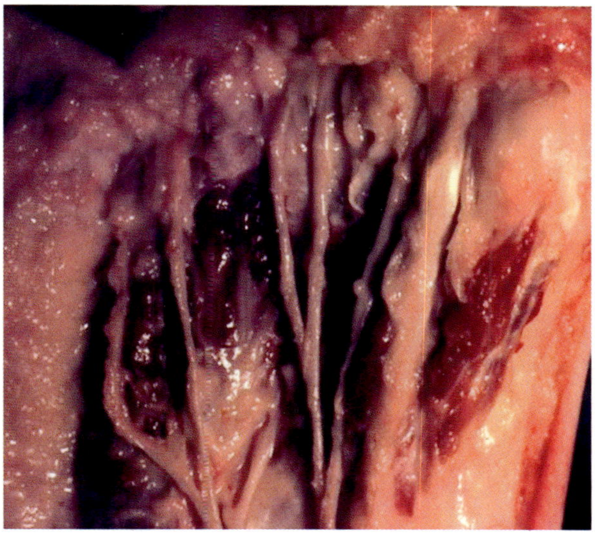

Figure 130 - Anatomical specimen showing interdigital nerves, a continuation of the medial and lateral branches of the posterior tibial nerve

injection of an anesthetic in the space in which the neuroma is suspected may be useful to confirm the diagnosis [192].
The initial treatment is conservative and consists of changes to the shoe (if particularly narrow), orthotics with a metatarsal pad just proximal to the metatarsal head, use of anti-inflammatories, injection of anesthetic and cortisone [194].
Nevertheless, only 30% respond favorably to conservative treatment, for which surgical treatment is required and is resolutive in about 90% of cases. Although several arthroscopic or open removal techniques have been described, with dorsal and plantar access. Normally, a minimally invasive open technique with dorsal access is to be preferred.
Surgical technique: incision from the web space proximal to about 1.5 cm. The two metatarsal heads are spread apart with the use of a retractor. The neuroma is highlighted, the transverse ligament is separated and after dissection and section of the terminal branches, the nerve is tractioned and sectioned as proximally as possible. The suture of the skin and compression bandage for two weeks with the possibility of loading is the principle of postoperative management (fig. 131) [194].

Tarsal tunnel syndrome and other nerve compressions

It represents an intrinsic or extrinsic compression neuropathy of the posterior tibial nerve or its branches at the level of the tarsal tunnel (fig. 132): the calcaneal branches and the medial plantar and lateral plantar [190, 195, 196]. The roof of the tarsal tunnel is formed by the flexor retinaculum and the floor by the bone component.
The main causes are bruises, previous sprains, fractured bone fragments, exostoses, excessive pronation, and tingling [190, 195, 196]. The patient complains of burning pain in the sole that affects one or both nerve branches. Pain may radiate proximally and be accentuated at night. A retromalleolar positive Tinel sign is present [190, 195]. Radiographs allow evaluating skeletal problems, which a CT will better highlight. A MRI can be useful to highlight possible ganglia, lipomas, venous changes. If no clear signs of compression are detected, it is advisable to avoid surgical treatment and favor a conservative treatment with anti-inflammatory, neurotrophic and orthotics to correct malalignment of the foot such as valgus or varus of the hindfoot. It is better to avoid cortisone injection. Local anesthetic injections may be useful to confirm the diagnosis [195]. Insoles may be useful in order to address foot deformities.
If the symptoms persist, surgical treatment is necessary and must respect these essential points: perform a wide incision to expose the nerve from the healthy proximal part, isolate the calcaneal branches and open distally until the medial and lateral plantar is visualized, separate the flexor retinaculum and fascial slings of the abductor hallucis muscles, use the tourniquet, preserve the skin and the nerve from tractions, apply a compressive dressing and a removable brace for two weeks until the wound is healed [190, 195].
Recovery times are long and sometimes associated to persistence of pain and positivity to the Tinel sign. It is important to avoid aggressive rehabilitation therapy and limit active mobilization and use of non-steroidal anti-inflammatory drugs and nonconstrictive shoes [195].
The most common causes of failure are due to poor exposure or incomplete release.
Another nerve compression may occur at the superficial peroneal nerve, the deep peroneal nerve, and the sural nerve [190].
Superficial peroneal nerve entrapment is mostly due to a lateral distortion or a blunt trauma at the

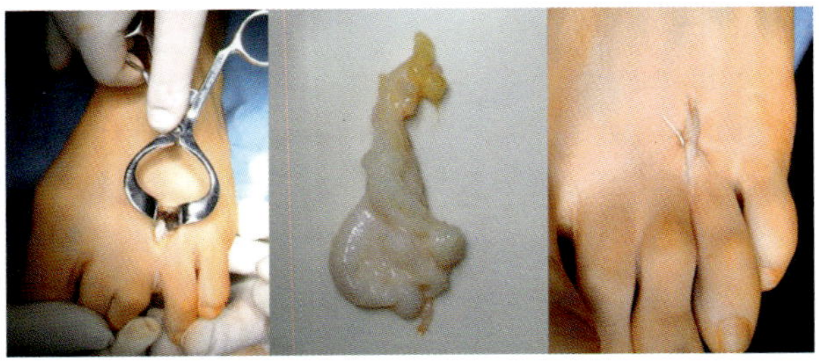

Figure 131 - Morton's neuroma surgical treatment: a dorsal incision at the third intermetatarsal web space is performed. The two metatarsal heads are spread apart with the use of a retractor. The neuroma is highlighted and sectioned as proximally as possible. Skin suture is performed with two reabsorbable stiches

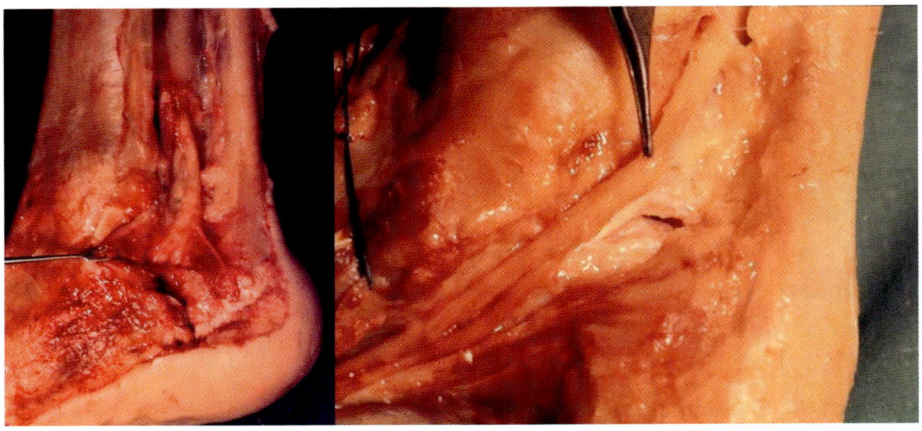

Figure 132 - Anatomical specimen showing, on the left side, the posterior tibial nerve, artery, and vein; on the right side, calcaneal branches and medial plantar and lateral plantar nerves are highlighted

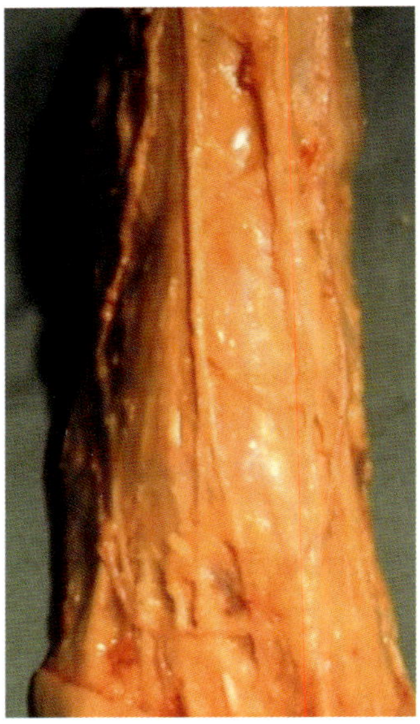

Figure 133 - Anatomical specimen showing the superficial peroneal nerve (left) and the saphenous nerve (right)

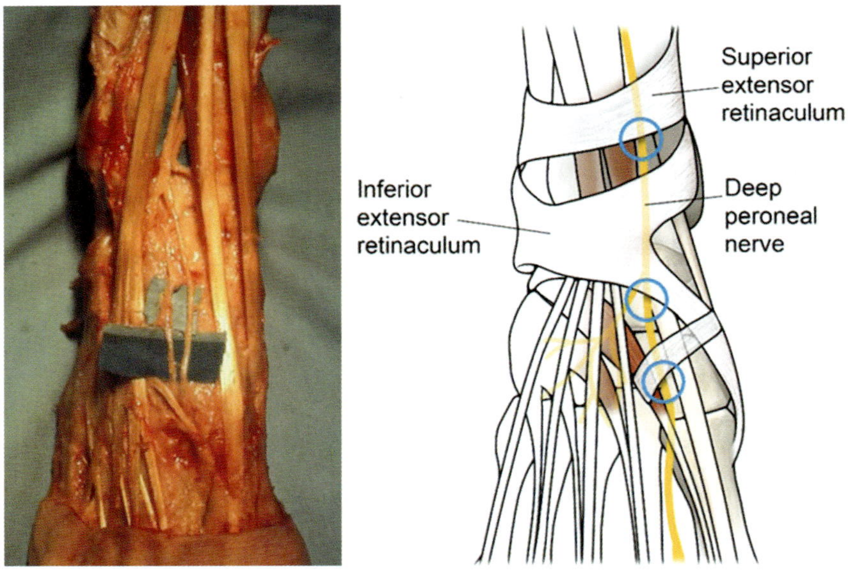

Figure 134 - On the left side, anatomical specimen showing the deep peroneal nerve. On the right side, the nerve root is highlighted

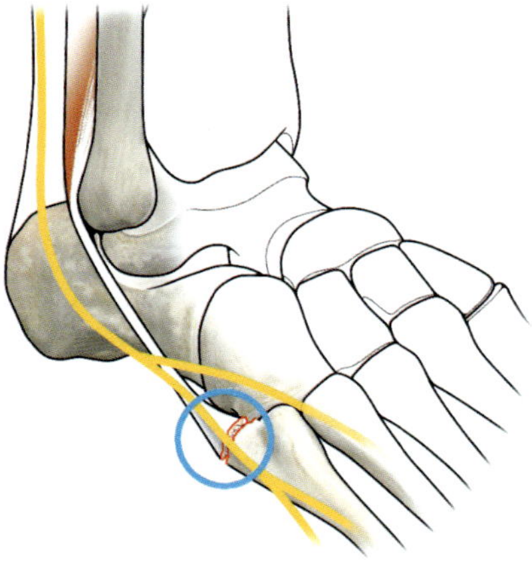

Figure 135 - Sural nerve entrapment due to a fifth metatarsal fracture

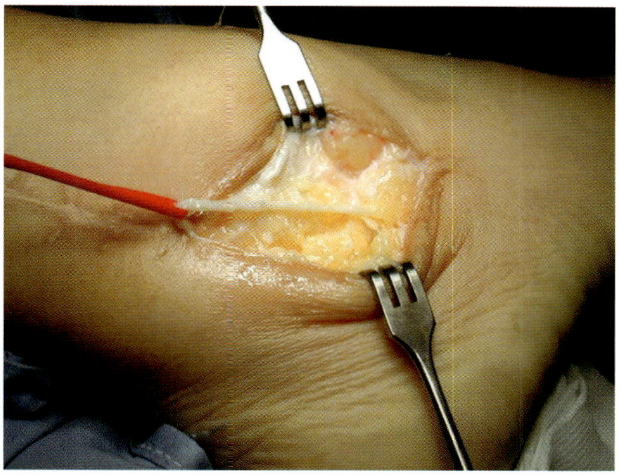

Figure 136 - Sural nerve neurolysis

emergence point of the fascia (fig. 133) [190, 197]. Deep peroneal nerve entrapment (fig. 134) is frequently caused by a dorsal osteophyte at talonavicular joint or due to a cuneiform prominence. Other risk factors are represented by ankle sprains or shoe constriction especially if in presence of a cavus foot, direct trauma caused by cleats along the nerve course, or repetitive shots to the ball with predisposing factors for deep peroneal nerve entrapment [190, 198].

Sural nerve entrapment (fig. 135) may be caused by ankle sprains, Achilles tendonitis with posterolateral swelling, or fifth metatarsal fractures. Pain is referred along the nerve course, in some cases together with paresthesia [190, 199, 200].

Palpation and compression may produce proximal and distal pain along the nerve course.

Some tests aimed at nerve distension can make the symptoms worse. An injection of anesthetic can be useful to identify the compression point. X-rays may show bone morphology alterations causing compression.

Treatment is usually conservative with anti-inflammatory drugs, topical cryotherapy, physical therapy, and steroid injections [190, 199, 200]. In case of a painful mechanical compression caused by fibrous or bony tissue, surgical neurolysis is required (fig. 136) [190].

Heel pain syndrome

There are many causes of heel pain. Serum negative arthritis, calcaneal stress fractures, bursitis, plantar fasciitis, plantar fascia ruptures, lumbosacral radiculopathy and nerve entrapment for the fifth finger abductor muscle (fig. 137) [201, 202].

The plantar fascia originates from the medial tubercle of the tuberosity of the calcaneus, has a thickness of up to 4 mm and medially posterior, with the fascia of the abductor muscle, it has the function of cushioning the loads on the bones and joints. Plantar fasciitis is the consequence of repeated traumas that affect the insertion of the fascia on the calcaneum with the possibility of microlesions at the level of the fibers that penetrate the bony part. These lesions repair and then reproduce, due to repeated traumas leading to a chronic injury. Sometimes the fascia can be affected by inflammation and pain even at the midfoot level.

X-rays may show a typical spur, a bony outgrowth from the calcaneal tuberosity (fig. 138).

The fascia tears are rare and mostly caused by a click or a fall after a jump.

The differential diagnosis of heel pain should be made with radiculopathy, tarsal tunnel syndrome, calcaneal fractures, seronegative enthesopathy, entrapment of the first branch of the lateral plantar nerve. In plantar fasciitis, the pain is particularly marked on palpation in the medial side of the calcaneal tuberosity or the center of the heel. Tensioning the band by flexing the fingers dorsally increases pain [201, 202].

In stress fractures, the pain is exacerbated by pressure along the medial and lateral heel wall. In case of entrapment of the first branch of the lateral plantar nerve, the site of tenderness is at the level of the passage between plantar and medial skin at about 5 cm from the posterior edge of the heel where the nerve flows between the abductor of the big toe and the square of the plant. An injection of an anesthetic in the case of plantar fasciitis and nervous entrapment eliminates pain. Radiographs in standard projection, ultrasound, bone scan, MRI and EMG studies are the tests that contribute to the diagnosis in the various forms of heel pain. The treatment of plantar fasciitis is usually conservative and consists in reducing the symptoms through the use of anti-inflammatories, hot and cold baths, ice by freezing water in a round performing, gastrocnemius stretching by a simple gentle wall stretch, deep massages, shock waves, 2 cm heel, taping [201, 202].

In the case of excessive pronation or supination,

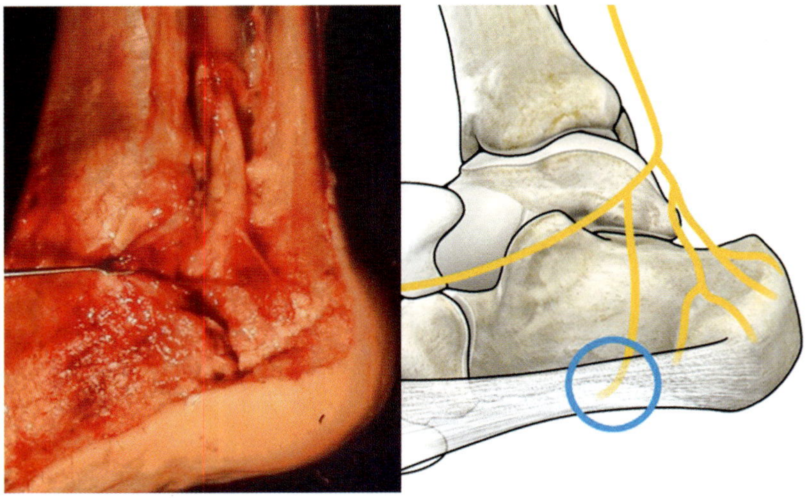

Figure 137 - On the left, anatomical specimen showing branches of the plantar nerves. The point of maximum tenderness and pain is highlighted on the right, usually caused by an involvement of the first branch of the medial plantar nerve

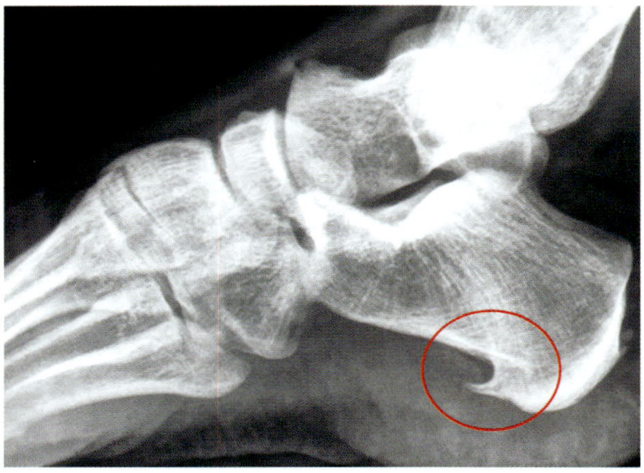

Figure 138 - Inferior calcaneal spur located on the inferior aspect of the calcaneus, a typical response to chronic plantar fasciitis

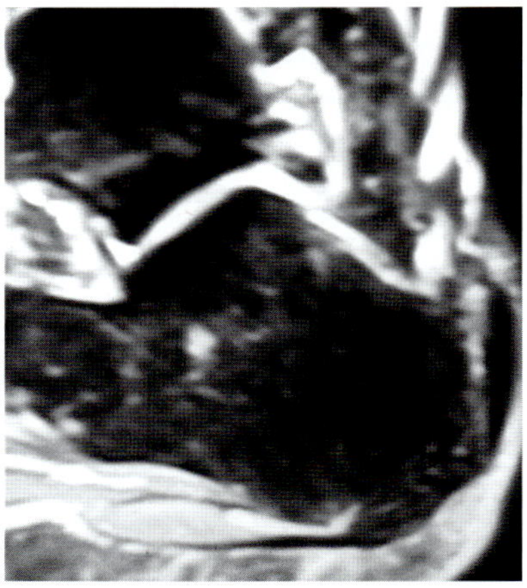

Figure 139 - Plantar fascia breakage highlighted by the MRI

Figure 140 - Open (left side) and percutaneous (right side) plantar fasciotomy

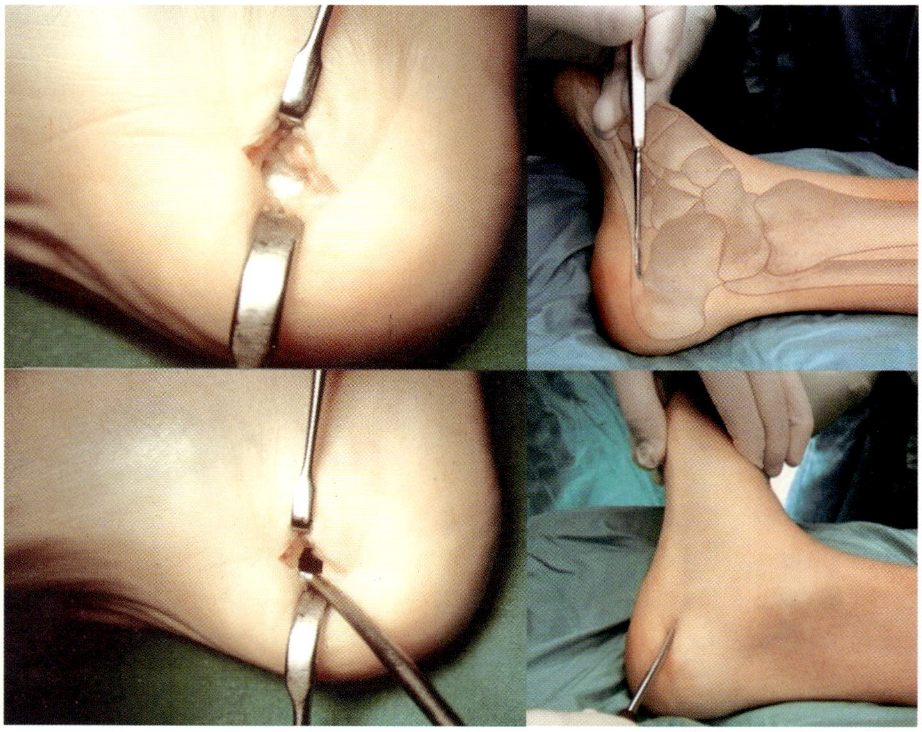

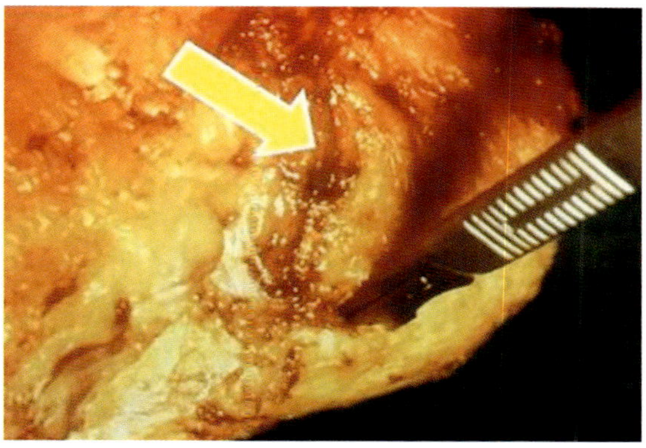

Figure 141 - Care must be taken in order not to damage the lateral plantar artery (yellow arrow)

orthotics can be useful stabilizing the hindfoot in a neutral position with the posterior case associated with a supinator or pronator forefoot wedge depending on the type of deformity.

Attention should be paid to local cortisone injections because although effective in reducing pain, they are frequently associated with fascia breakage and plantar fat atrophy (fig. 139) [203].

The risk appears to be related to the dose and type of cortisone and appears to be higher with the use of too flexible footwear.

In the case of poor results of the described conservative treatment, before proceeding with the surgical treatment (usually after a month) a shock wave treatment can be started to stimulate the repair process with increased vascularization [204]. Usually, three treatments are performed at intervals of one week using a low energy protocol that does not require the use of anesthesia and does not interrupt sports activities. The results of the literature show 70% success [205]; according to other authors a percentage of 40% is higher than placebo [203, 206].

If after a conservative treatment performed for 4/6 months no results are obtained, surgical treatment is indicated. This consists of plantar fasciotomy which can be performed endoscopically, percutaneously, with mini incisions and with traditional open access (fig. 140).

For the percutaneous treatment, after identifying the insertion point of the fascia to the calcaneus with a K-thread, keeping the fingers in dorsal flexion, the section of the medial part of the fascia is performed with a tenotome. Care must be taken

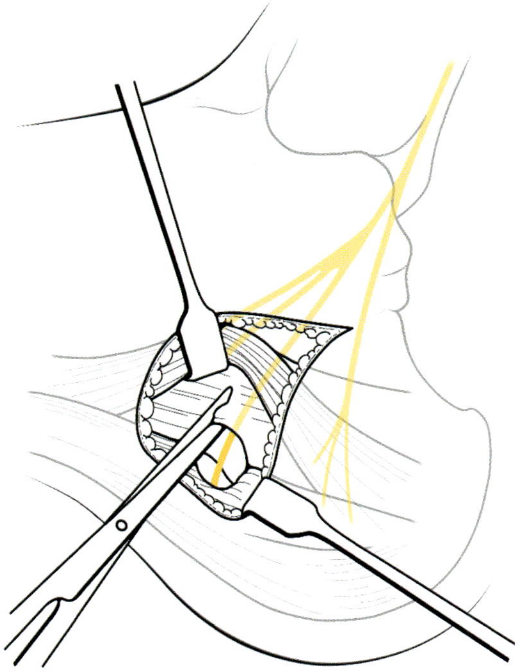

Figure 142 - Surgical lateral calcaneal nerve branch release

not to enter too distally so as not to dissect the lateral plantar artery that runs about 1 cm later, so a mini-incision of about 1.5 cm may be recommended medially about 5 cm from the tuberosity of the calcaneus at the point of the passage (fig. 141). After having removed a bit of fat, the plantar fascia is evident due to its insertion into the heel. A scissor is inserted between the fascia and the bone and the medial part of the fascia is selected with the scalpel. The wound is sutured with resorbable points. A brace or a Walker boot is then applied for three weeks without load, after that load and physical therapy. Activity resumes after 8/12 weeks.

When necessary, it is possible to associate a lateral calcaneal nerve branch release (fig. 142): an oblique medial incision is made towards the sole. The incision requires that the fascia of the abductor muscle of the big toe is incised. The muscle is then spread apart at the top. The medial edge of the plantar fascia is identified and a small 5x5 mm square of the plantar fascia is removed, then incision of the deep fascia of the abductor where the first branch of the lateral plantar runs in the square of the plant. When a plug is present it is removed, then suture and compressive dressing. The postoperative protocol is the same as the simple fasciotomy [204].

Foot deformities in soccer

Main foot deformities that can create problems in soccer practice are represented by flatfoot, cavus foot, posterior calcaneal tuberosity prominences, navicular or first metatarsal base prominences, hallux valgus, hallux rigidus, fifth toe varus and hammer toes [207].

Flat foot, due to its characteristic excessive pronation, can lead to a lateral pain at the sinus tarsal level caused by talo-calcaneal impingement, and medial pain along the posterior tibialis tendon, especially if associated with a prominent or accessory navicular, to pain in the plantar fascia and at the mid-foot level due to the protrusion of the talar head in the coxa pedis with distraction of the glenoid rim [208, 209].

Flat foot also may causes first ray insufficiency resulting in second metatarsalgia due to overloading of the second ray, possible metatarsal-phalangeal instability and second metatarsal stress fracture, especially in women [208, 210].

Treatment in the symptomatic forms is mostly conservative with the use of orthotics with a posterior shell stabilizing the hindfoot in neutral position and a supinator wedge at the forefoot level to compensate for the first metatarsal elevation.

Surgical treatment may be limited to the removal of an accessory navicular or a prominent navicular resection (fig. 143). In other cases a calcaneal osteotomy can be performed in order to restore the correct hindfoot axis through an oblique incision lateral to the heel of 3 cm and a fixation with a cannulated screw (figg. 144, 145).

Cavus foot, due to its increased plantar arch, is a foot characterized by a prevalent or persistent supination compared to what happens in a normal foot. Main features are represented by a dorsiflexed and varus hindfoot, a plantar flexed forefoot, and subsequent elevation of the plantar arch frequently toes claw deformity [211]. Due to the fixed cavus deformity of the first ray, a so-called tripod effect is produced, characterized by internal rotation of the foot with varus deviation of the heel (fig. 146). This functional alteration can lead to a metatarsalgia involving the first ray and may cause instability and frequent ankle sprains or stress fractures of the fifth metatarsal.

Furthermore, the compensation of the dorsiflexed and varus hindfoot and the plantar flexed forefoot leads to a greater dorsiflexion of the tibio-tarsal area with anterior impingement (fig. 147) and an increase traction at the level of the Achilles tendon insertion which increases the calcaneal pitch (fig. 148) [211].

A severe cavus foot is usually associated with a toe claw deformity which determines a dorsal compression of the foot at the apex of the vault, a dorsal compression at the level of the fingers proximal joints and at the apex of the fingers for the contrast with the shoes. These conditions can create tendon inflammatory reactions, exostoses formation in the back of the foot and forefoot callosities. Metatarsalgia is common due to overloading.

Even in cavus foot the treatment is mainly conservative with the use of orthotics with a 10 mm heel rise, a stabilizing shell in a neutral position on the back, a pronator wedge on the forefoot so as to discharge the first metatarsal head [211].

Selective functional metatarsalgia is usually treated with dedicated insoles.

In case of back pain, surgery is indicated with a bony resection of the calcaneal posterior apophysis (figg. 149, 150), of the base of the fifth metatarsal or dorsally at the level of the cuneiform.

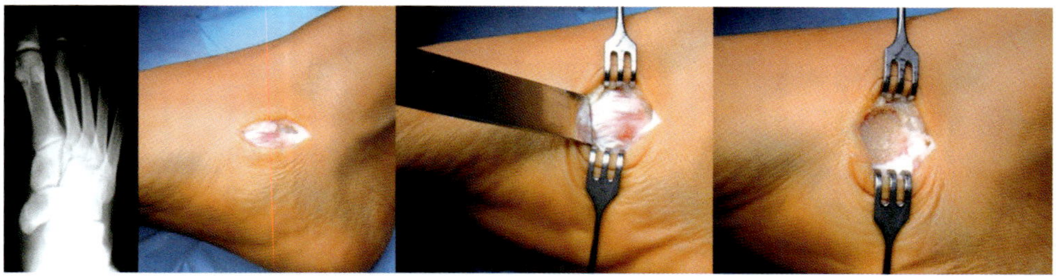

Figure 143 - The X-ray on the left shows a prominent navicular. An incision is performed at the level of the navicular tuberosity and a prominence resection is performed

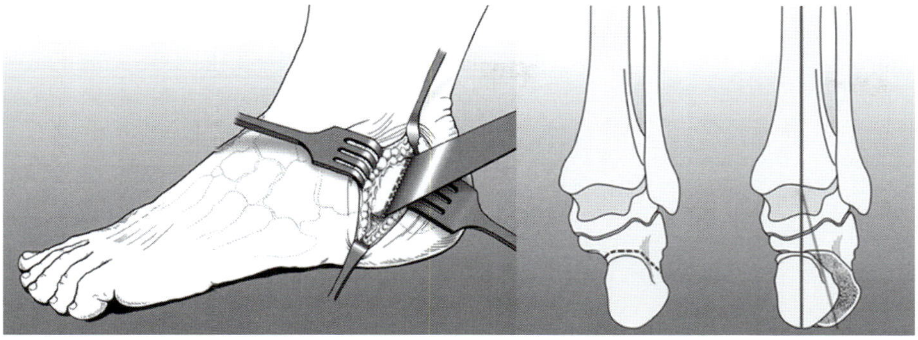

Figure 144 - Calcaneal osteotomy is performed through an oblique incision lateral to the heel; a medial translation of the calcaneal tuberosity allows for the hindfoot correction

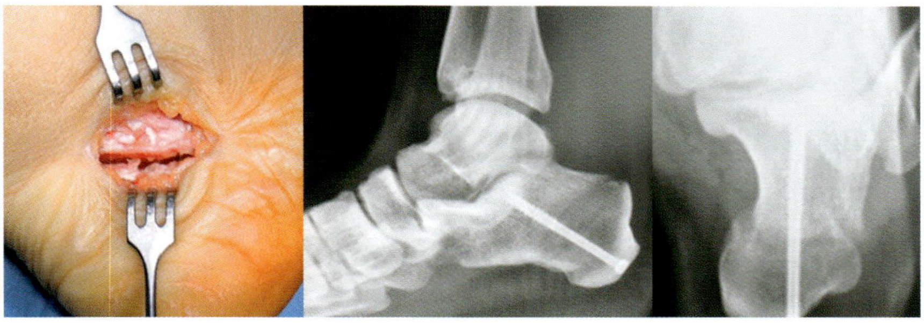

Figure 145 - Surgical procedure: oblique incision lateral to the heel, osteotomy and medial translation of the calcaneal tuberosity fixed with a cannulated screw

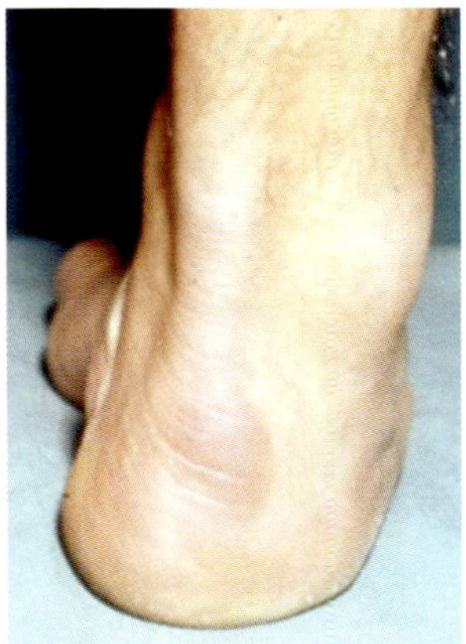

Figure 146 - Posterior view of a cavus foot hindfoot: due to the fixed cavus deformity of the first ray, a so-called tripod effect is produced, characterized by internal rotation of the foot with varus deviation of the heel

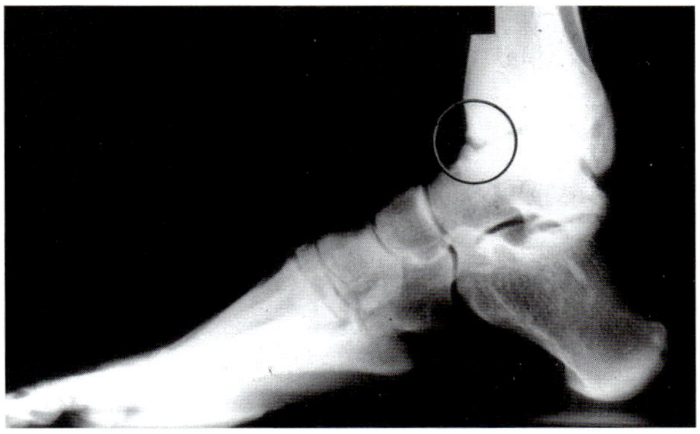

Figure 147 - Anterior ankle impingement caused by the excessive dorsiflexion of ankle joint in order to compensate for the dorsiflexed and varus hindfoot and the plantar flexed forefoot

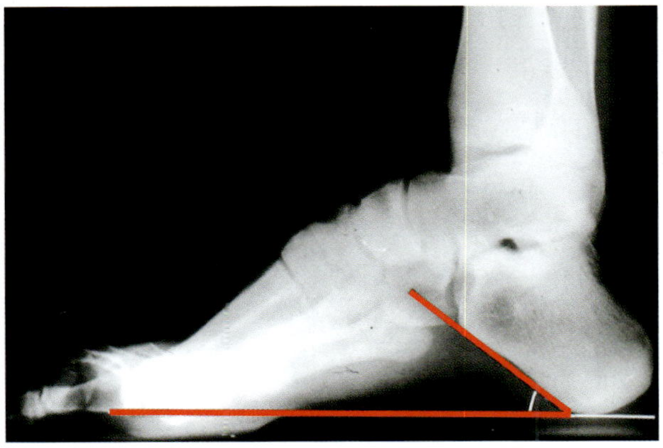

Figure 148 - An increase traction at the level of the Achilles tendon insertion that increases the Calcaneal pitch

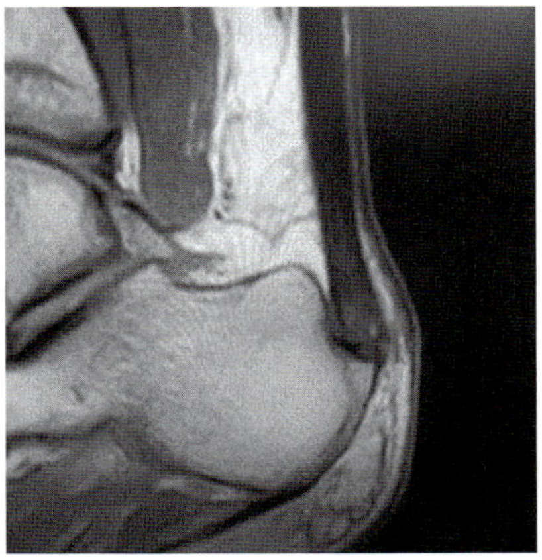

Figure 149 - Calcaneal posterior apophysis due to a bony prominence of the posterior tuberosity seen at the MRI

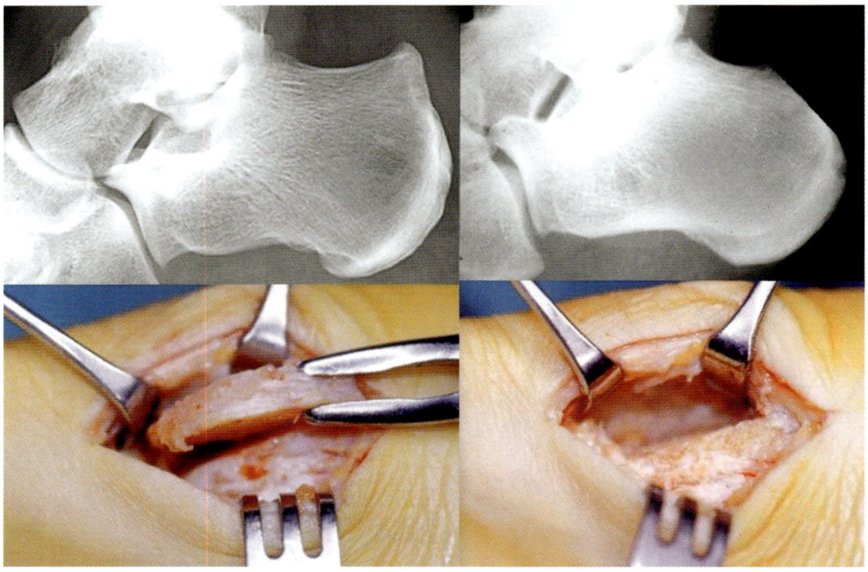

Figure 150 - Surgical procedure: the calcaneal posterior tuberosity resection is performed through a lateral incision. X-rays above show the prominence pre-operatively and the tuberosity aspect after the procedure

The first metatarsal overload can be treated with a proximal or distal metatarsal head dorsiflexion osteotomy (fig.151).

Toe deformity, if reducible, is treated with a shortening osteotomy of the first phalanx, while if structured with a proximal inter-falangeal arthrodesis.

Hallux valgus, due to the first metatarsal deviation in varus and the simultaneous big toe valgus deviation, creates a prominence of the metatarsal head with pain, bursitis, and possible ulceration.

For the functional insufficiency of the first ray, metatarsalgia of the second metatarsal and subsequent metatarso-phalangeal joint instability may occur.

In the event of failure of the conservative treatment (dedicated footwear and silicone orthosis), a minimally invasive extra-articular surgical treatment can correct all the anatomo-pathological alterations of the hallux valgus by means of a distal osteotomy fixed with a 2 mm Kirschner wire. The 1 cm incision allows to assess the direction and amount of displacement required (figg. 152, 153) (video 3).

In the case of interphalangeal valgus deformity an Akin osteotomy may be indicated (fig.154) [212].

Similarly to hallux valgus deformity, there may be a fifth toe varus: if conservative treatment is not effective, surgery is needed and consists of a linear osteotomy and a head displacement, which reduces the fourth inter-metatarsal space [213] (fig. 155).

Hallux rigidus is a relatively frequent condition, and represents the consequence of traumas, sprains, or fractures. It is characterized by a reduced range of motion, mainly in dorsiflexion. The pain is more pronounced in the phase of pushing the foot. The first metatarso-phalangeal joint shows a dorsal prominence on the first metatarsal head. The most frequent findings in the post-traumatic forms are a narrowing of the articular space and diffuse osteophytes formation. Based on these characteristics, different grades, from zero to three, have been proposed [214] (fig. 156).

MRI allows to evaluate metatarsal head or sesamoids osteochondral lesions, and alteration of the soft tissues.

Conservative treatment usually aims to correct foot pronation (when present) by using dedicated plantar orthosis; a toe spreader made of silicone may reduce the pressure between the first and second metatarsal. When pain persists, surgical treatment is necessary in order to increase range of motion and reduce pain. The type of treatment is different depending on the grade of arthritis [214].

In grade zero, with stiffness without arthritis, plantar release with a detachment of the glenoid rim from the phalanx base is able to eliminate the conflict between the medial sesamoid and the phalanx base and therefore improve dorsi-flexion (fig. 157).

From grade one to three a cheilectomy (fig. 158) or a SERI osteotomy (fig. 159) can be used [212].

The SERI technique should be performed with an oblique osteotomic line from distal to proximal in order to obtain a shortening of 3 mm and a plantar flexion able to decompress the joint and improve the results (figg. 159, 160).

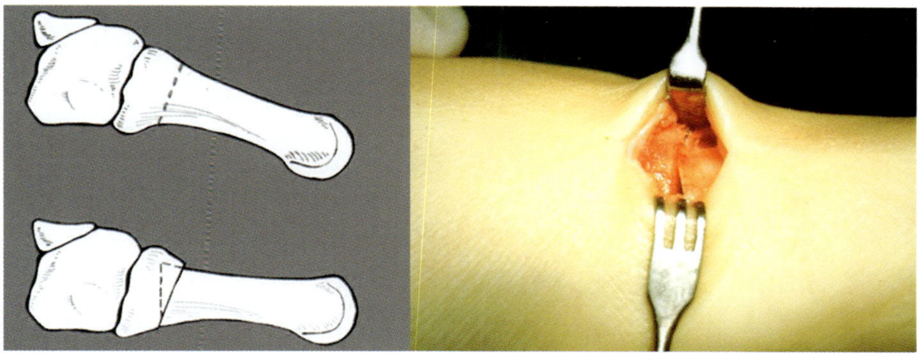

Figure 151 - A proximal metatarsal dorsiflexion osteotomy is performed by plantarflexing the metatarsal base

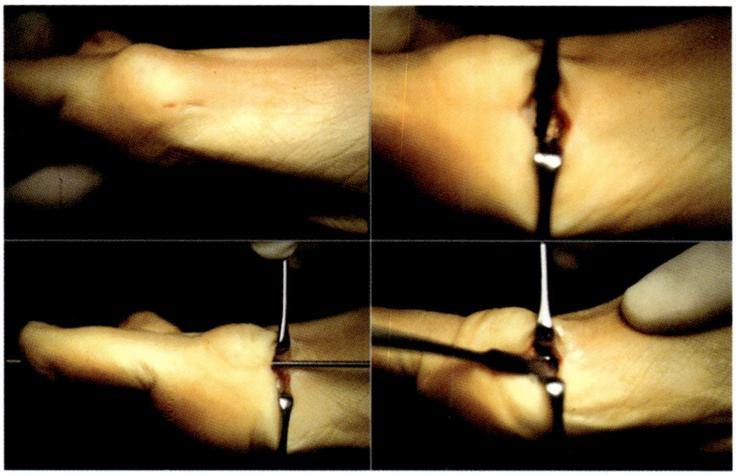

Figure 152 - Surgical procedure. Above, on the left, incision. Above, on the right, osteotomy. Below, on the left, a 2 mm Kirschner wire is inserted in a proximal to distal way. Below, on the right, the head translation and the Kirschner wire insertion on the metatarsal diaphysis

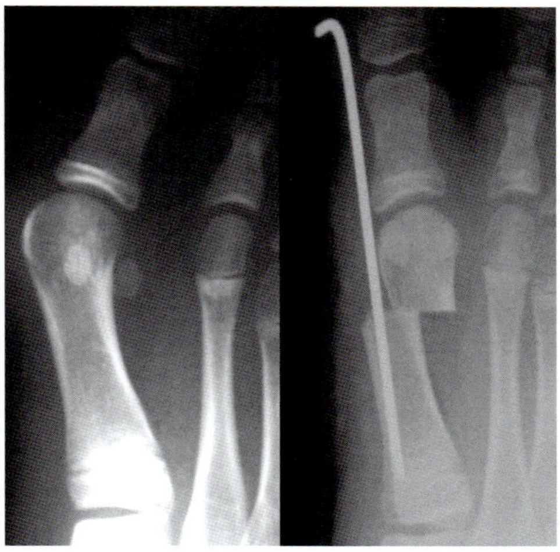

Figure 153 - On the left, X-ray showing a valgus deformity in a 16 years old male soccer player. On the right, correction after a distal metatarsal osteotomy stabilized with a Kirshner Wire

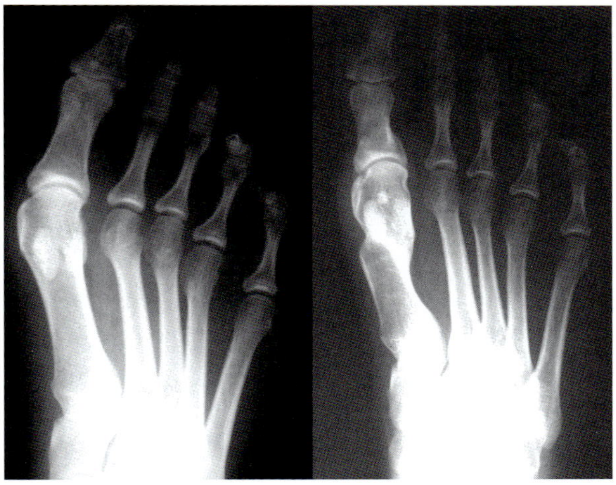

Figure154 - On the left, X-ray showing a valgus deformity associated to an interphalangeal valgus deformity in a 26 years old female soccer player. On the right, correction achieved at 1 year follow-up after a distal metatarsal osteotomy associated to a phalangeal Akin osteotomy

VIDEO 3

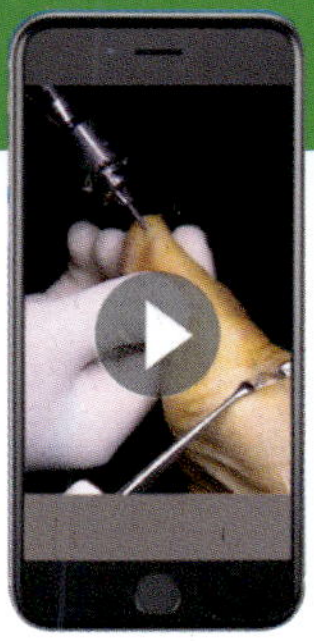

SERI technique for hallux valgus correction

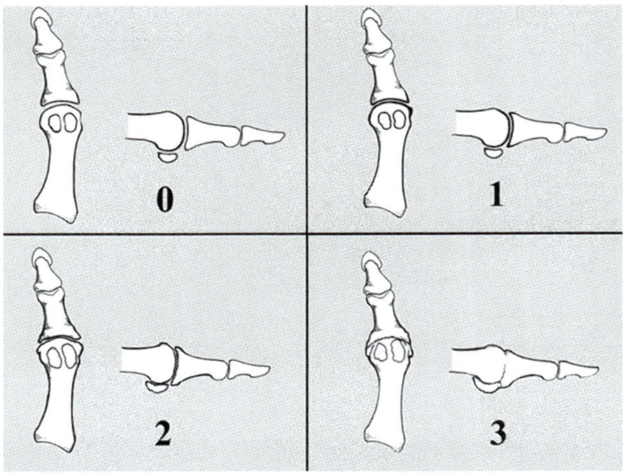

Figure 156 - Hallux rigidus classification based on articular space narrowing and osteophytes

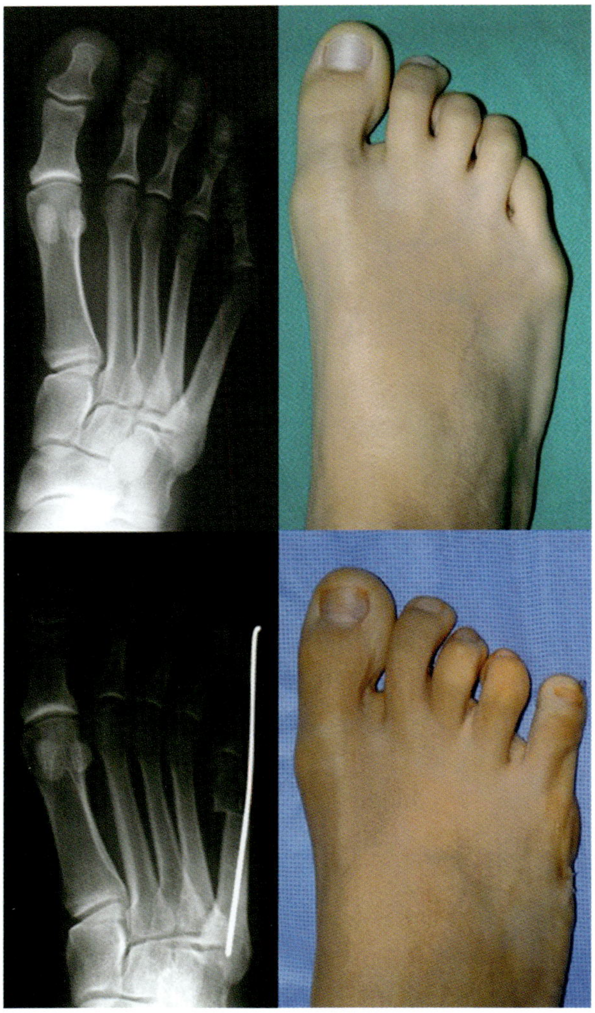

Figure 155 - Above, radiographic and clinical aspect of a varus fifth toe. Below, the X-ray shows the distal osteotomy stabilized with a Kirchner Wire, the picture on the right shows the correction achieved

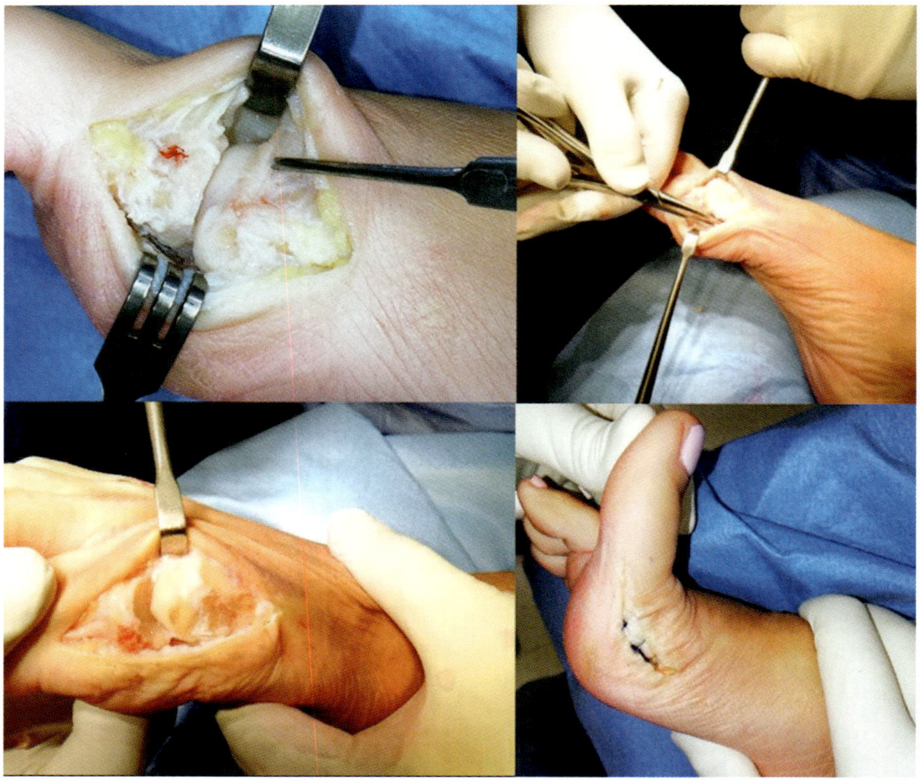

Figure 157 - Surgical procedure. An incision is performed on the first MPJ, a capsulotomy is performed. The osteophytes are identified and removed. A plantar release with a detachment of the glenoid rim from the phalanx base is able to eliminate the conflict between the medial sesamoid and the phalanx base and therefore improve dorsiflexion

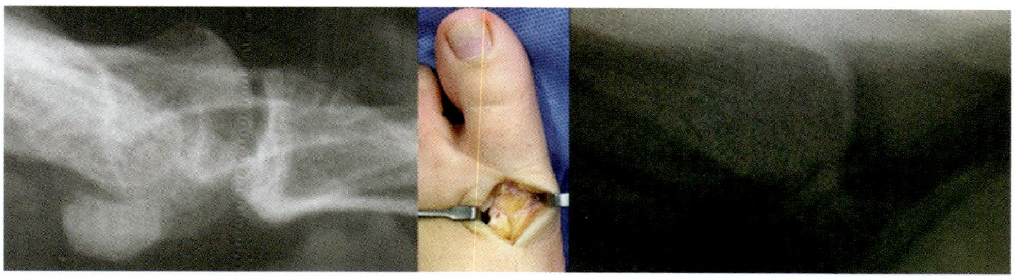

Figure 158 - On the left side, the X-ray shows a dorsal metatarsal prominence. Through a dorsal incision, a cheilectomy is performed (figure in the middle); on the right side, the X-ray shows a proper MTP joint profile

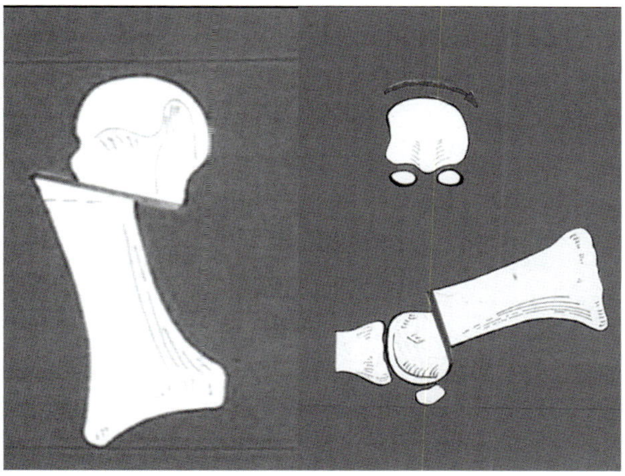

Figure 159 - An oblique osteotomic line from distal to proximal is able to provide a shortening and a plantar flexion of the metatarsal head able to decompress the joint

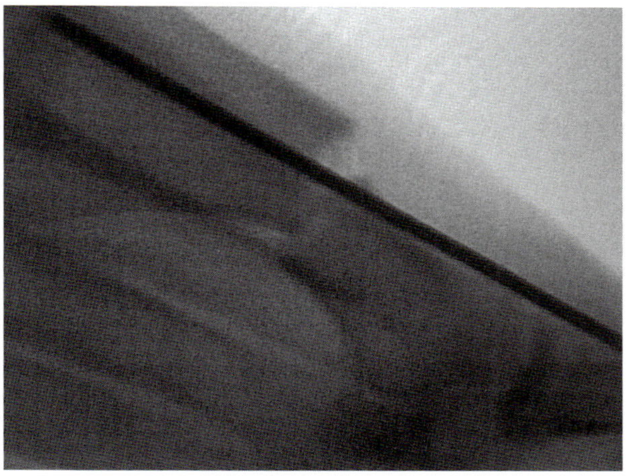

Figure 160 -Plantar flexion of the metatarsal head. A Kirschner wire stabilizes the osteotomy

In grade three the use of a bioabsorbable implant may be useful. After performing a massive release with osteophytes removal, the bioabsorbable polylactic-acid (PLLA) implant is inserted and works as a spacer improving range of motion and, with a slow reabsorption, producing a fibrous tissue in the joint (figg. 161, 162). If the movement is not sufficient, a dorsiflexion osteotomy of the first phalanx according to Moberg can be associated (fig. 163). Post-operative protocol is generally characterized by the use of a talus shoe from two to four weeks depending on the type of surgery performed [214].

Foot dermatology and nails pathologies

Nail pathologies are usually related to microtraumatic events: one of the most common is represented by the subungual hematoma and the ingrown nail (onychocryptosis). The subungual hematoma more frequently involves the first and the second toe. It may be caused by a direct trauma for a contrast, a kick against the ground, or a foot-step [215].

When pain is important as in the case of a large hematoma, drilling may be necessary to reduce the pressure under the nail. It is important to inform the soccer player that when the new nail underneath grows, the old one will fall spontaneously and therefore it is better not to remove it before its total detachment (fig. 164).

Ingrown nail (fig. 165) is a common condition in soccer player due to predisposing causes, such as the shape of the distal phalanx, which may contribute to the formation of a nail with more curved edges, but mainly because of microtraumas favored by narrow shoes, tight socks, too short cutting of the nails, or conflict with the second finger. The most affected side is the big toe. The clinical examination shows swelling, erythema, hypertrophy, and granulation of the nail fold. Purulent exudate is present in case of paranychial infection

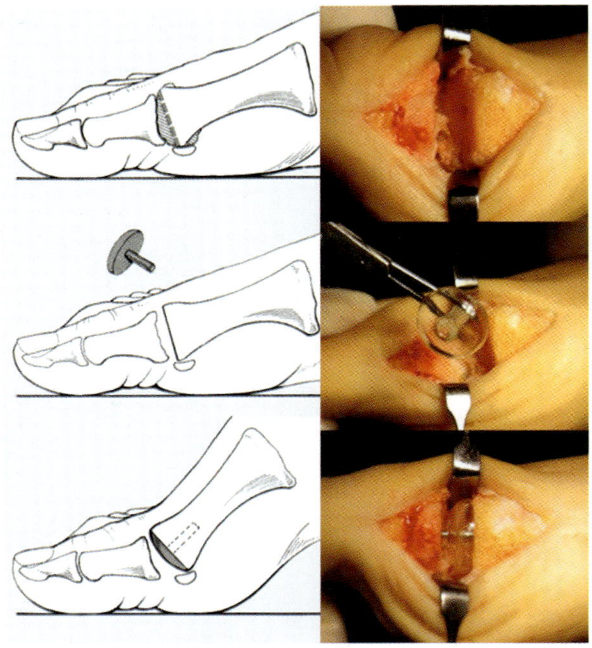

Figure161 - Surgical procedure. After performing a massive release with osteophytes removal, the bioabsorbable poly-lactic-acid (PLLA) implant is inserted and stabilized with a Kirshner Wire

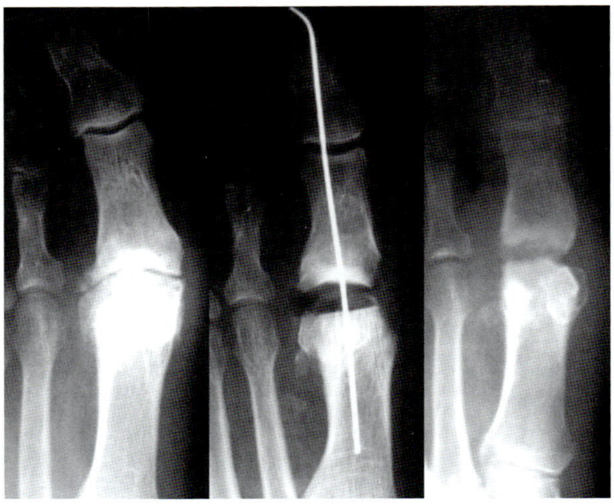

Figure 162 - On the left side, X-ray showing a grade III hallux rigidus. In the middle, post-operative X-ray, after a PLLA implant insertion. The device works as a spacer improving range of motion and, with a slow reabsorption, it produces a fibrous tissue in the joint. On the right side, the joint line is visible at 1 year follow-up on the X-rays

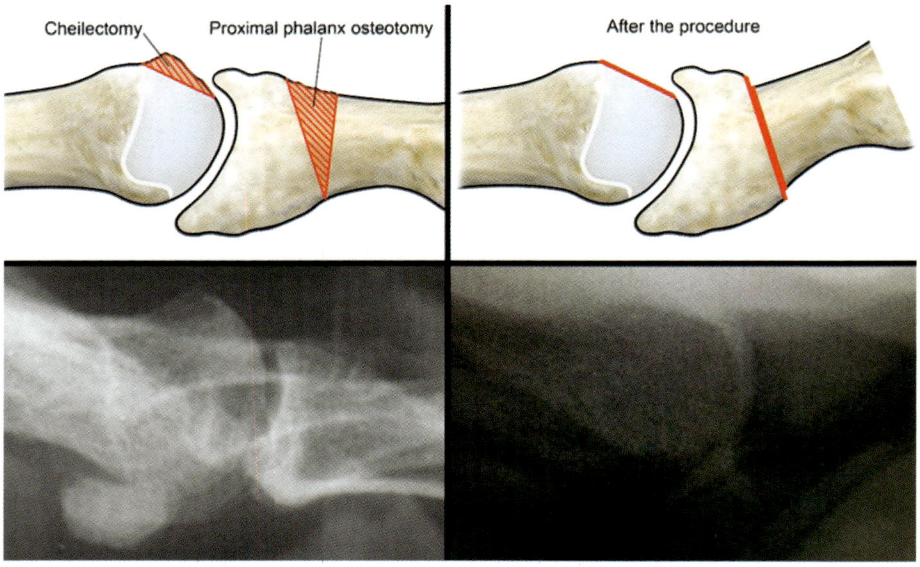

Figure 163 - Cheilectomy procedure associated to a Moberg dorsiflexion osteotomy of the first phalanx

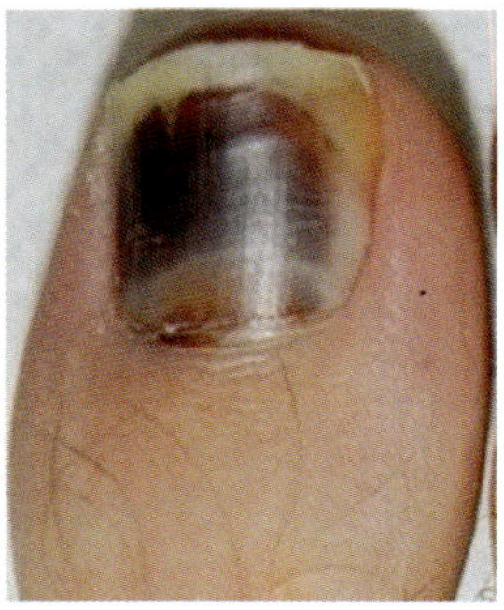

Figure 164 - Massive subungual hematoma occurred after a direct trauma

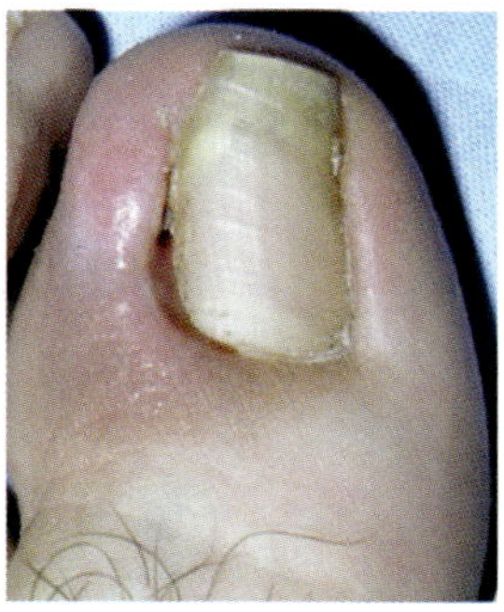

Figure 165 - Ingrown nail on the toe medial aspect

[216]. X-rays can exclude the presence of a sub-nail exostosis.

The most widely used treatments are the partial nail avulsion with reduction of the nail edge (fig. 166), the partial matricectomy that can be performed with various techniques, and the partial phenolization of the matrix with three applications of 3OS of 88% phenol, after having removed the nail edge [217].

The most common skin lesions are represented by corns, calluses, blisters, warts, and black heel [218, 219].

Corns are the result of both friction and localized pressure. They are more frequent at the mid-tarsal level. After the area of superficial hyperkeratosis is removed, a nail, which causes the tenderness, is clearly visible in the center. Removing the core in the center shows an immediate resolution of the pain [220].

Soft corn are more common in the fourth web space. When conservative treatment using spacer fails surgery is necessary with partial or complete excision of the distal portion of the proximal phalanx.

Calluses represent the most frequent pathologies in the foot and develop in hyperpressure areas or at the level of a bony prominence [22]. Calluses differ from corns and warts for more diffuse margins: they do not have a core center like corns and does not have a capillary dotting like wart.

Calluses are not usually as painful as corns and warts. The treatment consists in podological treatments, orthoses, or dedicated insoles. Surgical treatment is indicated to correct a deformity which causes the hyperkeratosis or when ulcers or infections are present [221].

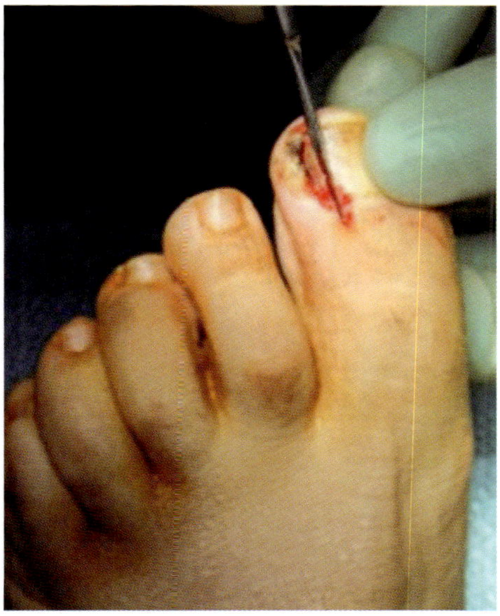

Figure 166 - Surgical emi-matricectomy

Painful blisters are caused by frictional forces that separate epidermal cells from the spinous layer [221]. They occur in an anatomical region where there is a thick corneal stroma and where the skin is moister. They contain a liquid content rich in aminoglycosides and nucleosides and usually reform in 2-3 days. The treatment consists in draining, trying to maintain the epidermal roof in order to reduce discomfort and prevent infections. After decompression, an advanced dressing is recommended.

In case of pain and in the need of resuming sport activity as soon as possible, a local anesthetic such as lidocaine can be used. The use of cold red laser may improve healing.

Blister containing blood should be evacuated and associated with an antibiotic treatment if cellulite is also present. Relapse prevention should be performed using cotton or wool socks and dedicated shoes [221].

Plantar warts are a skin infection caused by papilloma virus type 1 and type 2. They present several clinical aspects such as numerous small papillae, an isolated lesion measuring from 2 to 5 mm in size or in a mixed form [221, 222].

It is important to differentiate warts from corns and other pathologies.

The most important clinical sign to distinguish a wart is the presence, below the hyperkeratosis, of deep capillary dotting detectable by red-brown to black speectles, not present in the case of corns. One of the most effective treatments is cryotherapy after removing the area of hyperkeratosis, by two cycles of 10-second each with liquid nitrojen with an interval of 10 seconds [221, 222].

The black heel appears clinically as a dark red or black dot speckle of the foot.

It is produced by repeated traumas. The pigmentation is due to the collection of dried blood in the corneal stroma. The treatment is very simple and consists in removing the corneal stroma [223].

Bibliography

1. Chomiak J, Junge A, Peterson L, Dvorak J. Severe injuries in football players. Am J Sports Med.2000;28(5 Suppl):S58-S68.
2. Feria-Arias E, Boukhemis K, Kreulen C, Giza E. Foot and Ankle Injuries in Soccer. Am J Orthop (Belle Mead NJ). 2018 Oct;47(10).
3. Nery C, Raduan F, Baumfeld D. Foot and Ankle Injuries in Professional Soccer Players: Diagnosis, Treatment, and Expectations. Foot Ankle Clin. 2016 Jun;21(2):391-403.
4. Hawkins RD, Fuller CW. A prospective epidemiological study of injuries in four English professional football clubs. Br J Sports Med 1999;33:196–203.
5. Ekstrand J, Gillquist J. Soccer injuries and their mechanisms: a prospective study. Med Sci Sports Exerc 1983;15:267–70.
6. Cloke DJ, Ansell P, Avery P, Deehan D. Ankle injuries in football academies: a three-centre prospective study. Br J Sports Med. 2011;45(9):702-708.
7. Cloke DJ, Spencer S, Hodson A, Deehan D. The epidemiology of ankle injuries occurring in English Football Association academies. Br J Sports Med. 2009;43(14):1119-1125.
8. Dvorak J, Junge A, Derman W, Schwellnus M. Injuries and illnesses of football players during the 2010 FIFA World Cup. Br J Sports Med. 2011;45(8):626-630.
9. Fousekis K, Tsepis E, Vagenas G. Intrinsic risk factors of noncontact ankle sprains in soccer: a prospective study on 100 professional players. Am J Sports Med. 2012;40(8):1842-1850.
10. Gaulrapp H, Becker A, Walther M, Hess H. Injuries in women's soccer: a 1-year all players prospectivefield study of the women's Bundesliga (German premiere league). Clin J Sports Med. 2010;20(4):264-271.
11. Morgan BE, Oberlander MA. An examination of injuries in major league soccer. The inaugural season. Am J Sports Med. 2001;29(4):426-430.
12. Jain N, Murray D, Kemp S, Calder J. Frequency and trends in foot and ankle injuries within an English Premier League Football Club using a new impact factor of injury to identify a focus for injury prevention. Foot Ankle Surg. 2014;20(4):237-240.
13. Dvorak J, Junge A. Football injuries and physical symptoms. A review of the literature. Am J Sports Med 2000;28:S3–9.
14. Giza E, Fuller C, Junge A, Dvorak J. Mechanisms of foot and ankle injuries in soccer. Am J Sports Med. 2003;31(4):550-554.
15. Oztekin HH, Boya H, Ozcan O, Zeren B, Pinar P (2009) Foot and ankle injuries and time lost from play in professional soccer players. Foot (Edinb) 19(1):22–28.
16. Andersen TE, Floerenes TW, Arnason A, Bahr R. Video analysis of the mechanisms for ankle injuries in football. Am J Sports Med. 2004 Jan-Feb;32(1 Suppl):69S-79S.
17. Tucker AM. Common soccer injuries. Diagnosis, treatment and rehabilitation. Sports Med. 1997;23(1):21-32.
18. Espregueira-Mendes J, van Dijk CN, Neyret P, Cohen, M, Della Villa S, Pereira H, Oliveira JM. Injuries and Health Problems in Football. Berlin: Springer. (2017).
19. McKeon PO, Hertel J. Systematic review of postural control and lateral ankle instability, part I: can deficits be detected with instrumented testing? J Athl Train. 2008;43:293–304.
20. Munn J, Sullivan SJ, Schneiders AG. Evidence of sensorimotor deficits in functional ankle instability: a systematic review with meta-analysis. J Sci Med Sport. 2010;13:2–12.
21. McHugh MP, Tyler TF, Tetro DT, Mullaney MJ, Nicholas SJ. Risk factors for noncontact ankle sprains in high school athletes the role of hip strength and balance ability. Am J Sports Med. 2006;34:464–70.
22. Trojian TH, McKeag DB. Single leg balance test to identify risk of ankle sprains. Br J Sports Med. 2006;40:610–3.
23. de Noronha M, Refshauge KM, Herbert RD, Kilbreath SL. Do voluntary strength, proprioception, range of motion, or postural sway predict occurrence of lateral ankle sprain? Br J Sports Med. 2006;40:824–8.
24. Pope R, Herbert R, Kirwan J. Effects of ankle dorsiflexion range and pre-exercise calf muscle stretching on injury risk in army recruits. Aust J Physiother. 1998;44:165–72.
25. Emery C, Meeuwisse W. The effectiveness of a neuromuscular prevention strategy to reduce injuries in youth soccer: a cluster-randomised controlled trial. Br J Sports Med. 2010;44:555–62.
26. Waterman BR, Belmont PJ, Cameron KL, DeBerardino TM, Owens BD. Epidemiology of ankle sprain at the United States Military Academy. Am J Sports Med. 2010;38:797–803.
27. Arnason A, Sigurdsson SB, Gudmundsson A, Holme I, Engebretsen L, Bahr R. Risk factors for injuries in football. Am J Sports Med. 2004;32:5S–16S.
28. Engebretsen AH, Myklebust G, Holme I, Engebretsen L, Bahr R. Intrinsic risk factors for acute ankle injuries among male soccer players: a prospective cohort study. Scand J Med Sci Sports. 2010;20:403–10.
29. Tyler TF, McHugh MP, Mirabella MR, Mullaney MJ, Nicholas SJ. Risk factors for noncontact ankle sprains in high school football players the role of previous ankle sprains and body mass index. Am J Sports Med. 2006;34:471–5.
30. Milgrom C, Shlamkovitch N, Finestone A, Eldad A, Laor A, Danon YL, et al. Risk factors for lateral ankle sprain: a prospective study among military recruits. Foot Ankle Int. 1991;12:26–30.
31. Beynnon BD, Renström PA, Alosa DM, Baumhauer JF, Vacek PM. Ankle ligament injury risk factors: a prospective study of college athletes. J Orthop Res. 2001;19:213–20.
32. Baumhauer JF, Alosa DM, Renström PA, Trevino S, Beynnon B. A prospective study of ankle injury risk factors. Am J Sports Med. 1995;23:564–70.
33. McGuine TA, Keene JS. The effect of a balance training program on the risk of ankle sprains in high school athletes. Am J Sports Med. 2006;34:1103–11.
34. Pefanis N, Papaharalampous X, Tsiganos G, Papadakou E, Baltopoulos P. The effect of Q angle on ankle sprain occurrence. Foot Ankle Spec. 2009;2:22–6.
35. Pefanis N, Karagounis P, Tsiganos G, Armenis E, Baltopoulos P. Tibiofemoral angle and its relation to ankle sprain occurrence. Foot Ankle Spec. 2009.
36. McGuine TA, Hetzel S, Wilson J, Brooks A. The effect of lace-up ankle braces on injury rates in high school football players. Am J Sports Med. 2012;40:49–57.
37. LaBella CR, Huxford MR, Grissom J, Kim K-Y, Peng J, Christoffel KK. Effect of neuromuscular warm-up on injuries in female soccer and basketball athletes in urban public high schools: cluster randomizedcontrolled trial. Arch Pediatr Adolesc Med. 2011;165:1033–40.
38. Kofotolis ND, Kellis E, Vlachopoulos SP. Ankle sprain injuries and risk factors in amateur soccer players during a 2-year period. Am J Sports Med. 2007;35:458–66.
39. Surve I, Schwellnus MP, Noakes T, Lombard C. A fivefold reduction in the incidence of recurrent ankle sprains in soccer players using the Sport-Stirrup orthosis. Am J Sports Med. 1994;22:601–6.
40. Manganaro D, Alsayouri K. Anatomy, Bony Pelvis and Lower Limb, Ankle Joint. 2019 Aug 3. StatPearls [Internet]. Treasure Island (FL): StatPearls Publishing; 2019 Jan.

41. Woods C, Hawkins R, Hulse M, Hodson A. The Football Association Medical Research Programme: an audit of injuries in professional football: an analysis of ankle sprains. Br J Sports Med. 2003;37(3):233-238.
42. Kerkhoffs GM, Rowe BH, Assendelft WJ, Kelly KD, Struijs PA, van Dijk CN. Immobilisation for acute ankle sprain. A systematic review. Arch Orthop Trauma Surg. 2001;121(8):462-471).
43. Konradsen L, Holmer P, Sondergaard L. Early mobilizing treatment for grade III ankle ligament injuries. Foot Ankle. 1991;12(2):69-73.
44. Hintermann B. Medial ankle instability. Foot Ankle Clin. 2003;8(4):723-738.
45. Hopkinson WJ, St Pierre P, Ryan JB, Wheeler JH. Syndesmosis sprains of the ankle. Foot Ankle. 1990;10(6):325-330.
46. Murawski CD, Kennedy JG. Operative treatment of osteochondral lesions of the talus. J Bone Joint Surg Am. 2013;95(11):1045-1054.
47. Guney A, Akar M, Karaman I, Oner M, Guney B. Clinical outcomes of platelet rich plasma (PRP) as an adjunct to microfracture surgery in osteochondral lesions of the talus. Knee Surg Sports Traumatol Arthrosc. 2015;23(8):2384-2389.
48. Hatic SO, Berlet GC. Particulated juvenile articular cartilage graft (DeNovo NT Graft) for treatment of osteochondral lesions of the talus. Foot Ankle Spec. 2010;3(6):361-364.
49. van Eekeren IC, van Bergen CJ, Sierevelt IN, Reilingh ML, van Dijk CN. Return to sports after arthroscopic debridement and bone marrow stimulation of osteochondral talar defects: a 5- to 24-year follow-up study. Knee Surg Sports Traumatol Arthrosc. 2016;24(4):1311-1315.
50. Stiell IG, Greenberg GH, McKnight RD, Nair RC, McDowell I, Worthington JR. A study to develop clinical decision rules for the use of radiography in acute ankle injuries. Ann Emerg Med.1992;21(4):384-390.
51. Bachmann LM, Kolb E, Koller MT, Steurer J, ter Riet G. Accuracy of Ottawa ankle rules to exclude fractures of the ankle and mid-foot: systematic review. BMJ. 2003;326(7386):417.
52. Hayes R, Callaghan M. BET 2: Diagnostic value of ultrasound in determining lateral ligament injury of the ankle. Emerg Med J. 2019 Jan;36(1):56-57.
53. Martin RL, Davenport TE, Paulseth S, Wukich DK, Godges JJ, Altman RD, et al. Ankle stability and movement coordination impairments: ankle ligament sprains. J Orthop Sports Phys Ther. 2013;43:A1–A40.
54. Campbell SE, Warner M. MR imaging of ankle inversion injuries. Magn Reson Imaging Clin N Am.2008;16:1–18.
55. Prins JG. Diagnosis and treatment of injury to the lateral ligament of the ankle. A comparative clinical study. Acta Chir Scand Suppl. 1978;486:3.
56. Lin CF, Gross ML, Weinhold P. Ankle syndesmosis injuries: anatomy, biomechanics, mechanism of injury, and clinical guidelines for diagnosis and intervention. J Orthop Sports Phys Ther. 2006;36(6):372-384.
57. Chhabra A, Subhawong TK, Carrino JA. MR imaging of deltoid ligament pathologic findings and associated impingement syndromes. Radiographics. 2010;30(3):751-761.
58. Andrade R, Pereira H, Vilas-Boas JP, Espregueira-Mendes J, van Dijk CN. Injury of Ankle Ligaments. 2017. In: Injuries and Health Problems in Football (pp. 83-104). Springer, Berlin, Heidelberg.
59. Balduini FC, Vegso JJ, Torg JS, Torg E. Management and rehabilitation of ligamentous injuries to the ankle. Sports Med. 1987;4(5):364-380.
60. Ferkel RD, Chams RN. Chronic lateral instability: arthroscopic findings and long-term results. Foot Ankle Int. 2007;28:24–31.
61. van Dijk CN, Vuurberg G. Ankle ligament lesions. In: Volpi, editor. Football traumatology: new trends. 2nd ed. Cham: Springer; 2015. p. 333–42.
62. Lubberts B, D'Hooghe P, Bengtsson H, DiGiovanni CW, Calder J, Ekstrand J. Epidemiology and return to play following isolated syndesmotic injuries of the ankle: a prospective cohort study of 3677 male professional football players in the UEFA Elite Club Injury Study. Br J Sports Med. 2017.
63. Mulligan EP. Evaluation and management of ankle syndesmosis injuries. Phys Ther Sport. 2011;12:57–69.
64. Dubin JC, Comeau D, McClelland RI, Dubin RA, Ferrel E. Lateral and syndesmotic ankle sprain injuries: a narrative literature review. J Chiropr Med. 2011;10:204–19.
65. van Dijk C, Vuurberg G, Amendola A, Lee J. Anterior ankle arthroscopy: state of the art. J ISAKOS. 2016;1:105–15.
66. Harper MC, Keller TS. A radiographic evaluation of the tibiofibular syndesmosis. Foot Ankle. 1989;10(3):156-160.
67. Brown KW, Morrison WB, Schweitzer ME, Parellada JA, Nothnagel H. MRI findings associated with distal tibiofibular syndesmosis injury. AJR Am J Roentgenol. 2004;182(1):131-136.
68. Ogilvie-Harris DJ, Reed SC, Hedman TP. Disruption of the ankle syndesmosis: biomechanical study of the ligamentous restraints. Arthroscopy. 1994;10(5):558-560.
69. van Dijk CN, Longo UG, Loppini M, Florio P, Maltese L, Ciuffreda M, et al. Conservative and surgical management of acute isolated syndesmotic injuries: ESSKA-AFAS consensus and guidelines. Knee Surg Sports Traumatol Arthrosc. 2016;24:1217–27.
70. Jones CB, Gilde A, Sietsema DL. Treatment of syndesmotic injuries of the ankle. JBJS Rev. 2015;3:e1.
71. Del Buono A, Florio A, Boccanera MS, Maffulli N. Syndesmosis injuries of the ankle. Curr Rev Musculoskelet Med. 2013;6(4):313-319.
72. Schepers T. To retain or remove the syndesmotic screw: a review of literature. Arch Orthop Trauma Surg. 2011;131(7):879-883.
73. Naqvi GA, Cunningham P, Lynch B, Galvin R, Awan N. Fixation of ankle syndesmotic injuries: comparison of tightrope fixation and syndesmotic screw fixation for accuracy of syndesmotic reduction. Am J Sports Med. 2012;40(12):2828-2835.
74. Weening B, Bhandari M. Predictors of functional outcome following transsyndesmotic screw fixation of ankle fractures. J Orthop Trauma. 2005;19(2):102-108.
75. Colcuc C, Blank M, Stein T, et al. Lower complication rate and faster return to sports in patients with acute syndesmotic rupture treated with a new knotless suture button device. Knee Surg Sports Traumatol Arthrosc. 2017.
76. Hertel J. Functional anatomy, pathomechanics, and pathophysiology of lateral ankle instability. J Athl Train. 2002;37:364.
77. Freeman MA. Treatment of ruptures of the lateral ligament of the ankle. J Bone Joint Surg Br 1965;47:661-8.
78. Tropp H, Odenrick P, Gillquist J. Stabilometry recordings in functional and mechanical instability of the ankle joint. Int J Sports Med 1985;6:180-2.
79. Giannini S, Ruffilli A, Pagliazzi et al. Treatment algorithm for chronic lateral ankle instability. Muscles Ligaments Tendons J 2015;4:455-60.
80. Giannini S, Ceccarelli F, De Benedictis M, et al. Le lesioni capsulo-legamentose di caviglia. Il piede nello Sport 1998, pp. 127-141.
81. Wiltberger BR, Mallory TH. A new method for the reconstruction of the deltoid ligament of the ankle. Orthop Rev

1972;1:37-41.
82. Matsui K, Burgesson B, Takao M, et al. Minimally invasive surgical treatment for chronic ankle instability: a systematic review. Knee Surg Sports Traumatol Arthrosc 2016;24:1040-8.
83. Lui TH. Modified arthroscopic Brostrom procedure. Foot Ankle Surg 2015;21:216-9.
84. Guillo S, Archbold P, Perera A, et al. Arthroscopic anatomic reconstruction of the lateral ligaments of the ankle with gracilis autograft. Arthroscopy Tech 2014;3:e593-e8.
85. Guillo S, Cordier G, Sonnery-Cottet B, et al. Anatomical reconstruction of the anterior talofibular and calcaneofibular ligaments with an all-arthroscopic surgical technique. Orthop Traumatol Surg Res 2014;100:S413-7.
86. Bleakley CM, McDonough SM, MacAuley DC. Some conservative strategies are effective when added to controlled mobilisation with external support after acute ankle sprain: a systematic review. Aust J Physiother. 2008;54:7–20.
87. Petersen W, Rembitzki IV, Koppenburg AG, Ellermann A, Liebau C, Brüggemann GP, et al. Treatment of acute ankle ligament injuries: a systematic review. Arch Orthop Trauma Surg.2013;133:1129–41.
88. Hertel J. Sensorimotor deficits with ankle sprains and chronic ankle instability. Clin Sports Med. 2008;27:353–70.
89. Wikstrom EA, Naik S, Lodha N, Cauraugh JH. Bilateral balance impairments after lateral ankle trauma: a systematic review and meta-analysis. Gait Posture. 2010;31:407–14.
90. McKeon JMM, Bush HM, Reed A, Whittington A, Uhl TL, McKeon PO. Return-to-play probabilities following new versus recurrent ankle sprains in high school athletes. J Sci Med Sport. 2014;17:23–8.
91. Miyamoto W, Takao M, Yamada K, Matsushita T. Accelerated versus traditional rehabilitation after anterior talofibular ligament reconstruction for chronic lateral instability of the ankle in athletes. Am J Sports Med. 2014;42:1441–7.
92. Beynnon BD, Murphy DF, Alosa DM. Predictive factors for lateral ankle sprains: a literature review. J Athl Train. 2002;37:376.
93. Steib S, Hentschke C. Fatigue-induced alterations of static and dynamic postural control in athletes with a history of ankle sprain. J Athl Train. 2013;48:203.
94. Petrera M, Dwyer T, Theodoropoulos JS, Ogilvie-Harris DJ. Short-to medium-term outcomes after a modified Broström repair for lateral ankle instability with immediate postoperative weightbearing. Am J Sports Med. 2014:0363546514530668.
95. Maffulli N, Del Buono A, Maffulli GD, Oliva F, Testa V, Capasso G, et al. Isolated anterior talofibular ligament Broström repair for chronic lateral ankle instability 9-year follow-up. Am J Sports Med. 2013;41:858–64.
96. Calder JD, Bamford R, Petrie A, McCollum GA. Stable versus unstable grade II high ankle sprains: a prospective study predicting the need for surgical stabilization and time to return to sports. Arthroscopy. 2016;32:634–42.
97. Alt W, Lohrer H, Gollhofer A. Functional properties of adhesive ankle taping: neuromuscular and mechanical effects before and after exercise. Foot Ankle Int. 1999;20(4):238-245.
98. Garrick JG, Requa RK. Role of external support in the prevention of ankle sprains. Med Sci Sports.1973;5(3):200-203.
99. Sharpe SR, Knapik J, Jones B. Ankle braces effectively reduce recurrence of ankle sprains in female soccer players. J Athl Train. 1997;32(1):21-24.
100. Mohammadi F. Comparison of 3 preventive methods to reduce the recurrence of ankle inversion sprains in male soccer players. Am J Sports Med. 2007;35(6):922-926.
101. Steffen K, Emery CA, Romiti M, et al. High adherence to a neuromuscular injury prevention programme (FIFA 11+) improves functional balance and reduces injury risk in Canadian youth female football players: a cluster randomised trial. Br J Sports Med. 2013;47(12):794-802.
102. Junge A, Lamprecht M, Stamm H, et al. Countrywide campaign to prevent soccer injuries in Swiss amateur players. Am J Sports Med. 2011;39(1):57-63.
103. Michels F, Clockaerts S, Van Der Bauwhede J, Stockmans F, Matricali G. Does subtalar instability really exist? A systematic review. Foot Ankle Surg. 2019 Feb 18. pii: S1268-7731(19)30023-2.
104. Helgeson K. Examination and intervention for sinus tarsi syndrome. N Am J Sports Phys Ther. 2009 Feb;4(1):29-37.
105. Fraser JJ, Feger MA, Hertel J. Midfoot and forefoot involvement in lateral ankle sprains and chronic ankle instability. Part 1: anatomy and biomechanics. Int j sports phys ther. 2016 dec;11(6):992-1005.
106. Laird RC. Acute forefoot and midfoot injuries. Clin Podiatr Med Surg. 2015 Apr;32(2):231-8.
107. Mulcahy H. Lisfranc Injury: Current Concepts. Radiol Clin North Am. 2018 Nov;56(6):859-876. Epub 2018 Sep 17.
108. Frey C, Anderson GD, Feder KS. Plantarflexion injury to the metatarsophalangeal joint ("sand toe"). Foot Ankle Int. 1996; 17:576–581.
109. Childs SG. The pathogenesis and biomechanics of turf toe. Orthop Nurs 2006; 25(4):276–80.
110. George E, Harris AH, Dragoo JL, et al. Incidence and risk factors for turf toe injuries in intercollegiate football: data from the National Collegiate Athletic Association injury surveillance system. Foot Ankle Int 2014;35(2):108–15.
111. Kadakia AR, Molloy A. Current concepts review: traumatic disorders of the first metatarsophalangeal joint and sesamoid complex. Foot Ankle Int 2011;32(8): 834–9.
112. Clanton TO, Ford JJ. Turf toe injury. Clin Sports Med 1994;13(4):731–41.
113. McCormick JJ, Anderson RB. Turf toe: anatomy, diagnosis, and treatment. Sports Health 2010;2(6):487–94.
114. Clanton TO, Butler JE, Eggert A. Injuries to the metatarsophalangeal joints in athletes. Foot Ankle 1986;7(3):162–76.
115. Coker TP, Arnold JA, Weber DL. Traumatic lesions of the metatarsophalangeal joint of the great toe in athletes. Am J Sports Med 1978;6(6):326–34.
116. Anderson RB. Turf toe injuries of the hallux metatarsophalangeal joint. Tech Foot Ankle Surg 2002;1(2):102–11.
117. Richardson EG. Injuries to the hallucal sesamoids in the athlete. Foot Ankle 1987; 7(4):229–44.
118. Cavallo M, Natali S, Ruffilli A, Buda R, Vannini F, Castagnini F, Ferranti E, Giannini S. Ankle surgery: focus on arthroscopy. Musculoskelet Surg. 2013 Dec;97(3):237-45.
119. Tol JL, Slim E, van Soest AJ, van Dijk CN. The relationship of the kicking action in soccer and anterior ankle impingement syndrome. A biomechanical analysis. Am J Sports Med. 2002;30(1):45-50.
120. Sanders TG, Rathur SK. Impingement syndromes of the ankle. Magn Reson Imaging Clin N Am. 2008;16(1):29-38.
121. Ogilvie-Harris DJ, Gilbart MK, Chorney K. Chronic pain following ankle sprains in athletes: the role of arthroscopic surgery. Arthroscopy. 1997;13(5):564-574.
122. Mosier-La Clair SM, Monroe MT, Manoli A. Medial impingement syndrome of the anterior tibiotalar fascicle of the deltoid ligament on the talus. Foot Ankle Int. 2000;21(5):385-391.
123. Giannini S, Buda R, Mosca M, Parma A, Di Caprio F. Posterior ankle impingement. Foot Ankle Int. 2013 Mar;34(3):459-65.
124. Giza E, Mandelbaum B. Chronic footballer's ankle. In: Football Traumatology. Springer Milan, 2006:333-351.

125. Kuczinski A, Newman JM, Piuzzi NS, Sodhi N, Doran JP, Khlopas A, Beyer GA, Paulino CB, Mont MA. Trends and Epidemiologic Factors Contributing to Soccer-Related Fractures That Presented to Emergency Departments in the United States. Sports Health. 2019 Jan/Feb;11(1):27-31.
126. Coles CP, Tornetta P 3rd, Obremskey WT, Spitler CA, Ahn J, Mirick G, Krause P, Nana A, Rodriguez-Buitrago A; Orthopaedic Trauma Association's Evidence-Based Quality Value and Safety Committee. Ankle Fractures: An Expert Survey of Orthopaedic Trauma Association Members and Evidence-Based Treatment Recommendations. J Orthop Trauma. 2019 Sep;33(9):e318-e324.
127. Chun DI, Cho JH, Min TH, Park SY, Kim KH, Kim JH, Won SH. Diagnostic Accuracy of Radiologic Methods for Ankle Syndesmosis Injury: A Systematic Review and Meta-Analysis. J Clin Med. 2019 Jul 3;8(7). pii: E968.
128. Aiyer AA, Zachwieja EC, Lawrie CM, Kaplan JRM. Management of Isolated Lateral Malleolus Fractures. J Am Acad Orthop Surg. 2019 Jan 15;27(2):50-59.
129. Bartoníček J, Rammelt S, Tuček M. Posterior Malleolar Fractures: Changing Concepts and Recent Developments. Foot Ankle Clin. 2017 Mar;22(1):125-145.
130. Carter TH, Duckworth AD, White TO. Medial malleolar fractures: current treatment concepts. Bone Joint J. 2019 May;101-B(5):512-521.
131. van Zuuren WJ, Schepers T, Beumer A, Sierevelt I, van Noort A, van den Bekerom MPJ. Acute syndesmotic instability in ankle fractures: A review. Foot Ankle Surg. 2017 Sep;23(3):135-141.
132. Rammelt S, Pitakveerakul A. Hindfoot Injuries: How to Avoid Posttraumatic Varus Deformity? Foot Ankle Clin. 2019 Jun;24(2):325-345.
133. Razik A, Harris M, Trompeter A. Calcaneal fractures: Where are we now? Strategies Trauma Limb Reconstr. 2018 Apr;13(1):1-11.
134. Schepers T, Ginai AZ, Van Lieshout EM, Patka P. Demographics of extra-articular calcaneal fractures: including a review of the literature on treatment and outcome. Arch Orthop Trauma Surg. 2008 Oct;128(10):1099-106.
135. Mills HJ, Horne G. Fractures of the lateral process of the talus. Aust N Z J Surg. 1987 Sep;57(9):643-6.
136. Giannini S, Vannini F. Operative treatment of osteochondral lesions of the talar dome: current concepts review. Foot Ankle Int. 2004 Mar;25(3):168-75.
137. Berkowitz MJ, Kim DH. Process and tubercle fractures of the hindfoot. J Am Acad Orthop Surg. 2005 Dec;13(8):492-502.
138. Kim DH, Hrutkay JM, Samson MM. Fracture of the medial tubercle of the posterior process of the talus: a case report and literature review. Foot Ankle Int. 1996 Mar;17(3):186-8.
139. Tinner C, Sommer C. Fractures of the Lateral Process of the Talus. Foot Ankle Clin. 2018 Sep;23(3):375-395.
140. Giannini S, Cadossi M, Mosca M, Tedesco G, Sambri A, Terrando S, Mazzotti A. Minimally-invasive treatment of calcaneal fractures: A review of the literature and our experience. Injury. 2016 Oct;47 Suppl 4:S138-S146.
141. Ahmed A, Westrick E. Management of Midfoot Fractures and Dislocations. Curr Rev Musculoskelet Med. 2018 Dec;11(4):529-536.
142. Gorbachova T. Midfoot and Forefoot Injuries. Top Magn Reson Imaging. 2015 Aug;24(4):215-21.
143. Marshall D, MacFarlane RJ, Molloy A, Mason L. A review of the management and outcomes of tarsal navicular fracture. Foot Ankle Surg. 2019 Jun 12. pii:S1268-7731(19)30097-9.
144. Clements JR, Dijour F, Leong W. Surgical Management Navicular and Cuboid Fractures. Clin Podiatr Med Surg. 2018 Apr;35(2):145-159.
145. Cenatiempo M, Buzzi R, Bianco S, Iapalucci G, Campanacci DA. Tarsometatarsal joint complex injuries: A study of injury pattern in complete homolateral lesions. Injury. 2019 Jul;50 Suppl 2:S8-S11.
146. Rammelt S, Heineck J, Zwipp H. Metatarsal fractures. Injury. 2004 Sep;35 Suppl 2:SB77-86.
147. Bowes J, Buckley R. Fifth metatarsal fractures and current treatment. World J Orthop. 2016 Dec 18;7(12):793-800.
148. Hatch RL, Hacking S. Evaluation and management of toe fractures. Am Fam Physician. 2003 Dec 15;68(12):2413-8.
149. Brunet JA, Tubin S. Traumatic dislocations of the lesser toes. Foot Ankle Int.1997 Jul;18(7):406-11.
150. Boike A, Schnirring-Judge M, McMillin S. Sesamoid disorders of the first metatarsophalangeal joint. Clin Podiatr Med Surg. 2011 Apr;28(2):269-85, vii.
151. Mandracchia VJ, Mandi DM, Toney PA, Halligan JB, Nickles WA. Fractures of the forefoot. Clin Podiatr Med Surg. 2006 Apr;23(2):283-301, vi.
152. McBryde AM Jr, Anderson RB. Sesamoid foot problems in the athlete. Clin Sports Med. 1988 Jan;7(1):51-60.
153. Fitch KD. Stress fractures of the lower limbs in runners. Aust Fam Physician. 1984;13:511–5.
154. Kahanov L, Eberman LE, Games KE, Wasik M. Diagnosis, treatment, and rehabilitation of stress fractures in the lower extremity in runners. Open Access J Sports Med. 2015;6:87–95.
155. Welck MJ, Hayes T, Pastides P, Khan W, Rudge B. Stress fractures of the foot and ankle. Injury. 2017 Aug;48(8):1722-1726.
156. Gross CE, Nunley JA. Medial-sided stress fractures: medial malleolus and navicular stress fractures. Oper Tech Sports Med. 2014;22:296–304.
157. Ly PN, Fallat L. Hallux fractures: diagnosis and treatment. J Foot Surg. 1992 Jul-Aug;31(4):332-41.
158. Robertson GA, Wood AM. Return to sports after stress fractures of the tibial diaphysis: a systematic review. Br Med Bull. 2015 Jun;114(1):95-111.
159. Caesar BC, McCollum GA, Elliot R, Williams A, Calder JD. Stress fractures of the tibia and medial malleolus. Foot Ankle Clin. 2013 Jun;18(2):339-55.
160. Kor A, Saltzman AT, Wempe PD. Medial malleolar stress fractures. Literature review, diagnosis, and treatment. J Am Podiatr Med Assoc. 2003;93:292–7.
161. Robertson GA, Wood AM. Lower limb stress fractures in sport: Optimising their management and outcome. World J Orthop. 2017 Mar 18;8(3):242-255.
162. Sobczyk K, Moćko K, Sonecki L, Suchy G. Bilateral stress fracture of distal fibula and tibia--case report. Ortop Traumatol Rehabil. 2008 Mar-Apr;10(2):183-90.
163. Davis KW. Imaging pediatric sports injuries: lower extremity. Radiol Clin North Am. 2010 Nov;48(6):1213-35.
164. Srinivasan R. The Hallucal-Sesamoid Complex: Normal Anatomy, Imaging, and Pathology. Semin Musculoskelet Radiol. 2016 Apr;20(2):224-32.
165. Shimozono Y, Hurley ET, Brown AJ, Kennedy JG. Sesamoidectomy for Hallux Sesamoid Disorders: A Systematic Review. J Foot Ankle Surg. 2018 Nov -Dec;57(6):1186-1190.
166. Hossain M, Clutton J, Ridgewell M, Lyons K, Perera A. Stress Fractures of the Foot. Clin Sports Med. 2015 Oct;34(4):769-90.
167. Mandell JC, Khurana B, Smith SE. Stress fractures of the foot and ankle, part 2: site-specific etiology, imaging, and treatment, and differential diagnosis. Skeletal Radiol. 2017 Sep;46(9):1165-1186.

168. Hatch RL, Alsobrook JA, Clugston JR. Diagnosis and management of metatarsal fractures. Am Fam Physician. 2007 Sep 15;76(6):817-26.
169. Weinfeld SB, Haddad SL, Myerson MS. Metatarsal stress fractures. Clin Sports Med. 1997 Apr;16(2):319-38.
170. Thevendran G, Deol RS, Calder JD. Fifth metatarsal fractures in the athlete: evidence for management. Foot Ankle Clin. 2013 Jun;18(2):237-54.
171. Eisele SA, Sammarco GJ. Fatigue fractures of the foot and ankle in the athlete. J Bone Joint Surg Am. 1993;75:290–8.
172. Torg JS. Fractures of the base of the fifth metatarsal distal to the tuberosity. Orthopedics. 1990 Jul;13(7):731-7.
173. Matsuda S, Fukubayashi T, Hirose N. Characteristics of the Foot Static Alignment and the Plantar Pressure Associated with Fifth Metatarsal Stress Fracture History in Male Soccer Players: a Case-Control Study. Sports Med Open. 2017 Dec;3(1):27.
174. Saita Y, Nagao M, Kawasaki T, Kobayashi Y, Kobayashi K, Nakajima H, Takazawa Y, Kaneko K, Ikeda H. Range limitation in hip internal rotation and fifth metatarsal stress fractures (Jones fracture) in professional football players Knee Surg Sports Traumatol Arthrosc. 2018 Jul;26(7):1943-1949.
175. Fujitaka K, Taniguchi A, Isomoto S, Kumai T, Otuki S, Okubo M, Tanaka Y. Pathogenesis of Fifth Metatarsal Fractures in College Soccer Players. Orthop J Sports Med. 2015 Sep 18;3(9):2325967115603654.
176. Lee KT, Park YU, Young KW, Kim JS, Kim JB. The plantar gap: another prognostic factor for fifth metatarsal stress fracture. Am J Sports Med. 2011;39(10):2206-2211.
177. Ortiguera CJ, Fischer DA. A review of the current treatment for fracture of the proximal fifth metatarsal first described by Jones. Orthop Tech Rev. 2000;2:1–2.
178. DeLee JC, Evans JP, Julian J. Stress fracture of the fifth metatarsal. Am J Sports Med. 1983 Sep-Oct;11(5):349-53.
179. Ekstrand J, van Dijk CN. Fifth metatarsal fractures among male professional footballers: a potential career-ending disease. Br J Sports Med. 2013;47(12):754-758.
180. Shakked RJ, Walters EE, O'Malley MJ. Tarsal navicular stress fractures. Curr Rev Musculoskelet Med. 2017 Mar;10(1):122-130.
181. Gross CE, Nunley JA 2nd. Navicular Stress Fractures. Foot Ankle Int. 2015 Sep;36(9):1117-22.
182. Golano P, Fariñas O, Sáenz I. The anatomy of the navicular and periarticular structures. Foot Ankle Clin. 2004 Mar;9(1):1-23.
183. Khan KM, Brukner PD, Kearney C, Fuller PJ, Bradshaw CJ, Kiss ZS. Tarsal navicular stress fracture in athletes. Sports Med. 1994 Jan;17(1):65-76.
184. Saxena A, Fullem B, Hannaford D. Results of treatment of 22 navicular stress fractures and a new proposed radiographic classification system. J Foot Ankle Surg. 2000 Mar-Apr;39(2):96-103.
185. Fowler JRGJ, Boden BP, Pavlov H, Torg JS. The non-surgical and surgical treatment of tarsal navicular stress fractures. Sports Med. 2011;41:613–9.
186. Saxena A, Behan SA, Valerio DL, Frosch DL. Navicular Stress Fracture Outcomes in Athletes: Analysis of 62 Injuries. J Foot Ankle Surg. 2017 Sep -Oct;56(5):943-948.
187. Saxena A, Behan SA, Valerio DL, Frosch DL. Navicular Stress Fracture Outcomes in Athletes: Analysis of 62 Injuries. J Foot Ankle Surg. 2017 Sep -Oct;56(5):943-948.
188. Lorei MP, Hershman EB. Peripheral nerve injuries in athletes. Treatment and prevention. Sports Med. 1993 Aug;16(2):130-47.
189. Schon LC, Baxter DE. Neuropathies of the foot and ankle in athletes. Clin Sports Med. 1990 Apr;9(2):489-509.
190. Ferkel E, Davis WH, Ellington JK. Entrapment Neuropathies of the Foot and Ankle. Clin Sports Med. 2015 Oct;34(4):791-801.
191. Civinini F. Su d'un nervoso gangliare rigonfiamento alla pianta del piede. Lettera anatomica al Dr. Salomone Lampronti. Pistoia, Tip. Bracali, 1835.
192. Di Caprio F, Meringolo R, Shehab Eddine M, Ponziani L. Morton's interdigital neuroma of the foot: A literature review. Foot Ankle Surg. 2018 Apr;24(2):92-98.
193. Adams WR 2nd. Morton's neuroma. Clin Podiatr Med Surg. 2010 Oct;27(4):535-45.
194. Valisena S, Petri GJ, Ferrero A. Treatment of Morton's neuroma: A systematic review. Foot Ankle Surg. 2018 Aug;24(4):271-281.
195. Ahmad M, Tsang K, Mackenney PJ, Adedapo AO. Tarsal tunnel syndrome: A literature review. Foot Ankle Surg. 2012 Sep;18(3):149-52.
196. Doneddu PE, Coraci D, Loreti C, Piccinini G, Padua L. Tarsal tunnel syndrome: still more opinions than evidence. Status of the art. Neurol Sci. 2017 Oct;38(10):1735-1739.
197. Tzika M, Paraskevas G, Natsis K. Entrapment of the superficial peroneal nerve: an anatomical insight. J Am Podiatr Med Assoc. 2015 Mar;105(2):150-9.
198. Flanigan RM, DiGiovanni BF. Peripheral nerve entrapments of the lower leg, ankle, and foot. Foot Ankle Clin. 2011 Jun;16(2):255-74.
199. Pomeroy G, Wilton J, Anthony S. Entrapment neuropathy about the foot and ankle: an update. J Am Acad Orthop Surg. 2015 Jan;23(1):58-66.
200. Heaslet M, Patel D. Entrapment involving the lateral calcaneal branch of the sural nerve: a case study. J Am Podiatr Med Assoc. 2012 Jan-Feb;102(1):75-7.
201. Tu P. Heel Pain: Diagnosis and Management. Am Fam Physician. 2018 Jan 15;97(2):86-93.
202. Lareau CR, Sawyer GA, Wang JH, DiGiovanni CW. Plantar and medial heel pain: diagnosis and management. J Am Acad Orthop Surg. 2014 Jun;22(6):372-80.
203. Saxena A, Fournier M, Gerdesmeyer L, Gollwitzer H. Comparison between extracorporeal shockwave therapy, placebo ESWT and endoscopic plantar fasciotomy for the treatment of chronic plantar heel pain in the athlete. Muscles Ligaments Tendons J. 2013 Jan 21;2(4):312-6. Print 2012 Oct.
204. Bhatty UN, Khan SH, Zubairy AI. Managing the patient with heel pain. Br J Hosp Med (Lond). 2019 Apr 2;80(4):196-200.
205. Saxena A, Hong BK, Yun AS, Maffulli N, Gerdesmeyer L. Treatment of Plantar Fasciitis With Radial Soundwave "Early" Is Better Than After 6 Months: A Pilot Study. J Foot Ankle Surg. 2017 Sep - Oct;56(5):950-953.
206. Gollwitzer H, Saxena A, DiDomenico LA, Galli L, Bouché RT, Caminear DS, Fullem B, Vester JC, Horn C, Banke IJ, Burgkart R, Gerdesmeyer L. Clinically relevant effectiveness of focused extracorporeal shock wave therapy in the treatment of chronic plantar fasciitis: a randomized, controlled multicenter study. J Bone Joint Surg Am. 2015 May 6;97(9):701-8.
207. Sherman KP. The foot in sport. Br J Sports Med. 1999 Feb;33(1):6-13.
208. Giannini S, Catani F, Ceccarelli F, Girolami M, Benedetti MG. Kinematic and isokinetic evaluation of patients with flat foot. Ital J Orthop Traumatol. 1992;18(2):241-51.
209. Giannini S. Kenneth A. Johnson Memorial Lecture. Operative treatment of the flatfoot: why and how. Foot Ankle Int. 1998 Jan;19(1):52-8.
210. Benedetti MG, Berti L, Straudi S, Ceccarelli F, Giannini S. Clinicoradiographic assessment of flexible flatfoot in children. J Am Podiatr Med Assoc. 2010 Nov-Dec;100(6):463-71.

211. Giannini S, Ceccarelli F, Benedetti MG, Faldini C, Grandi G. Surgical treatment of adult idiopathic cavus foot with plantar fasciotomy, naviculocuneiform arthrodesis, and cuboid osteotomy. A review of thirty-nine cases. J Bone Joint Surg Am. 2002;84-A Suppl 2:62-9. PubMed PMID: 12479341.
212. Giannini S, Faldini C, Nanni M, Di Martino A, Luciani D, Vannini F. A minimally invasive technique for surgical treatment of hallux valgus: simple, effective, rapid, inexpensive (SERI). Int Orthop. 2013 Sep;37(9):1805-13.
213. Giannini S, Faldini C, Vannini F, Digennaro V, Bevoni R, Luciani D. The minimally invasive osteotomy "S.E.R.I." (simple, effective, rapid, inexpensive) for correction of bunionette deformity. Foot Ankle Int. 2008 Mar;29(3):282-6.
214. Giannini S, Ceccarelli F, Faldini C, Bevoni R, Grandi G, Vannini F. What's new in surgical options for hallux rigidus? J Bone Joint Surg Am. 2004;86-A Suppl 2:72-83.
215. Pingel C, McDowell C. Subungual Hematoma Drainage. 2019 May 18. StatPearls [Internet]. Treasure Island (FL): StatPearls Publishing; 2019 Jan.
216. Mayeaux EJ Jr, Carter C, Murphy TE. Ingrown Toenail Management. Am Fam Physician. 2019 Aug 1;100(3):158-164.
217. Di Chiacchio N, Di Chiacchio NG. Best way to treat an ingrown toenail. Dermatol Clin. 2015 Apr;33(2):277-82.
218. King MJ. Dermatologic problems in podiatric sports medicine. Clin Podiatr Med Surg. 1997 Jul;14(3):511-24.
219. Omura EF, Rye B. Dermatologic disorders of the foot. Clin Sports Med. 1994 Oct;13(4):825-41.
220. Hoffman PC, Lenet MD, Sherman M. Cutaneous horns: review of literature and case report. J Foot Surg. 1988 Mar-Apr;27(2):130-3.
221. Klein AW, Rish DC. Sports related skin problems. Compr Ther. 1992 Sep;18(9):2-4.
222. Witchey DJ, Witchey NB, Roth-Kauffman MM, Kauffman MK. Plantar Warts: Epidemiology, Pathophysiology, and Clinical Management. J Am Osteopath Assoc. 2018 Feb 1;118(2):92-105.
223. Conklin RJ. Common cutaneous disorders in athletes. Sports Med. 1990 Feb;9(2):100-19.
224. Myerson MS, Fisher RT, Burgess AR, Kenzora JE. Fracture dislocations of the tarsometatarsal joints: end results correlated with pathology and treatment. Foot Ankle. 1986 Apr;6(5):225-42.
225. Leardini A, O'Connor JJ, Giannini S. Biomechanics of the natural, arthritic, and replaced human ankle joint. J Foot Ankle Res. 2014; 7: 8.

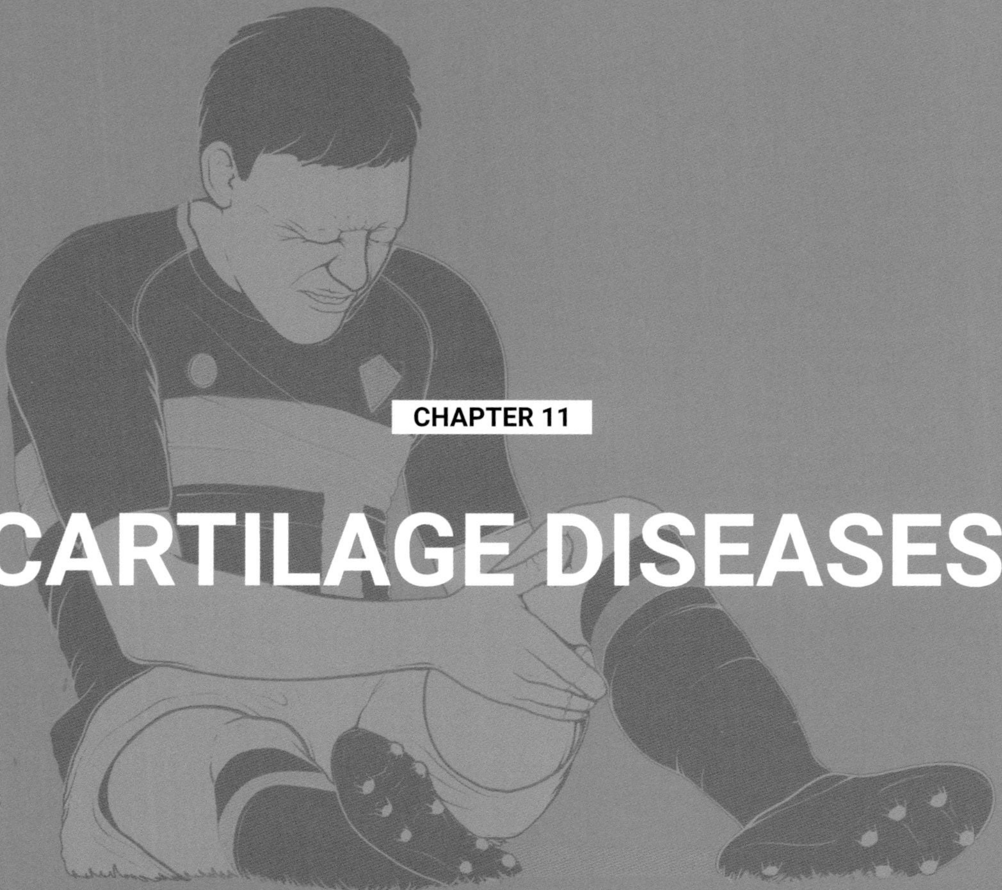

CHAPTER 11

CARTILAGE DISEASES

Roberto Buda [1]
Assunta Pandolfi [2]
Brunella Grigolo [3]
Luca Perazzo [4]
Matteo Parenti [5]
Danilo Bruni [1]

[1] Orthopedics and Traumatology Clinic (Director: R. Buda)
G. d'Annunzio University, Chieti-Pescara, Italy

[2] Department of Medical and Oral Sciences and Biotechnologies
G. d'Annunzio University, Chieti-Pescara, Italy

[3] Ramses Laboratory Manager
IRCCS Istituto Ortopedico Rizzoli, Bologna, Italy

[4] Regional Manager Medical Area FIGC SGS Emilia Romagna

[5] Department of Medicine and Aging Sciences
G. d'Annunzio University, Chieti-Pescara, Italy

Introduction

Soccer, the most popular sport in the world, is played by more than 300 million people. Increasing participation is associated with an increase in articular cartilage injuries in this high-impact sport, particularly at the competitive and world class level.

The incidence and the prevalence of articular cartilage lesions among athletes is considerably higher than in the general population. Treatment goals differ considerably between the professional and recreational athlete. High economic stakes and the generally short duration of a professional sports career influence the treatment selection for the professional athlete, while such parameters weigh differently in recreational sports and have much more limited influence in general population [1].

Traumatic or degenerative focal articular cartilage lesions may represent a serious injury in active sportsmen because they may cause serious reduction in sports performance. Furthermore, similarly to what happens for general population, they may lead to disabilities during daily life professional and recreational activities. This particularly counts for high-demanding sports such as basketball, American football, and soccer, where fast acceleration, deceleration, rotational, and pivoting movements are frequently executed in a non-repetitive fashion. Related symptoms such as pain, swelling, catching, giving way, and locking sensation make focal cartilage lesions an important reason to avoid further sports participation [2, 4]. Among professional athletes, the functional demand of the articular cartilage is even higher, so that articular cartilage lesions represent an even more significant issue to deal with [2]. After the menisci, the anterior cruciate ligament (ACL) and the ankle ligaments, the joint cartilage of the knee and ankle is the most frequently damaged structure in soccer players. Injures to the articular cartilage of the knee and ankle is recognized as the most important cause of functional disability in elite soccer players and may lead to early degenerative changes in these joints during, and after, a professional sports career [5].

Several surgical treatments for focal articular cartilage lesions in the general population have extensively proven to be effective, reproducible, and reliable. Consequently, evidence-based treatment algorithms have been designed and clinically applied [6, 7]. Anyway, treatment goals are considerably different between general population, recreational sportsmen, and professional sports players. Recreational players mainly hope for a rapid pain relief, functional recovery, and if possible, some further occasional sports participation. Conversely, professional players need a fast return to their previous, high-demanding, activity level without the blemish of having joint damage. Also, the generally short duration of the professional career makes a rapid recovery even more desirable for economic reasons and, not uncommonly, for legal implications.

This scenario depicts a complex clinical dilemma for the responsible physician and for the orthopaedic surgeon. Because of the excessive forces and the high mechanical load exposed to the regenerated cartilage and the wish for a fast rehabilitation, the treatment strategies for professional athletes might be different from those for recreational athletes. End-career contracts, high financial stakes, sports media pressures, and commitments towards the professional sports organization could also influence the process towards an optimal patient-specific treatment strategy. Therefore, understanding the need for good-quality cartilage regeneration in high-impact sports is necessary and should be the basis for a proper personalized treatment selection. Emphasis should be put on functionality during the sports career as well as on quality of life afterwards.

Existing articular cartilage repair techniques can return the athlete with articular cartilage injury to high-impact sports, but treatment does not produce normal articular cartilage, and this limits the success rate and durability of current cartilage repair in athletes. Novel scientific concepts and treatment techniques that apply modern tissue engineering technologies promise further advancement in the treatment of these challenging injuries in the high demand athletic population.

Epidemiology and pathophysiology

According to current literature, high-impact sport activities may produce elevated mechanical stresses to the articular cartilage, leading to temporary or permanent changes in cartilage and subchondral bone turnover and tridimensional architecture, and vascularity [8-10]. Defects of the joint cartilage have a very limited healing capacity. Therefore, injuries resulting from trauma or repetitive loading can lead to osteoarthritis over time.

High-impact sport activities, and particularly soccer, have been linked to increases in serum biomarker profiles as well as to changes in articular cartilage homeostasis [11, 12]. For this reason, exposing the articular cartilage to repetitive mechanical overloads could slow cartilage recovery instead of improving the biomechanical resistance, potentially leading to the development of full-thickness articular cartilage defects.

In soccer players, the intensity of high stresses and pivotal movements to the knee and the ankle is extreme, because of intense and demanding training programs and, for the elite soccer players, often 3 competitive games per week. Therefore, the documented high prevalence (35%; range, 18%-63%) of focal articular cartilage lesions among professional and recreational athletes, compared to a prevalence of 5% to 11% in the general population, is a logical result of the high-demanding professional career. This exemplifies the need for better understanding the impact and evaluation of treatment outcomes [2, 13-15].

Up to 60% of patients demonstrate significant cartilage damage on arthroscopic evaluation. In more than half of these patients, additional damage to the ligaments and menisci is present. The patella and the femoral condyle are most often affected, followed by injury to the tibial plateau. Anterior Cruciate Ligament (ACL) ruptures, which occur with up to a 3-fold higher probability in female athletes, have a 20% to 60% rate of chondral and osteochondral defects, increasing the risk for osteoarthritis up to 12 times in high-demand and pivoting athletes.

Injury of articular cartilage surfaces occurs in 36% of soccer athletes, which is more than twice than that in the general population. Higher injury rates are noted in competitive matches than during practice, in athletes with body mass index (BMI) over 30, and in certain playing positions. Besides BMI, age, female gender, duration of symptoms, defect location and size, number of previous interventions, and sensorimotor capability are additional important factors affecting return to sports. Most of current literature studies have investigated this issue in the knee but there is little evidence for the hip or ankle. To date, there is no published data on the epidemiology of hip and ankle focal articular cartilage lesions in athletes.

Articular cartilage injury in soccer athletes may occur in two separate pathways. Chronic repetitive loading of the articular cartilage during sports activity can lead to progressive articular cartilage degradation with accumulation of catabolic enzymes and cytokines, fragmentation of collagen and aggrecans, and resultant fissuring and progressive breakdown of the articular surface. The sports-associated chronic biochemical and metabolic changes are similar to the changes described in early osteoarthritis (OA) and contribute to the progressive joint degeneration observed in athletes. The high demands on the joint observed in impact athletes lead to a high incidence of cartilage abnormalities in asymptomatic athletes. Continued high-intensity loading, particularly in association with additional joint pathology, such as meniscal deficiency, joint instability or tridimensional alignment abnormality, can cause symptoms and lead to

rapid progression of cartilage injury. These results are supported by the up to 12-fold increased risk of knee OA in soccer athletes, particularly at the elite level.
Normal articular cartilage has the ability to adjust to the level of activity with an intrinsic biofeedback-like response. Increasing weight-bearing activity in athletes increases the volume and thickness of articular cartilage, and in the healthy athlete, there is a positive linear dose-response relationship between repetitive loading activities and articular cartilage function. However, this dose-response curve reaches a threshold after which there is maladaptation and articular cartilage injury develops. High-impact joint loading above this threshold decreases cartilage proteoglycan content, increases levels of degradative enzymes and causes chondrocyte apoptosis. If the integrity of the functional weight-bearing unit is lost, either through acute sports-related injury or chronic microtrauma, a chondropaenia results, consisting in loss of articular cartilage volume and stiffness, increased contact pressures, and development or progression of articular cartilage defects. Without intervention, chondropaenia contributes to the deterioration of articular cartilage function in athletes and can ultimately progress to OA and the inability to further participate in the sport.
Besides a chronic pathway, acute traumatic athletic cartilage injury in soccer players can frequently occur in association with other joint injuries, such as ligament or meniscal tears or fractures and dislocations. Depending on the force on the joint, acute traumatic cartilage injury may present with a spectrum of severity, such as (1) acute macroscopic chondral and osteochondral defects, or (2) a less obvious ultrastructural injury to the articular cartilage with disruption of chondral collagen and the proteoglycan network, as well as direct cell damage and apoptosis that may lead to gradual degradation of the articular cartilage. Irrespective of their origin, articular cartilage injuries in soccer athletes will often limit the athlete's ability to play sport. Besides causing loss of playing time, progressive articular cartilage degeneration and OA, which occurs in up to 32% of soccer players, is a major cause for disability and retirement from the sport.
The rationale for management of cartilage defects is based on understanding the pathophysiology underlying chondral lesions. The relative avascularity of articular cartilage prevents a physiological inflammatory response to cartilage injury and limits spontaneous repair of articular cartilage injury. Repetitive loading of the injured articular cartilage during sports activity leads to cellular degeneration, accumulation of catabolic enzymes and cytokines, disruption of collagen ultrastructure, and progressive macroscopic breakdown of the articular surface. Owing to the detrimental effect of high-impact articular loading, articular cartilage surface restoration should withstand the substantial mechanical joint stresses of up to 20 times body weight generated during high-impact, pivoting sports. Goals of treatment are to reduce pain, increase mobility, improve knee function, and ideally allow the player to return to sport at the pre-injury level. Several surgical techniques have achieved successful return to sport after articular cartilage repair with variable durability. Unfortunately, anyway, surgery does not produce completely normal hyaline articular cartilage. All coexisting joint pathologies, such as instability, malalignment, or meniscal deficiency, must be corrected to produce a successful and lasting cartilage repair. Concomitant pathology must be addressed to the initial surgery or subsequently in a staged approach. The simultaneous approach reduces the need for prolonged, repeated rehabilitation and absence from sport, and does not delay return to sport. Importantly, rehabilitation is critical for the success of any cartilage repair procedure and new concepts for cartilage rehabilitation in the athlete continue to develop.
Evidence-based treatment selection for the treatment of focal articular cartilage lesions in the general and recreational sports population is mainly based on the size of the lesion and the involvement of the subchondral bone. Clinical outcomes relevant for this population, such as pain reduction and functional improvement, were taken into account when developing these algorithms, where the goal was supposed to be resumption of daily life activities and working ability. However, a return to the preinjury sports activity level is much more important when dealing with high-level soccer players.

In addition, articular cartilage repair in these patients not only requires a regenerative product that can withstand the previously mentioned excessive shear stresses, cutting movements, rotations, pivoting movements during the career but should also be capable of allowing a normal function after this. Finally, when dealing with professional and recreational players at the beginning of their career, the responsible physician should also take the need for long-term performance of the regenerated cartilage into account. With this in mind, the better structural repair after ACI and OAT and the decrease in treatment success over time after microfracture are reasons to consider ACI or OAT as a first-line treatment option for these young sportsmen.

Bone marrow stimulation techniques, such as microfractures or microperforations, and transplantation methods, such as autologous chondrocyte implantation (ACI) and osteochondral autologous trans-plantation (OAT), are the most frequently applied treatment options for the surgical restoration of focal articular cartilage lesions in soccer players.

Reparative techniques

First-generation microfracture procedure still represents the most frequently used cartilage repair technique in athletes and uses pluripotent bone marrow-derived mesenchymal stem cells (MSC) which subsequently produce a mixed fibrocartilage repair tissue that contains varying amounts of type II collagen.

Broadly accepted indications for microfractures are cartilage lesion of grade 3-4, area of the cartilage lesion <10 mm^2 for the ankle and <20 mm^2 for the knee, depth <5 mm for both joints, healthy subchondral bone, normal alignment and stability for both joints. In selected patients, microfractures are an accepted technique also for degenerative lesions, whether alternative procedures are not a viable option.

The purpose of the microfracture technique is to develop micropenetrations into the subchondral bone of the debrided focal cartilage defect in order to allow bone marrow, consisting of multipotent stromal cells (MSCs), to enter the intra-articular space (figg. 1, 2). This should form a clot in the cartilage defect populated with MSCs and growth factors that eventually lead to functional fibrocartilaginous tissue [16, 17].

According to current literature, after microfracture, knee function improves in 58-95% of athletes and activity scores improve significantly. In total, 44-95% of athletes returned to competition after microfracture, 57% at the pre-injury level. Best results are with surgery within 12 months of injury, in athletes younger than 40 years and lesion size ≤200 mm [18]. After initial functional improvement, there was deterioration of knee function in 47-80% of athletes 18-36 months post surgery, but knee function still remained better than before surgery after 10 years. The exact reason for the functional decline is not known but insufficient volume of cartilage repair, limited integration of new material to the surrounding cartilage or subchondral bone changes may contribute.

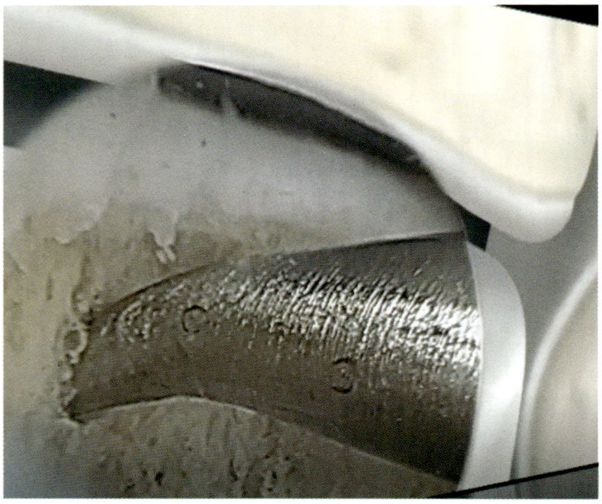
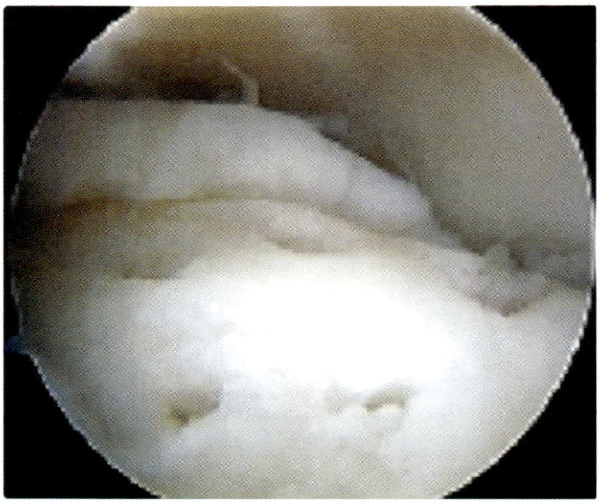

Figures 1-2 - Arthroscopic microfractures on full thickness cartilage lesion of the talus

Biological substitutive techniques

The concept of using cartilage cells (chondrocytes) in the repair of articular cartilage defects was first reported in humans in 1994 [19]. Autologous chondrocyte transplantation is a two-stage technique for hyaline-like repair of full-thickness articular cartilage lesions in the knee. It has provided long-term functional improvement for up to 20 years and functional MRI, using dGemric technology, showing repair tissue quality similar to the surrounding normal cartilage 18 years after implantation. Prospective multicenter studies in athletes, including soccer players, have been published, showing good to excellent results in 72-96% athletes, with improved activity scores in 82-100% [5]. Between 33% and 96% returned to high-impact athletics, while 60-80% were at the same skill level. Return to sport was better for competitive soccer athletes (83%) and adolescent athletes (96%), and 87% of returning athletes maintained their ability to perform 52 months after surgery. Athletes with single lesions, age <25 years, and short preoperative intervals had the best rate of return to sport.

In ACI original technique, as clinically described by Brittberg et al., autologous chondrocytes are harvested from a non-weight-bearing anatomical site in the knee, generally represented by the upper lateral portion of the femoral trochlea, expanded in vitro, and reimplanted in a second surgical procedure [19]. Limitations of this first-generation technique included its invasiveness, prolonged postoperative rehabilitation, and graft delamination from periosteal hypertrophy. Sport-specific rehabilitation has been successful, reducing the time to return to sport to as low as 10 months; substitution of the periosteum with a collagen membrane has reduced the risk for hypertrophy and delamination while maintaining the excellent clinical results of the first-generation technique.

Through the years, this technique has evolved into different variations, all aiming at a more reliable biological response, improved ease of surgical use, and a better clinical outcome. Second-generation autologous cartilage transplantation techniques use biodegradable scaffolds to temporarily support the chondrocytes until they are replaced by matrix components synthesized from the implanted cells. Scaffolds may be based on carbohydrates, protein polymers, artificial polymers, or composite polymer matrices. The biomatrix seeded with chondrocytes reduces surgical invasiveness and demonstrated improved knee function scores, KOOS sports and activity scores, minimal graft hypertrophy, and hyaline-like repair tissue.

One of the most popular evolutions of ACI technique is the matrix-associated chondrocyte implantation (MACI), which reduces donor site morbidity by avoiding the use of a periosteal suture flap to improve primary graft stability. Moreover, the implantation of cultured cells in 3-dimensional matrices reduces the surgery-related morbidity and follows a faster and easier rehabilitation, as it can be performed by a mini-arthrotomy or even arthroscopically [20]. Arthroscopic MACI has been described and showed improvement of knee function in 90% of athletes/patients, with improvement persisting to 5 years. Better results were seen in patients younger than 30 years and athletes participating in higher level competitive sports.

Osteochondral autograft transplantation (OAT) restores hyaline cartilage by harvesting cylindrical osteochondral grafts from areas of limited weight-bearing and transfers them into small to midsize (1-4 cm^2) defects of weight-bearing cartilage in the knee or ankle joint using a press-fit technique. Prospective studies have evaluated this technique in athletes and demonstrated up to 95% good or excellent results, with significantly improved knee function scores after 26-36 months [21, 22]. Return to athletic activity was reported in 61-93%, as early as 4-9 months postoperatively. Some athletes showed a decrease of athletic activity after 7 years [22]. Longer preoperative symptoms and age >30 years were associated with decreased return to sport. Donor site morbidity may occur immediately after surgery, but this appears to resolve.

Osteochondral allografts (i.e. from cadavers) avoid donor site morbidity and restore hyaline cartilage in large and deep chondral and osteochondral lesions. To optimize chondrocyte viability, matrix composition and mechanical properties, hypothermically stored cartilage grafts should be implanted within 14-21 days of graft harvest. The best function and fastest incorporation is observed for thin grafts (<15 mm). Osteochondral allograft transplantation in athletes allowed 88% to return to sport and 79% to their pre-injury level [23]. Better outcomes were seen in athletes younger than 25 years and in those with symptoms for less than 1 year. Besides osteochondral allograft and autograft, synthetic bilayer scaffolds have been developed that mimic the anatomy of osteochondral plugs. However, the results in the high demand athletic population have not yet been established [24].

Regenerative techniques

To address the limitations of existing cartilage repair technology, the continued scientific and clinical evolution aims to provide complex and individualized treatment options to treat articular cartilage injury in the soccer player. These evolving technologies aim to achieve hyaline cartilage repair of higher quality, faster progression of cartilage repair rehabilitation with quicker return to sports and more consistent durability of high-impact sports participation. Since injuries to articular cartilage of the knee present one of the most common causes of permanent disability in athletes, management of articular cartilage in this high- demand population has important long-term implications.

Platelet-rich plasma (PRP) has been used safely; its proposed healing properties are attributed to the increased concentrations of autologous growth factors and secretory proteins that may enhance recruitment, proliferation, and differentiation of cells involved in tissue regeneration [25]. While the few studies evaluating platelet aggregates in the treatment of chondral lesions or OA report decreased pain in the post injection period if compared with hyaluronic acid [26], these do not allow for comparative analysis of clinical effectiveness. There is currently insufficient evidence for PRP to be recommended in key guidelines, but well-designed randomized controlled trials are being conducted to test the clinical utility of PRP in this setting. Besides injections of growth factor combinations, injections of individual growth factors, such as transforming growth factor β3 and bone morphogenetic protein 7, to induce chondrogenic marker gene expression for type II/IX collagen, cartilage oligomeric matrix protein, and aggrecan with both qualitative and quantitative improvement of joint articular cartilage or repair tissue, have been tested; controlled clinical studies are pending.

New technologies have been developed to overcome the limitations of first-generation marrow stimulation technologies. These second-generation technologies are based on marrow-derived MSC and use modern tissue engineering technologies, such as growth factors and scaffolds, to increase and facilitate chondrogenic differentiation for both qualitative and quantitative improvement of repair cartilage tissue [27]. Clinical evaluation of these mesenchymal augmentation and scaffold stimulation technologies has been encouraging. Bone marrow aspirate concentrate (BMAC) uses a one-step surgery with concentrated MSC, aspirated from the pelvis and injected under a collagen I/III matrix. Early clinical results show improved cartilage repair compared with microfractures in animal models and significant improvement of joint function in humans [28]. BMAC may be particularly useful in the treatment of lesions of the tibia plateau where access is often limited by location. Clinical evidence demonstrating efficacy is evolving, but while BMAC offers an interesting therapeutic perspective, its clinical data, specifically in the athletic population, are still limited.

Using advanced tissue engineering technology, a new two-step technique that uses autologous chondrocytes seeded in a bovine collagen gel/sponge scaffold has been developed. The three-dimensional (3D) construct is incubated under defined hydrostatic pressure in a specifically designed bioreactor, stimulating the chondrocytes to produce cartilage matrix proteins and form a firm sponge-like neocartilage containing both active chondrocytes and extracellular matrix (ECM; NeoCart, Histogenics, Waltham, Usa). Implantation is performed using a novel bioadhesive that facilitates a minimally invasive surgical approach. Clinical trials showed good cartilage fill, peripheral integration, and pain relief in 86%

of patients up to 2 years after implantation. MRI T2 mapping demonstrated hyaline cartilage in 57% [29]. A larger prospective, randomized comparison of this technique with microfractures is currently being completed.

Repair of focal articular cartilage defects using allograft cartilage fragments has been recently described (DeNovo, Zimmer, Warsaw, Usa). Hyaline cartilage fragments are obtained from juvenile donor joints and contain viable juvenile chondrocytes that possess significantly (up to ×100) higher metabolic activity than adult chondrocytes. The small cartilage particles are moulded to the size of the recipient cartilage defect and implanted using fibrin glue fixation and a minimally invasive arthrotomy. Preliminary results from a prospective, multicenter case series, with follow-up of 25 patients of up to 24 months, demonstrated improved IKDC and KOOS scores as well as good cartilage repair tissue fill of the defects on MRI [30]. Larger, intermediate-term prospective clinical evaluation is currently under way using this technique to further evaluate the long-term results of this technique.

Although articular cartilage is generally thought to have poor self-renewal capacity, articular cartilage lesions undergo perfect regeneration in the womb [31, 32]. Scar-free fetal healing occurs in many tissue types and continues to inspire the design of regenerative environments to aid in healing of adult tissues. In articular cartilage, one of the most intriguing discoveries of the past decade is the existence of cartilage progenitor cells (CPCs) in the tissue. These progenitor cells are distinguishable from resident chondrocytes by their migratory behaviour, multidifferentiation capacity, and colony forming potential. In young healthy cartilage, the outgrowth of CPCs can form abundant neocartilage. Interestingly, CPCs may also be present in adult tissue, and repair tissue from late stage OA cartilage and their migration can be stimulated by mechanical damage, possibly through the release of chemoattractants from apoptotic cells.

With the identification of progenitor cells in articular cartilage comes the hope that these cells could be harnessed to heal damaged cartilage. If this approach were successful, it would eliminate the extensive cell culturing and expensive regulatory complexities required for cell-based therapies. A successful application of CPCs, however, will require a biomaterial which induces migration, but also has the optimal biomechanical, immunological and biochemical 3D environment to control the fate of the regenerating cells. This material should, furthermore, be injectable, adherent to the lesion surface and have tunable biostability/ degradability. Indeed, the field is turning increasingly towards acellular biomaterials with boosted bioactivity and functionality. Scaffolds based on decellularised cartilage ECM represent one fruitful way to incorporate some of the vast complexity of the native chondrocyte microenvironment into a scaffold. Other options are materials with cues for cell migration and adhesion and growth factor binding which are anti-inflammatory, antioxidant, and/or antiangiogenic. Although, to date, there is not a single biomaterial which incorporates all of the above properties, combinations of polymeric systems, called interpenetrating networks, can increase the overall functionality of the material.

Two-step technique

Autologous chondrocyte implantation (ACI) has been successfully used for the treatment of osteochondral lesions of the talus and the knee. This technique permits the repair of osteochondral lesions of the knee and the ankle with a high percentage of hyaline-like cartilage tissue and over the years it has also been applied to different joints, such as the hip, the elbow, and the shoulder. Although no severe complications have been reported to date, one of the main problems of this surgical strategy is related to the harvesting of the cartilage slice from a healthy knee, the so-called donor-site morbidity effect. In addition, it has been shown that knee cartilage differs in composition from ankle cartilage and theoretically also from other joints, having a lower level of proteoglycan synthesis and less active chondrocytes. These different characteristics might explain why the ankle is less affected by progressive osteoarthritis than the knee. This could mean that cartilage that is harvested from the knee may not represent the ideal solution to be cross implanted in different joints. In order to avoid damage to a healthy knee due to the harvesting of cartilage, and to utilize cartilage with the appropriate characteristics for implantation in an ankle joint, it may be reasonable to use the detached osteochondral fragments for chondrocyte cultures. For these reasons, Sandro Giannini and Roberto Buda have investigated the ability of the chondrocytes harvested from detached osteochondral fragment to proliferate and to serve as a viable source of cells for ACI in the repair of ankle and knee cartilage defects [33, 34].

At the beginning of this procedure, a standard arthroscopy of the ankle or of the knee was performed, which permitted fragment removal, a mild osteochondral shaving, and an accurate measurement of the lesion size. The detached fragments obtained from the injury site were collected and processed for chondrocyte isolation, and the cells thereby obtained were used for real-time polymerase chain reaction (PCR) and the PicoGreen proliferation tests.

The chondrocyte so obtained were implanted 30 days after harvesting using a Hyalograft-C membrane as a scaffold (Fab Advanced Biopolymers, Abano Terme, Padova, Italy). In both groups, the second arthroscopic step was performed using traditional anteromedial and anterolateral arthroscopic portals. The lesion was accurately shaved and sized. The chondrocytes were directly supported on an autoadhesive hyaluronan patch, which was arthroscopically positioned over the lesion. Fibrin glue was used to improve the stability of the transplanted matrix. Should the lesion have a depth >5 mm, cancellous bone grafting is required before scaffold implantation.

Recent papers have demostrated that the use of cartilage regenerative surgical procedures, such as MACI, as salvage procedures for young, active patients affected by chondral and osteochondral lesions in osteoarthritic knees, led to a limited improvement, with the majority of patients experiencing failure at long-term follow-up. Although a minor subpopulation experienced favorable and stable improvement, the use of MACI for such a challenging indication remains questionable until responding patients can be profiled. Despite ACI techniques have currently been nearly completely abandoned, they have represented an important step forward in developing new surgical strategies to treat cartilage lesions in young active patients [35].

One-step technique

Sandro Giannini, Roberto Buda and Brunella Grigolo have developed a one-step technique to transplant the entire bone-marrow cellular pool instead of isolated and expanded mesenchymal stem cells, so allowing the cells to be processed directly in the operating room, avoiding the need for a laboratory phase [36, 37, 38, 39]. The procedure can be performed arthroscopically using the same instrumentations and surgical tools previously used for ACI; furthermore, autologous platelet-rich fibrin (PRF) can be added in order to provide additional growth factors to the construct.

The technique has been successfully used to treat classical talar dome lesions in the posteromedial or anterolateral region of the talar dome, lesions of the medial/lateral femoral condyle, and patella-femoral joint in the knee and tibial plafond in the ankle. The greatest success achieved in repairing these lesions arthroscopically has occurred combining the cell, scaffold and growth factors trilogy in the surgical repair. Thanks to technical improvements, regenerative medical technologies have quickly moved forward from traditional ACI, overpassing the problems related to high costs and the need for two surgical steps. Conversely, bone marrow derived cells transplantation (BMDCT) represents a technique which has demonstrated its ability to provide a repair of the lesion by hyaline cartilage in a one-step procedure. Furthermore, its versatility to be combined with platelet gel and bioengineered scaffolds improves the potential to support multipoint mesenchymal cells growth and chondrogenic differentiation. Through this one-step technique, the complete bone-marrow cellular network is transplanted, instead of previously selected, isolated and expanded stem cells. So, Mesenchymal Stem Cells are implanted with all the mononuclear bone marrow derived cells and with high regenerative potential factors and cytokines present in the naive micro ambient.

For the ankle, the one-step arthroscopic treatment

VIDEO 1

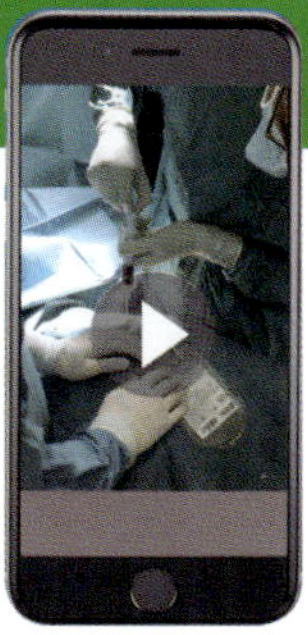

Arthroscopic bone marrow derived cell transplantation in osteochondral lesion of the talus

VIDEO 2

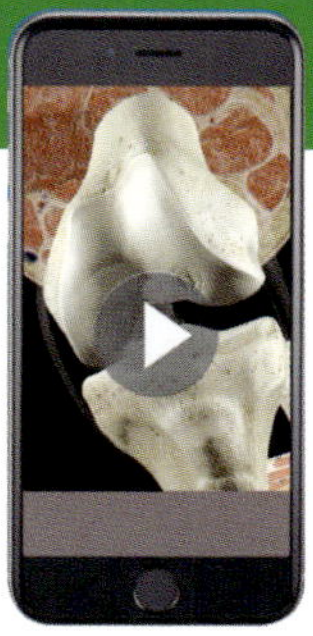

Arthroscopic bone marrow derived cell transplantation in osteochondral lesion of the knee

is indicated for focal grade 3-4 osteochondral lesions of the talar dome or tibial plafond according to the International Cartilage Repair Society (ICRS) classification These lesions have an area of 1 cm x 1 cm and a maximum depth of 5 mm. Should a lesion with a depth of more than 5 mm be detected, autologous bone grafting is recommended. Patients older than 60 years, patients with degenerative joint disease, rheumatoid arthritis, kissing lesions are not candidate for this technique. Malalignment and joint instability have to be addressed and corrected in the same surgical procedure (video 1).

For the knee, the procedure is indicated in patients with grade 3-4 ICRS osteochondral lesions involving the femoral condyle or the patella-femoral joint, with clinical symptoms such as pain, swelling, locking, or giving-way (video 2).

The first phase of the surgical procedure consists of PRF gel production. The PRF gel is produced with an automatic system the day before the operation or the same day; 120 ml of venous blood are harvested with a size 16 needle connected to a bowl previously prepared with anticoagulant solution. The bowl is inserted into the Vivostat System (Vivolution A/S, 3460, Birkeroed, Denmark) and processed. At the end of the processing cycle, a syringe containing 6 ml of PRF is extracted and stored at -35°C or used immediately. If stored, the solution must be slowly heated to normal ambient temperature for 30 minutes before use.

The bone marrow is aspired from the posterior iliac crest after standard sterile surgical field preparation, with the patient in a prone position and already under spinal or general anesthesia. The equipment for bone marrow harvesting, concentration and implantation was developed at Rizzoli Orthopedic Institute in collaboration with Novagenit (Mezzolombardo, Trento, Italy).

A bone marrow needle (11 G x 100 mm) is inserted 3 cm deep into the iliac crest bone and a total of 60 ml of bone marrow is collected and placed in a bag preloaded with 500 UI of epsodilave in 10 ml of saline solution. Multiple aspirations are performed through the same skin incision, collecting 5 ml of bone marrow each time, using different locations to maximize the collection of stroll cells and reduce the dilution arising from peripheral blood aspiration.

The bone marrow volume is reduced by eliminating the plasma cells and the red blood cells, increasing stroll cells concentration. A cell separator-concentrator (Res-Q, ThermoGenesis, Rancho Cordova, CA) is positioned in the operating room and in 12 minutes it provides 6 ml of concentrated cells. The patient is then positioned supine with a tourniquet applied. A standard knee or ankle arthroscopy is performed. The cartilage lesion is inspected and a flipped cannula is inserted into the lesion to enable insertion of the surgical tools and to retract the surrounding fat pad from the operative field. The lesion is derided until it results in an area with regular healthy cartilage margins for biomaterial implantation.

The lesion is sized and measured with a probe. A hyaluronic acid membrane (Hyalofast, Fidia Ad-

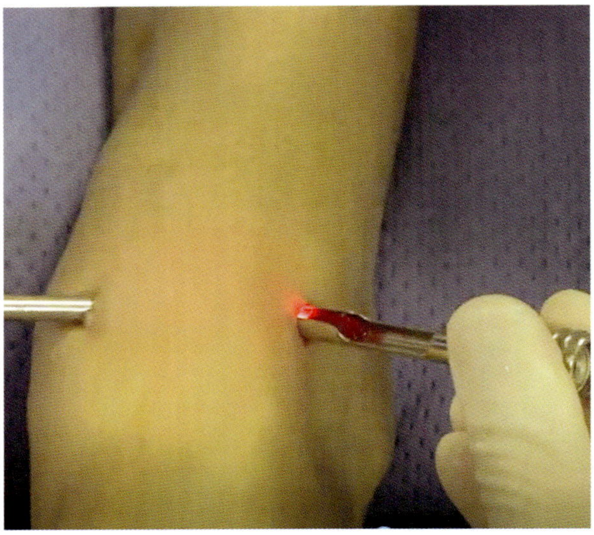

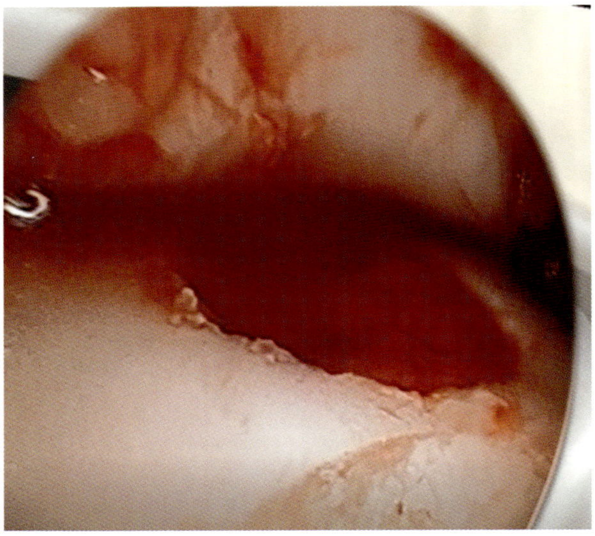

Figures 3-4 - Arthroscopic positioning of the cell-loaded matrix

vanced Biopolymers, Italy) or a collagen membrane (IOR-G1, Novagenit, Mezzolombardo, Trento, Italy) are used for cell support. Approximately 2 ml of concentrated marrow and 1 ml of PRF are loaded onto the membrane and lastly absorbed thanks to its highly hydrophilic structure. The bio construct is accurately clipped according to the size and the shape of the lesion previously determined. The cannula is then inserted through the arthroscopic access closer to the lesion using a tracer, then the tracer is removed and the joint irrigation is stopped. The joint is completely dried and the biomaterial is applied in the window cut out of the cannula and guided to the edge of the lesion (figg. 3, 4). The cannula is removed and the material is finely tuned to perfectly adhere to the lesion using a probe. The PRF is applied to cover the lesion, providing additional growth factors and improving immediate stability of the implant. The joint is cycled to several flexion/extension movements to check implant stability throughout complete range of motion. Skin accesses are closed and a standard medication is applied.

Bone marrow aspirate intra-articular injection

Mesenchimal stem cells contained in the bone marrow are a promising option for the treatment of knee, hip, and ankle osteoarthritis. MSCs are multipotent cells that exhibit strong self-renewal abilities, combined with a differentiation capacity to form chondrocytes, adipocytes, and osteocytes. These cells also have very important local paracrine effects to alter their local micro-environment to conditions which are favourable for regeneration and repair [40, 41, 42].

Bearing in mind the limitations of BMAC concentration technique, we try to find a new solution to have a simple, fast, well-tolerated procedure avoiding high costs, long hospitalization, complications, or adverse effects.

Intra-articular injection of bone marrow is a simple, minimally invasive, and efficient delivery procedure that could be done in day surgery without overnight stay (video 3). A large number of preclinical studies have proved the beneficial effects of intra articular delivery of MSCs on cartilage morphology and histology, showing a better tissue repair and less cartilage destruction.

In accordance with this, a growing number of clinical trials revealed that MSC therapy via intra-articular injection reduce pain and improve articular cartilage regeneration and physical function by stimulating cartilage regeneration.

Our technique consists in the intra-articular injection of 3 ml of bone marrow aspirate mixed with a pre-filled syringe of high molecular weight highly purified sodium hyaluronate. The hyaluronic acid acts as a vehicle for mesenchymal stem cells within the joint affected by OA.

With the patient in a prone position on the operating table, the posterior iliac crest was surgically prepped and draped in the usual fashion. A combination of conscious sedation and local anesthe-

VIDEO 3

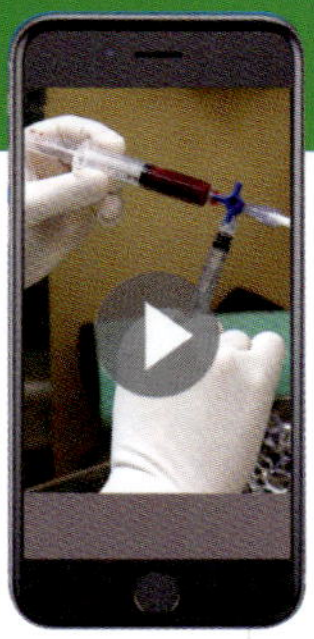

Intra-articular injection of bone marrow aspirate

sia (1% lidocaine) was used. Prior to aspiration, an 11-Gauge Bone Access Needle (Medtronic, Inc) and a 10 ml syringe are flushed with heparin (5,000 U/20ml) and then filled with 1 ml heparin solution.

Using a stab incision, the bone access needle is inserted and advanced through the periosteum of the anterior superior iliac spine. After the periosteum is pierced, the driver and stylet are removed and the 10 ml syringe is used to aspirate 3 ml of bone marrow. There was extra care to hold the needle still throughout the procedure in order to reduce peripheral blood contamination (hemodilution) [43].

When the harvest procedure is completed, the wound is treated and the patient is turned in supine position. Meanwhile, the 3 ml of bone marrow aspirate is mixed with hyaluronic acid using a 3-way stopcock luer lock connector. For the knee joint 3 ml of HA are used, but for the ankle joint the quantity is reduced to 1.5 ml. Final product is collected in a 20 ml syringe.

Injections were performed using an anterolateral approach to the knee joint by the same physician without anesthesia or other drugs, in order to prevent any interaction with the bone marrow. Immediately following injection, the knee joint was passively moved throughout its range of motion to disseminate the fluid throughout the joint.

Mean duration of bone marrow aspirate intra-articular injection procedure was approximately 15 minutes.

The patients were allowed full weight bearing and instructed to return to light activity as tolerated avoiding oral NSAIDs and corticosteroids. Within four weeks patients were allowed to return to full activities. There was no other therapeutic intervention (bracing, physical therapy, etc).

Literature review

The ability to return to soccer presents a critical aspect for successful treatment of articular cartilage injury in the soccer player [44]. Research studies by the Fédération Internationale de Football Association (FIFA) Medical Assessment and Research Center (F-MARC) have identified articular cartilage injuries as a serious knee injury that can be associated with inability to play. Because return to sports presents a key measure of successful outcome for injured players, many papers have been published regarding the ability to return to sport following articular cartilage repair, with a special focus on soccer players and the factors that can influence their ability to return to competition. Among these papers, the largest majority of them focuses on knee cartilage lesions and reports on ankle joint are a minority.

Mithoefer et al. reported on twenty studies describing 1,469 athletes including soccer players treated for articular cartilage injuries of the knee with microfracture, ACI, OAT, and osteochondral allograft transplantation. They concluded that defect size <2 cm^2 was associated with a significantly higher rate of return to high-impact athletics after microfracture and OAT and supports the established indications of these two techniques for smaller defects. Moreover, they stated that return to sports participation can be successfully achieved by all techniques.

Andrade et al. [45] performed a systematic literature review to explore the available scientific literature on the prevalence of articular cartilage and/or osteochondral lesions in soccer players' knees, and overview the surgical procedures and functional outcomes and return to sports. The authors collected data on a total of 217 articular cartilage and/or osteochondral lesions, where the medial and lateral femoral condyles were the most common sites of lesion. The surgical procedures investigated were mosaicplasty, microfracture,

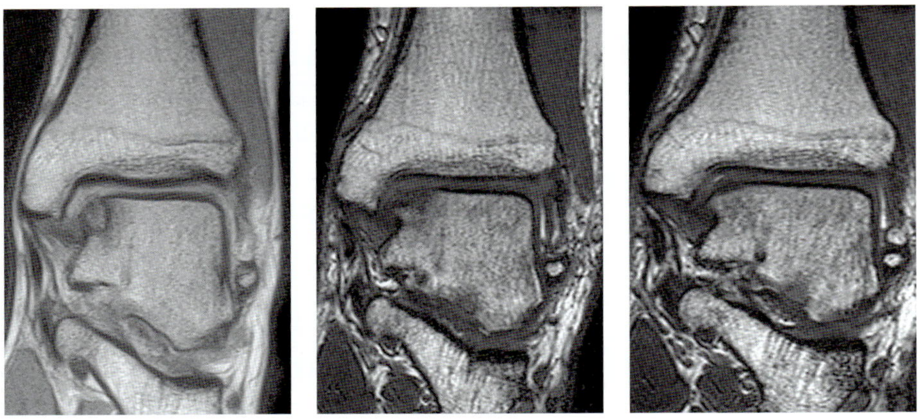

Figures 5-6-7 - MRI aspect of the lesion at time 0, 24 months and 48 months follow-up

autologous chondrocyte implantation, and chondral debridement. They found that no definitive conclusion could be reached in respect to the best current surgical technique for articular cartilage and osteochondral lesions. They also concluded that microfracture and mosaicplasty can provide a faster return to competition and faster clinical and functional results, whereas autologous chondrocyte implantation and/or matrix-induced autologous chondrocytes implantation procedures can enhance longstanding clinical and functional results.

Buda et al. [46] reported on a total of 140 athletes who underwent a "one-step" arthroscopic bone marrow-derived cell transplantation repair of osteochondral lesions of the talus. Among these patients, 46 were soccer players, with a mean age of 29 years and focal osteochondral lesions of the talar dome classified as chronic type II-IIA (>1.5 cm^2 in area, respectively <5 or >5 mm deep), according to the Giannini's classification [47]. The authors reported that AOFAS score improved from 58.7 ± 13.5 preoperatively to 90.6 ± 8.6 ($P < 0.005$) at 24 months, and to 90.9 ± 10.7 at 48 months and that Halasi score was 6.88 ± 1.8 preinjury, 4.08 ± 1.7 preoperatively, and 5.56 ± 2.0 at final follow-up. Also MRI evaluation demonstrated constant improvement overtime (figg. 5, 6, 7). Moreover, they reported that at the final follow-up, all the patients (beside 1 failure and 3 lost) were able to return to activity and 72.8% were able to resume sports at preinjury level. Basing on these findings, the authors concluded that "one-step" BMDCT repair of OLT had good clinical results that were durable over time in athletes, permitting a return to sports at preinjury level in the majority of patients. The preoperative presence of impingement and articular degeneration were the main negative prognostic factors.

Although an increasing number of reports are currently being published on this specific topic, literature on clinical effectiveness of bone-marrow aspirate concentrate (BMAC) injections for cartilage lesions is still scarce and based on small patients' series, enabling the possibility to highlight definitive conclusions.

Mautner et al. [48] investigated whether autologous orthobiologic tissue source affects pain and functional outcomes in 76 patients with symptomatic knee osteoarthritis (OA) who received microfragmented adipose tissue (MFAT) or bone marrow aspirate concentrate (BMAC) injection. At a minimum follow-up of 6 months, both groups demonstrated significant subjective and objective clinical improvement without any significant difference when comparing postprocedure scores between groups.

A systematic review of recent human studies recently published (Law et al.) [49], demonstrated no significant adverse events in 841 patients who reportedly received cellular products for mixed orthopaedic clinical conditions. The authors reported that pain and functional limitation generally improved, though no differences were seen over controls where present. The authors concluded that support in literature is strongest for the use of bone marrow aspirate concentrate (BMAC) injections for the treatment of knee pain respect to any other orthopaedic clinical condition, even if applications of the use of BMAC and peripheral blood-derived MSCs for the treatment of hip pain, tendon pain, and disc pain have all been reported. For these reasons, the authors also concluded that further research is strongly required, with large randomized controlled trials. Themistocleous et al. (50) recently evaluated the clinical efficacy and safety of an intra-articular injection of concentrated bone marrow aspirate as a treatment option for osteoarthritis of the knee in a single-center series of 121 patients retrospectively evaluated. The authors concluded that a single intra-articular injection of BMAC is a safe and reliable procedure that results in clinical improvement of knee OA, with a significant reduction of self-reported pain and a mean Oxford Knee Score improvement from 20.20 to 32.29 (P <0.001) at a mean final follow-up of 11 months.

Basing on current literature, translational studies have demonstrated good clinical efficacy of BMAC both concomitant with cartilage restoration procedures, at defined time points after surgery, and as isolated injections. Early clinical data suggests BMAC may help stimulate a more robust hyaline cartilage repair tissue response. Numerous questions remain regarding BMAC usage, including cell source, cell expansion, optimal pathology, and injection timing and quantity. Anyway, further investigation is required to determine the exact mechanisms of action, duration of efficacy, optimal frequency of treatments, and regenerative potential, expecially for the ankle joint.

Bibliography

1. Bekkers JE, de Windt TS, Brittberg M2, Saris DB. Cartilage Repair in Football (Soccer) Athletes: What Evidence Leads to Which Treatment? A Critical Review of the Literature. Cartilage. 2012 Jan;3(1 Suppl):43S-9S.

2. Flanigan DC, Harris JD, Trinh TQ, Siston RA, Brophy RH. Prevalence of chondral defects in athletes' knees: a systematic review. Med Sci Sports Exerc. 2010;42(10):1795-801.

3. Messner K, Maletius W. The long-term prognosis for severe damage to weight-bearing cartilage in the knee: a 14-year clinical and radiographic follow-up in 28 young athletes. Acta Orthop Scand. 1996;67(2):165-8.

4. Piasecki DP, Spindler KP, Warren TA, Andrish JT, Parker RD. Intraarticular injuries associated with anterior cruciate ligament tear: findings at ligament reconstruction in high school and recreational athletes. An analysis of sex-based differences. Am J Sports Med. 2003;31(4):601-5.

5. Mithoefer K, McAdams TR, Scopp JM, Mandelbaum BR. Emerging options for treatment of articular cartilage injury in the athlete. Clin Sports Med. 2009;28(1):25-40.

6. Bekkers JE, Inklaar M, Saris DB. Treatment selection in articular cartilage lesions of the knee: a systematic review. Am J Sports Med. 2009;37 Suppl 1:148S-55S.

7. McAdams TR, Mithoefer K, Scopp JM, Mandelbaum BR. Articular cartilage injury in athletes. Cartilage. 2010;1(3):165-79.

8. Buckwalter JA, Mankin HJ. Articular cartilage: degeneration and osteoarthritis, repair, regeneration, and transplantation. Instr Course Lect. 1998;47:487-504.

9. Goldring MB, Goldring SR. Osteoarthritis. J Cell Physiol. 2007;213(3):626-34.

10. Willick SE, Hansen PA. Running and osteoarthritis. Clin Sports Med. 2010;29(3):417-28.

11. Kim HJ, Lee YH, Kim CK. Biomarkers of muscle and cartilage damage and inflammation during a 200 km run. Eur J Appl Physiol. 2007;99(4):443-7.

12. Savage T, Niehoff A, Bruggemann L, Muller M, Zaucke F, Eckstein F, et al. The use of biomarkers to assess the response of cartilage to exercise. Br J Sports Med. 2011;45(4):326.

13. Curl WW, Krome J, Gordon ES, Rushing J, Smith BP, Poehling GG. Cartilage injuries: a review of 31,516 knee arthroscopies. Arthroscopy. 1997;13(4):456-60.

14. Hjelle K, Solheim E, Strand T, Muri R, Brittberg M. Articular cartilage defects in 1,000 knee arthroscopies. Arthroscopy. 2002;18(7):730-4.

15. Steadman JR, Rodkey WG, Rodrigo JJ. Microfracture: surgical technique and rehabilitation to treat chondral defects. Clin Orthop Relat Res. 2001;(391 Suppl):S362-9.

16. Williams RJ III, Harnly HW. Microfracture: indications, tech- nique, and results. Instr Course Lect. 2007;56:419-28.

17. Brittberg M, Lindahl A, Nilsson A, Ohlsson C, Isaksson O, Peterson L. Treatment of deep cartilage defects in the knee with autologous chondrocyte transplantation. N Engl J Med. 1994;331(14):889-95.

18. Ekstrand J, Hägglund M, Kristenson K, et al. Fewer ligament injuries but no preventive effect on muscle injuries and severe injuries: an 11-year follow-up of the UEFA Champions League injury study. Br J Sports Med 2013;47:732–7.

19. Brittberg M, Lindahl A, Nilsson A, Ohlsson C, Isaksson O, Peterson L. Treatment of deep cartilage defects in the knee with autologous chondrocyte transplantation. N Engl J Med. 1994;331(14):889-95.

20. Bedi A, Feeley BT, Williams RJ III. Management of articular cartilage defects of the knee. J Bone Joint Surg Am. 2010;92(4): 994-1009.

21. Kish G, Modis L, Hangody L. Osteochondral mosaicplasty for the treatment of focal chondral and osteochondral lesions of the knee and talus in the athlete. Rationale, indications, technique, and results. Clin Sports Med 1999;18:45–66.
22. Marcacci M, Kon E, Delcogliano M, et al. Arthroscopic autologous osteochondral grafting for cartilage defects of the knee: prospective study results at a minimum 7-year follow-up. Am J Sports Med 2007;35:2014–21.
23. Krych AJ, Robertson CM, Williams RJ III. Return to athletic activity after osteochondral allograft transplantation in the knee. Am J Sports Med 2012;40:1053–9.
24. Hindle P, Hendry JL, Keating JF, et al. Autologous osteochondral mosaicplasty or TruFitTM plugs for cartilage repair. Knee Surg Sports Traumatol Arthrosc 2014;22:1235–40.
25. Foster TE, Puskas BL, Mandelbaum BR, et al. Platelet-rich plasma: from basic science to clinical applications. Am J Sports Med 2009;37:2259–72.
26. Kon E, Mandelbaum B, Buda R, et al. Platelet-rich plasma intra-articular injection versus hyaluronic acid viscosupplementation as treatments for cartilage pathology: from early degeneration to osteoarthritis. Arthroscopy 2011;27:1490–501.
27. Neumann K, Dehne T, Endres M, et al. Chodrogenic differentiation capacity of human mesenchymal progenitor cells derived from subchondral corticospongious bone. J Orthop Res 2008;26:1449–56.
28. Gobbi A, Karnatzikos G, Sankineani SR. One-step surgery with multipotent stem cells for the treatment of large full-thickness chondral defects of the knee. Am J Sports Med 2014;42:648–57.
29. Crawford DC, DeBerardino TM, Williams RJ III. NeoCart, an autologous cartilage tissue implant, compared with microfracture for treatment of distal femoral cartilage lesions: an FDA phase-II prospective, randomized clinical trial after two years. J Bone Joint Surg Am 2012;94:979–89.
30. Kon E, Filardo G, Berruto M, et al. Articular cartilage treatment in high-level male soccer players: a prospective comparative study of arthroscopic second-generation autologous chondrocyte implantation versus microfracture. Am J Sports Med 2011;39:2549–57.
31. Farr J, Tabet SK, Margerrison E, et al. Clinical, radiographic, and histological outcomes after cartilage repair with particulated juvenile articular cartilage: a 2-year prospective study. Am J Sports Med 2014;42:1417–25.
32. Namba RS, Meuli M, Sullivan KM, et al. Spontaneous repair of superficial defects in articular cartilage in a fetal lamb model. J Bone Joint Surg Am 1998;80:4–10.
33. Buda R, Vannini F, Cavallo M, Grigolo B, Cenacchi A, Giannini S. Osteochondral lesions of the knee: a new one-step repair technique with bone-marrow-derived cells. J Bone Joint Surg Am. 2010 Dec;92 Suppl 2:2-11.
34. Giannini S, Buda R, Grigolo B, Vannini F, De Franceschi L, Facchini A. The detached osteochondral fragment as a source of cells for autologous chondrocyte implantation (ACI) in the ankle joint. Osteoarthritis Cartilage. 2005 Jul;13(7):601-7.
35. Andriolo L, Reale D, Di Martino A, Zaffagnini S, Vannini F, Ferruzzi A, Filardo G. High Rate of Failure After Matrix-Assisted Autologous Chondrocyte Transplantation in Osteoarthritic Knees at 15 Years of Follow-up. Am J Sports Med. 2019 Jul;47(9):2116-2122.
36. Giannini S, Buda R, Vannini F, Cavallo M, Grigolo B. One-step Bone Marrow-Derived Cell Transplantation in Talar Osteochondral Lesions. Clin Orthop Relate Res 2009; 467: 3307-3320.
37. Buda R, Castagnini F, Cavallo M, Ramponi L, Vannini F, Giannini S. "One-step" bone marrow-derived cells transplantation and joint debridement for osteochondral lesions of the talus in ankle osteoarthritis: clinical and radiological outcomes at 36 months. Arch Orthop Trauma Surg 136: 107-116.
38. Buda R, Vannini F, Cavallo M, Grigolo B, Cenacchi A, Giannini S. Osteochondral lesions of the knee: a new one-step repair technique with bone-marrow-derived cells. J Bone Joint Surg Am. 2010 Dec;92 Suppl 2:2-11.
39. Baldassarri M, Perazzo L, Ricciarelli M, Natali S, Vannini F, Buda R. Regenerative treatment of osteochondral lesions of distal tibial plafond. European Journal of Orthopedic Surgery & Traumathology. Eur J Orthop Surg Traumatol (2018) 28: 1199.
40. Kim JD, Lee GW, Jung GH, Kim CK, Kim T, Park JH, Cha SS, You YB. Clinical outcome of autologous bone marrow aspirates concentrate (BMAC) injection in degenerative arthritis of the knee. Eur J Orthop Surg Traumatol. 2014 Dec;24(8):1505-11.
41. Pittenger MF, Mackay AM, Beck SC, Jaiswal RK, Douglas R, Mosca JD, Moorman MA, Simonetti DW, Craig S, Marshak DR. Multilineage potential of adult human mesenchymal stem cells. Science. 1999 Apr 2;284(5411):143-7.
42. Lee EH, Hui JH. The potential of stem cells in orthopaedic surgery. J Bone Joint Surg Br. 2006 Jul;88(7):841-51.
43. Peters AE, Watts AE. Biopsy needle advancement during bone marrow aspiration increases mesenchymal stem cell concentration. Front Vet Sci. 2016 Mar 14;3:23.
44. Mithoefer K, Della Villa S. Return to sport after articular cartilage repair in the football (soccer) player. Cartilage. 2012; 3(Suppl. I) 57S-62S.
45. Andrade R, Vasta S, Papalia R, Pereira H, Oliveira JM, Reis RL, Espregueira-Mendes J. Prevalence of articular cartilage lesions and surgical clinical outcomes in football (soccer) players' knees: a systematic review. Arthroscopy. 2016 Jul;32(7):1466-77.
46. Vannini F, Cavallo M, Ramponi L, Castagnini F, Massimi S, Giannini S, Buda R. Return to sports after bone marrow-derived cell transplantation for osteochondral lesions of the talus. Cartilage. 2017 Jan;8(1):80-87.
47. Giannini S, Buda R, Faldini C, Vannini F, Bevoni R, Grandi G, et al. Surgical treatment of osteochondral lesions of the talus (OLT) in young and active patients: guidelines for treatment and evolution of the technique. J Bone Joint Surg Am. 2005;87(Suppl 2):28-41.
48. Mautner K, Bowers R, Easley K, Fausel Z, Robinson R. Functional outcomes following microfragmented adipose tissue versus bone marrow aspirate concentrate injections for symptomatic knee osteoarthritis. Stem Cells Transl Med. 2019 Jul 21.
49. Law L, Hunt CL, van Wijnen AJ , Nassr A, Larson AN, Eldrige JS, Mauck WD, Pingree MJ, Yang J, Muir CW, Erwin PJ, Bydon M, Qu W. Office-based mesenchymal stem cell therapy for the treatment of musculoskeletal disease: a systematic review of recent human studies. Pain Med. 2018 Dec 29.
50. Themistocleous GS , Chloros GD, Kyrantzoulis IM, Georgokostas IA, Themistocleous MS, Papagelopoulos PJ, Savvidou OD. Effectiveness of a single intra-articular bone marrow aspirate concentrate (BMAC) injection in patients with grade 3 and 4 knee osteoarthritis. Heliyon. 2018 Oct 18;4(10):e00871.

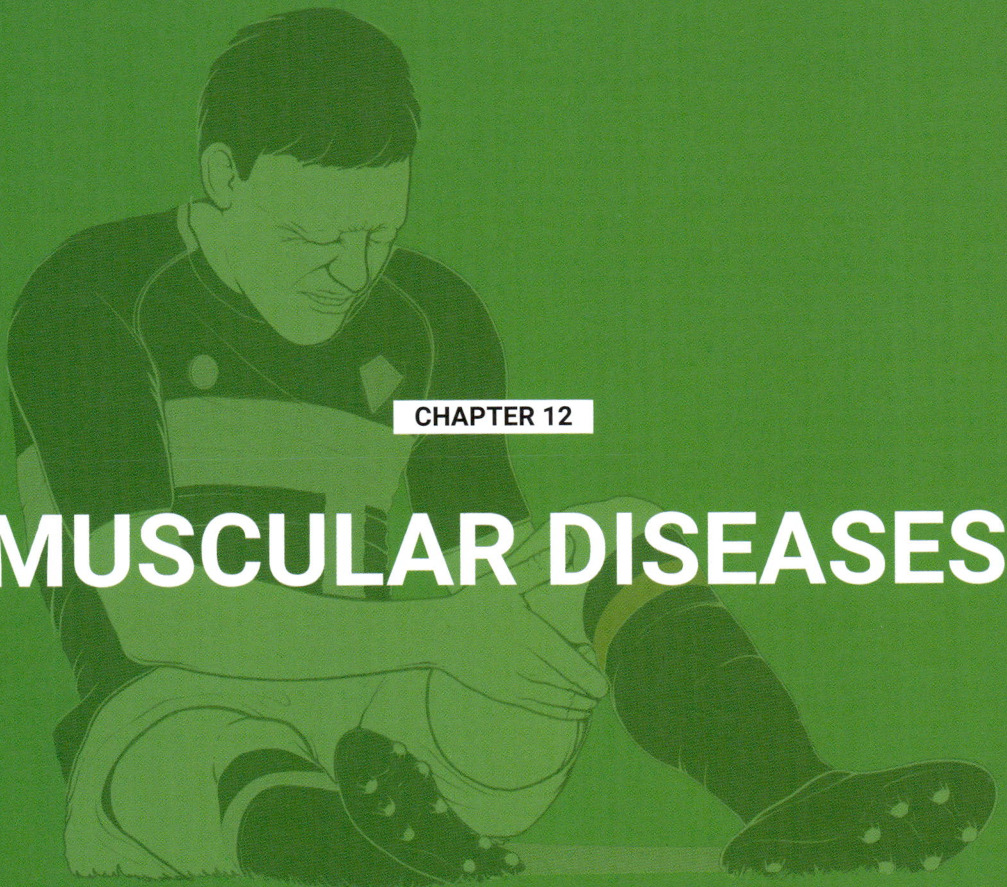

CHAPTER 12

MUSCULAR DISEASES

Gianni Nanni
Luca Bini
Riccardo Di Miceli
Giovanbattista Sisca

Medical Staff Bologna Football Club 1909

Isokinetic Medical Group, Bologna, Italy
FIFA Medical Centre of Excellence

Introduction

The most common lesions in soccer are muscle injuries, which account for about 40% of all lesions throughout the season.

According to Ekstrand, the injury rate in professional European soccer is 2.8/1,000 hours of exposure and above all 1.37/1,000 hours in training and 8.7/1,000 in matches [1]. In a team in the top division (Serie A) of Italian professional soccer the injury rate is 5.2/1,000 hours of exposure and above all 3.8/1,000 in training and 14.6/1,000 in matches. These figures include all muscle injuries, even those that did not prevent activity completely but allowed the player to carry out differentiated training, albeit not fully at the trainer's disposal (fig. 1).

The rate of muscular lesions seems to be lower, both in matches and in training, when playing on synthetic grass than on natural grass.

Muscular lesions caused by direct trauma (tears and contusions) are less common than those caused by indirect trauma and account for only 4% of all muscle injuries; the rate of direct trauma lesions, 0.19/1,000 hours' exposure, is eight times lower than that of indirect trauma lesions.

Types of lesions

Muscle tears occur after contact with the studs of opponents' boots or sharp surfaces around the playing field, such as advertising panels. The muscle belly needs to be sutured and, in more severe cases, the player cannot play for two or three months. With regard to direct trauma muscle lesions, the most common ones are contusions usually caused by contact with an opponent or with a hard structure on the pitch, such as the goalposts. They are divided into mild, moderate or severe (fig. 2). By far the most affected muscle group is the quadriceps (60% of cases) in particular the vastus lateralis and the vastus intermedius. The lesion may be greater if the bruise occurs on a relaxed muscle rather than a contracted one. Recovery times, if there are no complications, range from a few days for mild contusions to 15-20 days for more severe ones.

Unlike indirect traumas, not caused by direct contact, the likelihood of continuing to train and play is very high, at least for mild or moderate injuries. The most feared complication following muscle contusion, albeit rare, is circumscribed intramuscular bone calcification, also erroneously called myositis ossificans. This is usually caused by inappropriate treatment with heat or massage in the early days after the onset of a muscle hematoma and takes a long time to resolve, even months before the player gets back into training with the team. It is characterised by a sudden unexpected sharp pain and swelling in the involved muscle which takes on a wood-like texture upon palpation and is functionally impotent. It does not usually require surgery unless it involves or irritates a nerve fibre or restricts movement of a nearby joint, due to the extent of the bone calcification itself. In that case, if the scintigraphy test result is negative, the calcification is removed when it is fully mature. Indomethacin may be used to reduce the inflammation and calcification in the muscle involved, especially if taken at onset of the complication.

One rare and feared complication of direct muscle trauma, which occurs within hours of a contusion, is compartment syndrome. This should be closely monitored and, in severe cases, treated surgically promptly to avoid irreversible ischemic damage.

Indirect muscle lesions are, instead, more com-

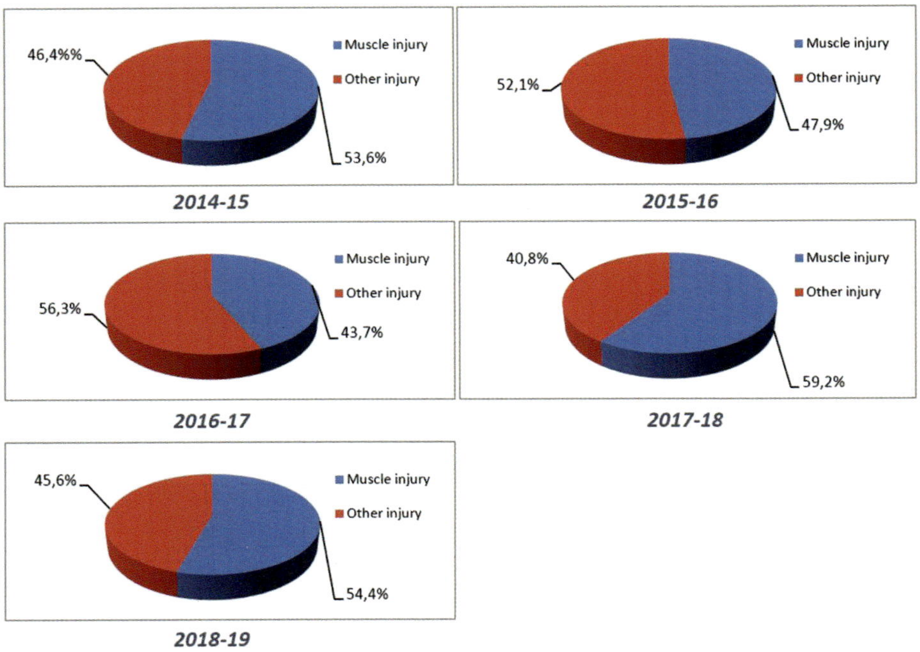

Fig. 1 - Muscle lesion rate over five seasons (2014-2019) in a professional Italian soccer team of serie A

mon (96% of all muscle lesions) and are the cause of lost days in about 30% of professional players and 20% of amateur players. According to Ekstrand et al., in a soccer team of 25 players there should be about 15 muscle lesions a year and by far the most affected muscles are the hamstrings (12.8% of all injuries and 37% of muscle lesions), and especially the long head of the biceps femoris; these are followed by the adductors, especially the long adductor (9.2% of all injuries and 23% of all muscle lesions), rectus femoris (5% of all injuries and 19% of all muscle lesions), the triceps surae (4.5% of all injuries and 13% of all muscle lesions) [1].
According to a paper published in 2013, which took into account 31 professional European soccer teams in the 2011/2012 season, each season a team should expect an average of 5 hamstring lesions and 3 rectus femoris lesions and thus have an average injury burden of 130 days [2]. Between 2001 and 2014 a mean increase in hamstring lesions of 2.3% a year, especially during training (4% a year) was recorded in professional soccer [3]. In that period, an increased intensity in training was observed in professional clubs. Trainers are more demanding with regard to the players' performance and in the same club players are more competitive with each other because of the high number of players at the club's disposal.
Fortunately, this trend is not supported by data on recent seasons, which show a tendency to have fewer hamstring lesion recurrences with regard to professional soccer. Should epidemiological data

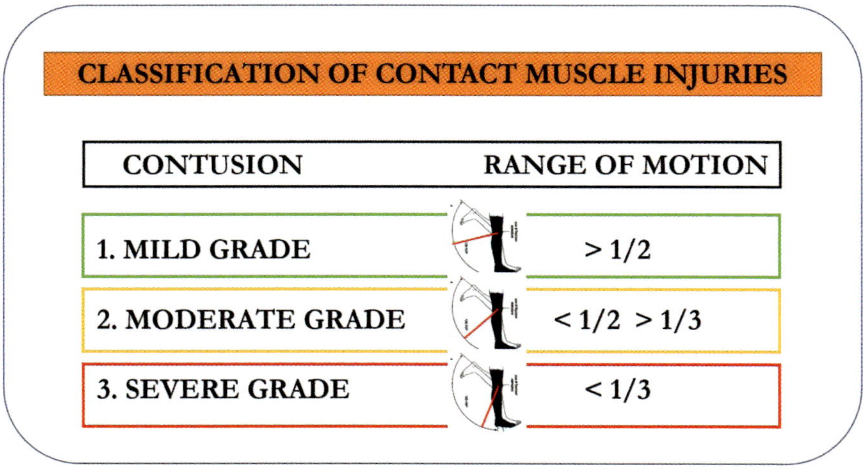

Fig. 2 - Classification of direct trauma muscle lesions (contusions) according to ability, after trauma, to move actively the corresponding joint (e.g. the knee for the quadriceps, the hip for the gluteus and the ankle for the triceps surae)

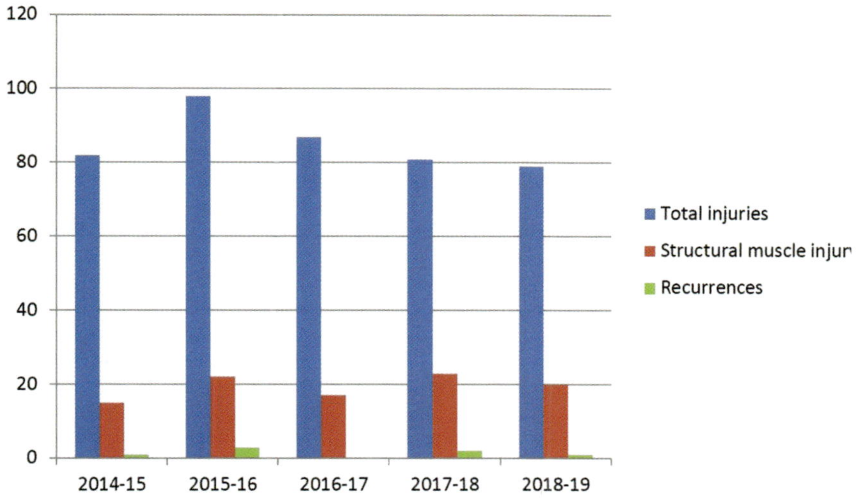

Fig. 3A - Number of indirect trauma muscle lesions and recurrences over the last five seasons in a professional Italian soccer team of serie A

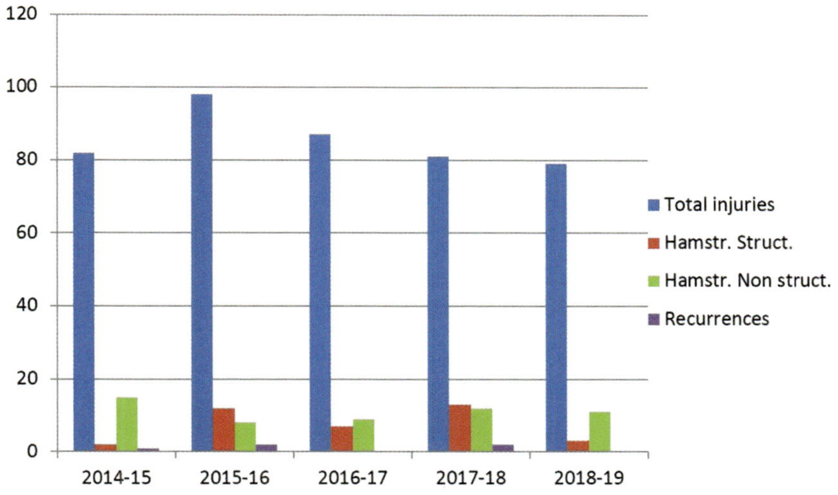

Fig. 3B - Number of indirect trauma hamstring muscle lesions and recurrences over the last five seasons in a professional Italian soccer team of serie A

continue to support this trend, we shall finally be able to claim that, despite increased intensity in the game and high workloads, health workers and technical staff are working correctly both on prevention and rehabilitation (figg. 3a, 3b).

Rectus femoris lesions are slightly more common in the dominant limb, whereas there is no prevalence in the dominant limb with regard to the other muscles. Concerning more severe hamstring lesions, grades 3B and 4 are more common in the dominant limb, whereas there is no difference in frequency between dominant and non-dominant limb with regard to absolute number of lesions. The number of muscle lesions seems to increase towards the end of each match half and especially in the last half hour of the match. Hamstring lesions are more frequent in midfielders and forwards, whereas the goalkeeper is less affected by lower limb muscle lesions. Quadriceps lesions are more common during the preparation period of the season before the championship begins, whereas lesions to other muscles increase during the season [4] (fig. 4).

Non-contact lesions are divided into two groups: non-structural and structural. The former, divided into 4 subgroups, 1A, 1B, 2A, and 2B, includes injuries that do not display anatomical lesions of the muscle fibres. They are characterised by an increase in the muscle tone of some muscle fascicles or the entire muscle belly in 1B (DOMS, Delayed Onset Muscle Soreness), accompanied by pain and a heavy feeling in the muscle. They can occur during sports activity and at rest in 1A, 2A, and 2B, or some hours after activity in 1B (DOMS). They can also occur either after fatigue or with repeated changes in type of ground (1A), altered neuromuscular control caused by problems in the spine and/or pelvis (2A), or due to incorrect function of the neural or muscular structures that ensure normal interaction between agonist and antagonist mus-

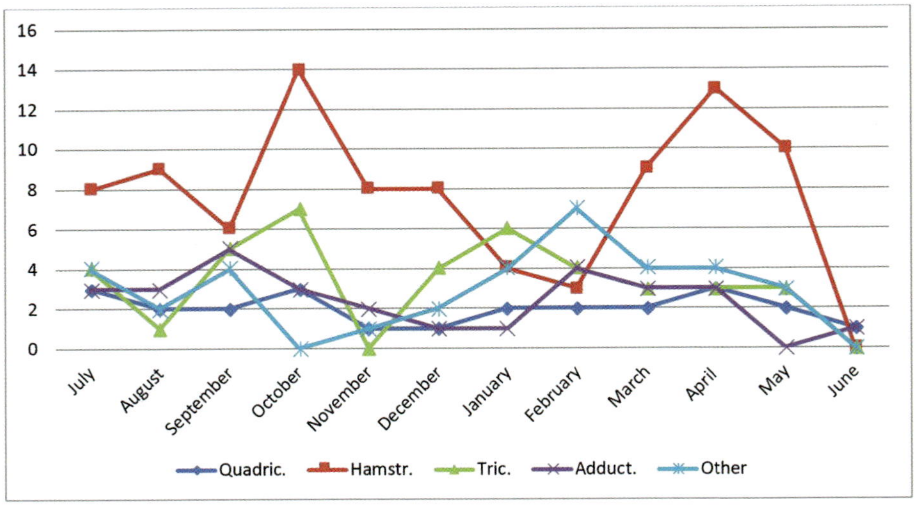

Fig. 4 - Muscle lesion trend over the last five seasons in a professional Italian soccer team of serie A

cles (2B). Conversely, DOMS (1B) occurs following intensive eccentric work.

As already said, these injuries never present anatomical lesions of the muscle fibre, and usually resolve if promptly diagnosed and correctly treated; they have a good prognosis which ranges from 3 to 15 days' rest. Nevertheless, precisely because these injuries are often underestimated and recovery times are accelerated, they account for over 50% of loss of training and matches in professional soccer.

Conversely, structural injuries always present an anatomical lesion that might involve a few fibres within the muscle fascicle (3A or minor partial lesion), multiple muscle fascicles with a rupture of up to 50% of the muscle belly surface in that section (3B or moderate partial lesion), multiple muscle fascicles with a rupture of more than 50% of the muscle belly surface in that section (4 or subtotal lesion) or a rupture of the entire muscle belly or tendon avulsion (4 or total lesion) [5] (fig. 5).

For a correct prognosis of structural injuries it is not enough to know the extent of the lesion and the muscle involved by the lesion itself, but additional information is needed about the region, within the muscle, where the lesion occurred (proximal, medial, distal), and the tissue, besides muscle tissue, that has been damaged by the lesion, and whether it is a primary lesion of the muscle or a recurrence. Indeed, with regards to the lesion site, prognosis varies depending on whether the lesion is proximal (where a hamstring or rectus femoris lesion is more severe from a prognostic point of view), or distal (where a medial gastrocnemius or soleus lesion is worse). Furthermore, a lesion involving the epimysium, also called myofascial lesion, has a much better prognosis than that of a lesion of similar entity of the myotendinous junction and

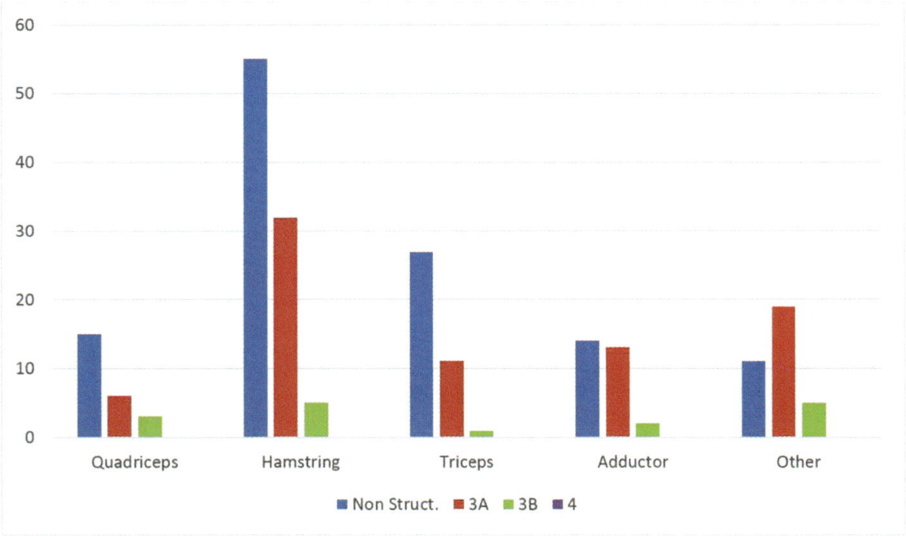

Fig. 5 - Non-structural and structural injury rate in the main lower limb muscles in a professional Italian soccer team of serie A, over the last five seasons

even more than that of a lesion involving only part of the central tendon or the free tendon.

Recurrences in muscle lesions

Recurrences of muscle lesions are usually more complex to treat and tend to have a longer prognosis than that of a primary lesion. By recurrence we mean a new muscle lesion that occurs in the same muscle as a previous lesion, even in a different area of the muscle, within two months of return-to-play (RTP). The general rate of recurrence in soccer ranges from 12% to 16%. Thus, of 100 soccer players that suffer a muscle lesion, between 12 and 16 of them have a recurrence.

In soccer, recurrences are more common in the hamstring, ranging from 16% to 30%. The rate of recurrence in the adductors is 18%, in the quadriceps (especially the rectus femoris) 17%, and in the triceps sural 13% (fig. 6).

They are more common in non-professional and recreational soccer players, with respective rates of 24% and 48%, whereas in professional soccer the recurrence rate is about 16%. Non-professionals, and to a greater extent recreational players, take less care of their injuries which inevitably leads to a greater risk of recurrence. To reduce the risk of recurrence it is very important to avoid early RTP after a muscle lesion before completing all the phases of the recovery program. The risk of accelerating RTP is always high because of environmental pressures and those of other professionals that interact with the player (trainer, club management, team-mates, agents and mass media etc.).

Clinical examination

From a clinical point of view structural injuries present precisely located pain upon palpation. In more severe lesions a depression or hollow can be felt in the acute phase, which is replaced by a hematoma during the first hours after injury. There is always an immediate functional deficit, especially types 3B and 4 lesions, making it impossible to continue with the match or training. Contraction against resistance is possible but painful in smaller lesions, and impossible in more severe 3B and 4 lesions. Stretching the injured muscle, which may be possible in smaller 3A lesions, can never match its counterpart muscle in the healthy limb and should be performed under the pain threshold.

The player always remembers the moment when the injury occurred and the technical movement that caused it. Ultrasound, preferably performed 48-72 hours after injury, is always positive in types 3B and 4 lesions. In type 3A lesions, especially small ones, ultrasound, even performed with power Doppler, might be negative. When there is a clinical suspicion of a lesion, nuclear magnetic resonance (NMR) might be necessary to dispel any doubts about whether the injury is structural or non-structural. NMR might be positive even on the first day after the lesion and should be performed to study muscles that are difficult to assess by ultrasound, such as the iliopsoas, the obturator muscles, or the intrinsic foot muscles, or the subscapularis in the upper limb (figg. 7, 8) (video 1). With regard to non-structural injuries the player

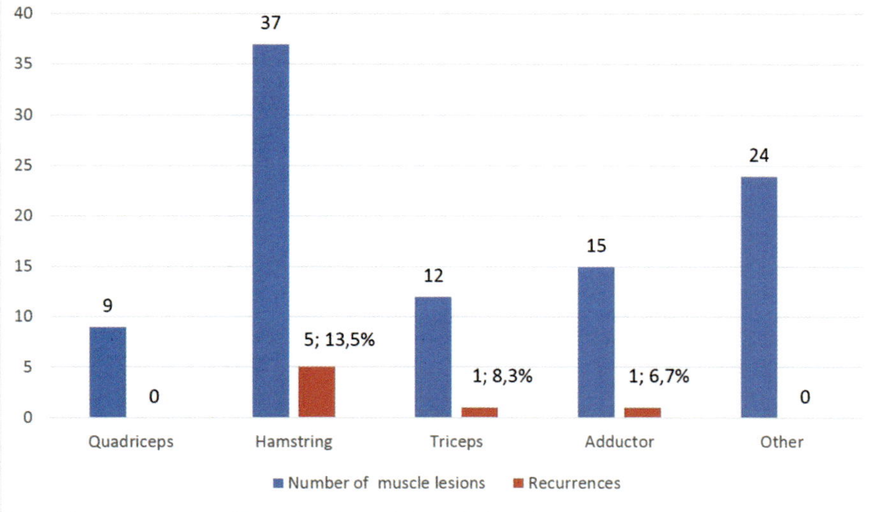

Fig. 6 - Injury recurrence rate in the main lower limb muscles in a professional Italian soccer team of serie A, over the last five seasons

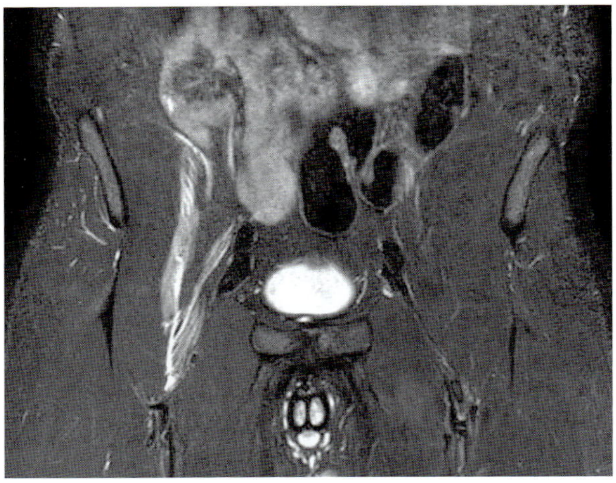

Fig. 7 - Nuclear magnetic resonance of a moderate partial lesion of the right iliopsoas in a professional soccer player. The injury occurred following an additional function imposed on the iliopsoas, which, besides acting as a hip stabiliser while the player was in the air, also had to flex and externally rotate the hip when kicking the ball to avoid being overtaken by it, as it could have happened in the video 1

VIDEO 1

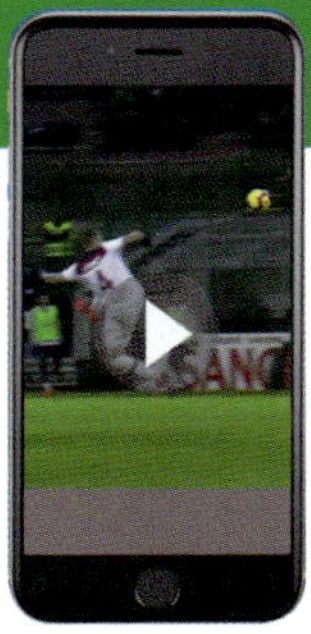

Additional function of iliopsoas

reports pain or heaviness in the muscle that occurs when playing; it might be present at rest and it often does not cause immediate functional impairment and the player cannot connect it to a precise moment or technical movement during a match or training. The onset of DOMS is typical at rest, some hours after play. Upon palpation of the muscle affected by a non-structural lesion, some stiff and painful fascicles can be felt; stretching can help to improve the muscle, except in 2A where it has no effect. In 1B or DOMS the entire muscle is stiff and painful. In non-structural lesions ultrasonography is usually negative. At most a hyperechoic image might be present, always negative with power Doppler, which resolves after 3-5 days.

NMR is always negative for lesions. An area of oedema might be present inside the muscle in some cases and, if so, despite being completely benign, the lesion will take a few days longer to resolve.

Risk factors

The risk factors for muscle lesions are usually divided into modifiable and non-modifiable. A single risk factor is unlikely to explain the occurrence of a muscle lesion. It is often the interaction of multiple risk factors that predispose a player to muscular lesions. Age is a non-modifiable risk factor. Players over 26 years old seem to be at twice the risk of triceps surae lesion compared with younger players [6]. The risk seems to increase for other muscle groups, especially the hamstrings, only when combined with other risk factors, such as reduced strength, especially eccentric strength, and reduced length of muscle fascicles [7]. Otherwise

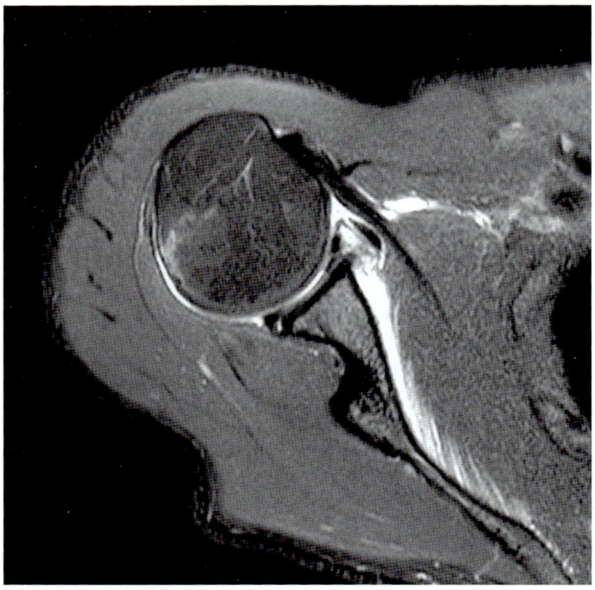

Fig. 8 - Nuclear magnetic resonance of a moderate partial lesion to the right subscapularis muscle in a professional soccer player

age does not seem to increase the risk of lesion in hamstrings, adductors and rectus femoris [6, 7].
The most important non-modifiable risk factor is certainly a history of previous muscle lesions. It is not only a risk factor for the same muscle that has previously suffered a lesion, but also for other muscle groups [6]. In soccer the risk of suffering a lesion in the same muscle can be three times higher, and even six times higher for the hamstrings (8). Injury recurrence in the same muscle can be caused by incorrect healing and the presence of scar tissue inside the muscle or incomplete recovery following the primary injury due to early RTP. Conversely, for other muscle groups biomechanical adjustment to functional alterations might explain the increased risk of injury.
Stature also seems to be a risk factor for rectus femoris lesions, although there are few papers on this topic; shorter players in particular carry a greater risk of injury to this muscle compared with taller players [9].
Modifiable risk factors include poor muscle extensibility and poor joint flexibility, although the literature presents contrasting opinions on this topic. Poor hip joint flexibility in professional players is a risk factor for adductor and hip flexor muscle lesions [10].
Reduced muscular strength seems to be an important risk factor for muscle lesions. At the beginning of the season players with reduced eccentric strength in the hamstrings carry a 4-5 times greater risk of hamstring injury throughout the season compared with players without a strength deficit [7]. The outcome of the isokinetic assessment of the hamstrings:quadriceps (H:Q) ratio is controversial; a low ratio seems to be correlated to a slightly higher risk of hamstring injury. Adductor strength deficit as an absolute value or as a reduced ratio between adductors and abductors is a risk factor for adductor lesions and generally for groin pain. Professional soccer players with reduced adductor strength carry a four times greater risk of these lesions compared with others [11]. Reduced eccentric strength of the quadriceps seems to increase by five times the risk of lesions in the same muscle and in particular the rectus femoris [12].
Recent studies have shown how muscle fascicle length in the long head of the biceps femoris of professional soccer players is an important risk factor to bear in mind. If the length is less than 10.6 cm the player has a four times greater risk of a lesion in the same muscle compared with players with longer muscle fascicles. The reason for this is that the more sarcomeres the muscle has in series the more it is protected during eccentric contraction, following which most indirect trauma muscle lesions occur [13].
Another important modifiable risk factor is the number of matches played in a season. The international and national championship calendar, both at club and national level, is particularly intense and compels players to play matches close together without having time to recover. Recent scientific studies have unequivocally highlighted that players that play matches less than six days apart carry a higher risk of suffering indirect muscle trauma and that this risk is five times greater in the period when the calendar includes two matches a week compared with periods when only one match is played a week [14]. Furthermore, these players often have to make long and frequent journeys, including intercontinental flights, change frequently habits and dietary patterns, and return only two days before their next match. The international bodies that govern soccer should, with support from doctors on their boards, better organise the calendar of various competitions both at club and international level, bearing in mind the players' health and therefore determine a number of matches that allows appropriate recovery times between one match and another.

How to prevent lesions

Is it possible to achieve adequate prevention of muscle lesions in soccer players? Is it easy to propose and adopt prevention programs in football clubs, especially professional ones? Unfortunately, the answer is no; although in recent years several technical staff and club managers and players themselves have begun to understand the importance of giving time and space, in their training programs, to group and personal work protocols, aimed at reducing injuries. This implies that the player should be appropriately assessed at the start of the season, using specific tests, both clinical and instrumental, and an accurate medical history to identify the main risk factors and design the best program to reduce modifiable factors and check and compensate for non-modifiable ones. Involving not only other players, but the other professionals that interact with the player as well, is a determining factor to achieve the objective of reducing the injury rate and number of days off in a soccer team.

A prevention program with the Nordic Hamstring Exercise, for hamstring muscle injury, has been found to reduce these lesions by about half in soccer players [15] and a program including strength exercises, especially eccentric strength, for the adductors, such as the Copenhagen adductor strengthening exercise, can reduce the rate of adductor muscle lesions by 41%.

Programs including exercises to improve muscles that stabilize the spine and pelvis are also considered important, albeit with less scientific evidence, in the prevention of lower and upper limb muscular lesions.

Indeed, just consider the greater biomechanical load, by transfer of function, on the rectus femoris or hamstrings in a player with a weak iliopsoas or gluteus maximus; besides their normal function of kicking the ball or running, the former also have the function of stabilizing the pelvis by compensating for the reduced readiness of the latter to perform this action [16].

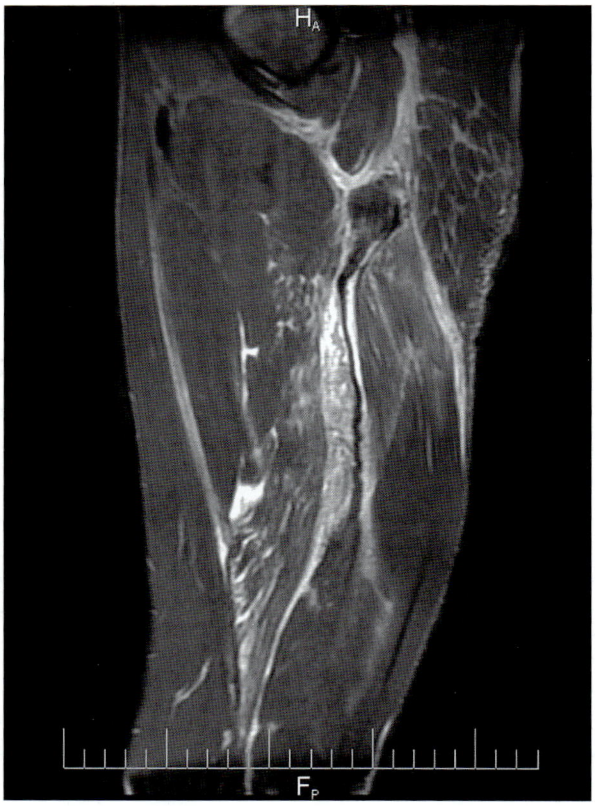

Fig. 9 - Nuclear magnetic resonance of a right conjoint tendon of the hamstrings detachment in a professional soccer player

FIFA 11+, a program of exercises performed during pre-training or pre-match warm-up lasting about twenty minutes, systematically adopted, can reduce general lesions in non-professional and recreational soccer by 20%-50% and by 51% for hamstring injuries with the introduction of the Nordic Hamstring Exercise into the program.

To prevent injuries overall and muscle lesions in particular, the player's workload should be constantly monitored especially with regard to running and high intensity exercises in general.

With the advent and use of GPS we can monitor precisely acute workloads in relation to chronic workloads, the latter being the average monthly workload. The acute workload should not be more than 1.3 times the chronic workload in order to stay within a safety range. Indeed higher values, especially >1.5 times, increase the risk of injury [17].

Dynamics of muscle injuries

In soccer, structural non-contact muscle lesions occur mostly after eccentric contractions with high-intensity rapid movements. Specific technical movements, such as kicking, abrupt changes in speed or direction, sliding up to the ball, braking, accelerating, jumping or landing from a jump, tackling, receiving and controlling the ball, are movements indicted after a muscle injury has occurred. However, these movements that are very often made during training and matches without consequences, can be altered by unforeseen events that compromise their correct execution, thus increasing the demand for eccentric strength, and often requiring an additional function of the muscle. One of the movements that carries the highest risk for the hamstrings is sliding up to the ball, especially with a flexed hip, and an unforeseen object interrupts the sliding of the heel which digs into the playing field (tuft of grass, hole, or another player's boot). The hamstrings, in particular at the proximal third, bear a further eccentric load due

to increased hip flexion at the moment of impact between the foot and object (fig. 9) (video 2).
Another movement indicted in hamstring lesions is running into an opponent and making contact at pelvis level. In that case the hamstrings of the weight-bearing leg, already involved in the run, have to add another function, i.e. that of stabilizing the pelvis, which has been moved laterally by the opponent, in an illegal attempt to block the player's run (video 3).
Sometimes, while running, a player may have to control a ball that has arrived after an uneven bounce on the playing field or has been passed by a teammate at a higher or lower speed than expected, or has changed direction due to the wind. In that case, if the player has to control this ball while running fast, receiving a long pass or making an extended sprint, and he has to flex the trunk slightly forwards to get the ball, that is when the added eccentric demand of the hamstrings can lead to injury (video 4).
Another potentially dangerous technical movement for the hamstrings is trying to control a ball coming from above and behind, with the knee extended during the run. In that case the middle or distal third of the hamstrings are at a greater risk (video 5).
Semimembranosus lesions which occur during a stretching movement, which is not necessarily made at high speed, are rare but not impossible injuries in soccer players, but they are very common in dancers. In soccer this can happen, for example, when a player is running at low-medium speed and an opponent hits, often involuntarily, the player's heel while the knee is extended in the final phase of the stride before the foot touches the ground, thus causing a forward movement of the limb in the air, with added eccentric demand on the hip

VIDEO 2

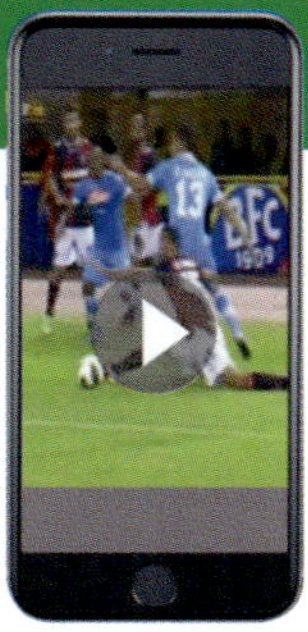

The arrow indicates the player being injured; the bar shows the moment of injury

VIDEO 3

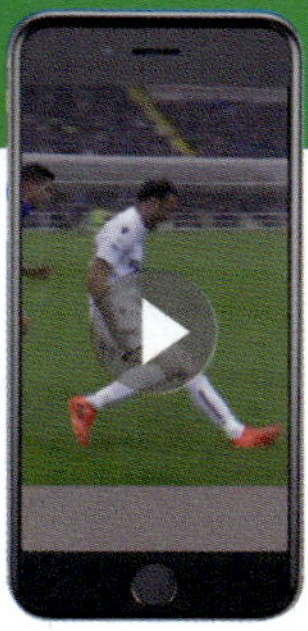

The arrow indicates the player being injured; the bar shows the moment of injury

VIDEO 4

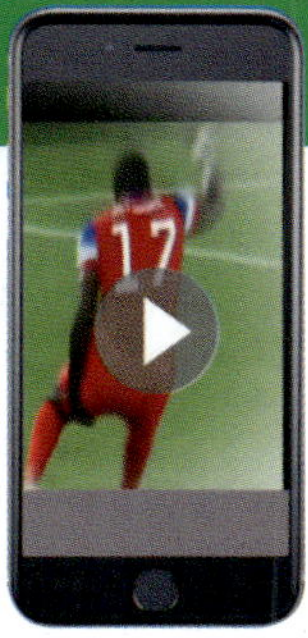

The arrow indicates the player being injured; the bar shows the moment of injury

VIDEO 5

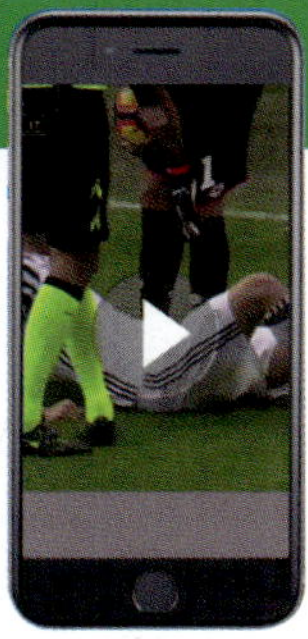

The arrow indicates the player being injured; the bar shows the moment of injury

extensors.
With regards to the rectus femoris, the riskiest movement is kicking the ball. This is obviously a common technical gesture for the soccer player but, if an unexpected event alters the motor pattern during movement, it might result in injury. An unforeseen event might be a slipping of the foot on the ground slightly forwards with respect to the ball, so as to hit the ball with the player's body too far over the ball. To get the right trajectory on the ball with the appropriate strength and accuracy, the player is obliged to lift the trunk slightly and extend the hemipelvis of the leg in the air that is striking the ball, thus requiring an eccentric contraction from the rectus femoris, especially at proximal third level, before hitting the ball itself.
Another unforeseen event that can occur while kicking the ball with the top of the foot is having to win a tackle with an opponent who was not expected to stop the action. The slight flexion movement of the knee of the kicking limb requires eccentric strength that might be enough to cause a rectus femoris lesion, in this case more commonly in the middle or distal third of the muscle itself.
The rectus femoris can also be injured, especially in the proximal third, when using the inside of the foot to stop a ball with an unexpected change in trajectory height of the ball itself because of hitting uneven ground before being controlled by the player. The ball tends to rise or slightly accelerate and the player with one leg in the air has no choice, in order to control the ball, but to extend the hip slightly and therefore require an unforeseen eccentric contraction of the rectus femoris of the leg that is stopping the ball.
A rectus femoris lesion can also be caused by other movements, such as accelerating or decelerating while running when an opponent unexpectedly tries to unbalance the player in action by pushing the pelvis, laterally in the former case and posteriorly in the latter; this forces the rectus femoris to assume the added function of pelvis stabilizer. Pulling a player's shirt also brakes his action and causes a modest hip extension in the leg with the foot on the ground. Hip extension following an unforeseen event, with increased eccentric demand of the rectus femoris in the weight-bearing leg, also occurs when a player goes to tackle an opponent but the latter has control of the ball and, realizing this, the player stops suddenly, partially to protect himself from being hit by the ball, as it can be seen in the film (video 6).
The rectus femoris can also be injured during the push-off or landing phase of a jump when an opponent prevents the normal expected movement by altering the motor pattern and unbalancing the player performing the action.
In some cases instead of having a lesion of the proximal myotendinous junction of the rectus femoris or direct tendon avulsion, there is an indirect tendon avulsion with a subtle and deceptive symptomatology which can delay diagnosis. In that case the player reports pain and noise at the hip and a moving sensation of the hip joint itself during play. The player feels immediate pain on the lateral side around the tensor fasciae latae. At rest, the symptoms and functional deficit resolve abruptly in about 7-10 days, thus leading the player and his staff into a false sense of security. What remains from a clinical point of view is still a clear positive rectus femoris stretch test compared with the healthy limb. This should indicate caution and an early RTP will inevitably lead to a recurrence that will delay recovery time, which is usually estimated at forty days before returning to training after the primary lesion. Follow-up X-rays after 6-8 months with the player back in full activity will reveal asymptomatic calcification along the tendon reflex, above all if the avulsion caused a detachment of small bone fragments at the time of injury (fig. 10).

VIDEO 6

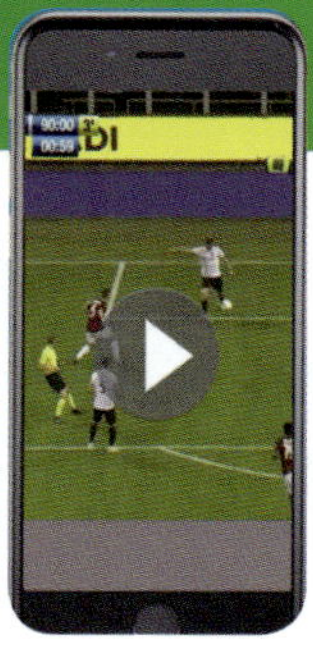

The arrow indicates the player being injured; the bar shows the moment of injury

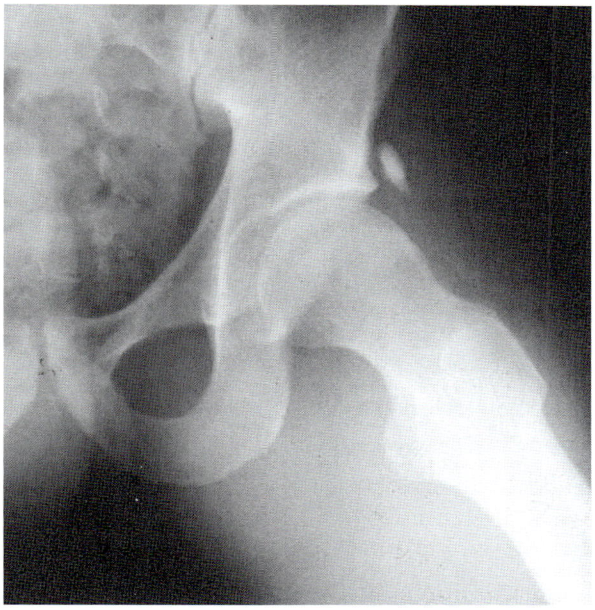

Fig. 10 - X-ray of the pelvis in a professional soccer player who had suffered a left rectus femoris tendon detachment eight months earlier

With regard to the adductor group, the adductor longus is by far the most commonly affected. Over 90% of muscle lesions to the groin affect this muscle. The movements at risk are usually those performed with the hip extended, abducted and externally rotated and include kicking, tackling, changing direction, receiving a pass, intercepting the ball, and jumping over an opponent or an obstacle. Even in these cases the presence of an unforeseen event during the movement can be taken into account as an important element to explain an injury that occurs following a movement that is commonly performed in training or matches. Even the slightest slide on a weight-bearing leg can be an unforeseen event during a change of direction, especially at high speed, which leads to further eccentric load of the adductor longus on the same side. Likewise, receiving a ball that is slightly more forward than expected can stretch the adductors in the weight-bearing leg and produce an added function with further demand for eccentric contraction and subsequently an impossibility to fulfil the new functional demand. Furthermore, even a legal challenge by an opponent while performing an inside kick can unbalance the body slightly forwards with respect to the ideal line of the ball with the weight-bearing leg being too far forwards of the ball and thus with the need to externally rotate and further extend the hip of the kicking leg. This causes further eccentric load on the adductors of the kicking leg, and impossibility to bear the load with a lengthening of the muscle. A technical movement that can put the adductors of the weight-bearing leg at risk is trying to stop the opponent from crossing by using the other leg with knee extended to get the ball and that the opponent with his arm stops the trunk and pelvis from flexing forward, thus requiring further eccentric strength from the adductors of the weight-bearing limb (video 7).

A change in direction while running is also a movement that can put certain muscles at risk, such as the obturator externus and the obturator internus, which are less frequently involved by soccer lesions. This can happen to an obturator of the weight-bearing leg when in changing direction the player further rotates the pelvis, for example, by following and marking an opponent from behind, who suddenly changes direction internally with a more acute angle than expected. The player that is marking and does not expect the opponent's sudden change in direction towards the same side as the weight-bearing leg is forced to rotate noticeably with the pelvis towards the same side by internally rotating the pelvis towards the weight-bearing leg and obliges the obturators to bear a sudden eccentric contraction. It is virtually a more abrupt and wider internal rotation movement of the pelvis towards the leg in contact with the ground (video 8).

Concerning muscle lesions of the triceps surae,

VIDEO 7

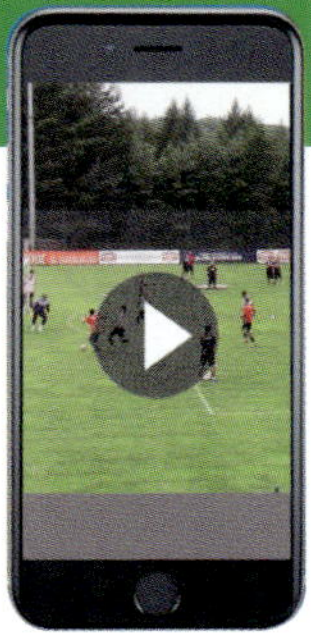

The arrow indicates the player being injured; the bar shows the moment of injury

VIDEO 8

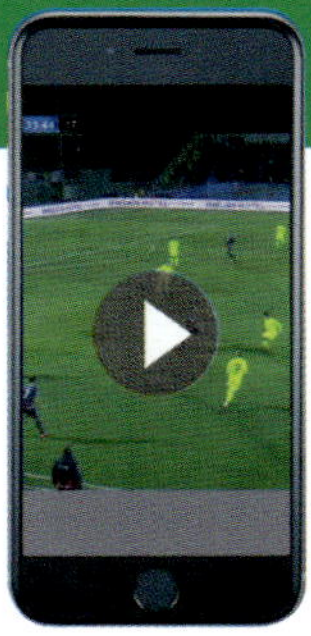

The arrow indicates the player being injured; the bar shows the moment of injury

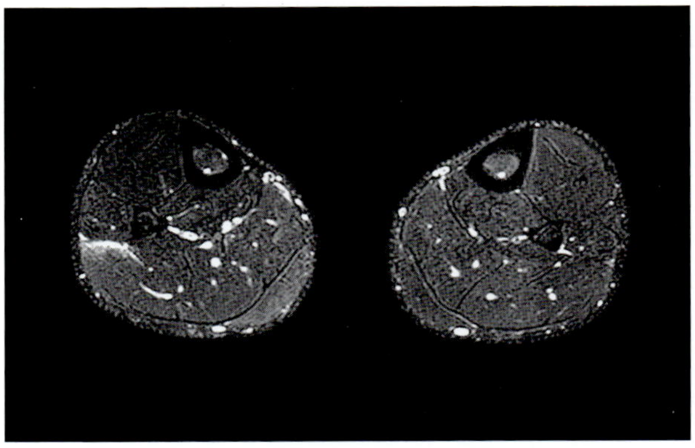

Fig. 11 - Nuclear magnetic resonance of a 3A soleus lesion in a professional soccer player with negative ultrasonography

we should distinguish between those involving the medial gastrocnemius and especially the distal myotendinous junction (very rare are those involving the lateral gastrocnemius) and those of the soleus.

A medial gastrocnemius lesion can occur following a sprint, a change in direction, acceleration or deceleration or kicking the ball. In that case the lesion can affect the weight-bearing leg at the moment of striking the ball, or the ball-striking leg when the foot hits the ground after kicking. An unforeseen event when performing this action might be uneven ground under the forefoot, which imposes a slight increase in dorsal flexion of the ankle and therefore a demand for eccentric strength with a longer muscle, or an always possible push or hold by the opponent that forces the player into weight bearing with more dorsal flexion in order to get free or not decrease running speed. The player feels an acute shooting pain that does not allow the action to be continued.

Conversely, in the case of soleus lesions, at least minor ones (3A), which are far more common in soccer players than more severe structural lesions (3B and 4), pain appears gradually throughout the match. It does not necessarily stop the player from finishing the match or training session. It can increase with the player at rest and produce a limp. Its onset can be subtle and deceptive on the lateral side of the triceps and suggest a problem with the lateral gastrocnemius (very rare) and then move medially to the centre of the muscle over the following hours or days.

Ultrasonography is often negative because of the small size of the lesion and power Doppler is of little use, especially if the lesion is deep in the soleus. Conversely, NMR is very useful in these cases because, particularly with STIR sequences with fat suppression, it will show the small lesion and enable us to classify it correctly and treat the player (fig. 11). Failing that, since symptoms tend to subside completely at rest, the player and staff are induced to resume training. However, after a few steps of running the problem reappears in the form of a cramping pain that forces the player to stop. This situation can last for several weeks unless the injured player rests and undergoes appropriate treatment, instead of making futile and frustrating attempts to resume activity before time. This lesion is favoured by plyometric exercise or close, intense sessions of bounding. The movement that causes the lesion is hard to investigate given the characteristics of its onset, so it is the unforeseen event that favours the injury.

Treatment

The treatment of muscle lesions in soccer players is mostly conservative but recovery must be complete before returning to work with the team. A hurried or incomplete recovery could lead to complications or recurrences that significantly delay definitive and safe RTP. The best treatment for contusions or structural lesions is to apply ice (better directly on the pitch), an elastic-compression bandage and rest for the limb, with the use of crutches for a few days in severe cases. Ice and cryotherapy machines should be used at regular intervals, even in the dressing room for a few hours after the injury [18]. After the acute phase it is important to mobilize the limb as soon as possible, from 2 to 5 days after the injury, depending on the severity of the lesion, by cautious movements while following the no-pain rule. The only massage treatment allowed is lymphatic drainage, to enable faster reabsorption of the hematoma. If the hematoma is large, it can be aspirated under ultrasound guidance in a sterile field. Anti-inflammatory drugs and painkillers can only be used in rare, particularly painful cases, and only for two or three days after injury. Subsequently, when muscle mobilization exercises are started, these drugs should not be used because they raise the pain threshold and prevent the physiotherapist and player from working in safety.

After the acute phase, the rehabilitation protocol is divided into three progressive steps, each of which has to achieve precise functional objectives before moving on to the next one. The first step is aimed at resolving predisposing factors (hypo-extensibility of antagonist muscles, minor intervertebral defects at thoracolumbar spine level, and asymmetric movements in the sacroiliac joints), resolving pain in daily living movements, recovering over 90% of the extensibility in the injured muscle, and enabling the injured muscle to work with loads of not less than 50% of theoretical maximum load. In this step work is carried out in the gym and the player is assisted by a physiotherapist.

The functional objective of the second step is complete recovery of extensibility in the injured muscle, recovery of strength in the injured muscle, especially eccentric strength, and the recovery of sport-specific aerobic parameters (S2: aerobic threshold, S4: anaerobic threshold). In soccer, the minimum parameters for professional players are: S2 = 11.5 km/h, and S4 = 13.8 km/h. These values are to be considered minimum being low enough for modern soccer. The professional team we assessed was in Serie A of the Italian championship and did not take part in European tournaments and had a mean value of S2 = 12.8 km/h and S4 = 15.2 km/h.

The choice of eccentric exercises with the correct progression of loads is fundamental for the optimal recovery of the player. To avoid recurrences, the injured muscle should be able to develop and shift peak torque at longer lengths, thus arranging sarcomeres in series thanks to stimulation by eccentric exercise. In the tension-length diagram of the muscle the curve should shift towards the right [19] (fig. 12).

There are now several papers in the literature that advocate achieving this objective during rehabilitation and maintaining it once the player has made a full return to playing with the team [20, 21].

Another parameter to achieve is the recovery of optimum weight and percentage of optimal fat mass, which in the soccer player should not exceed 10%. In this step the work is carried out partially in the gym with the physiotherapist and partially on the field with the fitness coach.

The third and final step involves the consolidation of the extensibility and strength of the injured muscle, recovery of sport-specific technical move-

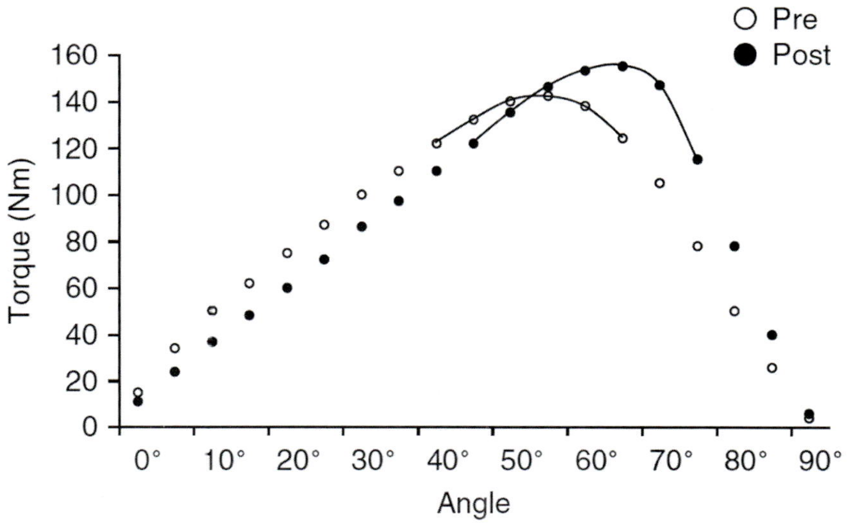

Fig. 12 - Length-tension diagram of the muscle before (pre) and after (post) strengthening by eccentric exercises (from Brughelli et al. [19])

ments, recovery of high-intensity sports parameters for soccer, and reliability and movement-specific strength with respect to the movement that caused the injury. Work in this step is carried out mainly, but not exclusively, on the field with the help of the fitness coach. In the gym, the physiotherapist continues consolidating the optimal characteristics of the injured muscle and should monitor the muscle carefully until the end of the field session and before starting the next session the day after. In this step the risk of a recurring injury in the same muscle is higher than it is in the other steps, especially if the fundamental rules of rehabilitation are not followed, such as the no-pain rule and that of progressive loading, both with regards to athletic performance and technical movements.

It is necessary to understand what is meant by recovery of high-intensity sports parameters in soccer. Before returning to work with the team and being at the manager's disposal, the injured player, during the rehabilitation sessions on the field, should have achieved the average parameters for match playing and not only those for training, which, as it can be seen in the figure 13 are much lower than the former (fig. 13).

To reduce the recurrence rate of muscle lesions, more common in match playing than in training by about six times according to some authors, we should think in terms of RTP and not be content with return-to-training (RTT), during the rehabilitation period. RTT is certainly easier to achieve and less risky, but it exposes the player to greater risks having been put back at the manager's disposal, who will try to use him as soon as possible thinking that he has recovered.

During the third step of rehabilitation, achieving another functional objective, that of reliability and movement-specific strength, is as important as it is risky, but fundamental before allowing the player back to work with his team. It concerns making the injured muscle reliable and resilient, not only with regard to the specific technical movements of soccer, but also and above all in relation to the movement that caused the lesion. This should be tested and exercised several times during the rehab sessions on the field and unexpected situations should be introduced so as to prepare the muscle for the movement and situation that caused the injury, which will certainly crop up again once the player is back working with team. Failing this, the player would feel held back psychologically from making that movement which caused the injury or would make it less freely and less effectively, by using biomechanical compensations which might carry the risk of injuring other muscles or structures such as joints, bones, and tendons.

It is key that the injured muscle has made a full recovery of extensibility and strength and that the player has achieved the required sport-specific parameters and optimal weight and percentage of fat mass parameters before doing reliability and movement-specific exercises, in order to avoid the risk of recurrence in this delicate phase of recovery.

To reduce the likelihood of setbacks during recovery, it is necessary to look out for any red lights, which prevent the player from going on to the next step. Between the first and second step, pain reported by the player when performing the strength exercises in this phase, or when running at low speed on the treadmill, should be seen as a red light; between the second and third step, the stretch test of the injured muscle being still positive, compared to the contralateral one, should be seen as a red light against moving on to the next step. Moreover, advancing from the third step to returning to the team is strongly discouraged if the player reports any difference in the muscle compared to the contralateral one during or after being on the field.

Clinical and ultrasound monitoring during the recovery of an injured muscle is very important to assess the progress of scarring, any complications and to reassure those who have to decide about progressive loading and moving on to the next step.

We believe that NMR is not important to decide if and when a player has completed his recovery and can be ready for RTP. NMR can still be positive weeks or months after RTP without the occurrence of new problems even through the player has resumed activity with the team without functional limitations [18]. Ultrasound, which is performed within 48 hours of injury, should be repeated at the start of the first step of rehabilitation, before doing exercises on the field (be-

		Distance	Dist high vel	Dist vel >25	Dist max acc	Dist max dec
training	min	1691	99	0	27	5
training	average	4570	868	40	90	88
training	max	8228	2655	178	153	151
	match	**11486**	**2605**	**271**	**261**	**282**

Distance ▶ **total meters traveled during training or match**
Dist high vel ▶ **meters covered above 15 km/h**
Dist vel >25 ▶ **meters covered above 25 km/h**
Dist max acc ▶ **meters covered above 3 m/s²**
Dist max dec ▶ **meters covered under -3 m/s²**

RTT ▶ RTP

RTT ▶ Return to Training **RTP ▶ Return to Play**

Fig. 13 - Total distance run and distance run under high-intensity work in training and in matches. Parameters recorded in a professional Italian soccer team of serie A

ginning of the second step) and certainly before the third step, which is the riskiest. Ultrasound should show an advanced stage of maturity and stability of the scar and the power Doppler should be negative. A final ultrasound scan, before returning to work with the team, should confirm biological healing, besides clinical healing of the injured muscle, despite the intense work expected in the final step before RTP.

The choice of extensibility and strength exercises for the bi-articular muscles, especially in the first and second step, is made according to the site of the lesion (proximal, middle or distal), and should take into account the prevalent articular movement that involves the injured muscle fibres (video 9, 10, 11, 12, 13, 14) . It would be useful to have a film of the injury or at least understand in the player's words what movement caused the lesion. It would also be useful to know which of the strength exercises proposed activates one muscle more than another in the same muscle group. With regards to this, however, there are not many papers in the literature, the only ones being about the hamstrings (long head of the biceps femoris versus the semitendinosus) or the quadriceps [22].

If there are no complications, the prognosis varies according to the lesion grade, the muscle, the lesion site and the type of tissue involved by the

VIDEO 9

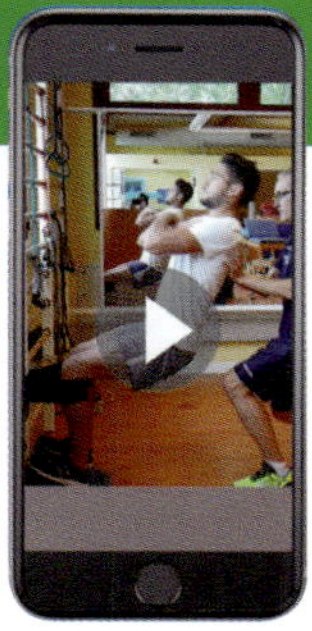

Eccentric muscle exercise for the rectus femoris with prevalent hip movement

VIDEO 10

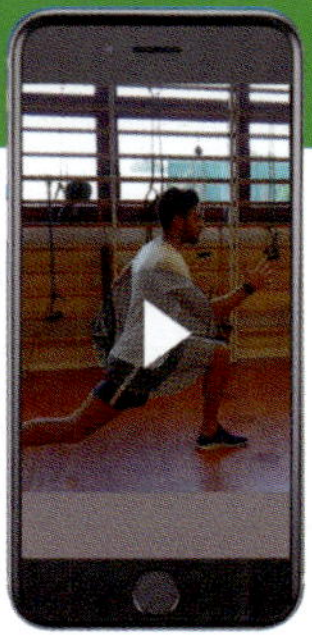

Eccentric muscle exercise for the rectus femoris with prevalent hip movement

lesion besides muscular tissue. It usually ranges from 15 to 30 days for a structural 3A lesion, 30 to 45 days for a 3B lesion and up to 2 months for a type 4 lesion.

My experience as doctor of a professional soccer team has enabled me to follow some cases, often unexplainable, of players who did not stop playing after suffering a structural injury, or who resumed full activity way too soon. These injuries involved certain muscles, such as the obturators, the adductors or the semitendinosus, but the lesion was myofascial, or in the middle third and of type 3A entity. This never happened for major lesions or myotendinous junction lesions or even if the lesion involved the tendon and never for the biceps femoris, semimembranosus or triceps surae. The unexplainable cases included only one that involved the rectus femoris with a middle third 3B lesion. It also involved the intramuscular (central) tendon. This player never stopped playing, and made a significant contribution to winning the Serie B championship and had no recurrences in following years. He never underwent therapy outside our centres or regenerative infiltrative therapy. RTP in players affected by very rare muscle lesions, such as the tensor fascia lata, gluteus medius and gluteus minimus, was respectively five, three and two days without complications or recurrence.

Complications

The complications that can occur after a non-contact trauma muscle lesion and that can delay recovery times are, in order of frequency:

- scarring;
- intramuscular fluid collection;
- intramuscular fluid cyst;
- muscle calcification;

VIDEO 11

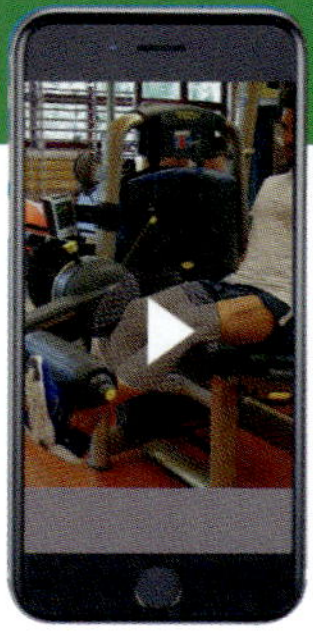

Eccentric muscle exercise for the rectus femoris with prevalent knee movement

VIDEO 12

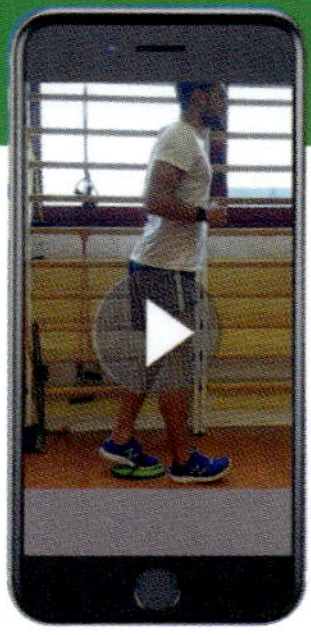

Eccentric muscle exercise for the hamstrings with prevalent hip movement

VIDEO 13

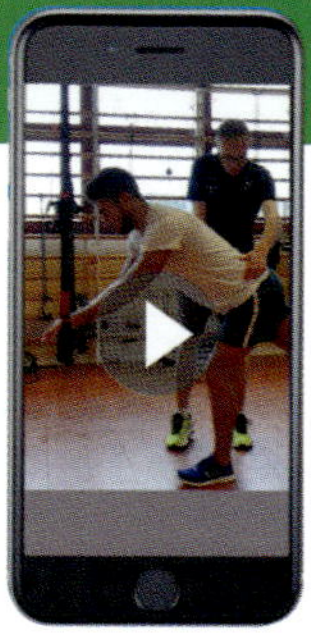

Eccentric muscle exercise for the hamstrings with prevalent hip movement

VIDEO 14

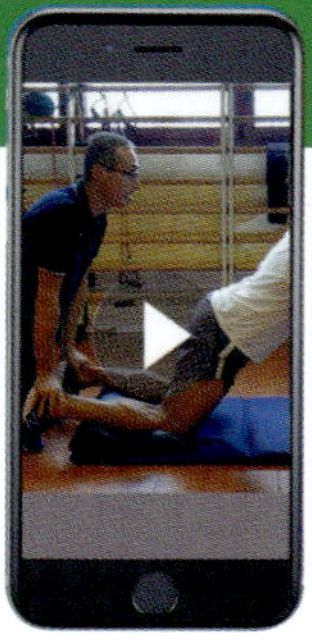

Eccentric muscle exercise for the hamstrings with prevalent knee movement (Nordic Hamstring Exercise)

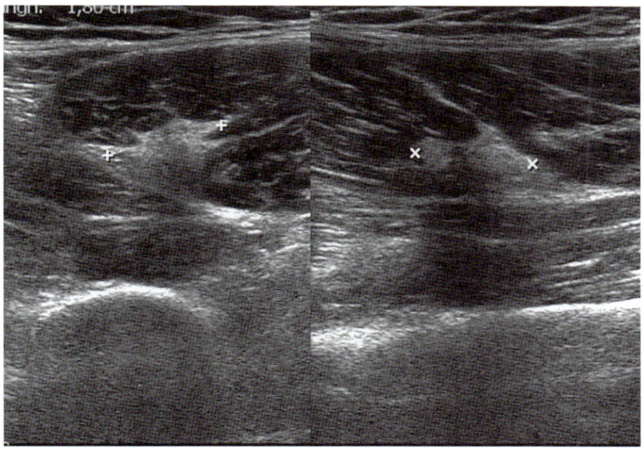

Fig. 14 - Ultrasound of muscle: scar tissue of the rectus femoris in a professional soccer player

- circumscribed intramuscular bone calcification;
- vein thrombosis;
- muscle hernia.

Scarring is the most common one. It occurs after treating a muscle lesion too cautiously, remaining too long without appropriate movement stimulation, or, conversely, after undergoing exercises with excessive load, too early and not appropriate for the rehabilitation phase and biological characteristics of the scar tissue that is forming. An excessive deposit of collagen fibre with respect to the elastic tissue and muscle fibrils makes the scar tissue excessively stiff, impairing normal sliding of the fascia inside the muscle or with nearby muscles and tissues (fig. 14). In this case the most indicated treatment methods are percutaneous scar release using special fibrolysis hooks (followed by eccentric exercises of the injured muscle), which is very operator dependent but also very effective, and shockwave therapy for soft tissues. Before treatment an ultrasound study of the area to be treated is performed.

Intramuscular fluid collection consists of serosanguinous fluid that separates the epimysium between two adjacent muscles. It usually occurs between the medial gastrocnemius and soleus muscle, after a triceps surae lesion or between the rectus femoris and vastus intermedius in quadriceps lesions, often caused by the insufficient application of an elastic compression bandage or massages that are too energetic, deep and traumatic in the first 7-10 days after injury. In this case the most effective treatment is lymphatic drainage massage or ultrasound-guided fluid aspiration, followed by the application of an elastic bandage or stocking, which should be kept in place as long as possible throughout the day, for at least a week. After aspirating the fluid, it might be indicated to inject a vial of cortisone under ultrasound guidance to reduce the risk of fluid reforming (fig. 15).

An intramuscular cyst is a collection of fluid, but in this case it occurs inside the muscle belly, probably between two perimysiums. The causes are the same. Aspirating the fluid or injecting cortisone into the cyst is hardly ever indicated, unless the cyst grows to a size that prevents the player from performing normal sports activity. It is useful to wear an elastic bandage during training and matches.

Muscle calcification usually occurs inside an area of scar tissue that is poorly vascularized. If it is painful, the treatment of choice is shockwave therapy. A few sessions are enough to solve the problem. When a player feels heaviness of the muscle or sharp pain inside the muscle itself and is wary about continuing his run, if at high intensity, or after a specific technical movement, then the onset of one of these complications should be suspected.

As already mentioned, circumscribed intramuscular ossification, or inappropriately called myositis ossificans, is a direct trauma or contact lesion. It is very rare in indirect structural traumas and, as in those caused by direct trauma, it is helped by the application of heat or trauma massages in the early days after injury (fig. 16).

Vein thrombosis is a very rare complication that occurs after an injury to the medial gastrocnemius, especially if treated by too little weight bearing on the affected limb.

Muscle hernia is rare but it does not usually cause major problems for the player. It is more evident when the muscle is relaxed and disappears when the muscle contracts. It is more common in the

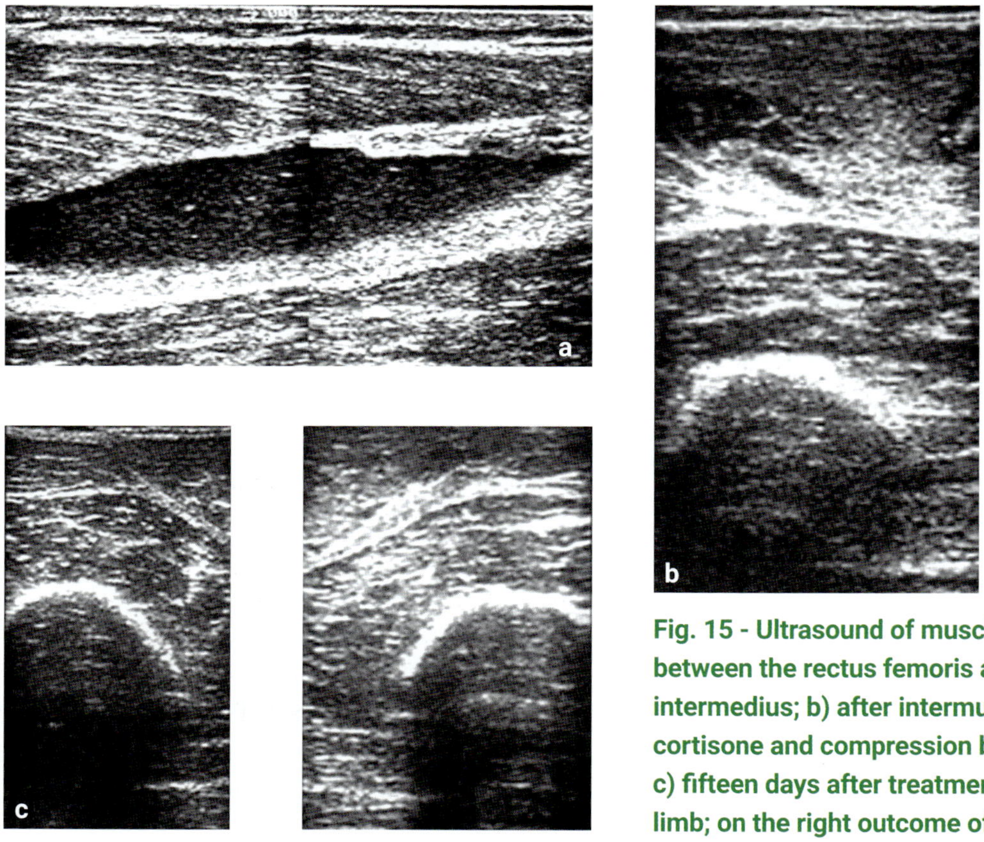

Fig. 15 - Ultrasound of muscle: a) fluid collection between the rectus femoris and vastus intermedius; b) after intermuscular injection with cortisone and compression bandage for five days; c) fifteen days after treatment: on the left healthy limb; on the right outcome of fluid collection

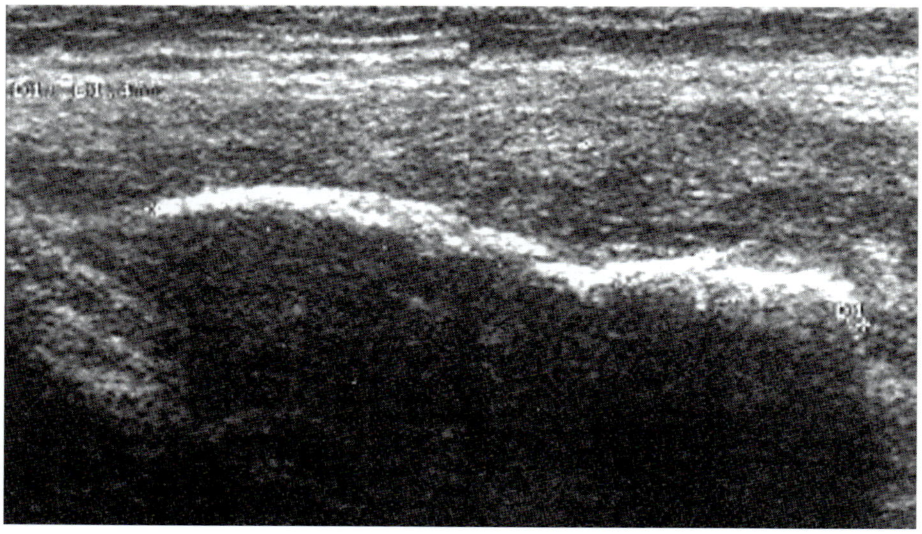

Fig. 16 - Ultrasound of muscle: circumscribed intramuscular ossification of the quadriceps two years after a direct trauma in a fully active player, without pain

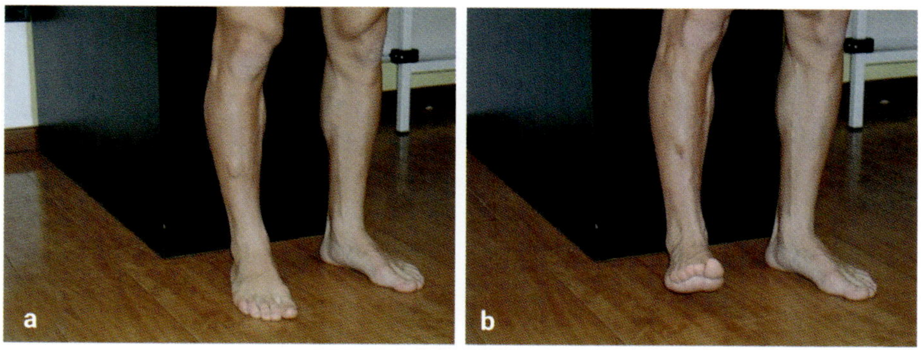

Fig. 17 - Muscle hernia of right tibialis anterior: a) muscle relaxed b) muscle contracted

tibialis anterior and quadriceps (fig. 17). False muscle hernia can occur after a total muscle lesion and, unlike a true hernia, it is more evident during muscle contraction and tends to decrease or disappear when the muscle is relaxed (fig. 18).

Other treatments

Some muscle lesions in soccer players require surgical treatment. They are type 4 lesions with avulsion of the rectus femoris proximal tendon or the conjoint tendon of the hamstrings, especially if the gap is greater than two centimetres [23, 24]. These injuries can heal with conservative treatment, but there would be functional deficit, such as reduced muscular strength and the development of scar tissue, which might include or compress peripheral nerve fibres and be responsible of disabling pain such as Hamstring Syndrome. Furthermore, healing times, if surgery is performed within two weeks of injury, are shorter than those of injuries treated conservatively. That would suggest a preference for surgical treatment in soccer players. Conversely, indication for surgery is controversial with regards to type 4 lesions of the adductor longus or adductor magnus. For these injuries there are papers in the literature that show similar results for both surgical and conservative treatment, both in terms of functional recovery and recovery time [25]. Postoperative prognosis ranges from three to four months for the adductors, four to five months for the rectus femoris, and five to six months and over for the hamstrings, taking into account RTP as the final objective.

In recent years regenerative therapy, by injecting platelet-rich plasma (PRP) into the injured muscle, has been adopted with the aim of qualitatively improving scarring, reducing complications and accelerating healing and RTP. The scientific evidence found in the literature is not yet clear and unequivocal, but even with the help of this therapy with growth factors, an optimal result cannot be achieved without a correct rehabilitation protocol that involves reaching the functional goals of each step.

In the 1980's some German authors, in particular Hans-Wilhelm Müller-Wohlfahrt introduced injecting a substance called Actovegin into the treatment of injured muscles and obtained excellent results both in non-structural and structural injuries. His experience as doctor of a very important German club and of the German national team enabled him to treat a large number of professional soccer players using this method without having adverse effects and sometimes with miraculous results.

However, the papers published in the literature by this author's group have a low level of evidence [18]. Nevertheless, even according to these authors healing and RTP cannot be achieved without following a precise rehabilitation protocol that includes the various phases of progressive return to work with the team.

The treatment of non-structural injuries is totally different: besides reducing the work load, de-contracting massages, heat, TENS, spine and pelvis manipulation in 2A, extensibility exercises for stiff muscles, usually the antagonists of those injured,

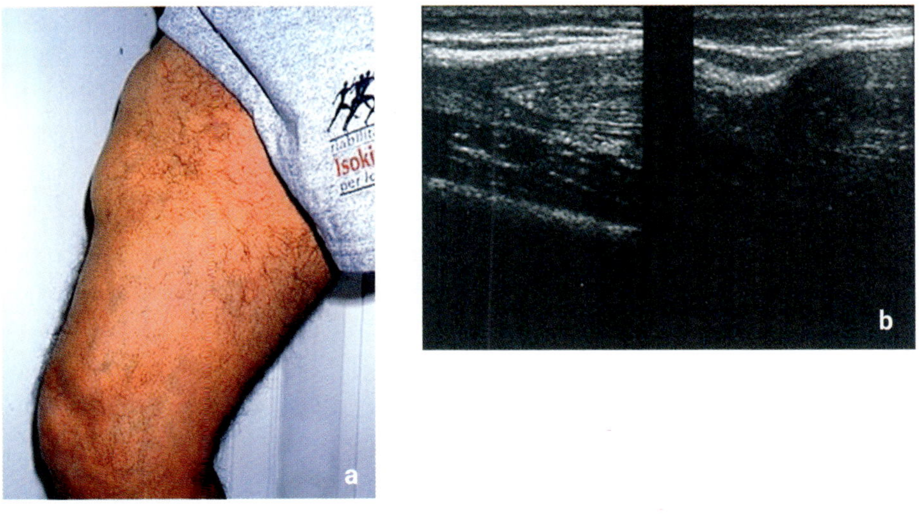

Fig. 18 - False muscle hernia of the rectus femoris:
a) muscle contracted
b) ultrasound of false hernia with muscle first relaxed and then contracted

eccentric toning exercises for weaker muscles, and aerobic exercises in the swimming pool, exercise bike, treadmill or cross trainer.
There is scientific evidence that immerging the lower limbs in water at a temperature of 8-10 degrees for 10 minutes after training and matches can prevent the post-exercise pain typical of DOMS. This practice, or the use of a cryotherapy chamber, rather than a cryosauna, after exercise are techniques already widely used in professional soccer, but the level of evidence is still low. The cryotherapy chamber reaches very low temperatures, requires the presence of special staff during its use, and requires the use of gloves to protect the hands and special socks to protect the feet.

Muscle lesions in young soccer players

There are few epidemiological studies for youth soccer and the ones that are available use different definitions of injury, classification and concepts of exposure times. Professional soccer clubs should implement the data collection of young players' injuries and promote epidemiological studies that enable a greater number of risk factors to be identified in order to reduce the injury rate in this category. Indeed, an injury in a young player often produces emotional stress, which, being accentuated by family expectations and pressure from the trainer and teammates, could have a negative effect on the psychological growth and maturation with repercussions not only on the player's sporting life.
The literature shows that, of all injuries, muscle lesions are the most common with rates that range from 26% to 46% and the rates of muscle lesions range from 0.42 and 1.47 per 1,000 hours of exposure and that most of these injuries occur during training rather than matches. The quadriceps account for between 21% and 46%, the hamstrings 13% and 35%, and the adductors about 18% of muscle injuries. Thus, in youth soccer, quadriceps muscle injuries seem to be the most common lesions in the lower limbs.
A recent study on young Spanish athletes of all kinds, but soccer players in particular (Valle et al.), revealed fewer hamstring injuries on the whole, but slightly more semimembranosus and semitendinosus lesions, compared with adult athletes [26]. The hamstring lesions were more frequent in the final part of the season when the number of matches was greater. Hamstring injuries were already present, although rarely, at the age of 9 but were mostly in 15-17-year-olds.
In the youth sector of a high level English professional team, an epidemiological study on a single season showed that muscle lesions accounted for 46% of all lesions and a prevalence in the quadriceps muscles. A wider study on 38 English teams over two consecutive seasons showed a 31% rate of muscle lesions in the youth sector with a slight prevalence during training rather than matches. Another wider study over five years of English youth soccer (8-16 years old) conducted by Clocke et al., on Premiership teams, found a mean annual rate of muscle lesions of 0.52 per 1,000 hours of activity and that midfielders suffered the most injuries, followed by defenders and then forwards [27]. This study also showed that the quadriceps muscles were those most frequently affected. The risk of injury during a match increased towards the end of half time and for all of the second half. There were two peaks in the injury rate throughout the season (january and september) and the injury rate in the hamstrings, adductors and quadriceps only differed slightly according to age.
Conversely, the rate of severe lesions increased according to the age of the player. The mean inactivity time after injury was 13 days and 27% of injuries had a recurrence.
In a study of Portuguese youth soccer (age 12-19 years old) over four seasons of a top team, muscle lesions accounted for 26% of all lesions. Of these muscle lesions, 41% occurred in the first three months of the season with a rate of 0.75/1000 hours of exposure. Also in this study the most frequently affected muscle was the quadriceps (46%), followed by the hamstrings (36%), adductors (18%) and the triceps surae (6.25%). Mean recovery times for the quadriceps, adductors and hamstrings were 24.7, 19.5 and 15.4 days respectively. The hamstrings had the highest recurrence rate over the 12 months after injury (21%) [28].
A study of the youth sector in Barcelona performed over a single season included a population of 139 young players. The percentage of muscle lesions was 48% of the total and the rate

was 1.47/1,000 hours of exposure, 0.89/1,000 hours in training and 6.47/1000 hours in matches. The under fourteen category had a lower rate of muscle lesions, whereas the higher age group players had a higher rate of hamstring and adductor injuries. In the under 16 players the most affected muscle group was the hamstrings and had a higher injury burden, 109 days, compared with the higher age group, 50 days. The injuries sustained during matches were more frequent in the last 15 minutes of the second half; this rate was three times greater than that of any other time in the match. There was no important prevalence in role and few recurrences were recorded (3.5%) with respect to professional soccer.

In this study the under 14 players did not suffer structural injuries to the hamstrings, whereas they had a high rate of adductor lesions with a rather high injury burden, 175 days [29].

We carried out a study on three consecutive seasons (from 15/7/2015 to 30/5/2018) in the youth sector (age 13-20 years old) of a top italian professional soccer club which showed that muscle lesions accounted for 38.1% of all injuries, with a rate of 1.97/1,000 hours of exposure. Structural lesions (29.37%), thus with a muscle fibre lesion, had a rate of 0.58/1000 hours' exposure, whereas non-structural lesions (70.6%) had a rate of 1.39/1,000 hours' exposure. Muscle lesions were more prevalent in the older categories, under 19 and under 17, and thus more severe. The hamstrings were the most frequently involved by muscle lesions; the rate of hamstring lesions was 36.25%, followed by rectus femoris (24.37%) and adductors (15%). Mean number of days lost was 16.08 with an injury burden of 101.31 days per 1000 hours' exposure for structural injuries and 55.36 for non-structural injuries. Our study also confirms that the thigh muscles are those most affected, but with a prevalence in the hamstrings over the quadriceps.

Comparing different age categories, in the under 14 group the number of hamstring injuries was three times greater than that of quadriceps injuries, but nearly all of them were non-structural; in the under 15 group the number of injuries was more or less similar in thigh muscle groups. In the under 17 and under 19 groups the number of hamstring injuries was double that of quadriceps injuries, and in the under 16 group the number of muscle lesions was lower overall.

Compared with adult soccer, in youth soccer there are further difficulties in designing effective injury prevention programs in general and in muscles in particular. The reason is that within the same team and same age group there are players with different degrees of biological maturity and anthropometric characteristics. Indeed, as it occurs in growing young people in the general population, also in growing soccer players of the same age group there can be differences in psycho-physical development, which do not always correspond to the players' chronological age. In the youth categories the likelihood that the chronological age matches biological age is very low and therefore to reduce injury players should be divided into classes of biological maturity with similar anthropomorphic characteristics and not purely according to their age.

Another reason why it is more difficult to design prevention programs in young players is that, unlike professional soccer players, they also go to school and have less time to dedicate to recovery, correct diet, and personalised exercise programs. However, they have to undergo rigorous training sessions, which are more and more required by modern soccer, even in this age group.

Using GPS to monitor exercise, especially high intensity exercise, should help to keep a good ratio between acute and chronic load, with the same concepts used for adult professional players, thus enabling trainers of young players to avoid putting them through training sessions that are too intense and too stressful with the risk of injury.

Muscle lesions in female soccer players

Concerning female soccer, there are still not enough epidemiological studies in the literature on injuries, and in particular muscular lesions, although the number of women playing soccer is growing worldwide. In Italy by 30 June 2017 there were 23,665 women soccer player members of Federcalcio (12,747 under 18) and in the 2017/18 season the number of clubs in the various championships was 677. Among these clubs, 12 played in Serie A and 57 in Serie B.

Most muscle lesions, even in women's soccer, occur by indirect trauma and more often during matches rather than training.

Larruskain et al. who compared the injuries of men and women over five seasons in a first division Spanish soccer team, found that hamstring lesions were 1.93 times more common in men than in women, whereas quadriceps lesions were 2.25 times more frequent in women [30].

In a study of 165 women soccer players (mean age 22 years old) of 9 teams in the German national championship, muscle injuries accounted for only 15.21% of the total number of injuries, and half of these occurred in matches. In this study, direct trauma injuries were more frequent than they were in most studies including those on men's soccer, which accounted for about 14% of all muscle lesions [31].

The conclusions of a study carried out on a single season including 173 players from 12 teams belonging to the Norwegian first division were different; muscle lesions accounted for 34% of the total number of injuries and those of the hamstrings far exceeded those of the quadriceps.

A study on 123 adult women soccer players in 8 Swedish teams over a single season showed that muscle injuries accounted for 32.3% of all injuries and slightly more of these occurred in matches. In this study the number of hamstring lesions was higher than that of quadriceps lesions.

Younger players seem to have a lower rate of injuries compared with older ones. A study on 25,397 Spanish women players, half of whom were under 18, showed a 14% rate of muscle lesions over a single season.

A study by FIFA on seven international women's soccer tournaments including 184 matches and 6,072 hours reported 8% of muscle lesions.

However, on the whole, women players have a higher rate of quadriceps injuries compared with men, but the latter suffer more injuries in the hamstrings and adductors compared with women players.

As in youth soccer, also in women's soccer the FIFA 11+ preventive exercise protocol has shown it can reduce the rate of injuries in general and muscle injuries in particular [32].

Bibliography

1. Ekstrand J, Hagglund M, Walden M. Epidemiology of muscle injuries in professional football (soccer). Am J Sports Med. 2011; 39(6):1226-1232.

2. Ekstrand J, Askling C, Magnusson H et al. Return to play after thigh muscle injury in elite football players: implementation and validation of the Munich muscle injury classification. Br J Sports Med 2013;47:769-774.

3. Ekstrand J, Walden M, Hagglund M. Hamstring injuries have increased by 4% annually in men's professional football, since 2001: a 13-year longitudinal analysis of the UEFA Elite Club injury study. Br J Sports Med 2016;50:731-737.

4. Hagglund M, Walden M. Ekstrand J. Risk factors for lower extremity muscle injury in professional soccer: the UEFA Injury Study. Am J Sports Med 2013;41:327-35.

5. Mueller-Wohlfahrt HW, Hansel L, Mithoefer K et al. Terminology and classification of muscle injuries in sport: a consensus statement. Br J Sports Med 2012;47:342-50.

6. Hagglund M, Walden M, Magnusson H et al. Injuries affect team performance negatively in professional football:an 11-year follow-up of the UEFA Champions League injury study. Br J Sports Med 2013;47:738-42.

7. Timmins RG, Bourne MN, Shield AJ et al. Short biceps femoris fascicles and eccentric knee flexor weakness increase the risk of hamstring injury in elite football (soccer): a prospective cohort study. Br J Sports Med 2016;50(24):1524-1535.

8. Arnason A, Sigurdsson SB, Gudmundsson A et al. Risk factors for injuries in football. Am J Sports Med 2004;32(suppl 1):S5-16.

9. Orchard J. Intrinsic and extrinsic risk factors for muscle strains in Australian football. Am J Sports Med 2001;29:300-3.

10. Bradley PS, Portas MD. The relationship between preseason range of motion and muscle strain injury in elite soccer players. J Strength Cond Res 2007;21:1155-9.

11. Whittaker JL, Small C, Maffey L et al. Risk factors for groin injury in sport:an updated systematic review. Br J Sports Med 2015;49(12):803-9.

12. Fousekis K, Tsepis E, Poulmedis P et al. Intrinsic risk factors of non-contact quadriceps and hamstring strains in soccer: a prospective study of 100 professional player. Br J Sports Med 2011;45:709-14.

13. Timmins R, Shield AJ, Williams MD et al. Biceps femoris long head architecture:a reality and retrospective injury study. Med Sci Sports Exerc 2015;47:905-13.

14. Bengtsson H, Ekstrand J, Walden M et.al. Muscle injiury rate in professional football is higher in matches played within 5 days since the previous match: a 14-year prospective study with more than 130000 match observations. Br J Sports Med 2018; 52(17):1116-1122.

15. Al Attar WS, Soomro N, Sinclair PJ et al. Effect of injury prevention programs that include the Nordic hamstring exercise on hamstring injury rates in soccer players: a systematic review and meta-analysis. Sports Med 2017; 47(5): 907-916.

16. Schuermans J, Danneels L, Tiggelen DV et al. Proximal neuromuscular control protects against hamstring injuries in male soccer players: a prospective study with electromyography time-series analysis during maximal sprinting. Am J Sports Med 2017;45: 1315-25.

17. Gabbett TJ. The training-injury prevention paradox: should athletes be training smarter and harder? Br J Sports Med 2016; 50: 273-80.

18. Ueblacker P, Haensel L, Mueller-Wohlfahrt HW. Treatment of muscle injuries in football. J of Sports Sciences 2016 vol.34, n.24, 2329-2337.

19. Brughelli M, Cronin J. Altering the length-tension relationship with eccentric exercise. Sports Med 2007;37(9): 807-826.

20. Fyfe JJ, Opar DA, Williams MD, Shield AJ. The role of neuromuscular inhibition in hamstring strain injury recurrence. J Electromyogr Kinesiol. 2013 Jun;23(3):523-30.

21. Tyler TF, Schmitt BM, Nicholas SJ et al. Rehabilitation after hamstring- strain injury emphasizing eccentric strengthening at long muscle lengths: results of long-term follow-up. J of Sport Rehabilitation 2017,26, 131-140.

22. Tsaklis P, Malliaropoulos N, Mendiguchia J et al. Muscle and intensity base hamstring exercise classification in élite female track and field athletes: implications for exercise selection during rehabilitation. J Sports Med. 2015; 6: 209-217.

23. Harris JD, Griesser MJ, Best TM et al. Treatment of proximal hamstring ruptures - a systematic review. International J of Sports Medicine 2011, 32(7),490-495.

24. Ueblacker P, Müller-Wohlfahrt HW, Hinterwimmer S et al. Suture anchor repair of proximal rectus femoris avulsions in elite football players. Knee Surgery, Sports Traumatology, Arthroscopy 2015, 23(9), 2590-2594.

25. Ueblacker P, English B, Muller-Wohlfahrt HW. Nonoperative Treatment and return to play after complete proximal adductor avulsion in high-performance athletes. Knee Surg Sports Traumatol Arthrosc. 2016 Dec;24(12):3927-3933.

26. Valle X, Malliaropoulos N, Parraga Botero JD et al. Hamstring and other thigh injuries in children and young athletes. Stand J Med Sci Sports 2018 del; 28(12):2630-2637.

27. Cloke D, Shah T et al. Thigh muscle injuries in young soccer: predictors of recovery. Am J Sports Med 2012 feb;40(2) 433-9.

28. Diniz P, Cardoso D, Ferreira D et al. Is there a specific distribution of thigh muscle injuries in Youth football? Football Medicine Outcome abstract book 2018.

29. Raya-Gonzales J, Suarez-Aronnes L, Larruskain J. Muscle injuries in the accademy of a Spanish professional football club: A one- year prospective study. Apunts 2018; 53(197):3-9.

30. Larruskain J, Lekne JA, Díaz N et al. A comparison of injuries in elite male and female football players: A fine-season prospective study. Stand Med Sci Sports 2018 Jan;28(1):237-245.

31. Faude O, Junge A, Kindermann W et al. Injuries in female soccer players: a prospective study in the German national league. Am J Sports Med 2005 nov; 33(11): 1694-700.

32. Owoeye OB, Akinbo SR, Tella BA, Olawale OA. Efficacy of the FIFA 11+ Warm-Up Programme in Male Youth Football: A Cluster Randomised Controlled Trial. J Sports Sci Med. 2014 May 1;13(2):321-8.

CHAPTER 13

TENDON DISEASES

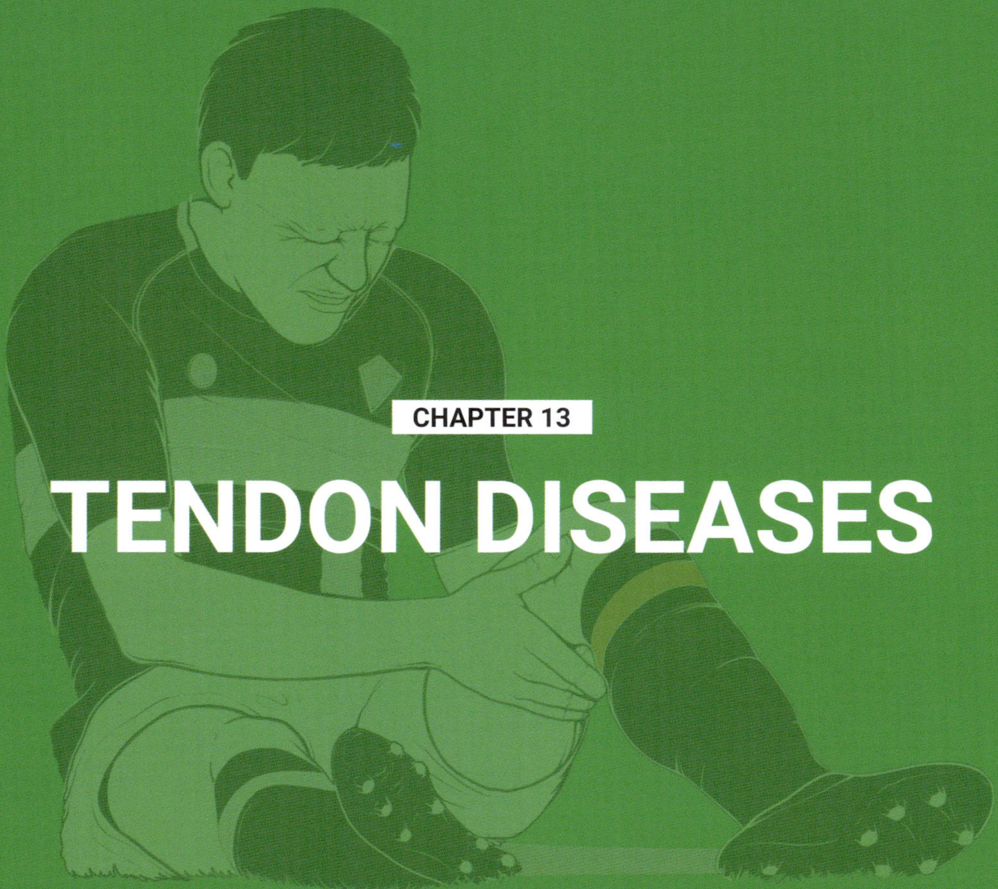

Antonio Mazzotti [1]

Antonio Oliva [1]

Sandro Giannini [2]

Cesare Faldini [1, 2]

[1] 1st Orthopaedic and Traumatologic Clinic (Director: C. Faldini)
IRCCS Istituto Ortopedico Rizzoli, Bologna, Italy

[2] IRCCS Istituto Ortopedico Rizzoli, Bologna, Italy
University of Bologna, Italy

Introduction

Tendons are fibrous structures made principally of collagen, located between muscle and bone, whose role is to transmit the force generated by the muscle to the skeleton so as to produce movement and maintain physiological posture.
Tendons are remarkably resistant to the force of traction and can bear great loads without becoming deformed so as to transmit the force generated by muscles without dissipating it [1].
Tendon injuries represent 30-50% of all sport injuries and, given the increase in sport activity within the population, the risk of such injuries is increasing [2].
Tendon injuries are frequent in soccer as it exposes tendons to extrinsic risk factors for tendinopathy such as overload, overuse and acute traumas. Professional soccerers present around two injuries per season, resulting in a seasonal average of a loss of 37 days every 300 [3]. Inadequate preparation, as well as eccessive loads with inadequate rest periods, can contribute to increasing the overall risk, especially during periods of particularly intense and heavy training during the competitive season [4].
Overload tendinopathies cause swelling and pain in the affected tendon, reducing resistance to force and functionality of the limb during exercise [5].
Clinically, it is possible to distinguish between acute tendinopathies (developed within the 2 weeks before observation), subacute (developed within the previous 2 to 6 weeks) and chronic (over 6 weeks).
Based on the location of the disease, tendinopathies can be classified into insertional, located at the osteo-tendinous junction (enthesopathy) and non-insertional, located along the course of the tendon or at the musculotendinous junction.
In clinical practice, the term "tendinopathy" defines an array of pathologies with different etiopathogenisis, varying from lesions with a prevailing inflammatory component (acute lesions), to lesions of a prevailing degenerative nature such as tendinosis (chronic lesions) [6].
The term "tendinitis", widely used in the past, is no longer used today as it presumes the presence of an inflammatory process that is not always present, particularly in chronic lesions [7].

Physiopathology of tendinopathies

Structure

Tendons are composed of hypocellular tissue belonging to the dense connective tissue histology group, made principally of parallel collagen fibres, cells (tenocyte, tenoblast), and extracellular matrix (ECM).
Based on shape, you can identify long and short tendons (rounded or flattened).
Some structures facilitate the sliding of the tendon in relation to the adjacent layers of tissue, peritendinous sheaths, synovial sheaths, reflection pulleys.
In healthy tendons 65-80% of the tendon mass is made of type I collagen, whose elementary unit is tropocollagen synthesised inside tenocytes and formed by two alpha-1 chains and one alpha-2 chain united in a triple-helix structure.
The tropocollagen is secreted by tenocytes in the extracellular matrix where, via cross-links, they form, fibrils, fibers and fibers fascicles [8]. This fiber fascicles structure allows the tendon to bear very high loads in traction.

Risk factors

The main risk factors for tendinopathies are:

- age;
- genetics;
- mechanical factors (overuse, overload, trauma);
- obesity, diabetes, hormones;
- drugs, medication;
- alcohol, smoking.

Age

One of the main risk factors of tendon pathology is age. As age increases, tendons undergo qualitative and quantitative extracellular matrix changes affecting collagenic and non-collagenic components. Not only are there degenerative matrix changes, but also changes in cellular and vascular components.

The main age-related biochemical changes are degeneration of the tenocytes and collagen fibres, reduction in the number and activity of the tenoblasts, the accumulation of fats, calcium deposits and ground substance (glycosaminoglycan). An ageing tendon is weaker than its younger counterpart and more predisposed to suffering from overload or breaking [9].

Sports injuries in older athletes are more frequently associated to overuse than acute lesions and generally have a degenerative cause [10].

Genetics

Specific genetic mutations have been associated with a higher rate of tendon injuries [11, 12].

Above all, we are dealing with genes codifying for structural proteins like collagen, factors involved in the remodelling of the matrix such as metalloproteinases or factors involved in the apoptotic process [13].

The strongest link with tendon pathology was found in subjects with mutations of the gene that codifies for type V (COL5A1) collagen. Although only contributing minimally to the composition of the tendon, it is an important factor for the aggregation of type I collagen (the main type of collagen in tendons) in fibrils [14].

Moreover, some studies have shown a correlation between the ABO blood group and the tendency for tendon injuries, particularly between the blood group 0 and the spontaneous breaking of the Achilles tendon [15, 16, 17, 18].

Mechanical factors

Excessive mechanical loads on the tendon or micro traumas repeated over time can determine the rupture of fibres and thus tendinopathy [19]. Lack of exposure to adequate levels of physiological stress for a prolonged period can also paradoxically lead to a predisposition to overload lesions [20]. A tendon which has not been subjected to loads of a certain intensity can become incapable of responding to increased solicitation. In this context, the lack of use, or inadequate use of a tendon can lead to an imbalance between the activity of the matrix metalloproteinases and that of the respective inhibitors (metalloproteinases tissue inhibitors), thus leading to degeneration of the tendon. This triggers a healing process in the damaged tendon which repairs the suffered damage. If during this phase, however, the excessive load training continues, the entity of the damage can exceed the capacity of the tendon to heal, thus leading to acute injuries or tendinopathy. As such, it is fundamental to plan work carefully for athletes with tendinopathy in its initial phases.

As well as excessive mechanical loads, other factors can influence the onset of a tendinopathy, like, for example, inadequate basic technique in amateur athletes [5] or inadequate athletic equipment [21]. Intrinsic factors can also alter the load that tendons undergo, like, for example, the state of the muscles, ligaments, bones, and peritendinous tissue [22].

The other factors

The incidence of tendinopathy has risen in obese individuals, in whom there is a reduced sensitivity to insulin, as in patients affected by type 1 or type 2 diabetes mellitus [23].

Risk factors for tendinopathy also include drugs such as fluorochinolones [24], as well as substances such as alcohol and smoking which can influence the pathology, producing hypoxic and microvascular damage.

Physiopathology of tendon lesions

Inflammation

Inflammation plays an important role in the pathogenesis of tendinopathy, above all in the initial phase when the pathology is not yet clinically evident [25].

The role of the inflammatory response in the pathogenesis of tendinopathy is limited to the initial phase of the pathology and this has been demonstrated by the fact that numerous studies have shown no biochemical or histologic evidence of inflammation in tendon biopsies from patients with chronic tendon pathology [26, 27]. Therefore it has been hypothesised that the inflammatory process precedes fibrotic and degenerative changes which are typical of tendinopathies [28].

In the acute phase it is possible to find signs of inflammation deriving from the notable release of cytokines and immunomodulant factors responsible for phenomena such as cellular proliferation or degradation of the extracellular matrix [29].

The phase in which we find the initial production and release of cytokines can be considered the prelude to the condition in which it becomes clinically evident [30]. When the quantity of inflammatory cells becomes significant, there is an imbalance between pro-inflammatory factors responsible for the degradation of the extracellular matrix and protective factors, causing the beginning of symptoms of pain due to the release of substance P, glutamate, and the production of COX2 and PGE2 [30, 28, 31].

In the absence of the initial inflammatory phase, the healing process and the changes that characterise chronic tendinopathies cannot occur [30]. The mechanism that leads to the acute inflammatory phase degenerating into chronic tendinopathy is not yet clear, however [19].

Changes in matrix, collagen, cells, vessels

In a tendon affected by tendinopathy, macroscopically, you can observe the transition from the characteristic bright white colour to a grey-brown colour; histologically, this corresponds to the degeneration of the collagen fibres that appear thinner with the loss of their characteristic orientation in parallel fasci, to hypercellularity with rounded-nucleus tenocytes and increased vascularisation [32, 33].

Sometimes the tendon degeneration can lead to the deposit of fibrin, calcification or fat accumulation [34].

The main structural and biochemical changes include: upregulation of the mRNA of type I and III collagen, with a notable increase in type III collagen in the ECM compared to a healthy tendon, increased levels of fibronectin, tenascin C, GAGs, aggrecan and biglycan [33].

There are also changes in activity of various enzymes such as matrix metalloproteins (MMPs), disintegrins, ADAMs, ADAMTSs, and TIMPs metalloproteinases that contribute to the weakening of the tendon matrix [35, 36].

In Achilles tendinopathy, downregulation of MMP-3 and upregulation of MMP-2 and VEGF were also observed [37, 33].

Role of hypoxia and ROS (Reactive Oxygen Species)

There is still debate about the reasons for which tendinopathy becomes chronic, but as well as injuries and repeated mechanical stress, it has been suggested that hypoxia can also lead to a predisposition to chronicity [38]. The increase in demand for oxygen by tenocytes during functional overload, added to individual susceptibility, causes a state of hypoxia that determines the production of oxygen radicals (ROS). These are one of the most important stimulations for the release of VEGF and inflammation factors [39, 40, 41].

The term "reactive oxygen species" (ROS) includes all the free radicals deriving from oxygen that contain one or more unpaired electrons. ROS can be involved in tendinopathies or in stress reactions: in fact, they influence the synthesis, the structure and integrity of the connective tissues [42]. During the cyclical work of the tendon, the period of maximum tensile load is associated with ischemia, and the relaxation phase with perfusion; the return to normal oxygenation of the tissue can result in a sudden increase in the production of ROS [43].

For these reasons, following intense training sessions, there is a possibility of potential re-oxygenation damage, caused by the increase in the production of ROS to sub-lethal levels inside the tendon [43].

Types of degeneration

The degeneration process of the tendon can be considered as a failure of the matrix to adapt and remodel due to an imbalance between the synthe-

sis process and destruction of the matrix caused by excessive mechanical load and stress factors [35].
The imbalance between metalloproteinases and tissue inhibitors of metalloproteinases (TIMPs) plays an important role in the degenerative process.
Various types of tendon degeneration have been observed through electron microscope studies [44], among which:
• hypoxic degeneration;
• hyaline degeneration;
• mucoid or myxoid degeneration (large mucoid patches and vacuoles between thin, fragile collagen fibers);
• fibrinoid degeneration (fibrinoid material deposit within collagen fibers);
• lipoid degeneration (lipid cells interspersed within collagen fibers);
• calcification (calcific deposit within collagen fibers);
• fibrocartilaginous and bony metaplasia.

Failure of healing process hypothesis
Tendinopathies can be considered as a failure of the healing process.
According to this model, the inflammatory process which appears following an acute injury and which would normally determine the resolution of said injury, turns towards an inefficient response which results in degenerative changes in the tendon [45] with proliferation and apoptosis of the tenocytes, destruction of the collagen fibres, and an increase in the non-collagen component of the matrix [46, 47].
The degenerative process is not therefore the elementary lesion of the tendinopathy but the consequence of the failure of the healing process, presumably resulting from constant inappropriate mechanical stimuli [31].

Healing principles

Tendons are capable of healing through a repair process brought about by tendon cells and the surrounding extracellular matrix. The formation of scar tissue begins immediately after tendon damage. This process can be divided into three stages:
• inflammation;
• cellular proliferation;
• matrix remodelling.
The first phase (inflammation) starts with the forming of hematoma immediately after the injury. Blood cells such as platelets, neutrophils, monocytes, and erythrocytes are attracted to the site of the damage by the release of pro-inflammatory cytokines. Fibroblasts begin synthesising components of the matrix such as type III collagen, and the secretion of angiogenic factors promotes the formation of a new vascular network responsible for the initial stabilization of the damage site [48, 49, 50].
After a few days, a new phase begins: that of cellular proliferation accompanied by the synthesis of numerous matrix components such as proteoglycans, collagens (above all type III) which are present, however, in a non-organised way. During this phase, as well as an increase in cellularity, there is also the reabsorption of a great quantity of liquid at the site of damage [48, 51].
The remodelling phase can be further divided into two sub-phases: this begins 6-8 weeks after injury and can last around 1-2 years depending on the age and condition of the patient. The first sub-phase, that of consolidation, is characterised by the reduction in cellularity, the production of matrixes, and the substitution of type III collagen with type I collagen, in order to help the tissue become more fibrous. The collagen fibres begin to form, following the main axes of the tendons, thus restoring the rigidity and traction strength of the tendon [52, 29].
After about 10 weeks, the maturation phase begins, where collagen fibrils increase the number of crosslinks thus ensuring a continued increase in strength [53]. The tendon healing process is made up of two overlapping mechanisms: extrinsic and intrinsic healing. The extrinsic healing process starts first and involves the invasion of inflammatory cells at the site of damage, with the initial synthesis of matrix components. The intrinsic healing process, on the other hand, contributes to the repair of damage through local stem cell action [54].
The healed tendon, however, seldom reaches the mechanical capacity of a healthy tendon [48, 54].
The reduced strength of scar tissue compared to never-damaged tendon tissue is attributable to the changed layout of the collagen fibres and

the presence of type III collagen (smaller diameter) compared to type I collagen, most present in healthy tendons. Consequently, in order to cope with this reduced mechanical strength, the tendon becomes rigid and loses elasticity, thus reducing its functional capacity compared to that of a healthy tendon [32].

Conservative treatment

The management of tendinopathies can vary depending on clinical history, the entity of the condition, severity of symptoms, functional demands or the level of activity of the athlete.
Conservative measures are the mainstay of most tendinopathy treatments, while surgery is necessary for recurrent cases, or in clear surgical lesion cases [6].

Training with eccentric exercise

Eccentric exercise muscle training is characterised by exercises in which the muscle and tendon are lengthened while under tension. This type of exercise has been much studied and used as a form of treatment for tendinopathies [55].
Numerous studies have demonstrated that eccentric exercise can have a favourable impact on tendinopathies. This has been observed while evaluating various outcomes such as improvement in strength, improvement in the tendon's appearance via medical imaging, and through evaluating various ECM remodelling biochemical and histologic markers [56, 57].
Eccentric exercise favours the production of type I collagen and the increase in fibril density, even although the mechanism by which this takes place at a molecular level is not yet clear [58]. Moreover, the mechanical load causes the expression of various genes such as those that codify for the proteins scleraxis and tenomodulin associated with the proliferation of new tenocytes and the production of matrix components [59, 60].
One particular type of eccentric exercise, defined "heavy slow resistance", using heavy loads with slow repetition, has proved extremely effective in the treatment of patellar tendinopathy [57].
The effectiveness of eccentric training demonstrated by numerous studies, the low cost of the therapy, and evidence of improvement in ECM at a cellular and molecular level have all led to eccentric exercise often being considered as first-line therapy in the management of tendinopathies [6].
The most widely used protocol is the Alfredson protocol which recommends 3 series of 15 repetitions, twice a day for 12 weeks [61]. It has been shown that 12 weeks of eccentric exercise following the Alfredson protocol determines an increase in the levels of type I collagen carboxyterminal propeptide (PICP), a marker of type I collagen synthesis [58].

NSAIDs

The action mechanism of NSAIDs can be explained by the blocking of the production of prostaglandin by the cyclooxygenase enzyme. Prostaglandins are molecules deriving from arachidonic acid that play an important role in the development of acute inflammation. Thanks to their rapid analgesic effect, these drugs are one of the most popular choices [67, 68], and are administered both topically and orally [62, 63].
Despite the usefulness of NSAIDs in the reduction of pain and inflammation, these drugs have no impact on the course of the chronic pathology because there is no clear evidence of inflammation in tendons affected by chronic pathologies [64, 65]. Moreover, these drugs do not accumulate in sufficient quantity to influence the gene transcription in tendon tissue [66].
There is, however, evidence that these drugs can have a negative impact on tendon healing, reducing the proliferation and differentiation of tenocytes and promoting the differentiation of mesenchymal stem cells in adipocytes [67, 68].
In conclusion, NSAIDs can be relatively useful in relieving acute pain but much evidence indicates that this class of drugs has no effect, or even a damaging effect, in the management of tendinopathies [6].

Corticosteroids

Corticosteroids (CCS) are synthetic drugs similar to the particular class of steroid hormones produced by the adrenal gland. These powerful anti-inflammatory molecules have been studied in numerous clinical trials in patients with tendinopathy [69, 70].

Despite the fact that the inflammatory process does not play a central role in the pathogenesis of tendinopathies, numerous studies have shown how steroid therapy has a significant impact on pain relief and on the return to activity in short-term treatment [71].
It is thought that the positive effect of CCS on pain and function may be due to a reduction in the inflammatory process in the peritendinous tissues [57]. However, there is still potential risk of iatrogenic tendon breakage and atrophy of the surrounding soft tissues in the event of repeated use of CCS.
According to a 2015 review, there is no evidence to support routine use of therapy with injections that include CCS in the treatment of painful Achilles tendon [72].
In conclusion, despite the fact that CCS have proven effective in the reduction of symptoms of pain in numerous tendinopathies, clinicians should be very careful not to abuse this class of drugs when managing tendinopathies, as there is still a lack of evidence on longterm benefits and the potential risk of adverse effects [6].

Nitric oxide

The treatment of tendinopathies with nitric oxide (NO) has become increasingly popular over the last few years [73]. The most common treatment method in this areas provides the transdermal release of nitroglycerine at the site of injury by the local application of slow release transdermal patches to be kept in place for 24 hours.
The nitroglycerine is converted into biologically active nitric oxide (NO) by the endogenous nitric oxide synthase enzyme [73]. The effects of nitric oxide (NO) at a cellular and molecular level include the increase of the proliferation of tenocytes and collagen synthesis; in fact, inhibiting the nitric oxide synthase enzyme, it reduces the area of healing of the tendon, as seen under the microscope, and reduces the mechanical load required to break of the tendon [74].
Numerous randomised clinical trials have studied the effectiveness of the topical use of nitroglycerine in patients with tendinopathy; however, results are discordant [75, 76]. Two meta-analyses have concluded that, despite the need for further studies, there is sufficient evidence to support the local use of patches with low doses of nitroglycerine (0,72 mg/day) for short term relief from pain caused by tendinopathy [77, 78].
Studies on the effectiveness of long term treatment of tendinopathy using nitroglycerine patches have not, however, demonstrated positive effects on pain symptoms and the return to functionality [79]. The topic use of nitroglycerine can cause various side effects, including headaches, skin rashes, flushing, and profuse sweating [76]. These potential side effects, along with contradictory results regarding short term effects and the lack of effectiveness in long term treatment, have limited the use of nitroglycerine patches as a first line therapy in the management of tendinopathies [6].

Prolotherapy

Prolotherapy is an acronym that derives from "proliferation-therapy". In the field of tendon pathology, this term refers to the injection of an irritant in or around the affected tendon [80].
The effect of the irritant promotes inflammation and triggers a regenerative response that allows the healing of the damaged ECM in chronic tendinopathy. There are various irritants that can be injected in varying concentrations, although most of these contain dextrose, fenol-glycerol-glucose, or morrhuate sodium. Although the action mechanism is not yet clear, it is thought that dextrose in hypersmolar concentrations can act by dehydrating and destroying cells, the fenol-glycerol-glucose by local irritation to tissue, and morrhuate sodium as a chemotactic agent for inflammation cells and mediators [80]. Moreover, these irritant solutions can also bring about sclerosis of small vessels and nociceptor fibres in pathological tendons.
Various studies have tried to evaluate the effectiveness of prolotherapy in patients with tendinopathy, however, the meaningfulness of most of these studies is limited by the small size of samples analysed or by the absence of appropriate control groups [81, 82]. Therefore, despite the fact that prolotherapy offers the possibility of a relatively safe and cheap treatment, further randomised control trials are necessary before using this treatment as a first choice in the management of tendinopathies [6].

Platelet Rich Plasma

Platelet Rich Plasma (PRP) is an autologous blood product made of plasma enriched with platelets in much higher concentrations that those found in blood, generally at least four times the base value [83]. In the last few years, the popularity of PRP as a treatment aimed at quickening healing in numerous musculoskeletal conditions has greatly increased, and numerous potential applications of PRP have been studied, including the treatment of tendinopathies.

Platelets are a very important element in the healing of load-induced tissue lesions as, inside them, they contain a large quantity of growth factors and cytokines, among which, the transforming growth factor beta (TGF-β), interleukins (ILs), fibroblast growth factors (FGFs), growth factors deriving from platelets (PDGFs), vascular endothelium growth factors (VEGFs), connective tissue growth factors (CTGF), as well as others [83].

When released locally into the site of the injury, these factors favour healing of the tissues [52]. Moreover, recent large scale studies in bioinformatics and genomic analysis have demonstrated the role of PRP in the induction of local inflammatory response in tissues [83].

There are different methods and protocols for the production of PRP; each of these determines the formation of a product with a different composition in growth factors, leukocytes and cytokines, and with different release kinetics. This diversity contributes to the difficulty in evaluating the effectiveness of this treatment, as there is not yet a standardized procedure for the use of PRP in the various musculoskeletal pathologies it is used. In fact, the optimum concentration of platelets to be used to maximize biological impact has not yet been defined.

There is also diversity in injection techniques: some authors suggest the use of ultrasound to guide the needle with precision into the degenerated tendon area, others prefer to practise the peppering technique of injection, injecting the PRP circumferentially to the lesion to obtain an increased release area.

Finally, there is also debate about the optimum volume to inject and the number of injections to be carried out as, in some studies, only one injection is carried out while, in others, two or three are administered and at varying intervals [84].

Numerous studies have analysed the effectiveness of PRP in the treatment of patients with tendinopathy, but with conflicting results [85, 86]. The more encouraging results were obtained in the treatment of lateral epicondylitis: it was shown that the administration of PRP was almost twice as effective as corticosteroids [85]. However, a recent meta-analysis has shown that PRP injections in patients with tendinopathy bring about no significant improvement compared to placebos after 6 months of follow-up, even although a mild positive impact was observed in patients affected by tendinopathy of the rotator cuff [87]. Other more detailed clinical studies are necessary, carried out selectively on the various anatomical sites to be treated, to learn more about the effectiveness of PRP as a treatment for tendinopathies [6].

Hyaluronic acid

Recently, hyaluronic acid has been taken into consideration as a treatment for tendinopathies thanks to its anti-inflammatory and lubricant properties [88].

Hyaluronic acid is a polisaccaride with high molecular weight (between 100 kDa e 10 MDa), which is found mainly in the ECM where it carried out various functions in different parts of the body. This polisaccaride maintains the viscoelasticity of liquid connective tissues such as in sinovial joints and in the vitreous body of the eye. Moreover, it guarantees the lubrification of anatomical structures such as muscles and joints. The intra-articular injections of hyaluronic acid are widely used in the treatment of osteoarthrosis [89].

The use of hyaluronic acid in tendinopathy can improve the flowing capacity of tendons and reduce adherence, thus limiting the proliferation of fibroblasts and stabilising type III collagen (increased in pathological tendons) [90, 91 92]. Moreover, hyaluronic acid would seem to inhibit the expression of factors involved in NF-kB signalling (important factor in inflammatory process), with a dose related effect [93, 94]. Studies describe therapeutic protocols using hyaluronic acid for tendinopathies that involve one or two injections at the site of tendon degeneration, preferably ecography-guided, as described for the injections of PRP [95, 96]. In vivo and in vitro, studies show encouraging results on the use of hyaluronic acid in tendinopathies; however, other studies are necessary to validate this as a first line treatment in the management of tendinopathies [88].

Surgical treatment

Conservative treatment in patients affected by tendinopathies fails in a third of all cases [2]. In this case, patients reduce their level of sporting activity or evaluate the possibility of surgical treatment.
The aim of surgical treatment in patients with tendinopathy is to remove the degenerated areas of the tendon or to induce the healing process through low level controlled damage, applied to the degenerated areas of the tendon. The principal of this treatment is the same as prolotherapy or PRP.

Percutaneous longitudinal tenotomy

In this procedure, the surgeon carries out one or more incisions parallel to the longitudinal axis of the tendon to promote tissue regeneration, increase blood flow and create a good environment for the healing process [97]. This procedure is relatively simple and can be carried out in day surgery with only local anaesthetic [50].
Ultrasound can be used to identify the degenerated areas of the tendon and where incisions should be made. Possible complications are rare and, however, there is no long term morbidity [50].

Percutaneous ultrasonic microtenotomy

Percutaneous ultrasonic microtenotomy has recently been adopted as treatment for tendinopathy. This is a minimally invasive technique that uses the ultrasound's energy to debride the pathological tissue using a needle which is inserted into the tendon [6].
A case series of 20 patients with recurring lateral epicondylitis has shown improvement in pain symptoms and functionality in 95% of patients treated with this technique, after one year [98]. The follow-up of these patients has shown the effectiveness of this treatment after 3 years with 100% of patients showing increased diameter of the tendon and 95% showing the resolution of tendon hypervascularity [99].
Although studies regarding the effectiveness of this technique are limited to lateral epicondylitis, percutaneous ultrasonic microtenotomy represents a potential treatment in all cases of non-responsive tendinopathy [6].

Tendoscopy

The first endoscopic procedure in tendons was described by Wertheimer et al. [100] in the treatment of tenosynovitis of the posterior tibialis muscle tendon. In 1997, Niek van Dijk et al. [101] published a report on endoscopic procedures on the Achilles tendon, the anterior tibialis tendon and the peroneus muscle tendon in 40 patients, naming the procedure "tendoscopy".
Endoscopic surgery allows a minimally invasive approach with a lower rate of complications compared to open surgery, such as less scarring, less post-operative pain, fewer complications of the wound, and speedier healing [102, 103].
Surgical treatment is recommended in patients who don't respond to conservative treatment over a period of 6 months, and endoscopic was successfully carried out obtaining results comparable to those of open surgery in the excision of degenerated tissues, debriding of adherences, removal of thickened peritenon, and stimulation of the healing process in chronic tendinopathy [102].
Today, compared to the first descriptions of endoscopy in 1995 by Wertheimer et al. and in 1997 by Niek van Dijk et al., orthopaedic surgeons have extended the use of endoscopy to other tendons in the foot and ankle, including the tibialis posterior tendon, extensor digitorum longus muscle tendon, extensor hallucis longus muscle tendon, flexor hallucis longus muscle tendon, and flexor digitorum longus muscle tendon.
In general, studies show good results and tendoscopy seems to be an effective diagnostic and therapeutic procedure for a variety of conditions. Moreover, it can be converted into open surgery when necessary [104].
Until now, there is little evidence (grade C) to support endoscopy as a treatment for tendinopathy of the Achilles, flexor hallucis longus, and peroneus tendons. There is insufficient evidence (Grade I) for the other tendons of the foot and ankle [105]. Moreover, there are no clear guidelines about the indications and modality of use for this technique.

Main tendinopathies in soccer

Patellar tendinopathy

Patellar tendinopathy is a clinical condition characterised by pain at the level of the inferior pole of the patella or at the level of the proximal portion of the patellar tendon [7].

This condition is very common in sports that require jumps, such as volleyball, basketball, and soccer and, as such, it is commonly known as "jumper's knee" [106, 107]. In fact, sports that require a high frequency and intensity of jumping put repetitive stress on the knee extensor muscles. Symptoms can sometimes be so severe as to result in functional impotence with subsequent absence from sporting activity for the sportsman [108, 109].

Epidemiology

There is a 45% prevalence of patellar tendinopathy among professional volleyball players, and a 32% among professional basketball players [110]. Only a few studies have investigated the prevalence of this condition in soccer. In this sport, jumping is less frequent and most injuries to the patellar tendon are due to repetitive stress to the knee extensor mechanism. Overload injuries constitute a significant problem in soccer and represent about a third of total injuries [111].

There is a 2.4% prevalence of patellar tendinopathy among professional soccerers in any single season [110], with a rate of 0.12 injuries for every 1,000 hours played per year. During the soccer season, 2,4% of players miss training or games because of patellar tendinopathy, with absences from the field being brief on the whole, less than one week, but with a high rate of recurrence.

The prevalence of patellar tendinopathy is relatively higher among young players, with players between 15 and 17 years at maximum risk [112].

Risk factors and physiopathology

Risk factors for patellar tendinopathy can be intrinsic and extrinsic.

Intrinsic risks include:

• masculine sex [106];
• tall stature [106];
• high BMI or abdominal circumference [113, 106, 114, 115];
• reduced dorsiflexion of the ankle [116];
• patella anomalies (malalignment of the patella, high riding patella, excessive patellar laxity) [117];
• weakness or insufficient distensibility of the quadriceps and hamstring [118];
• asymmetry of the lower limbs [118];
• flat foot [118].

Extrinsic factors include:

• hours of training (incidence 1,2/1,000 h) [100, 119, 120];
• high frequency of training with weights and jumps (there is a raised incidence rate of patellar tendinopathy during the pre-championship period when work loads are heavy) [110].

The most commonly held theory is that patellar tendinopathy is caused by a combination of extrinsic and intrinsic factors.

The term "stiffness" indicates the link between the force applied to a tissue and the resulting shift, and it is one of the most useful mechanisms in the evaluation of tendon function both in passive and active conditions [121, 122]. The stiffness parameter has been widely used to evaluate changes in tendon mechanical properties after training in the presence of pathologies. Professional soccer athletes display heightened patellar tendon stiffness values compared to the control group [123]. A patellar tendon with heightened stiffness results in better transmission of force during contraction [123]. This can be explained by the well-documented phenomenon of the adaptation of tendons to training [124, 125].

Artificial grass playing fields do not represent a heightened risk for patellar tendinopathies [110].

Clinical aspects

Clinically, patellar tendinopathy can be identified by pain in correlation to activity localised at the inferior pole of the patella and at the proximal portion to the patellar tendon [7].

Pain is insidious and worsens when sporting activity increases. At the beginning, it starts after physical activity but can progress until it is present during any activity at all or even when at rest [126].

Examination reveals swelling in correspondence with the insertion site of the path of the tendon, with the patient experiencing pain on palpation. One can check for Bassett's sign: the patient complains of pain at the inferior pole of the patella when the leg is actively extended, with the pain diminishing in this point with the knee in flexion. A test to reproduce the symptoms associated with patellar tendinopathy is the “decline squat test”, where the patient effects a squat with the affected leg, so the knee bends 30° while keeping the other knee of the other leg straight [126].

Imaging

First choice imaging techniques for patellar tendinopathy are ultrasound and MRI [126]. Ultrasound is the first level instrumental exam; often in athletes with patellar tendinopathy there are areas of thinning and hypoechogenic areas visible with ultrasound.

MRI is reserved for patients with chronic or refractory tendinopathy and for patients needing surgery; with this method the thinning of the tendon can be observed, togheter with the presence of any edemas, and areas of heightened intensity in T1 weighed and T2 weighed signal sequence (fig. 1).

Classification

Blazina’s classification (1973) is still th most used today and is based on clinical characteristics. It includes four stages.

- Stage I: pain only following physical activity.
- Stage II: pain at the beginning of physical activity, disappearing with warm up and reappearing after physical activity.
- Stage III: constant pain at rest.
- Stage IV: complete rupture of the patellar tendon [126].

Differential diagnosis

The main conditions that can accompany a differential diagnosis with patellar tendinopathy are:

- patellofemoral syndrome;
- Hoffa’s disease;
- meniscopathy;
- cartilage lesions;
- referred pain [126].

Conservative treatment (see general section)

- Eccentric exercise;
- shock waves;
- CCS injections, PRP, hyaluronic acid, prolotherapy, cell-based therapy, aprotinin [126].

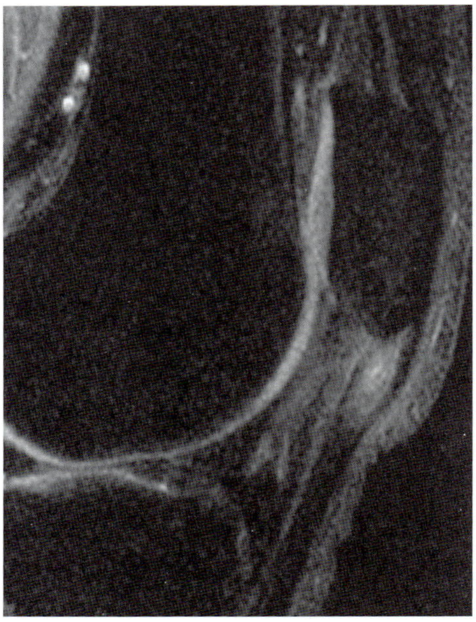

Figure 1 - MRI of a patellar tendinopathy showing edemas

Surgical therapy

Although conservative treatment succeeds in most patients with patellar tendinopathy, around 10% of all patients do not improve and require a surgical operation [52].

Surgery normally involves tenotomy of the patellar tendon, the excision of abnormal tissue, and the induction of the healing process through perforation and marginal resection of the inferior pole of the patella [126].

Open surgery

A longitudinal incision is made from the inferior pole of the patella to the tibial tubercle.

The paratenon is exposed and opened longitudinally to expose the patellar tendon. The surgeon makes a longitudinal incision, reaching the posterior degenerative tissue and carrying out the debridement of said tissue.

The distal 5 mm of the inferior pole of the patellar are removed, and with a drill, holes are made to produce a bleeding that promotes repair.

Finally, the tendon and the paratenon are suturated with absorbable stitches [126].

Arthroscopy

The procedure starts with diagnostic arthroscopy to exclude intra-articular pathologies.

It is particularly important to exclude chondral

lesions of the patella, which are frequently associated with patellar tendinopathy.
The inferior pole of the patella is identified and the adjacent synovial tissue is resected, exposing the degenerative tissue in the posterior zone of the proximal patellar tendon which is subjected to scarification until the normal tendon fibres can be seen.
The most distal 5 mm of the patella are resected using a burr.
Finally, the surgeon effects hemostasis and carries out articular lavage [126].
In medical literature, the results for open surgery and arthroscopy are comparable.

Post-surgery rehabilitation
Generally, the same rehabilitation protocol is used for open surgery and arthroscopy, consisting in complete load based on pain response.
Once the surgical wound has healed, generally around 10 days after surgery, patients begin a rehabilitation program which consists of eccentric exercise with squats on a sloping board as part of a muscle-strengthening program.
Patients can return to sporting activity when they have completed at least 3 months of rehabilitation and feel no pain during exercises [126].

Rupture of the patellar tendon
Injuries of the extensor apparatus have an incidence rate of 0.5-6%. They are potentially very serious lesions given that the extensor apparatus is essential for normal walking and any malfunction can cause significant disability [52].
Ruptures of the patellar tendon are often a result of direct or indirect trauma: they can be the final consequence of chronic patellar tendinopathy, micro traumas, or functional overload [127].
In general, these lesions appear in young (less than 40 years old), physically active patients and are normally caused by an indirect trauma to the knee, such as a sudden contraction of the quadricep with the knee in slight flexion (such as when jumping, sprinting, trying to avoid a fall etc.) [128].
Tendon ruptures in a patient subjecting himself to extreme stress during static phase are extremely rare [129]. The traction forces that act on the tendon are greater at the level of the osteotendinous junction than at the central portion: for this reason lesions in the latter site are rarer. Given the great force necessary to rupture a healthy tendon, most medical literature considers tendinopathy a necessary condition for even traumatic ruptures, above all in cases that involve the central region of the tendon [130].
Risk factors therefore overlap those of chronic patellar tendinopathy and early identification of tendinopathy in professional athletes can therefore be considered a fundamental factor in the prevention of tendon ruptures [110].

Clinical aspects
In general, patients complain of a sudden pain with functional impotence of the knee which can sometimes be associated with a fall following a rapid movement. In these cases, it is necessary to investigate a possible history of previous patellar tendinopathy and research possible risk factors or associated comorbidities.
During clinical inspection, the knee appears swollen and often the patella is indistinguishable because of the abundant edema. Palpation often reveals a discontinuity in the tendon with the patella in a very high position, especially in the case of a complete rupture. Active extension of the knee is impossible with complete lesions, however, in non-complete lesions, extension is partially conserved [131].

Imaging
An ultrasound exam can be useful in the diagnosis of an incomplete rupture with the advantage that, compared to other techniques, a dynamic evaluation can be carried out.
A two X-ray projection exam can show signs suggesting a tendon rupture such as: high patella (fig. 2), avulsion of the patellar tendon, or fracture of the tibial tuberosity.
MRI is the best instrument for the diagnosis of a ruptured tendon but cost and availability can limit its use [131].

Treatment
Incomplete ruptures with un-compromised function can be treated in a conservative way with 2-3 weeks of immobilization in position of complete

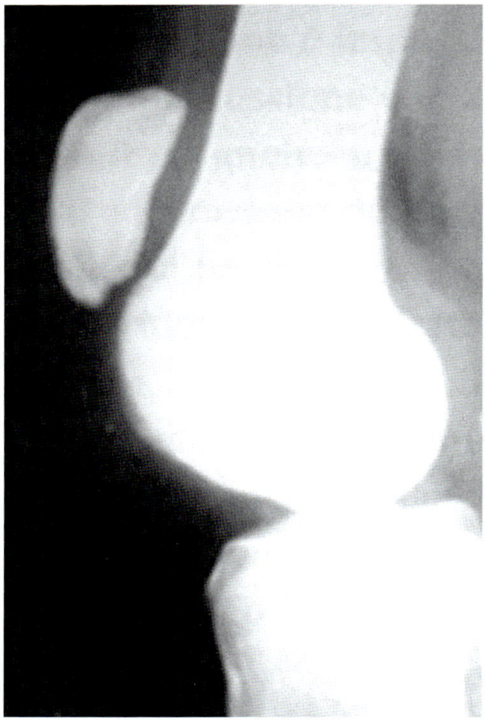

Figure 2 - High patella indicating patellar tendon rupture

extension [132]. In incomplete lesions with extension deficit or complete ruptures, surgical treatment is necessary.
Repair should be carried out as soon as possible, so as to ensure greater possibility of obtaining a suture without excessive tension [128]. During the acute phase, repair with only suture of the tendon is not recommended due to its high failure rate. The fact that most lesions occur at the bone insertion site facilitates transosseous suture of the tendon [131].
Normally, anterior approach through an incision on the median line is the best choice, followed by a precise dissection of the fibres of the retinaculum and the debridement of the tendon extremity. Microperforations of the inferior pole of the patellar are carried out to facilitate bleeding and, therefore, healing.
The tendon extremities are attached with two non-absorbable suture threads using the Kracow or similar techniques and three bone tunnels are created in the patella through which the threads are passed to create a transosseous suture.
The optimal position of the patella and the strength of the suture are evaluated by carrying out flexion of the knee [132].

In rare cases of rupture involving the central portion of the tendon, continuous stitches are used to reattach the extremities and patellar bone tunnels in order to contain the proximal fragment [133]. In these cases, some authors prefer to carry out additional distal bone tunnels at the level of the tibia through which to pass the suture and obtain greater stability [134].
Various techniques have been described for obtaining greater stability in the repair of patellar tendons, the most common of which uses an autograft with the semitendinosus [135], although there is no consensus in medical literature regarding the true necessity to resort to this technique [136].

Achilles tendinopathy

The elastic properties of the Achilles tendon are important for locomotion [137]. This tendon has the ability to withstand a load up to 12.5 greater than body weight [138]; despite this, many athletes suffer tendon injuries in this area [139].
Achilles tendinopathy is a clinical condition characterized by pain, swelling, and functional impotence. Depending on the anatomical site, it can be classified into insertional tendinopathy (near the heel insertion) and non-insertional (2-6 cm from the calcaneal insertion) [140]. This anatomical distinction presupposes differences also from the physiopathological point of view and therefore in the management of these conditions [141].
The definition "Achilles tendinopathy" includes both acute conditions, characterized by a greater inflammatory component, and chronic conditions such as tendinosis, characterized by a prevalent degenerative component [7, 142].
The Achilles tendinopathy is often difficult to treat and often has a negative prognosis [143, 144, 145] because of the tendency to become chronic or relapse [146] causing long periods of absence from the fields for affected athletes [147].

Epidemiology

Achilles tendinopathy is common among athletes, particularly among those who practice sports that require running and jumping like soccer [148]. It represents 96% of all sports injuries to the Achilles tendon [149, 150]. Many patients with this condition have histological features on Achilles tendon biopsy despite being totally asymptomatic [151]. The tendinopathy of the middle portion of the tendon represents 55-65%, while the insertional tendinopathy 20-25% of cases [152]. In the last 30 years the incidence of Achilles tendinopathy has increased due to the increase of sporting practice in the population. Achilles tendon disorders are responsible for 3.8% of time lost outside the fields for soccerers and are more common in older athletes.

In professional soccerers the risk of recurrence and reinjury is greater after short periods of abstention from the sporting activity. About a third of these injuries occur during the preseason, where workloads are more intense [149].

Risk factors and phisiopathology

Intrinsic factors:

- age;
- male sex;
- BMI;
- biomechanical anomalies (reduced tibio-tarsic and subtalar joint ROM; varus deformity of forefoot; pes cavus; leg length discrepancy; ankle instability; gastrocnemius-soleus complex dysfunction; excessive movement of the hindfoot in the frontal plane with excessive compensatory pronation [153, 154, 155, 156]).

Extrinsic factors:

- improper training with excessive loads on the tendon [19];
- previous injuries,
- environmental factors;
- type of footwear;
- drugs (steroids, fluoroquinolones, statins, aromatase inhibitors) [157].

The Achilles tendon, unlike the other tendons, does not run inside a proper and well-defined tendon sheath but is wrapped in a thin connective layer (peritenon).

Its vascularization is guaranteed by the posterior tibial artery and the peroneal artery; the tendon presents a characteristic critical area of hypovascularization at about 4-6 cm from the calcaneal insertion. For this reason, this area is more susceptible to ischemic suffering and to the development of degenerative phenomena.

Clinical aspects

The diagnosis of Achilles tendinopathy is mainly based on the history and physical examination [158]. A frequent symptom is morning stiffness or after physical inactivity. Pain can be a late symptom. Typically, pain is localized from 2 cm to 6 cm proximal to the heel insertion, particularly after exercise.

The discomfort increases at the beginning and at the end of physical activity, with an intermediate period of attenuated symptomatology. As the condition progresses, the pain appears after less and less physical effort, interfering a lot with the sport activity. In severe cases the pain occurs even during rest. For the clinical diagnosis we must first evaluate the hindfoot: look for any malalignment, deformity, tendon asymmetry, thickening, Haglund deformity, or previous scars. In the acute phase it is possible to find swelling of the Achilles tendon from 4 cm to 6 cm proximal to the calcaneal insertion. In the chronic phase, areas of swelling, thickening, nodularity, or crackling in the affected area can be found on palpation.

Dorsal or plantar flexion of the foot, both active and passive, can be painful. The evaluation of the painful arc of movement helps to distinguish clinically a tendon injury from a peritenon injury. In the latter, in fact, the area of palpable thickening or nodularity remains fixed during the flexion movements of the ankle, while it is mobile in intratendinous lesions [159].

The Royal London Hospital test is considered positive when the local palpation causes pain with the ankle in a neutral position or slightly plantar flexion, while the pain subsides or disappears completely when the patient carries the ankle in maximum dorsiflexion [158, 160].

Imaging

Evaluation with imaging techniques is very important for diagnosis and treatment planning. Radiographic examination is useful because it can show an associated bone anomaly or any calcifications.

The use of MRI or ultrasound allows to obtain more information on tendon morphology and it has great utility for preoperative planning (figg. 3, 4).

The MRI images on the sagittal and axial planes are useful to determine the percentage of involvement of tendon fibers; this is important because with an involvement of more than 50%, the tendon must be treated surgically.

Visa classification

The Victorian Institute of Sports Assessment questionnaire - Achilles (VISA-A) specifically measures the severity of Achilles tendinopathy [161]. This questionnaire investigates the parameters: pain, function, and activity. The scores are added up to give a total of 100. The score 100 indicates no symptomatology. In the clinic, the VISA-A questionnaire provides a valid, reliable and easy-to-use index of tendinopathy severity [162].

Differential diagnosis

- Peritenon pathology.
- Insertional tendinopathy.
- Retrocalcanear bursitis.
- Sever's disease.
- Ossification of the tendon.
- Osteomyelitis or neoplasia of tibia and calcaneus.
- Tendinopathy of the flexor hallucis longus.
- Tendinopathy of the posterior tibialis.
- Peroneal tendinopathy.
- Os trigonum.

Conservative treatment (see general section)

- Eccentric exercise is the cornerstone for conservative management of Achilles tendinopathy.
- ESWT.
- NSAIDs.
- Steroid injections (not recommended).
- PRP injection (no definitive conclusion possible).
- Sclerosis agents (no definitive conclusion possible).
- High-volume injections (no definitive conclusion possible).
- Autologous blood injections (no definitive conclusion possible).

Surgical treatment: minimally invasive stripping

In minimally invasive stripping for chronic Achilles tendinopathy four skin incisions are made, two proximal and two distal. The first two skin incisions of 5 mm are made medially and laterally to the proximal origin of the tendon. The other two incisions of 5 mm are made medially and laterally to the heel insertion but 1 cm distal to it.

The proximal portion of the tendon is released from the peritendinous adhesions by a mosquito through the proximal incisions. Ethibond num-

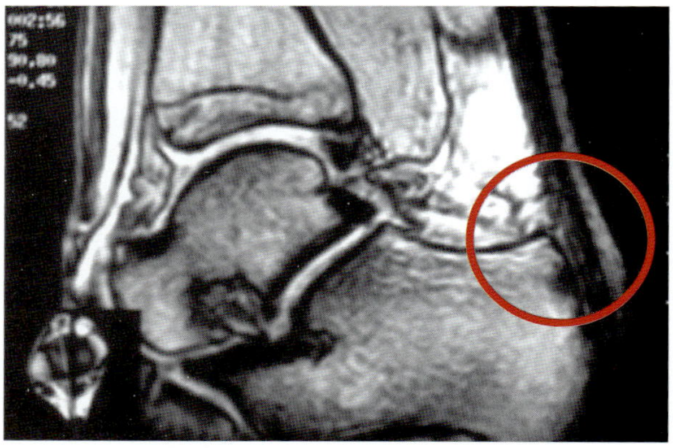

Figure 3 - MRI showing retrocalcaneal bursa involvement. Pain spreads from the bursa located between the Achilles tendon and the heel bone. Tendon shape is not affected

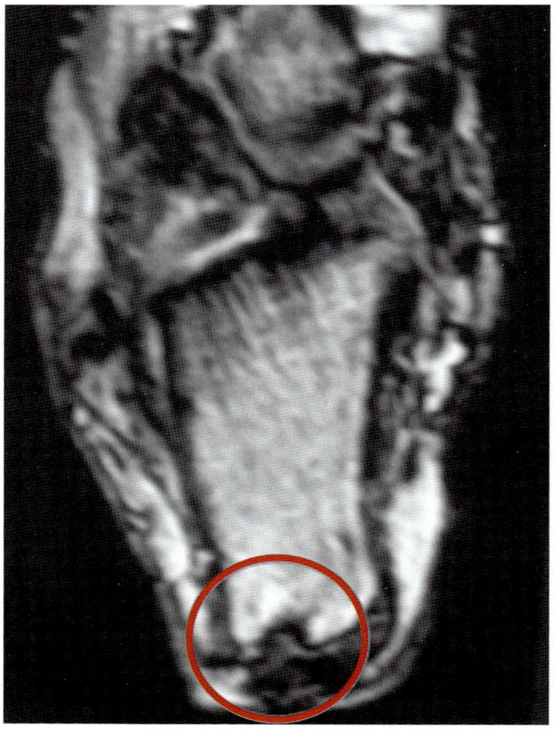

Figure 4 - MRI showing insertional inflammation

ber 1 suture thread is inserted through the proximal incisions and the thread is recovered from the distal incisions with a mosquito. The procedure is also repeated for the anterior side of the tendon.

The passage of the wire frees the tendon from the peritendinous adhesions, from the fat of the triangle of Kager, from the neovases typical of chronic tendinopathy and from the nerve fibers that from the peritenonium reach the tendon. The latter are considered important in the pathophysiology of pain in chronic tendinopathy [163].

Surgical treatment: percutaneous longitudinal tenotomy

Longitudinal incisions are made along the major axis of the tendon to promote tissue regeneration, increase blood flow and create a suitable environment for the healing process.

This technique can be used when there is no peritenon involvement and when the intratendinous lesion is less than 2.5 cm. The procedure can be performed under ultrasound guidance, which is able to confirm the precise location of the lesions. The blade of the scalpel enters the tendon at full thickness, longitudinal incisions are made with different angles of the scalpel and, maintaining the blade still, passive plantar flexion of the ankle is performed (fig. 5).

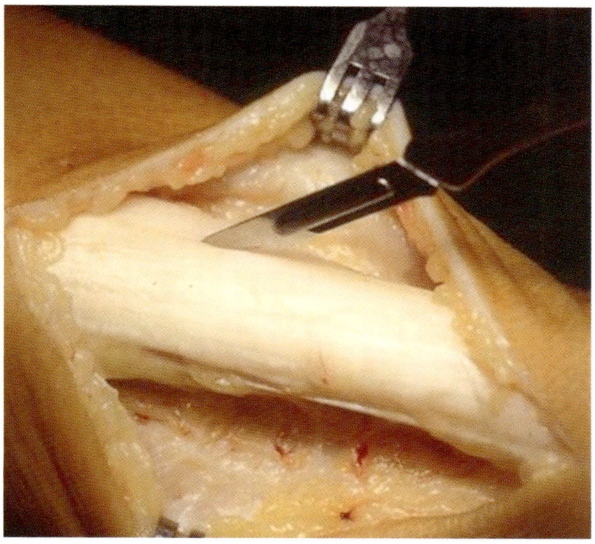

Figure 5 - Percutaneous longitudinal tenotomy

Open surgery

The most frequently used approach is through a posteromedial longitudinal incision. The skin, the subcutaneous fat, and the peritenon are incised, avoiding the sural nerve and the small saphenous vein that are localized laterally.

The pathological tissue can be identified because it generally has lost its shiny appearance and often contains disorganized bundles of fibers (fig. 6). This pathological tissue is removed. The remaining space can be repaired using a side-to-side suture or, in the case of major tissue loss, through a tendon augmentation or transfer.

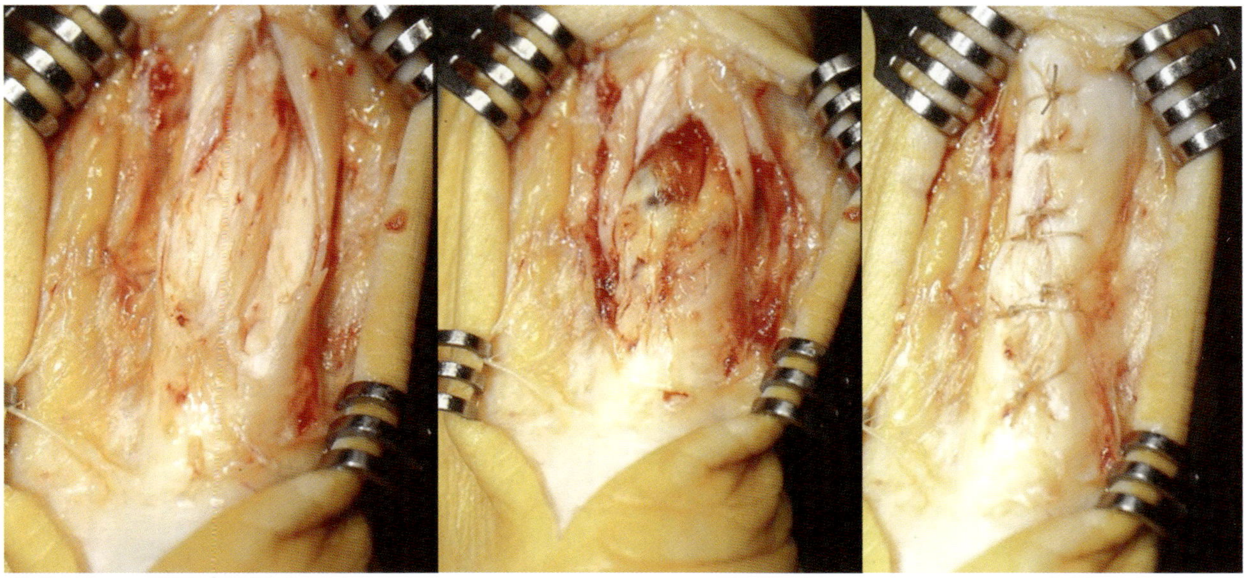

Figure 6 - Degenerated tendon appearance: pathological tissue together with longitudinal lesion and disorganized bundles of fibers. The pathological tissue is removed. The remaining space is repaired using a side-to-side suture

Rupture of Achilles tendon

The Achilles tendon is the strongest tendon in our body due to its ability to withstand the load [164]. Despite its resistance, it is one of the tendons most frequently affected by injuries [165, 166]. The incidence of rupture is between 7 and 37 per 100,000 people a year, most of which occur during physical activity in subjects between 30 and 40 years [167]. The Achilles tendon reaches its maximum tension during the eccentric phase of muscle contraction, a frequent mechanism in sports activities such as soccer [168].

Achilles tendon rupture is not a frequent occurrence, with an incidence rate among professional soccerers of 0.01/1,000 hours played [149]. However, it can be a dramatic event for the sportsman, as it can determine the end of the career, especially for the less young athletes [154, 146, 58, 169].

Achilles tendon ruptures can be partial or total and acute or chronic, if caused by direct trauma or degenerative lesions, respectively. Untreated tendinous ruptures within 4-6 weeks are generally defined as chronic [170]. Total Achilles ruptures are the most frequent and represent up to 35% of all tendon ruptures. They are more frequent in males between 30 and 50 years who practice sports without the correct training, defined by the anglo-saxon literature "week-end warriors".

Rupture is typically unilateral, with rates of contralateral tendon rupture up to 25%. In almost all cases, the rupture occurs in an area between 2 and 6 centimeters from the distal insertion of the tendon, which corresponds to the critical area of hypovascularization. This justifies the greater frequency of lesions on a degenerative basis. More rarely the cause of rupture is due to acute high-energy trauma or direct trauma.

The patient reports an acute feeling of weakness associated with pain and significant functional limitation. Patients often report the feeling of having been kicked from behind at the time of rupture [171].

The visit must include an accurate physical examination, with the patient prone and the feet protruding from the edge of the couch. The interruption in the tendon context should be investigated during palpation (fig. 7). The Thomson test evaluates tendon continuity and consists in compressing the muscular belly of the triceps which normally causes a slight ankle flexion of the ankle: in case of rupture of the Achilles tendon, no movement occurs.

The diagnosis of total rupture is clinical. In case of suspected partial injury the ultrasound examination will confirm the diagnosis (fig. 8). MRI is particularly indicated in chronic (inveterate) ruptures, to quantify the loss of substance between tendon stumps (fig. 9).

The treatment of total acute rupture of Achilles is generally surgical and can be performed with open surgery (fig. 10) or with percutaneous and minimally invasive techniques with the aim of carrying out a termino-terminal suture of the stumps (fig. 11).

In chronic (inveterate) ruptures, the termino-terminal suture is not always possible due to the significant loss of substance between the tendon stumps. Therefore, additive plastics are often performed with homologous tissues, autologous (triceps sura fascia, fascia lata, pes anserinus tendons, and patellar tendon) (fig. 12), synthetic (fig. 13) or local ten-

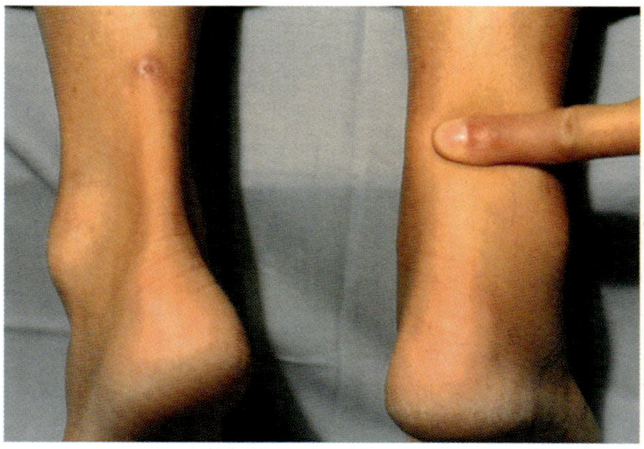

Figure 7 - The interruption of the Achilles tendon is clinically evident in case of complete rupture

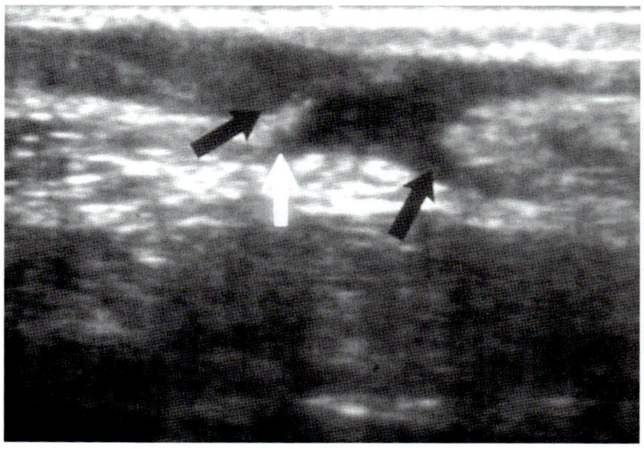

Figure 8 - Ultrasound examination showing the Achilles tendon rupture (arrows)

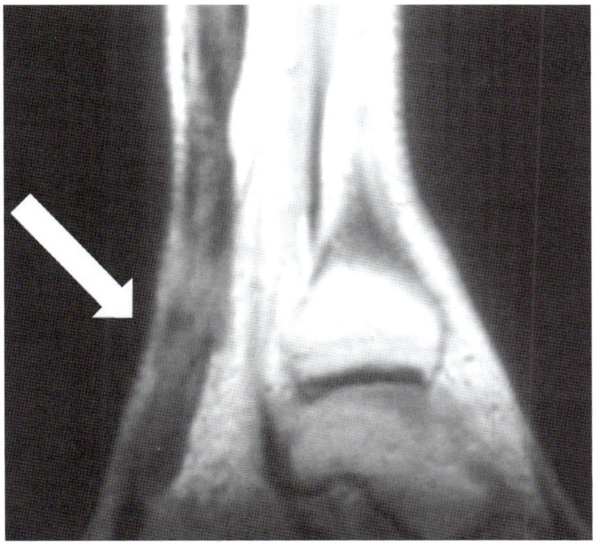

Figure 9 - Chronic and partial Achilles tendon rupture detected at the MRI

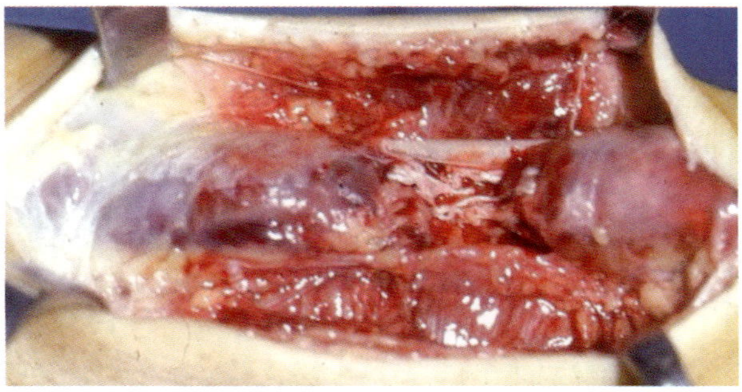

Figure 10 - Achilles tendon lesion in open surgery

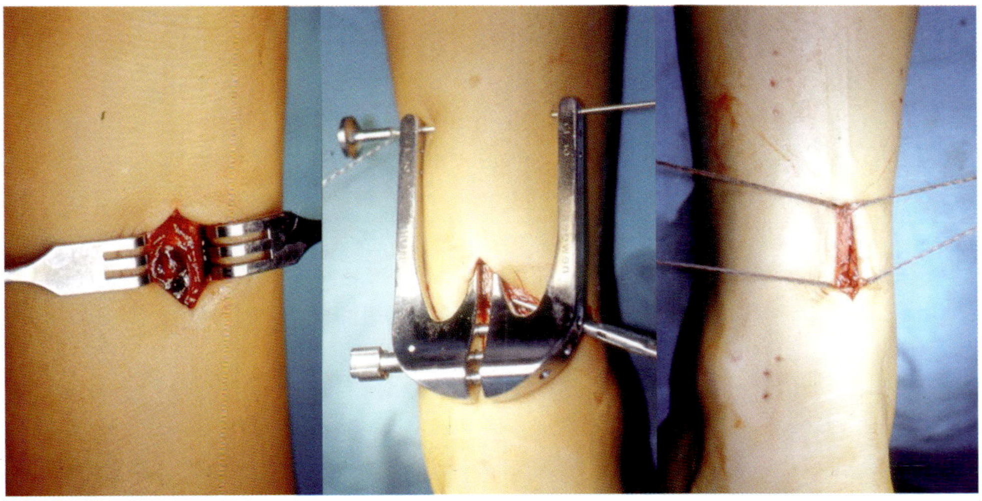

Figure 11 - "Achillon" minimally invasive techniques for Achilles tendon repair

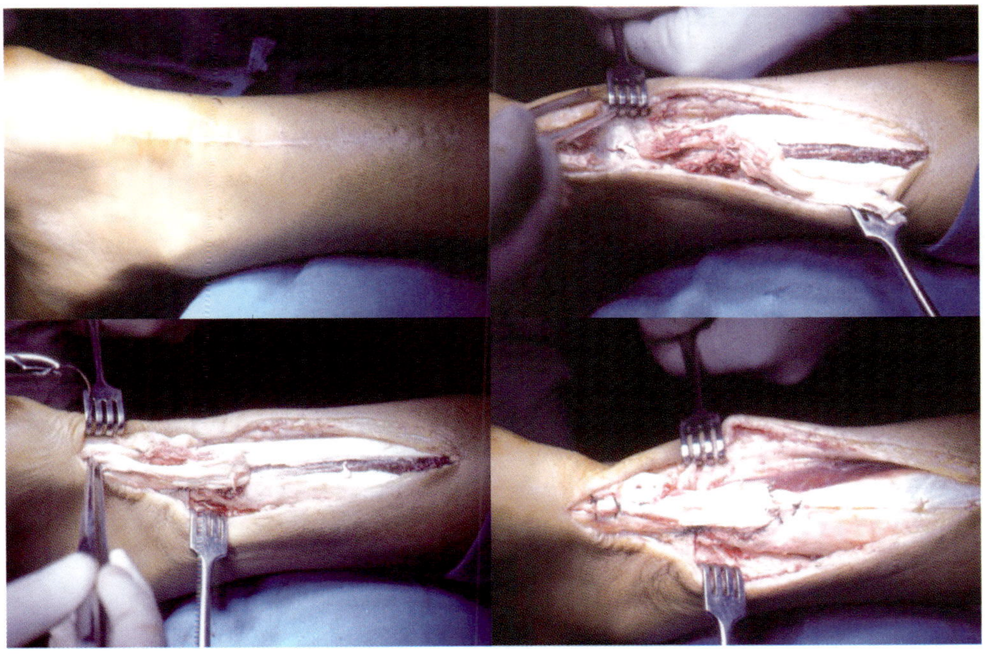

Figure 12 - Chronic rupture with tendon tissue loss. The muscle fascia is used to perform a reconstructive plastic procedure. The defect is then sutured side to side

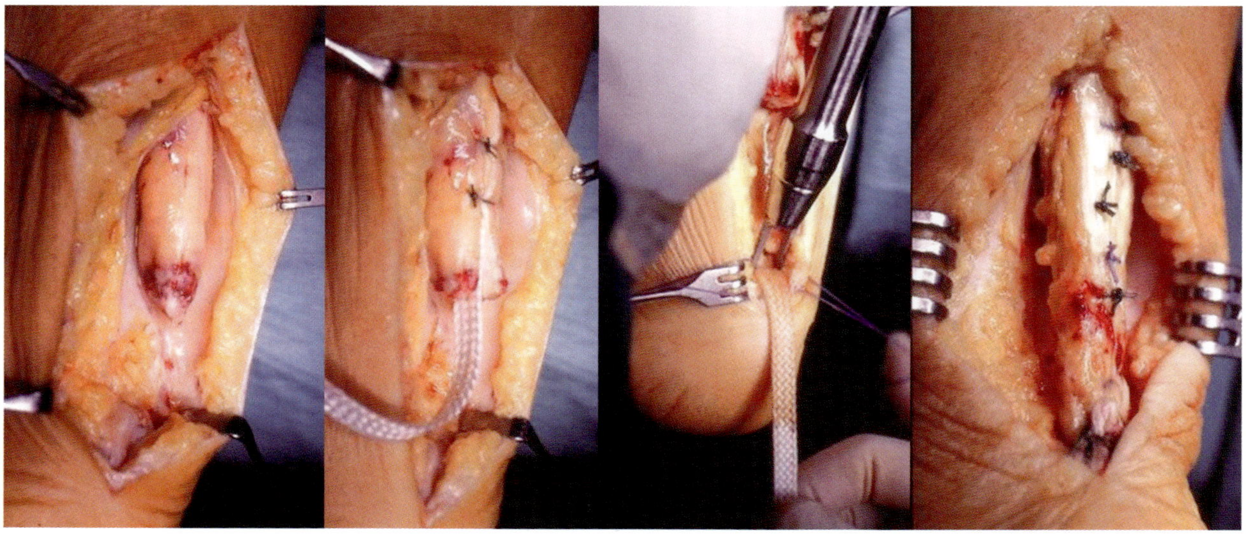

Figure 13 - Chronic rupture with severe and massive tendon tissue loss. Synthetic graft reconstruction

don transpositions using the flexor hallucis longus, the peroneus brevis or the plantaris.

Sports hernia (athletic pubalgia)

Sports hernia is a definition that describes different causes of groin pain. It can be described as anatomically localized pain in inguinal region in an athlete in the absence of a true hernia [172].

The term sport hernia includes a series of clinical conditions that gofrom chronic groin pain [173] to groin tendon ruptures secondary to functional pelvic instability [174]. However, due to the absence of a true hernia, the term "inguinal disruption" is preferred [175]. This is a clinical condition still not well characterized from a physiopathological point of view [173].

Epidemiology

Inguinal pain is an extremely common condition in soccer [176]. 5-15% of professional soccerers suffer from acute groin pain at least once during the season [177, 178]. Chronic inguinal pain is not as frequent and the diagnosis is often complex due to the variety of pathological conditions that can determine it [179]; however, it is more common in contact sports such as soccer than in sports where there is no physical contact such as swimming [176].

Sports hernia, together with the pathology of the adductor and gracilis and pubic osteitis, is the most frequent cause of chronic inguinal pain in professional soccerers [176].

Physiopathology and risk factors

The pubic symphysis acts as a fulcrum for the anterior pelvis and all the structures involved in the genesis of sports hernia have intimate relations with this fulcrum. The fibers of the abdominal rectum, of the conjoint tendon (fusion of the fibers of the internal and transverse oblique of the abdomen), and of the external oblique merge to constitute a single aponeurosis that is inserted to pubis. The latter joins with the pubic origin of the adductor and gracilis tendons.

The most commonly referred physiopathological mechanism in sports hernia is the increase in groin tension caused by repeated and excessive movements of torsion of the trunk, rotation, and flexion of the hip [175]. This tension can cause suffering and thinning of the inguinal structures which is manifested clinically with pain.

Furthermore, the loss of intra and extra-rotation of the hip can contribute to the etiology, given the correlation between loss of hip ROM and sports hernia in athletes [180]. Loss of hip movement can stress the pubic symphysis and lead to pelvic instability. Similarly, femoral-acetabular impingement of the hip can cause inguinal pain [181]. Standing on one leg, as it occurs in many sports, the adductor muscles work with the abdominal muscles to control and stabilize the pelvis while the hip rotates, adducts and flexes. The weakness of one of these muscular structures can lead to instability, stress or overload damage to the tendons of the muscles that are inserted into

the groin [182, 183]. Furthermore, the cause of pubic pain can also be attributed to a nerve compression of the iliohypogastric and genitofemoral nerve branches or to an inflammation of the conjoint tendon [184].
Risk factors include also a high BMI and the number of hours of sports practice [176].

Clinical aspects
Patients report pain in the groin located mainly at the pubic symphysis and irradiated to the tendons of the abdominal rectum or adductors.
Symptoms are aggravated by sporting activity such as kickingsprint, especially with rapid acceleration, and are relieved by rest [174, 185].
The cough can cause pain that can be radiated to the thigh or to the testicles due to the anatomical position of potentially compressed nerves [185].

British Hernia Society diagnostic criteria
According to the diagnostic criteria described by the British Hernia Society [175] at least three of the following five criteria must be met to diagnose sports hernia:
- pain described as dull or diffuse radiating to the medial aspect of the thigh, to the perineum, or to the contralateral side;
- tenderness on palpation of the pubic tubercle, to the insertion of the inguinal ligament;
- pain on palpation of the deep inguinal ring;
- pain on palpation of the tendon of the adductor longus;
- pain on palpation of the superficial inguinal ring or dilatation of the same.

Imaging
The first step in the instrumental diagnosis of sports hernia is represented by the radiograph of the pelvis and the hip to evaluate the bony structures and eventually exclude pathologies that can clinically simulate this condition [185]. However, the gold standard for diagnosis is represented by MRI, which is important in identifying any associated clinical conditions and for making differential diagnoses.
The most common finding is the relief of tension in the tendon of the abdominal rectum and a partial or total detachment of the tendon of the adductor longus [173, 185].
MRI has a sensitivity of 68% and a specificity of 100% for injuries to the tendon of the abdominal rectum and a sensitivity of 86% and a specificity of 89% for injuries to the tendon of the adductor longus [186]. It can also detect the presence of bone edema in the pubic symphysis.

Differential diagnosis
In the differential diagnosis should be considered [187, 188, 180, 184, 189, 185]:
- inguinal hernia;
- intra-abdominal pathological conditions;
- urogenital pathology;
- herniated disc symptomatology;
- femoral-acetabular impingement;
- entrapment and nerve compression symptomatology;
- pathology of the sacroiliac joint;
- piriformis pathology;
- ileopsoas pathology;
- pubic osteitis;
- soft tissue pathology.

Conservative treatment
The treatment of sports hernia is initially conservative, surgical options are considered only after 3-6 months without any clinical response [183, 190].
The first conservative approach in the management of this condition should include an intervention on the balance of the pelvis and on the loss of hip ROM. The exercises in this phase should aim at strengthening the gluteus medius and maximus, the abdominal muscles and the flexors of the hip to obtain greater stability of the pelvis. In athletes these exercises must be set to sport-specific mode as much as possible [175, 183].
Another rehabilitative protocol consists of a first resting phase with the subsequent gradual return to the activity, insisting on muscular reinforcement in particular through exercises from the supine to the vertical position [191].

Surgical treatment
Surgical treatment is considered after 3-6 months of conservative treatment failure. Surgical procedures for sports hernia can be performed with open, minimally invasive or laparoscopic access.

The purpose of surgical treatment is to strengthen the posterior wall of the inguinal canal through the use of synthetic meshes or through the plication of the fascia of the abdominal rectum with suture to the pubis and inguinal ligament. This procedure can be associated with tenotomy of the adductor muscles and with decompression of the genital branch of the genitofemoral nerve [184, 185, 192, 193]. For possible nerve involvement a radiofrequency denervation can also be practiced.

The return to sporting activity is usually expected about one month after the intervention [173].

When associated, it is recommended to treat the femoroacetabular impingement which, causing alteration of the hip ROM, might play a role in the genesis of tension in the inguinal structures.

Other foot and ankle tendon injuries

The foot and ankle are the anatomical sites most frequently injured in soccer [194]. A study carried out on professional English soccerers showed that around a third of athletes had at least one or more injuries to the foot or ankle during the competitive season (3-9/1,000 hours played) [195], above all to the lower dominant leg (79%), above all due to direct contact (59%) [196, 195]. Among all the injuries that involve the foot or ankle, lesions to the tendon make up between 2 and 23% of the total [197].

Tendon injuries to the foot and ankle therefore represent an important percentage of sports injuries, in terms of the impact due to lost play days for the professional player or lost working days for the amateur sportsman. Because of this, medical professional need to concentrate on the prevention and cure of such injuries.

Tendinopathies of the peroneal tendons

Peroneus tendinopathies are frequent and tenosynovitis, chronic lesions, and dislocation are the most common.

Etiology can be traumatic or degenerative. Usually the most common causes of peroneus tendinopathy are twisted ankles, peroneal tubercle hypertrophy, traumas to the external malleolus, or as a result of fractures to the heel. A modified anatomical profile of the heel can enter into conflict with the peroneus tendons [198].

There are, moreover, specific risk factors such as diabetes, neuropathy, dyslipidemia, corticosteroid therapy, and hyperuricemia. Peroneus tenosynovitis can appear at various levels along the length of the tendon, although the area most commonly involved is in proximity of the lateral surface of the heel. Typically, the patient feels pain in the posterior and lateral area of the foot, with painful swelling along the length of the tendon. The pain increases when a varus stress manoeuvre is applied.

Peroneus brevis tendinopathies are commonly found in the lower third of the fibula, while peroneus longus tendinopathies are lower and mainly found in the cuboid area [199, 200]. Peroneus brevis tendinopathies are usually due to lateral instability of the ankle, that over time, cause the development of micro-lesions or longitudinal fissures.

Classification

These lesions can be classified in four degrees in terms of severity:

- in grade 1 lesions, the tendon appears flattened or widened with no macroscopic lesions;
- in grade 2 lesions, there are longitudinal fissures of partial thickness of maximum length of 1 cm;
- in grade 3 and 4 lesions, there are full-thickness lesions of less than 2 cm length (grade 3) and more than 2 cm length (grade 4).

Clinical aspects

Normally, the most frequent clinical feature is the subjective sensation of a “click”. This is accompanied by swelling and pain when pressure is applied behind the external malleolus. The Sobel test consists in applying pressure in correspondence to the superior peroneal retinaculum, asking the patient to evert and dorsiflex the foot: in the case of a longitudinal tear you hear a “click”, while in the case of subluxation, you can hear a “snap” [201].

Another clinical aspect to consider is enthesopathy of the peroneus brevis which provokes pain only in the insertional site, miming other clinical possibilities such as avulsion fractures or stress fractures and apophysitis of the base of the fifth metatarsal bone.

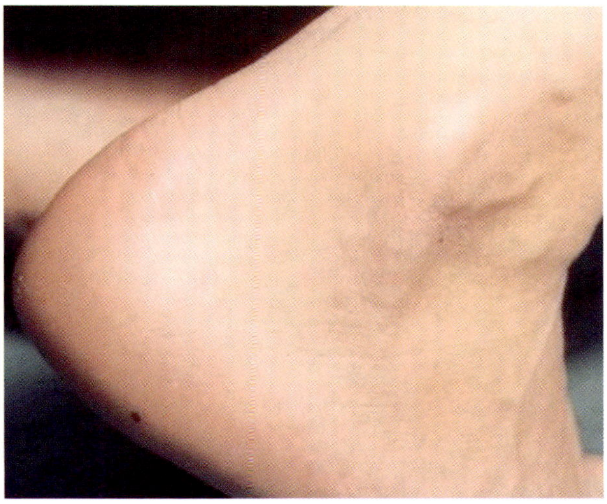

Figure 14 - Chronic peroneal tendons luxation: no swelling but the tendons appear to be anterior to the lateral malleolus posterior aspect

VIDEO 1

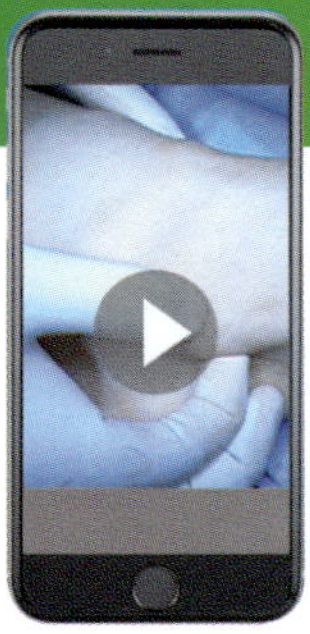

Clinical presentation: peroneal tendon manual dislocation

Lesions of the peroneus longus are rarer and normally occur as a result of a trauma from an inversion ankle sprain. Symptoms can be vague; usually there is pain localized behind the peroneal malleolus or at the plantar surface of the cuboid bone along the path of the tendon. This pain is aggravated by forced eversion and by plantar flexion against resistance of the first toe.

Luxations or subluxations of the tendon are often the result of sports injuries and are particularly prevalent in Alpine skiing, although there are also descriptions of congenital luxations [202]. They are usually the result of lesions to the osteofibrous tunnel at the distal fibula level where the tendons run and, in particular, of lesions of the superior peroneal retinaculum [203]. Luxations are usually classified as grade 4 within an anatomical-pathology framework.

Luxation classification

Eckert and Davis classification was modified by Oden.

- Grade I: the superior peroneal retinaculum is stripped from the peroneal malleolus and is dissected by the tendons that have migrated forwards between the bone and the periosteum.
- Grade 2: the superior peroneal retinaculum is lacerated and detached from the malleolus.
- Grade 3: the superior peroneal retinaculum is detached from the mallerous with avulsion of small bone fragment.
- Grade 4: complete tear to the superior peroneal retinaculum in posterior zone. In this case the retinaculum is under the subluxated tendon.

Luxation can be acute or chronic. In acute luxation, patients tell of a traumatic event and have swelling and local bruising with retromalleolar pain. In chronic luxation, there is a history of ankle instability with recurrent ankle sprains and there is little or no swelling and bruising (fig. 14) (video 1).

Imaging

MRI is the gold standard for diagnosis of these lesions and allows differential diagnosis between simple tendinitis and real lesions. It can identify longitudinal fissures, hypertrophy and other pathological alterations of these tendons with very high specificity, although sensitivity is around 75% [204].

When a break is suspected in the peroneus longus tendon, a standard X-ray can be useful. In particular, when the os peroneum is present, it points to the peroneus longus tendon and should it have an irregular position this indicates there is lesion to this tendon (fig. 15).

In the diagnosis process of luxation and subluxation, a standard X-ray will identify even minimal bone avulsion at the superior peroneal retinaculum level, while MRI can identify any other luxation or other tendon lesions there might be (fig. 16) [205].

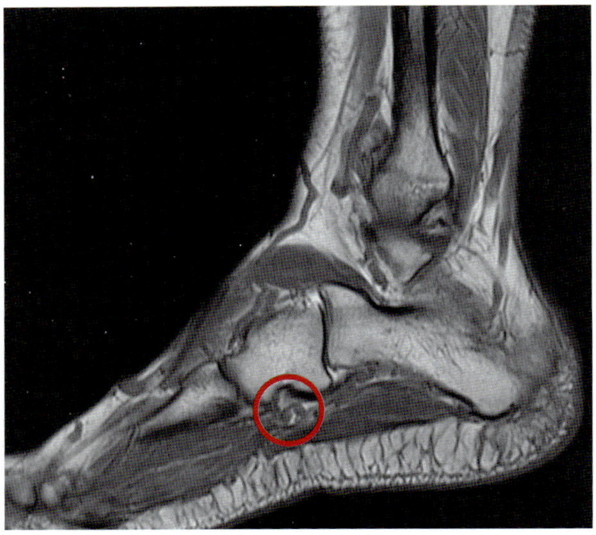

Figure 15 - Os peroneum normal aspect highlighted at the MRI. In a non-pathological condition the os peroneum should be located distally to the calcaneo-cuboid joint, under the cuboid bone

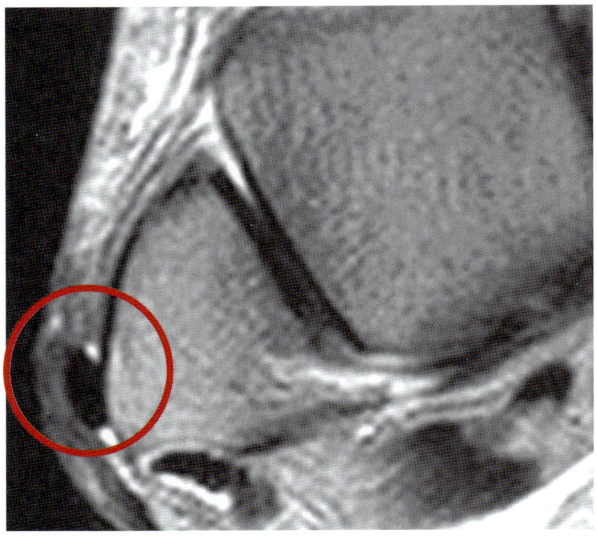

Figure 16 - MRI showing an anterior peroneal tendons luxation

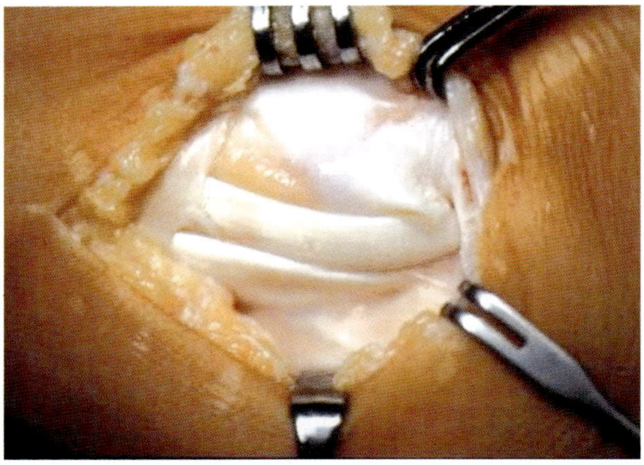

Figure 17 - Retinaculum chronic lesion associated with peroneal tendon luxation

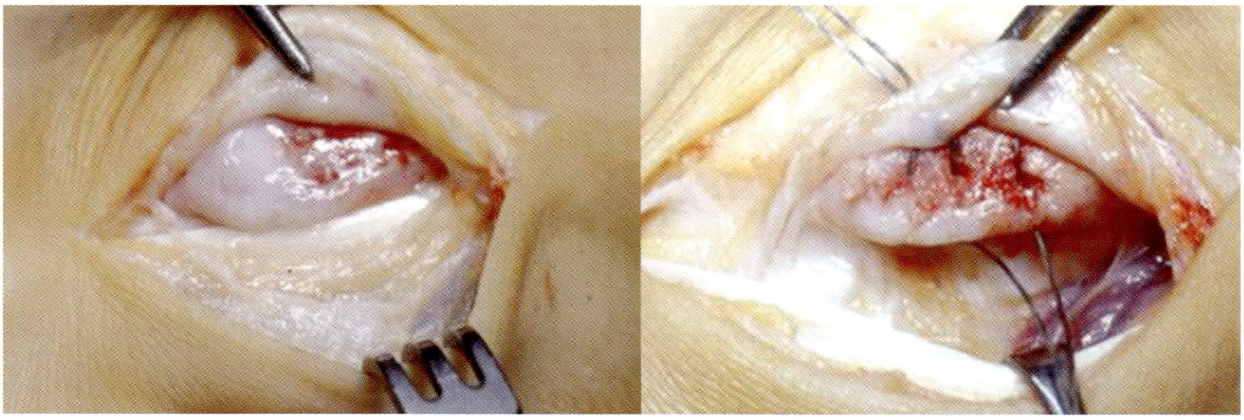

Figure 18 - Retinaculum lesion (on the left) repaired with a transosseous suture (on the right)

Treatment

For tendinopathies with no signs of lesions, the first line treatment is conservative with rest, use of orthesis, and rehabilitation. Should this fail, surgical treatment is required [206]. The type of surgical treatment depends on the kind of lesion; in the case of a single longitudinal fissure, removal or suture is indicated.

In the case of a tendon degeneration area, a peroneal tendon debridement and tubularization is required [207]. In the case of a lesion of the peroneus longus tendon, reconstruction is needed; but in the case of an irreparable lesion, tenodesis with the peroneus brevis is needed.

In case of acute luxation, conservative treatment consists in immobilization with the ankle in slight plantarflexion and slight inversion of the foot using a non-removable cast for 6 weeks. Because of the high rate of complications, surgical treatment with direct reinsertion of the peroneal retinaculum is often preferable.

In case of chronic luxation with serious retinaculum damage (fig. 17), surgical treatment consists of reconstruction of the retinaculum (fig. 18) and, if necessary, a peroneal groove deepening [208].

Tendinopathies of the posterior tibialis tendon

Tendinopathies of the posterior tibialis are often chronic and are generally caused by flatfoot deformity which puts the tendon under great strain. The posterior tibialis muscle has a limited sliding excursion, about 2 cm. For this reason, even small strains can prove injurious [209].

Repeated micro-traumas caused by persistent pronation of the foot can lead to a vast array of clinical manifestations relating to the anatomopathological aspects of the lesion and can vary from small fissures to complete rupture.

In other cases, primary lesions to the posterior tibialis tendon can lead to secondary flatfoot condition. In this case, the loss of functionality in the tendon causes the plantar arch to collapse [210].

Clinical aspects

Patients with chronic tendinopathy of the posterior tibialis complain of pain in the medial region, generally the retromalleolar or further away in the peri-insertional zone at the scaphoid.

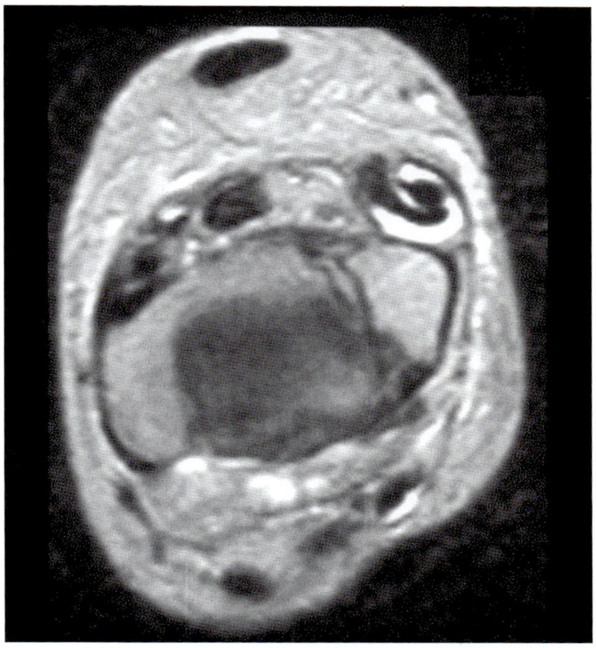

Figure 19 - Fluid surrounding the posterior tibialis tendon which appears hypertrophic at the MRI

Bearing in mind the pronation at the basis of the pathology, there are other changes to the walk with an insufficient push phase [211].

It's important to understand the history so as to identify the presence of inflammatory arthropathy, which is another possible cause. To diagnose tendinopathy of the posterior tibialis, a MRI will show the involvement of the tendon (fig. 19) [212].

Classification

Lesions of the posterior tibialis tendon can vary in severity. The first classification proposed for tendinopathy of the posterior tibialis was that of Rosemberg, based on MRI findings and providing four possible configurations.

- Type 1 lesion: hypertrophy of the tendon with longitudinal fissuring (fig. 20).
- Type 2 A lesion: partial lesion (involving less than 50% of the tendon) (fig. 21).
- Type 2 B lesion: subtotal lesion (involving more than 50% of the tendon) (fig. 22).
- Type 3 lesion: lesion with complete rupture of the tendon.

Treatment

Treatment can be conservative or surgical.

Conservative treatment consists of functional rest and use of implants to support the plantar arch, so

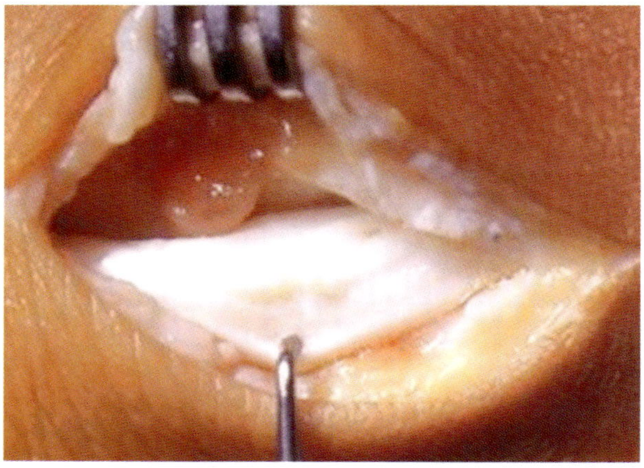

Figure 20 - Type 1 lesion showing some degrees of tendon hypertrophy together with a longitudinal fissuring

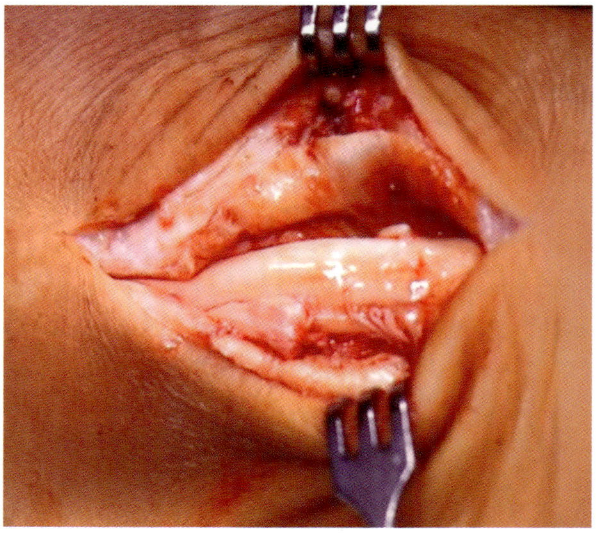

Figure 21 - Type 2 A lesion: less than 50% of the tendon is involved. Degenerated fibers and tendon hypertrophy

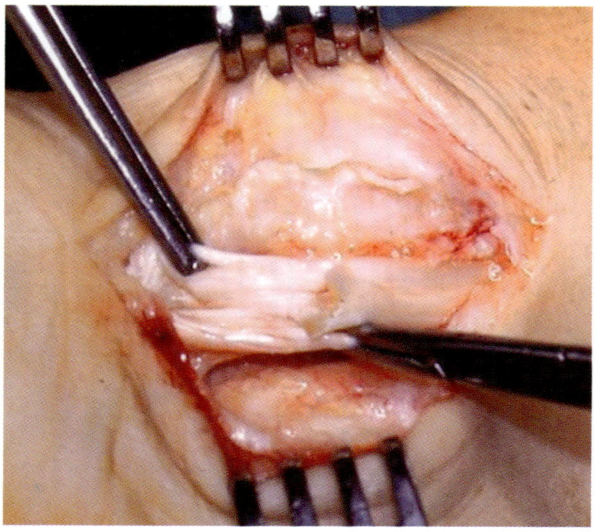

Figure 22 - Type 2 B lesion with subtotal lesion involving more than 50% of the tendon

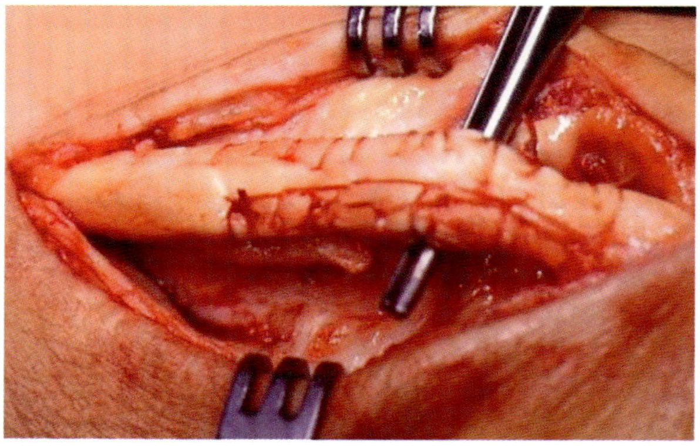

Figure 23 - Tenolysis and tendon suture with absorbable thread for a type 2 A lesion

as to discharge the stress that occurs at the level of the tendon [213].

Lesions of the posterior tibialis tendon are treated according to their grade/type. Grade 1 lesions generally require repair; if there are fibrous adhesions a tenolysis is carried out. If there is a lesion, it is sutured with absorbable thread [214].

In grade 2 lesions, the degenerated portion of the tendon is removed and the remaining portion is sutured (fig. 23).

If the remaining section is less than 50% of the tendon, a reinforcement with half of the flexor digitorum longus tendon is needed [215].

Grade 3 lesions, after the removal of the degenerated components, are generally treated by transferring the tendon of the flexor digitorum longus, which is fixed at the navicular level by a tunnel (video 2).

In presence of severe third or fourth grade lesions and associated sub-talar arthritis, a sub-talar joint arthrodesis may be required.

Rupture of the posterior tibialis tendon

The posterior tibialis tendon is frequently affected by inflammatory processes which, if not cured, can develop irreversible degeneration. These inflammatory processes are generally linked to a pronation of the foot deformity or physiological degenerative processes typical of the senile period which can provoke partial or total lesions.

On the other hand, acute lesions of the posterior tibialis tendon are rare and usually caused by sprain traumas, and can be associated with fractures of the surrounding bones [216].
From an etiopathogenetic point of view, sprain traumas in external pronation-rotation are the main cause of tendon lesions; in the case of fractures of the medial malleolus, there is an increased risk of lesions.
Total lesions resulting from direct trauma are rarer than sprain traumas.
Lesions of the posterior tibialis tendon in their acute phase are often mis-recognised. In most cases, they only become evident when the acute phase is over, through persistent pain or secondary changes of the morphology of the foot in flat foot.
Treatment of these lesions, be they partial or total, is generally surgical, with repair in isolated lesions or termino-terminal tenorrhaphy in the case of total ruptures [217].

Tendinopathies of the anterior tibialis tendon

The main tendinopathies of the anterior tibialis are insertional tendinopathies, stenosing tenosynovitis, hypertrophic tenosynovitis, and tendinosis. Symptoms can be vague and can extend from the the antero-medial region of the ankle to the midfoot [218].
Stenosing tenosynovitis is a rare pathology of difficult differential diagnosis. There is stenosing at the level of the bifurcated ligament (calcaneo-scaphoid and calcaneo-cuboid ligament) impeding the sliding of the tendon. Patient reports pain and bruising along the path of the tendon at the level of the instep and difficulty in carrying out flexion-extension movements of the foot [219].
Hypertrophic tenosynovitis can be seen in young sports patients who use shoes with high uppers and undergo repeated flexion-extension movements of the foot, or in older patients affected by deformities such as flatfeet or bursitis which alter the physiology of walking. This condition is characterised by phlogosis of the tendon sheath. There is secondary bruising at the distension of the sheath and, using your hands, it is possible to feel the movement of liquids. Pain is exacerbated by the dorsiflexion of the ankle [220].
Tendinoses are pathological degenerative conditions, most often complex and secondary to chronic inflammation, ageing, and repeated mechanical stress. In the absence of associated inflammatory processes, they are often paucisymptomatic and can present just a modest increase of the size of the tendon [221].

Treatment

First choice treatment of stenosing tenosynovitis is conservative, consisting in rest, immobilization and, if necessary, infiltration therapy. Should this fail, surgery is needed, consisting in tenolysis at the level of the bifurcated ligament [222].
In the case of hypertrophic tenosynovitis, treatment consists in the removal of risk factors, the use of anti-inflammatory drugs and, if necessary, orthotic implants to compensate for associated deformities. Should conservative therapies fail, synovectomy surgery is needed [223].

Rupture of the anterior tibialis tendon

Ruptures of the anterior tibialis tendon are rare and usually secondary to traumas in plantar flexion of the ankle and foot [224].
In the case of acute rupture, the patient reports pain with localized swelling and ecchymosis associated with difficulty in the dorsiflexion of the foot. In the case of acute lesions, a surgical operation is necessary and involves a termino-terminal suture of the tendon or a trans-bone re-insertion of the tendon [225].

VIDEO 2

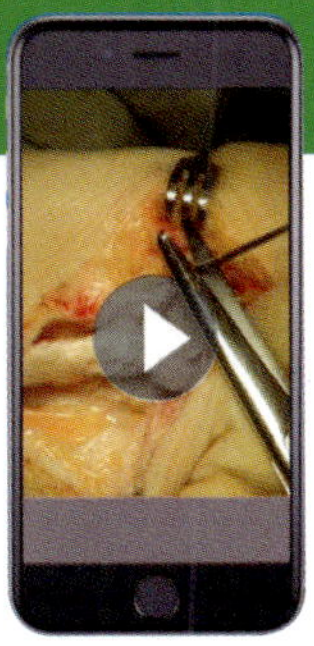

Flexor digitorum longus transfer

Bibliography

1. Canata GL, D'Hooghe P, Hunt KJ. Muscle and tendon injuries: Evaluation and management. Ed. Springer 2017.
2. Ackermann PW, Renström P. Tendinopathy in sport. Sports Health. 2012 May;4(3):193-201.
3. Ekstrand J, Hägglund M, Waldén M. Injury incidence and injury patterns in professional soccer: the UEFA injury study. Br J Sports Med. 2011 Jun;45(7):553-8.
4. Gabbett TJ, Kennelly S, Sheehan J, Hawkins R, Milsom J, King E, Whiteley R, Ekstrand J. If overuse injury is a 'training load error', should undertraining be viewed the same way? Br J Sports Med. 2016 Sep;50(17):1017-8.
5. Kibler WB, Chandler TJ, Pace BK. Principles of rehabilitation after chronic tendon injuries. Clin Sports Med. 1992 Jul;11(3):661-71.
6. Mead MP, Gumucio JP, Awan TM, Mendias CL, Sugg KB. Pathogenesis and Management of Tendinopathies in Sports Medicine. Transl Sports Med. 2018 Jan;1(1):5-13.
7. Mead MP, Gumucio JP, Awan TM, Mendias CL, Sugg KB. Pathogenesis and Management of Tendinopathies in Sports Medicine. Transl Sports Med. 2018 Jan;1(1):5-13.
8. Abat F, Alfredson H, Cucchiarini M, Madry H, Marmotti A, Mouton C, Oliveira JM, Pereira H, Peretti GM, Spang C, Stephen J, van Bergen CJA, de Girolamo L. Current trends in tendinopathy: consensus of the ESSKA basic science committee. Part II: treatment options. J Exp Orthop. 2018 Sep 24;5(1):38.
9. O'Brien M. Functional anatomy and physiology of tendons. Clin Sports Med. 1992 Jul;11(3):505-20.
10. Kannus P, Niittymäki S, Järvinen M, Lehto M. Sports injuries in elderly athletes: a three-year prospective, controlled study. Age Ageing. 1989 Jul;18(4):263-70.
11. Longo UG, Loppini M, Margiotti K, Salvatore G, Berton A, Khan WS, Maffulli N, Denaro V. Unravelling the genetic susceptibility to develop ligament and tendon injuries. Curr Stem Cell Res Ther. 2015;10(1):56-63.
12. Vaug hn NH, Stepanyan H, Gallo RA, Dhawan A. Genetic Factors in Tendon Injury: A Systematic Review of the Literature. Orthop J Sports Med. 2017 Aug23;5(8):2325967117724416.
13. John R, Dhillon MS, Sharma S, Prabhakar S, Bhandari M. Is There a Genetic Predisposition to Anterior Cruciate Ligament Tear? A Systematic Review. Am J Sports Med. 2016 Dec;44(12):3262-3269.
14. Wenstrup RJ, Florer JB, Brunskill EW, Bell SM, Chervoneva I, Birk DE. Type V collagen controls the initiation of collagen fibril assembly. J Biol Chem. 2004 Dec 17;279(51):53331-7.
15. Jozsa L, Balint JB, Kannus P, Reffy A, Barzo M. Distribution of blood groups in patients with tendon rupture. An analysis of 832 cases. J Bone Joint Surg Br. 1989 Mar;71(2):272-4.
16. Kujala UM, Järvinen M, Natri A, Lehto M, Nelimarkka O, Hurme M, Virta L, Finne J. ABO blood groups and musculoskeletal injuries. Injury. 1992;23(2):131-3.
17. Leppilahti J, Puranen J, Orava S. ABO blood group and Achilles tendon rupture. Ann Chir Gynaecol. 1996;85(4):369-71.
18. Maffulli N, Reaper JA, Waterston SW, Ahya T. ABO blood groups and Achilles tendon rupture in the Grampian Region of Scotland. Clin J Sport Med. 2000 Oct;10(4):269-71.
19. Leadbetter WB. Cell-matrix response in tendon injury. Clin Sports Med. 1992 Jul;11(3):533-78.
20. Gaida JE, Ashe MC, Bass SL, Cook JL. Is adiposity an under-recognized risk factor for tendinopathy? A systematic review. Arthritis Rheum. 2009 Jun 15;61(6):840-9.
21. Aicale R, Tarantino D, Maffulli N. Overuse injuries in sport: a comprehensive overview. J Orthop Surg Res. 2018 Dec 5;13(1):309.
22. Maffulli N, Benazzo F. Basic Science of Tendons Sports Med. Arthrosc. 2000; 8: 1–5.
23. Gaida JE, Ashe MC, Bass SL, Cook JL. Is adiposity an under-recognized risk factor for tendinopathy? A systematic review. Arthritis Rheum. 2009 Jun 15;61(6):840-9.
24. Stahlmann R. Clinical toxicological aspects of fluoroquinolones. Toxicol Lett. 2002 Feb 28;127(1-3):269-77.
25. D'Addona A, Maffulli N, Formisano S, Rosa D. Inflammation in tendinopathy. Surgeon. 2017 Oct;15(5):297-302.
26. Alfredson H, Forsgren S, Thorsen K, Lorentzon R. In vivo microdialysis and immunohistochemical analyses of tendon tissue demonstrated high amounts of free glutamate and glutamate NMDAR1 receptors, but no signs of inflammation, in Jumper's knee. J Orthop Res. 2001 Sep;19(5):881-6.
27. Legerlotz K, Jones ER, Screen HR, Riley GP. Increased expression of IL-6 family members in tendon pathology. Rheumatology (Oxford). 2012 Jul;51(7):1161-5.
28. Fedorczyk JM, Barr AE, Rani S, Gao HG, Amin M, Amin S, Litvin J, Barbe MF. Exposure-dependent increases in IL-1beta, substance P, CTGF, and tendinosis in flexor digitorum tendons with upper extremity repetitive strain injury. J Orthop Res. 2010 Mar;28(3):298-307.
29. Sharma P, Maffulli N. Biology of tendon injury: healing, modeling and remodeling. J Musculoskelet Neuronal Interact. 2006 Apr-Jun;6(2):181-90.
30. Ackermann PW, Domeij-Arverud E, Leclerc P, Amoudrouz P, Nader GA. Anti-inflammatory cytokine profile in early human tendon repair. Knee Surg Sports Traumatol Arthrosc. 2013 Aug;21(8):1801-6.
31. van Dijk CN, van Sterkenburg MN, Wiegerinck JI, Karlsson J, Maffulli N. Terminology for Achilles tendon related disorders. Knee Surg Sports Traumatol Arthrosc. 2011 May;19(5):835-41.
32. Rees JD, Wilson AM, Wolman RL. Current concepts in the management of tendon disorders. Rheumatology (Oxford). 2006 May;45(5):508-21.
33. Riley G. Tendinopathy--from basic science to treatment. Nat Clin Pract Rheumatol. 2008 Feb;4(2):82-9.
34. Milz S et al. Molecular composition and pathology of entheses on the medial and lateral epicondyles of the humerus: a structural basis for epicondylitis. Ann Rheum Dis. 2004 Sep;63(9):1015-21.
35. Sharma P, Maffulli N. Tendinopathy and tendon injury: the future. Disabil Rehabil. 2008;30(20-22):1733-45.
36. Mazzone MF, McCue T. Common conditions of the achilles tendon. Am Fam Physician. 2002 May 1;65(9):1805-10.
37. Alfredson H, Lorentzon M, Bäckman S, Bäckman A, Lerner UH. cDNA-arrays and real-time quantitative PCR techniques in the investigation of chronic Achilles tendinosis. J Orthop Res. 2003 Nov;21(6):970-5.
38. Dakin SG, Dudhia J, Werling NJ, Werling D, Abayasekara DR, Smith RK. Inflamm-aging and arachadonic acid metabolite differences with stage of tendon disease. PLoS One. 2012;7(11):e48978.
39. Yao L, Bestwick CS, Bestwick LA, Aspden RM, Maffulli N. Non-immortalized human tenocyte cultures as a vehicle for understanding cellular aspects to tendinopathy. Transl Med UniSa. 2011 Oct 17;1:173-94.
40. Millar NL, Murrell GA, McInnes IB. Alarmins in tendinopathy: unravelling new mechanisms in a common disease. Rheumatology (Oxford). 2013 May;52(5):769-79.
41. Oliva F, Barisani D, Grasso A, Maffulli N. Gene expression analysis in calcific tendinopathy of the rotator cuff. Eur

Cell Mater. 2011 Jun 20;21:548-57.
42. Karousou E, Ronga M, Vigetti D, Barcolli D, Passi A, Maffulli N. Molecular interactions in extracellular matrix of tendon. Front Biosci (Elite Ed). 2010 Jan 1;2:1-12.
43. Longo UG, Oliva F, Denaro V, Maffulli N. Oxygen species and overuse tendinopathy in athletes. Disabil Rehabil. 2008;30(20-22):1563-71.
44. Longo UG, Ripalda P, Denaro V, Forriol F. Morphologic comparison of cervical, thoracic, lumbar intervertebral discs of cynomolgus monkey (Macaca fascicularis). Eur Spine J. 2006 Dec;15(12):1845-51.
45. Longo UG, Ronga M, Maffulli N. Achilles Tendinopathy. Sports Med Arthrosc Rev. 2018 Mar;26(1):112-26.
46. Longo UG, Franceschi F, Ruzzini L, Rabitti C, Morini S, Maffulli N, Forriol F, Denaro V. Light microscopic histology of supraspinatus tendon ruptures. Knee Surg Sports Traumatol Arthrosc. 2007 Nov;15(11):1390-4.
47. Magra M, Maffulli N. Matrix metalloproteases: a role in overuse tendinopathies. Br J Sports Med. 2005 Nov;39(11):789-91.
48. James R, Kesturu G Balian G, Chhabra AB. Tendon: biology, biomechanics, repair, growth factors, and evolving treatment options. J Hand Surg Am. 2008 Jan;33(1):102-12.
49. Hoffmann A, Gross G. Tendon and ligament engineering: from cell biology to in vivo application. Regen Med. 2006 Jul;1(4):563-74.
50. Maffulli N, Longo UG, Denaro V. Novel approaches for the management of tendinopathy. J Bone Joint Surg Am. 2010 Nov 3;92(15):2604-13.
51. Oakes DA, McAllister DR. Failure of heat shrinkage for treatment of a posterior cruciate ligament tear. Arthroscopy. 2003 Jul-Aug;19(6):E1-4.
52. Sharma P, Maffulli N. Tendon injury and tendinopathy: healing and repair. J Bone Joint Surg Am. 2005 Jan;87(1):187-202.
53. Martin DE, Severns AE, Kabo JM. Determination of mechanical stiffness of bone by pQCT measurements: correlation with non-destructive mechanical four-point bending test data. J Biomech. 2004 Aug;37(8):1289-93.
54. Kajikawa Y, Morihara T, Sakamoto H, Matsuda K, Oshima Y, Yoshida A, Nagae M, Arai Y, Kawata M, Kubo T. Platelet-rich plasma enhances the initial mobilization of circulation-derived cells for tendon healing. J Cell Physiol. 2008 Jun;215(3):837-45.
55. Lorenz D, Reiman M. The role and implementation of eccentric training in athletic rehabilitation: tendinopathy, hamstring strains, and acl reconstruction. Int J Sports Phys Ther. 2011 Mar;6(1):27-44.
56. Gärdin A, Movin T, Svensson L, Shalabi A. The long-term clinical and MRI results following eccentric calf muscle training in chronic Achilles tendinosis. Skeletal Radiol. 2010 May;39(5):435-42.
57. Kongsgaard M et al. Corticosteroid injections, eccentric decline squat training and heavy slow resistance training in patellar tendinopathy. Scand J Med Sci Sports. 2009 Dec;19(6):790-802.
58. Langberg H, Ellingsgaard H, Madsen T, Jansson J, Magnusson SP, Aagaard P, Kjaer M. Eccentric rehabilitation exercise increases peritendinous type I collagen synthesis in humans with Achilles tendinosis. Scand J Med Sci Sports. 2007 Feb;17(1):61-6.
59. Gumucio JP, Phan AC, Ruehlmann DG, Noah AC, Mendias CL. Synergist ablation induces rapid tendon growth through the synthesis of a neotendon matrix. J Appl Physiol (1985). 2014 Dec 1;117(11):1287-91.
60. Schwartz AJ, Sarver DC, Sugg KB, Dzierzawski JT, Gumucio JP, Mendias CL. p38 MAPK signaling in postnatal tendon growth and remodeling. PLoS One. 2015 Mar 13;10(3):e0120044.
61. Alfredson H, Pietilä T, Jonsson P, Lorentzon R. Heavy-load eccentric calf muscle training for the treatment of chronic Achilles tendinosis. Am J Sports Med. 1998 May-Jun;26(3):360-6.
62. Mazières B, Rouanet S, Velicy J, Scarsi C, Reiner V. Topical ketoprofen patch (100 mg) for the treatment of ankle sprain: a randomized, double-blind, placebo-controlled study. Am J Sports Med. 2005 Apr;33(4):515-23.
63. Petri M, Hufman SL, Waser G, Cui H, Snabes MC, Verburg KM. Celecoxib effectively treats patients with acute shoulder tendinitis/bursitis. J Rheumatol. 2004 Aug;31(8):1614-20.
64. Khan KM, Cook JL, Bonar F, Harcourt P, Astrom M. Histopathology of common tendinopathies. Update and implications for clinical management. Sports Med. 1999 Jun;27(6):393-408.
65. Magra M, Maffulli N. Nonsteroidal antiinflammatory drugs in tendinopathy: friend or foe. Clin J Sport Med. 2006 Jan;16(1):1-3.
66. Heinemeier KM, Øhlenschlæger TF, Mikkelsen UR, Sønder F, Schjerling P, Svensson RB, Kjaer M. Effects of anti-inflammatory (NSAID) treatment on human tendinopathic tissue. J Appl Physiol (1985). 2017 Nov 1;123(5):1397-1405.
67. Fredriksson M, Li Y, Stålman A, Haldosén LA, Felländer-Tsai L. Diclofenac and triamcinolone acetonide impair tenocytic differentiation and promote adipocytic differentiation of mesenchymal stem cells. J Orthop Surg Res. 2013 Sep 2;8:30.
68. Zhang Y, Wang X, Qiu Y, Cornish J, Carr AJ, Xia Z. Effect of indomethacin and lactoferrin on human tenocyte proliferation and collagen formation in vitro. Biochem Biophys Res Commun. 2014 Nov 14;454(2):301-7.
69. Smidt N, van der Windt DA, Assendelft WJ, Devillé WL, Korthals-de Bos IB, Bouter LM. Corticosteroid injections, physiotherapy, or a wait-and-see policy for lateral epicondylitis: a randomised controlled trial. Lancet. 2002 Feb 23;359(9307):657-62.
70. Tonks JH, Pai SK, Murali SR. Steroid injection therapy is the best conservative treatment for lateral epicondylitis: a prospective randomized controlled trial. Int J Clin Pract. 2007 Feb;61(2):240-6.
71. Smidt N, Assendelft WJ, van der Windt DA, Hay EM, Buchbinder R, Bouter LM. Corticosteroid injections for lateral epicondylitis: a systematic review. Pain. 2002 Mar;96(1-2):23-40.
72. Kearney RS, Parsons N, Metcalfe D, Costa ML. Injection therapies for Achilles tendinopathy. Cochrane Database Syst Rev. 2015 May 26;(5):CD010960.
73. Andres BM, Murrell GA. Treatment of tendinopathy: what works, what does not, and what is on the horizon. Clin Orthop Relat Res. 2008 Jul;466(7):1539-54.
74. Murrell GA et al. Modulation of tendon healing by nitric oxide. Inflamm Res. 1997 Jan;46(1):19-27.
75. Berrazueta JR, Losada A, Poveda J, Ochoteco A, Riestra A, Salas E, Amado JA. Successful treatment of shoulder pain syndrome due to supraspinatus tendinitis with transdermal nitroglycerin. A double blind study. Pain. 1996 Jul;66(1):63-7.
76. Paoloni JA, Murrell GA, Burch RM, Ang RY. Randomised, double-blind, placebo-controlled clinical trial of a new topical glyceryl trinitrate patch for chronic lateral epicondylosis. Br J Sports Med. 2009 Apr;43(4):299-302.
77. Gambito ED, Gonzalez-Suarez CB, Oquiñena TI, Agbayani RB. Evidence on the effectiveness of topical nitroglycerin in the treatment of tendinopathies: a systematic review and meta-analysis. Arch Phys Med Rehabil. 2010

Aug;91(8):1291-305.
78. Garrick JG. Topical nitroglycerin decreases pain intensity in daily activities: a review. Clin J Sport Med. 2011 Nov;21(6):539-40.
79. Paoloni JA, Murrell GA. Three-year followup study of topical glyceryl trinitrate treatment of chronic noninsertional Achilles tendinopathy. Foot Ankle Int. 2007 Oct;28(10):1064-8.
80. Distel LM, Best TM. Prolotherapy: a clinical review of its role in treating chronic musculoskeletal pain. PM R. 2011 Jun;3(6 Suppl 1):S78-81.
81. Ryan M, Wong A, Taunton J. Favorable outcomes after sonographically guided intratendinous injection of hyperosmolar dextrose for chronic insertional and midportion achilles tendinosis. AJR Am J Roentgenol. 2010 Apr;194(4):1047-53.
82. Scarpone M, Rabago DP, Zgierska A, Arbogast G, Snell E. The efficacy of prolotherapy for lateral epicondylosis: a pilot study. Clin J Sport Med. 2008 May;18(3):248-54.
83. Hudgens JL, Sugg KB, Grekin JA, Gumucio JP, Bedi A, Mendias CL. Platelet-Rich Plasma Activates Proinflammatory Signaling Pathways and Induces Oxidative Stress in Tendon Fibroblasts. Am J Sports Med. 2016 Aug;44(8):1931-40.
84. de Vos RJ, van Veldhoven PL, Moen MH, Weir A, Tol JL, Maffulli N. Autologous growth factor injections in chronic tendinopathy: a systematic review. Br Med Bull. 2010;95:63-77.
85. Peerbooms JC, Sluimer J, Bruijn DJ, Gosens T. Positive effect of an autologous platelet concentrate in lateral epicondylitis in a double-blind randomized controlled trial: platelet-rich plasma versus corticosteroid injection with a 1-year follow-up. Am J Sports Med. 2010 Feb;38(2):255-62.
86. Thanasas C, Papadimitriou G, Charalambidis C, Paraskevopoulos I, Papanikolaou A. Platelet-rich plasma versus autologous whole blood for the treatment of chronic lateral elbow epicondylitis: a randomized controlled clinical trial. Am J Sports Med. 2011 Oct;39(10):2130-4.
87. Tsikopoulos K et al. The clinical impact of platelet-rich plasma on tendinopathy compared to placebo or dry needling injections: A meta-analysis. Phys Ther Sport. 2016 Jan;17:87-94.
88. Kaux JF, Samson A, Crielaard JM. Hyaluronic acid and tendon lesions. Muscles Ligaments Tendons J. 2016 Feb 13;5(4):264-9.
89. Zhang W et al. EULAR evidence-based recommendations for the diagnosis of knee osteoarthritis. Ann Rheum Dis. 2010 Mar;69(3):483-9.
90. Salti NI, Tuel RJ, Mass DP. Effect of hyaluronic acid on rabbit profundus flexor tendon healing in vitro. J Surg Res. 1993 Oct;55(4):411-5.
91. Akasaka T, Nishida J, Imaeda T, Shimamura T, Amadio PC, An KN. Effect of hyaluronic acid on the excursion resistance of tendon graft: a biomechanical in vitro study in a modified human model. Clin Biomech (Bristol, Avon). 2006 Oct;21(8):810-5.
92. Taguchi M, Zhao C, Sun YL, Jay GD, An KN, Amadio PC. The effect of surface treatment using hyaluronic acid and lubricin on the gliding resistance of human extrasynovial tendons in vitro. J Hand Surg Am. 2009 Sep;34(7):1276-81.
93. Neumann A, Schinzel R, Palm D, Riederer P, Münch G. High molecular weight hyaluronic acid inhibits advanced glycation endproduct-induced NF-kappaB activation and cytokine expression. FEBS Lett. 1999 Jun 25;453(3):283-7.
94. Moreland LW. Intra-articular hyaluronan (hyaluronic acid) and hylans for the treatment of osteoarthritis: mechanisms of action. Arthritis Res Ther. 2003;5(2):54-67.
95. Meloni F, Milia F, Cavazzuti M, Doria C, Lisai P, Profili S, Meloni GB. Clinical evaluation of sodium hyaluronate in the treatment of patients with sopraspinatus tendinosis under echographic guide: experimental study of periarticular injections. Eur J Radiol. 2008 Oct;68(1):170-3.
96. Muneta T, Koga H, Ju YJ, Mochizuki T, Sekiya I. Hyaluronan injection therapy for athletic patients with patellar tendinopathy. J Orthop Sci. 2012 Jul;17(4):425-31.
97. Maffulli N, Testa V, Capasso G, Bifulco G, Binfield PM. Results of percutaneous longitudinal tenotomy for Achilles tendinopathy in middle- and long-distance runners. Am J Sports Med. 1997 Nov-Dec;25(6):835-40.
98. Koh JS, Mohan PC, Howe TS, Lee BP, Chia SL, Yang Z, Morrey BF. Fasciotomy and surgical tenotomy for recalcitrant lateral elbow tendinopathy: early clinical experience with a novel device for minimally invasive percutaneous microresection. Am J Sports Med. 2013 Mar;41(3):636-44.
99. Seng C, Mohan PC, Koh SB, Howe TS, Lim YG, Lee BP, Morrey BF. Ultrasonic Percutaneous Tenotomy for Recalcitrant Lateral Elbow Tendinopathy: Sustainability and Sonographic Progression at 3 Years. Am J Sports Med. 2016 Feb;44(2):504-10.
100. Wertheimer SJ, Weber CA, Loder BG, Calderone DR, Frascone ST. The role of endoscopy in treatment of stenosing posterior tibial tenosynovitis. J Foot Ankle Surg. 1995 Jan-Feb;34(1):15-22.
101. Van Dijk CN, Sholten PE, Kort N. Tendoscopy (tendon sheath endoscopy) for overuse tendon injuries. Oper Tech Sports Med 1997;5:170-178.
102. Steenstra F, van Dijk CN. Achilles tendoscopy. Foot Ankle Clin. 2006 Jun;11(2):429-38, viii.
103. Lui TH. Treatment of chronic noninsertional Achilles tendinopathy with endoscopic Achilles tendon debridement and flexor hallucis longus transfer. Foot Ankle Spec. 2012 Jun;5(3):195-200.
104. Carreira D, Ballard A. Achilles tendoscopy. Foot Ankle Clin. 2015 Mar;20(1):27-40.
105. Cychosz CC, Phisitkul P, Barg A, Nickisch F, van Dijk CN, Glazebrook MA. Foot and ankle tendoscopy: evidence-based recommendations. Arthroscopy. 2014 Jun;30(6):755-65.
106. Lian OB, Engebretsen L, Bahr R. Prevalence of jumper's knee among elite athletes from different sports: a cross-sectional study. Am J Sports Med. 2005 Apr;33(4):561-7.
107. Gisslén K, Alfredson H. Neovascularisation and pain in jumper's knee: a prospective clinical and sonographic study in elite junior volleyball players. Br J Sports Med. 2005 Jul;39(7):423-8; discussion 423-8.
108. Cook JL, Khan KM, Kiss ZS, Griffiths L. Patellar tendinopathy in junior basketball players: a controlled clinical and ultrasonographic study of 268 patellar tendons in players aged 14-18 years. Scand J Med Sci Sports. 2000 Aug;10(4):216-20.
109. Fredberg U, Bolvig L. Significance of ultrasonographically detected asymptomatic tendinosis in the patellar and achilles tendons of elite soccer players: a longitudinal study. Am J Sports Med. 2002 Jul-Aug;30(4):488-91.
110. Hägglund M, Zwerver J, Ekstrand J. Epidemiology of patellar tendinopathy in elite male soccer players. Am J Sports Med. 2011 Sep;39(9):1906-11.
111. Pfirrmann D, Herbst M, Ingelfinger P, Simon P, Tug S. Analysis of Injury Incidences in Male Professional Adult and Elite Youth Soccer Players: A Systematic Review. J Athl Train. 2016 May;51(5):410-24.
112. Bode G et al. Patellar tendinopathy in young elite soccer-clinical and sonographical analysis of a German elite soccer academy. BMC Musculoskelet Disord. 2017 Aug 8;18(1):344.
113. Crossley KM, Thancanamootoo K, Metcalf BR, Cook JL, Purdam CR, Warden SJ. Clinical features of patellar tendinopathy and their implications for rehabilitation. J Orthop

Res. 2007 Sep;25(9):1164-75.
114. Lian Ø, Refsnes PE, Engebretsen L, Bahr R. Performance characteristics of volleyball players with patellar tendinopathy. Am J Sports Med. 2003 May-Jun;31(3):408-13.
115. Malliaras P, Cook JL, Kent PM. Anthropometric risk factors for patellar tendon injury among volleyball players. Br J Sports Med. 2007 Apr;41(4):259-63; discussion 263.
116. Malliaras P, Cook JL, Kent P. Reduced ankle dorsiflexion range may increase the risk of patellar tendon injury among volleyball players. J Sci Med Sport. 2006 Aug;9(4):304-9.
117. Witvrouw E, Bellemans J, Lysens R, Danneels L, Cambier D. Intrinsic risk factors for the development of patellar tendinitis in an athletic population. A two-year prospective study. Am J Sports Med. 2001 Mar-Apr;29(2):190-5.
118. van der Worp H, van Ark M, Roerink S, Pepping GJ, van den Akker-Scheek I, Zwerver J. Risk factors for patellar tendinopathy: a systematic review of the literature. Br J Sports Med. 2011 Apr;45(5):446-52.
119. Fu SC, Wang W, Pau HM, Wong YP, Chan KM, Rolf CG. Increased expression of transforming growth factor-beta1 in patellar tendinosis. Clin Orthop Relat Res. 2002 Jul;(400):174-83.
120. Stasinopoulos D, Stasinopoulos I. Comparison of effects of exercise programme, pulsed ultrasound and transverse friction in the treatment of chronic patellar tendinopathy. Clin Rehabil. 2004 Jun;18(4):347-52.
121. Fouré A, Nordez A, McNair P, Cornu C. Effects of plyometric training on both active and passive parts of the plantarflexors series elastic component stiffness of muscle-tendon complex. Eur J Appl Physiol. 2011 Mar;111(3):539-48.
122. Kongsgaard M, Nielsen CH, Hegnsvad S, Aagaard P, Magnusson SP. Mechanical properties of the human Achilles tendon, in vivo. Clin Biomech (Bristol, Avon). 2011 Aug;26(7):772-7.
123. Cristi-Sánchez I, Danes-Daetz C, Neira A, Ferrada W, Yáñez Díaz R, Silvestre Aguirre R. Patellar and Achilles Tendon Stiffness in Elite Soccer Players Assessed Using Myotonometric Measurements. Sports Health. 2019 Mar/Apr;11(2):157-162.
124. Bohm S, Mersmann F, Arampatzis A. Human tendon adaptation in response to mechanical loading: a systematic review and meta-analysis of exercise intervention studies on healthy adults. Sports Med Open. 2015 Dec;1(1):7.
125. Wiesinger HP, Kösters A, Müller E, Seynnes OR. Effects of Increased Loading on In Vivo Tendon Properties: A Systematic Review. Med Sci Sports Exerc. 2015 Sep;47(9):1885-95.
126. Figueroa D, Figueroa F, Calvo R. Patellar Tendinopathy: Diagnosis and Treatment. J Am Acad Orthop Surg. 2016 Dec;24(12):e184-e192.
127. Raschke D, Schüttrumpf JP, Tezval M, Stürmer KM, Balcarek P. Extensor-mechanism-reconstruction of the knee joint after traumatic loss of the entire extensor apparatus. Knee. 2014 Jun;21(3):793-6.
128. Saragaglia D, Pison A, Rubens-Duval B. Acute and old ruptures of the extensor apparatus of the knee in adults (excluding knee replacement). Orthop Traumatol Surg Res. 2013 Feb;99(1 Suppl):S67-76.
129. Zernicke RF, Garhammer J, Jobe FW. Human patellar-tendon rupture. J Bone Joint Surg Am. 1977 Mar;59(2):179-83.
130. Kelly DW, Carter VS, Jobe FW, Kerlan RK. Patellar and quadriceps tendon ruptures--jumper's knee. Am J Sports Med. 1984 Sep-Oct;12(5):375-80.
131. Rosso F, Bonasia DE, Cottino U, Dettoni F, Bruzzone M, Rossi R. Patellar tendon: From tendinopathy to rupture. Asia Pac J Sports Med Arthrosc Rehabil Technol. 2015 Aug 7;2(4):99-107.
132. Lee D, Stinner D, Mir H. Quadriceps and patellar tendon ruptures. J Knee Surg. 2013 Oct;26(5):301-8.
133. Hsu KY, Wang KC, Ho WP, Hsu RW. Traumatic patellar tendon ruptures: a follow-up study of primary repair and a neutralization wire. J Trauma. 1994 May;36(5):658-60.
134. Giles SN, Morgan-Jones R, Brown MF. The use of hinged Kirschner wires for fixation of patellar tendon rupture. Injury. 1999 Oct;30(8):539-40.
135. Kasten P, Schewe B, Maurer F, Gösling T, Krettek C, Weise K. Rupture of the patellar tendon: a review of 68 cases and a retrospective study of 29 ruptures comparing two methods of augmentation. Arch Orthop Trauma Surg. 2001 Nov;121(10):578-82.
136. Marder RA, Timmerman LA. Primary repair of patellar tendon rupture without augmentation. Am J Sports Med. 1999 May-Jun;27(3):304-7.
137. Muramatsu T, Muraoka T, Takeshita D, Kawakami Y, Hirano Y, Fukunaga T. Mechanical properties of tendon and aponeurosis of human gastrocnemius muscle in vivo. J Appl Physiol (1985). 2001 May;90(5):1671-8.
138. Komi PV, Fukashiro S, Järvinen M. Biomechanical loading of Achilles tendon during normal locomotion. Clin Sports Med. 1992 Jul;11(3):521-31.
139. Kujala UM, Sarna S, Kaprio J. Cumulative incidence of achilles tendon rupture and tendinopathy in male former elite athletes. Clin J Sport Med. 2005 May;15(3):133-5.
140. Chimenti RL, Cychosz CC, Hall MM, Phisitkul P. Current Concepts Review Update: Insertional Achilles Tendinopathy. Foot Ankle Int. 2017 Oct;38(10):1160-1169.
141. Longo UG, Ramamurthy C, Denaro V, Maffulli N. Minimally invasive stripping for chronic Achilles tendinopathy. Disabil Rehabil. 2008;30(20-22):1709-13.
142. Almekinders LC, Temple JD. Etiology, diagnosis, and treatment of tendonitis: an analysis of the literature. Med Sci Sports Exerc. 1998 Aug;30(8):1183-90.
143. Maffulli N, Kader D. Tendinopathy of tendo achillis. J Bone Joint Surg Br. 2002 Jan;84(1):1-8.
144. Alfredson H, Lorentzon R. Chronic Achilles tendinosis: recommendations for treatment and prevention. Sports Med. 2000 Feb;29(2):135-46.
145. Maffulli N, Walley G, Sayana MK, Longo UG, Denaro V. Eccentric calf muscle training in athletic patients with Achilles tendinopathy. Disabil Rehabil. 2008;30(20-22):1677-84.
146. Fredberg U, Bolvig L, Andersen NT. Prophylactic training in asymptomatic soccer players with ultrasonographic abnormalities in Achilles and patellar tendons: the Danish Super League Study. Am J Sports Med. 2008 Mar;36(3):451-60.
147. Sankey RA, Brooks JH, Kemp SP, Haddad FS. The epidemiology of ankle injuries in professional rugby union players. Am J Sports Med. 2008 Dec;36(12):2415-24.
148. Maffulli N, Wong J, Almekinders LC. Types and epidemiology of tendinopathy. Clin Sports Med. 2003 Oct;22(4):675-92.
149. Gajhede-Knudsen M, Ekstrand J, Magnusson H, Maffulli N. Recurrence of Achilles tendon injuries in elite male football players is more common after early return to play: an 11-year follow-up of the UEFA Champions League injury study. Br J Sports Med. 2013 Aug;47(12):763-8.
150. Järvinen TA, Kannus P, Maffulli N, Khan KM. Achilles tendon disorders: etiology and epidemiology. Foot Ankle Clin. 2005 Jun;10(2):255-66.
151. Singh A, Calafi A, Diefenbach C, Kreulen C, Giza E. Noninsertional Tendinopathy of the Achilles. Foot Ankle Clin. 2017 Dec;22(4):745-760.
152. Maffulli N, Via AG, Oliva F. Chronic Achilles Tendon Disorders: Tendinopathy and Chronic Rupture. Clin Sports

Med. 2015 Oct;34(4):607-24.
153. Clement DB, Taunton JE, Smart GW. Achilles tendinitis and peritendinitis: etiology and treatment. Am J Sports Med. 1984 May-Jun;12(3):179-84.
154. Kvist M. Achilles tendon injuries in athletes. Sports Med. 1994 Sep;18(3):173-201.
155. Nigg BM. The role of impact forces and foot pronation: a new paradigm. Clin J Sport Med. 2001 Jan;11(1):2-9.
156. Kannus P. Etiology and pathophysiology of chronic tendon disorders in sports. Scand J Med Sci Sports. 1997 Apr;7(2):78-85.
157. Kirchgesner T, Larbi A, Omoumi P, Malghem J, Zamali N, Manelfe J, Lecouvet F, Vande Berg B, Djebbar S, Dallaudière B. Drug-induced tendinopathy: from physiology to clinical applications. Joint Bone Spine. 2014 Dec;81(6):485-92.
158. Maffulli N, Oliva F, Loppini M, Aicale R, Spiezia F, King JB. The Royal London Hospital Test for the clinical diagnosis of patellar tendinopathy. Muscles Ligaments Tendons J. 2017 Sep 18;7(2):315-322.
159. Barnes SJ, Gey van Pettius D, Maffulli N. Angioleiomyoma of the Achilles tendon. Bull Hosp Jt Dis. 2003;61(3-4):137-9.
160. Maffulli N, Kenward MG, Testa V, Capasso G, Regine R, King JB. Clinical diagnosis of Achilles tendinopathy with tendinosis. Clin J Sport Med. 2003 Jan;13(1):11-5.
161. Kader D, Saxena A, Movin T, Maffulli N. Achilles tendinopathy: some aspects of basic science and clinical management. Br J Sports Med. 2002 Aug;36(4):239-49.
162. de Jonge S, van den Berg C, de Vos RJ, van der Heide HJ, Weir A, Verhaar JA, Bierma-Zeinstra SM, Tol JL. Incidence of midportion Achilles tendinopathy in the general population. Br J Sports Med. 2011 Oct;45(13):1026-8.
163. Maffulli N, Giai Via A, Oliva F.Minimally invasive stripping for chronic achilles tendinopathy in Minimally Invasive Surgery in Orthopedics, 2016.
164. Doral MN, Alam M, Bozkurt M, Turhan E, Atay OA, Dönmez G, Maffulli N. Functional anatomy of the Achilles tendon. Knee Surg Sports Traumatol Arthrosc. 2010 May;18(5):638-43.
165. Kernozek T, Gheidi N, Ragan R. Comparison of estimates of Achilles tendon loading from inverse dynamics and inverse dynamics-based static optimization during running. J Sports Sci. 2017 Nov;35(21):2073-2079.
166. Malagelada F, Clark C, Dega R. Management of chronic Achilles tendon ruptures-A review. Foot (Edinb). 2016 Aug;28:54-60.
167. Leppilahti J, Orava S. Total Achilles tendon rupture. A review. Sports Med. 1998 Feb;25(2):79-100.
168. Raikin SM, Garras DN, Krapchev PV. Achilles tendon injuries in a United States population. Foot Ankle Int. 2013 Apr;34(4):475-80.
169. Parekh SG, Wray WH 3rd, Brimmo O, Sennett BJ, Wapner KL. Epidemiology and outcomes of Achilles tendon ruptures in the National Football League. Foot Ankle Spec. 2009 Dec;2(6):283-6.
170. Maffulli N, Ajis A, Longo UG, Denaro V. Chronic rupture of tendo Achillis. Foot Ankle Clin. 2007 Dec;12(4):583-96, vi.
171. Singh D. Acute Achilles tendon rupture. Br J Sports Med. 2017 Aug;51(15):1158-1160.
172. Hopkins JN, Brown W, Lee CA. Sports Hernia: Definition, Evaluation, and Treatment. JBJS Rev. 2017 Sep;5(9):e6.
173. Rossidis G, Perry A, Abbas H, Motamarry I, Lux T, Farmer K, Moser M, Clugston J, Caban A, Ben-David K. Laparoscopic hernia repair with adductor tenotomy for athletic pubalgia: an established procedure for an obscure entity. Surg Endosc. 2015 Feb;29(2):381-6.
174. Garvey JF, Hazard H. Sports hernia or groin disruption injury? Chronic athletic groin pain: a retrospective study of 100 patients with long-term follow-up. Hernia. 2014;18(6):815-23.
175. Sheen AJ et al. 'Treatment of the sportsman's groin': British Hernia Society's 2014 position statement based on the Manchester Consensus Conference. Br J Sports Med. 2014 Jul;48(14):1079-87.
176. Paajanen H, Ristolainen L, Turunen H, Kujala UM. Prevalence and etiological factors of sport-related groin injuries in top-level soccer compared to non-contact sports. Arch Orthop Trauma Surg. 2011 Feb;131(2):261-6.
177. Nielsen AB, Yde J. Epidemiology and traumatology of injuries in soccer. Am J Sports Med. 1989 Nov-Dec;17(6):803-7.
178. Soligard T, Myklebust G, Steffen K, Holme I, Silvers H, Bizzini M, Junge A, Dvorak J, Bahr R, Andersen TE. Comprehensive warm-up programme to prevent injuries in young female footballers: cluster randomised controlled trial. BMJ. 2008 Dec 9;337:a2469.
179. Gilmore J. Groin pain in the soccer athlete: fact, fiction, and treatment.
Clin Sports Med. 1998 Oct;17(4):787-93, vii.
180. Rambani R, Hackney R. Loss of range of motion of the hip joint: a hypothesis for etiology of sports hernia. Muscles Ligaments Tendons J. 2015 Mar 27;5(1):29-32.
181. Strosberg DS, Ellis TJ, Renton DB. The Role of Femoroacetabular Impingement in Core Muscle Injury/Athletic Pubalgia: Diagnosis and Management. Front Surg. 2016 Feb 12;3:6.
182. Farber AJ, Wilckens JH. Sports hernia: diagnosis and therapeutic approach. J Am Acad Orthop Surg. 2007 Aug;15(8):507-14.
183. Larson CM, Pierce BR, Giveans MR. Treatment of athletes with symptomatic intra-articular hip pathology and athletic pubalgia/sports hernia: a case series. Arthroscopy. 2011 Jun;27(6):768-75.
184. Comin J, Obaid H, Lammers G, Moore J, Wotherspoon M, Connell D. Radiofrequency denervation of the inguinal ligament for the treatment of 'Sportsman's Hernia': a pilot study. Br J Sports Med. 2013 Apr;47(6):380-6.
185. Larson CM. Sports hernia/athletic pubalgia: evaluation and management. Sports Health. 2014 Mar;6(2):139-44.
186. Omar IM, Zoga AC, Kavanagh EC, Koulouris G, Bergin D, Gopez AG, Morrison WB, Meyers WC. Athletic pubalgia and "sports hernia": optimal MR imaging technique and findings. Radiographics. 2008 Sep-Oct;28(5):1415-38.
187. Suarez JC, Ely EE, Mutnal AB, Figueroa NM, Klika AK, Patel PD, Barsoum WK. Comprehensive approach to the evaluation of groin pain. J Am Acad Orthop Surg. 2013 Sep;21(9):558-70.
188. Hölmich P. Long-standing groin pain in sportspeople falls into three primary patterns, a "clinical entity" approach: a prospective study of 207 patients. Br J Sports Med. 2007 Apr;41(4):247-52.
189. Mullens FE, Zoga AC, Morrison WB, Meyers WC. Review of MRI technique and imaging findings in athletic pubalgia and the "sports hernia". Eur J Radiol. 2012 Dec;81(12):3780-92.
190. Kuikka L, Hermunen H, Paajanen H. Effect of pubic bone marrow edema on recovery from endoscopic surgery for athletic pubalgia. Scand J Med Sci Sports. 2015 Feb;25(1):98-103.
191. Becker LC, Kohlrieser DA. Conservative management of sports hernia in a professional golfer: a case report. Int J

Sports Phys Ther. 2014 Nov;9(6):851-60.
192. Paajanen H, Brinck T, Hermunen H, Airo I. Laparoscopic surgery for chronic groin pain in athletes is more effective than nonoperative treatment: a randomized clinical trial with magnetic resonance imaging of 60 patients with sportsman's hernia (athletic pubalgia). Surgery. 2011 Jul;150(1):99-107.
193. Jakoi A, O'Neill C, Damsgaard C, Fehring K, Tom J. Sports hernia in National Hockey League players: does surgery affect performance? Am J Sports Med. 2013 Jan;41(1):107-10.
194. Giza E, Fuller C, Junge A, Dvorak J. Mechanisms of foot and ankle injuries in soccer. Am J Sports Med. 2003 Jul-Aug;31(4):550-4.
195. Woods C, Hawkins R, Hulse M, Hodson A. The Football Association Medical Research Programme: an audit of injuries in professional football: an analysis of ankle sprains. Br J Sports Med. 2003 Jun;37(3):233-8.
196. Oztekin HH, Boya H, Ozcan O, Zeren B, Pinar P. Foot and ankle injuries and time lost from play in professional soccer players. Foot (Edinb). 2009 Mar;19(1):22-8.
197. Fong DT, Hong Y, Chan LK, Yung PS, Chan KM. A systematic review on ankle injury and ankle sprain in sports. Sports Med. 2007;37(1):73-94.
198. Dombek MF, Lamm BM, Saltrick K, Mendicino RW, Catanzariti AR. Peroneal tendon tears: a retrospective review. J Foot Ankle Surg. 2003 Sep-Oct;42(5):250-8.
199. Bruce WD, Christofersen MR, Phillips DL. Stenosing tenosynovitis and impingement of the peroneal tendons associated with hypertrophy of the peroneal tubercle. Foot Ankle Int. 1999 Jul;20(7):464-7.
200. Brandes CB, Smith RW. Characterization of patients with primary peroneus longus tendinopathy: a review of twenty-two cases. Foot Ankle Int. 2000 Jun;21(6):462-8.
201. Sobel M, Geppert MJ, Hannafin JA, Bohne WH, Arnoczky SP. Microvascular anatomy of the peroneal tendons. Foot Ankle. 1992 Oct;13(8):469-72.
202. Oden RR. Tendon injuries about the ankle resulting from skiing. Clin Orthop Relat Res. 1987 Mar;(216):63-9.
203. Ogawa BK, Thordarson DB, Zalavras C. Peroneal tendon subluxation repair with an indirect fibular groove deepening technique. Foot Ankle Int. 2007 Nov;28(11):1194-7.
204. Kijowski R, De Smet A, Mukharjee R. Magnetic resonance imaging findings in patients with peroneal tendinopathy and peroneal tenosynovitis. Skeletal Radiol. 2007 Feb;36(2):105-14.
205. O'Neil JT, Pedowitz DI, Kerbel YE, Codding JL, Zoga AC, Raikin SM. Peroneal Tendon Abnormalities on Routine Magnetic Resonance Imaging of the Foot and Ankle. Foot Ankle Int. 2016 Jul;37(7):743-7.
206. Ogawa BK, Thordarson DB. Current concepts review: peroneal tendon subluxation and dislocation. Foot Ankle Int. 2007 Sep;28(9):1034-40.
207. Redfern D, Myerson M. The management of concomitant tears of the peroneus longus and brevis tendons. Foot Ankle Int. 2004 Oct;25(10):695-707.
208. Jennings AG, Sefton GK. Dislocation of the peroneal tendons: A new operative treatment. Foot. 2000;10:78–80.
209. Smyth NA, Aiyer AA, Kaplan JR, Carmody CA, Kadakia AR. Adult-acquired flatfoot deformity. Eur J Orthop Surg Traumatol. 2017 May;27(4):433-439.
210. Richie DH Jr. Biomechanics and clinical analysis of the adult acquired flatfoot. Clin Podiatr Med Surg. 2007 Oct;24(4):617-44, vii.
211. Gluck GS, Heckman DS, Parekh SG. Tendon disorders of the foot and ankle, part 3: the posterior tibial tendon. Am J Sports Med. 2010 Oct;38(10):2133-44.
212. Lee MS, Vanore JV, Thomas JL, Catanzariti AR, Kogler G, Kravitz SR, Miller SJ, Gassen SC. Clinical Practice Guideline Adult Flatfoot Panel. Diagnosis and treatment of adult flatfoot. J Foot Ankle Surg. 2005 Mar-Apr;44(2):78-113.
213. Nielsen MD, Dodson EE, Shadrick DL, Catanzariti AR, Mendicino RW, Malay DS. Nonoperative care for the treatment of adult-acquired flatfoot deformity. J Foot Ankle Surg. 2011 May-Jun;50(3):311-4.
214. Rabbito M, Pohl MB, Humble N, Ferber R. Biomechanical and clinical factors related to stage I posterior tibial tendon dysfunction. J Orthop Sports Phys Ther. 2011 Oct;41(10):776-84.
215. Mosier-LaClair S, Pomeroy G, Manoli A 2nd. Operative treatment of the difficult stage 2 adult acquired flatfoot deformity. Foot Ankle Clin. 2001 Mar;6(1):95-119.
216. Wang D, SooHoo NF. Posterior tibiali tendon dysfunction. In: Foot and ankle disorders: an illustrated reference. Springer 2016. pp. 335-70.
217. Bluman EM, Myerson MS. Stage IV posterior tibial tendon rupture. Foot Ankle Clin. 2007 Jun;12(2):341-62, viii.
218. Grundy JR, O'Sullivan RM, Beischer AD. Operative management of distal tibialis anterior tendinopathy. Foot Ankle Int. 2010 Mar;31(3):212-9.
219. Beischer AD, Beamond BM, Jowett AJ, O'Sullivan R. Distal tendinosis of the tibialis anterior tendon. Foot Ankle Int. 2009 Nov;30(11):1053-9.
220. Taras J, Valentine B. Tenosynovitis. Current Orthopaedic Practice 2010. 21. 609-614.
221. Rees JD, Maffulli N, Cook J. Management of tendinopathy. Am J Sports Med. 2009 Sep;37(9):1855-67.
222. Markarian GG, Kelikian AS, Brage M, Trainor T, Dias L. Anterior tibialis tendon ruptures: an outcome analysis of operative versus nonoperative treatment. Foot Ankle Int. 1998 Dec;19(12):792-802.
223. Harkin E, Pinzur M, Schiff A. Treatment of Acute and Chronic Tibialis Anterior Tendon Rupture and Tendinopathy. Foot Ankle Clin. 2017 Dec;22(4):819-831.
224. van Acker G, Pingen F, Luitse J, Goslings C. Rupture of the tibialis anterior tendon. Acta Orthop Belg. 2006 Jan;72(1):105-7.
225. Anagnostakos K, Bachelier F, Fürst OA, Kelm J. Rupture of the anterior tibial tendon: three clinical cases, anatomical study, and literature review. Foot Ankle Int. 2006 May;27(5):330-9.

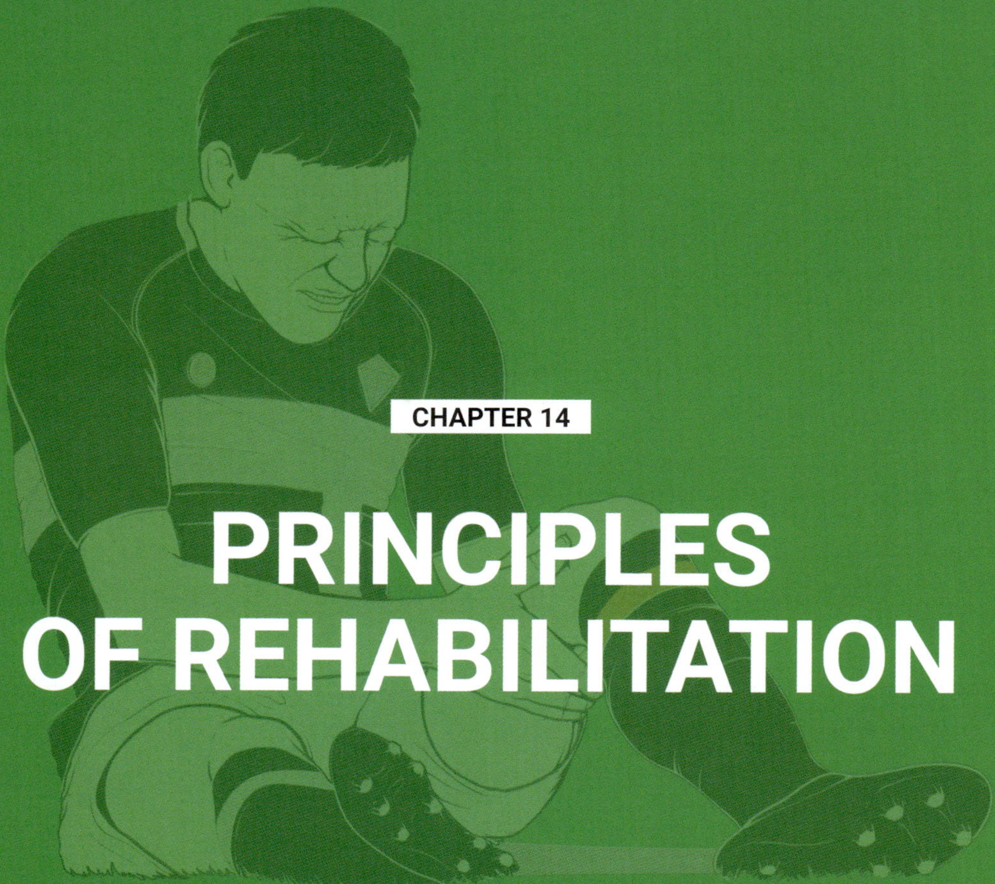

CHAPTER 14

PRINCIPLES OF REHABILITATION

Stefano Della Villa
Margherita Ricci
Matthew Buckthorpe
Francesco Della Villa

Education and Research Department
Isokinetic Medical Group, Bologna, Italy
FIFA Medical Centre of Excellence

Introduction

Soccer is the most commonly played sport in the world with more than 300 million players [1]. Unfortunately, soccer is also a complex contact sport, with substantial injury risk for professional players, but even higher risk for recreational players. Data from large prospective studies indicate that lower limb injuries are the most frequent problems, with muscles and joints (especially ankle and knee injuries) being the cause of most time loss [2] (fig. 1).

As such, the sport medicine community faces a large proportion of injured players each year. For example, a team of 25 male soccer players can expect up to fifteen muscles injuries every season [3], whilst a team of 25 female soccer players can expect to sustain up to two anterior cruciate ligament (ACL) injuries each season: female soccer players are in fact two to three times at higher risk to sustain an ACL injury.

A history of previous injury is the strongest risk factor for future injury [4]. Therefore, optimal functional recovery from primary injuries is a key aspect of injury prevention in soccer. It is essential to take soccer injuries seriously, as severe or repeated injuries can be detrimental for both the player's career and health. For example, athletes who sustain an ACL injury typically experience a reduction in career length [5] as well as a high rate of post traumatic knee osteoarthritis [6]. As such, the treatment of soccer-related musculoskeletal injuries is of paramount importance to maximize not only short-term goals, such as fast and safe return to play (RTP), but also long-lasting sports participation and long-term health.

Most injuries in soccer are non-surgical and/or conservatively treated and, even if surgical, many of the concepts utilised in the functional recovery process are similar to those used post-operatively. Although each individual injury is different, with its own specifics, most principles of rehabilitation are generalisable to all injuries. Thus, a thorough understanding of rehabilitation principles is essential and can maximize the medical care for all injury types.

The goal of this chapter is to explain the key aspects (principles) of rehabilitation following soccer injuries, both organizational and clinical aspects, which can be applied to soccer players to optimise outcomes following soccer injury. These principles can be translated in the day by day practice and virtually applied to all injuries to maximize the clinical approach to injured soccer players.

The milestones: overview of the principles

In order to give a logical progression to the chapter, in this section we will treat the milestones in delivering an optimal sport medicine and orthopedic rehabilitation service to the soccer player. In this chapter, soccer is considered as an example that can be easily translated also to other team sports or individual activity.

First, we must start from a clinical perspective. In general terms, rehabilitation should be personalized, progressive and supervised.

- Personalized: optimal rehabilitation should consider the needs of the individual patient, their baseline features (e.g. activity level), injury type, localization, and severity (e.g. structural hamstring injuries grade 3A) and of course their responses to injury (e.g. also emotive and psychological).
- Progressive: each rehabilitation process should

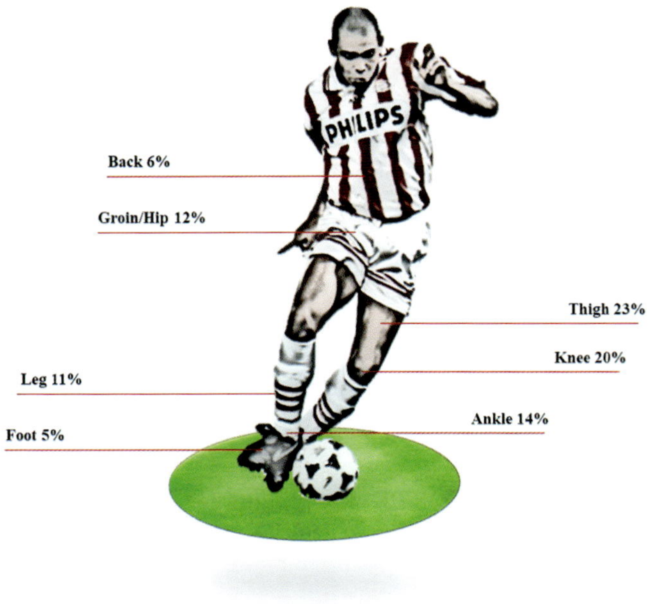

Figure 1 - Injury distribution according to anatomical regions in male and female soccer players. Lower limb injuries accounted for the clear majority of soccer injuries, with thigh, knee and ankle injuries being the most frequently injured districts

be based on the principle of specific adaptations to imposed demands. The increase in rehabilitation loads should be gradual (fig. 2B), respectful of Scott Dye's theory of the "Envelope of function" (fig. 2A) and based on specific criteria. Both overload and underload should be avoided to give the correct stimuli to the healing tissues (fig. 2A). The envelope of function theory was firstly introduced for knee related problems, but it can be considered as a logical general rule.

• Supervised: there is no doubt that the gold standard in the care of the injured athlete or soccer player should lie in an updated evidence-based practice delivered by a specialized team of care givers. We will explain better this concept in the subsequent paragraphs.

Given that the ultimate goal of rehabilitation is the optimal recovery from soccer injuries, we generally focus on both organizational and clinical pitfalls. By an organizational point of view, three main aspects should be highlighted in the delivery of high-quality soccer rehabilitation:

1. proper team;
2. proper facilities;
3. proper method.

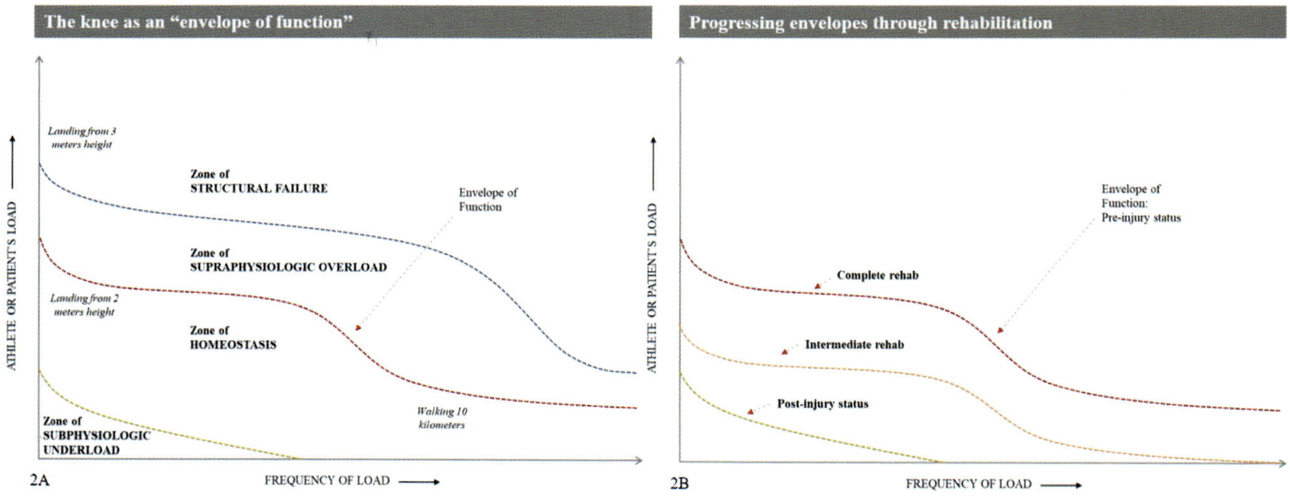

Figure 2

2A - The knee as a biologic transmission with an envelope of function. The amount of progressive load through rehabilitation should avoid both sub-physiologic underload and excessive supraphysiologic overload

2B - The injured athlete is progressing towards the envelope of function curve (red) but generally stands lower in graph, especially in the first phases of recovery, so progression should be gentle and well thought. The different phases of rehabilitation are associated with different thresholds of overload and structural failures, as well as underload (re-adapted from Dye et al [31])

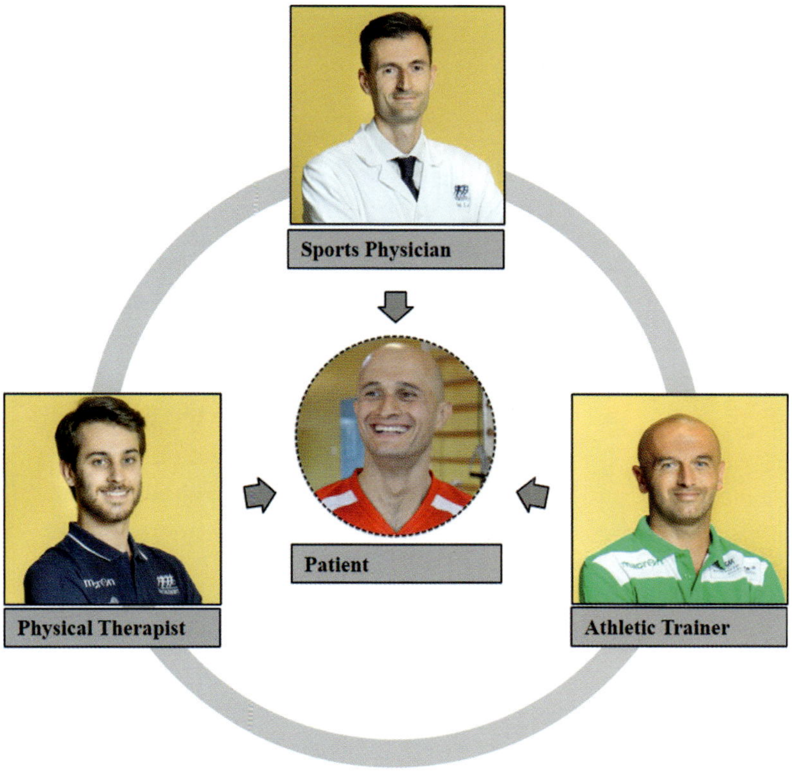

Figure 3 - Proper team. A proper Sports Medicine Team is composed at least by a Sports Physician, a Physical Therapist and an Athletic Trainer.
The "patient first" approach is highlighted in the picture as he/she stands in the center of the triangle

Proper team

Literature recommendations and the experience as a long lasting (30+ years) provider of sports rehabilitation service suggest that having a proper Sports Medicine Team is a key factor to achieve the best clinical outcomes. According to the Isokinetic Medical Group philosophy of care, the patient should be followed by the same Sports Medicine Team from the time of injury to the time of official RTP, hence the team composition should be properly thought to cover the specific skills of each phase of functional recovery.

A proper team consists at least of: (1) a Sport Medicine Physician, (2) a Physical Therapist and (3) an Athletic Trainer (fig. 3). The whole team efforts should be "patient-centered" and a "patient first approach" is needed (fig. 4). As clearly stated above in the introduction to this section, tailoring the progressive protocol on patient's need is one of the key basic principles. Getting inside the team, the Sports Physician, as discussed later in the text, should be the leading actor, guiding the team to achieve patient's goals. The same physician should consult on the same patient at each control consultation, giving the right direction (evolving over the course of rehabilitation) to functional recovery, based on objective, measurable parameters. The Physical Therapists and Athletic Trainers should be highly specialized but also consider the whole functional recovery process, without narrow views on just one single phase of the injury-to-recovery pathway. Other professional figures, external or internal to the rehabilitation center may be involved in the recovery to cover specific needs (e.g. Sport Psychologist to address excessive fear of poor readiness to return to play), but they must link with the Sports Physician.

In the case of patients requiring surgery, perfect communication between the surgical and rehabilitation team is recommended. This statement may appear obvious and logical but unfortunately in the day by day practice there is often a lack of this crucial organizational aspect. The Sports Physician is the person who is regularly in charge of communicating with the surgeon.

Proper facilities

A second organizational concept when dealing with soccer injuries is having the correct environment (facilities) in place to allow the caregivers (team) to fully complete their commitment on the patient. Again, this concept seems basic in nature, but the real application is exactly the opposite.

To complete an injury-to-recovery process of an

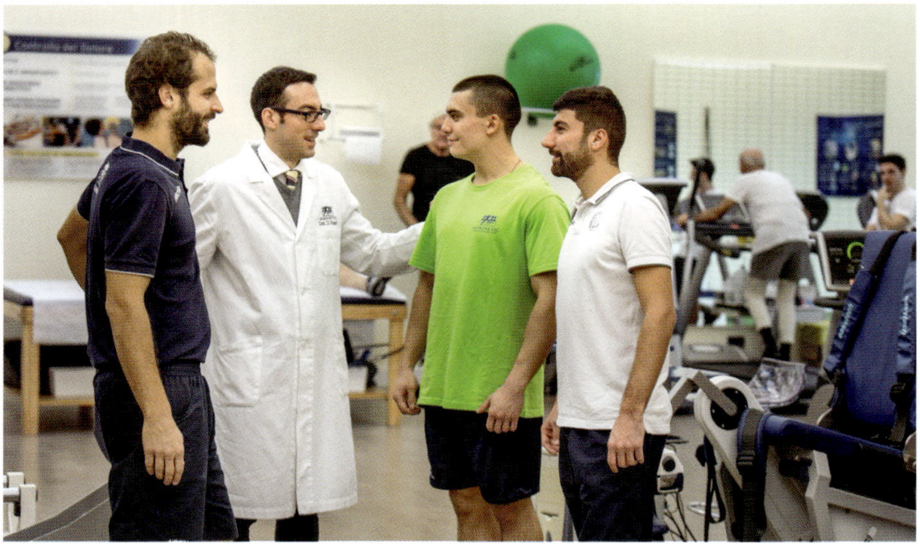

Figure 4 - Patient's centered approach. A patient's first approach is warranted. The only interest that should count is the patient's one. Here an example of patient's engagement with the Sports Medicine Team in a rehabilitation environment

injured soccer player the sport medicine team needs: medical offices, rehabilitation pools (for IPR, in-pool rehabilitation), rehabilitation gyms, biomechanics (movement) labs, and sports field (for OFR, on-field rehabilitation). Having such a broad number of different spaces (fig. 5) allows a real customized progression of loading, especially for, but not limited to, long-term injuries.

Beside medical offices, dedicated in our model to diagnosis, initial consultation, periodical follow up, and final evaluation, there are four main areas utilized in well-defined moments of the rehabilitation path.

Rehabilitation pools are important spaces, mainly dedicated (but not limited) to the first rehabilitation phases. Buckthorpe et al. recently underlined the benefit of IPR as applied to functional recovery after ACLR [7]. Given the property of the water, early range of motion (ROM) and strengthening exercises may be commenced earlier, together with a gradual resumption of the correct gait cycle. The use of different water depths (progressing from deep to shallow) allows a gradual and progressive increase in load. In intermediate phases of the functional recovery approach, movement pattern re-training

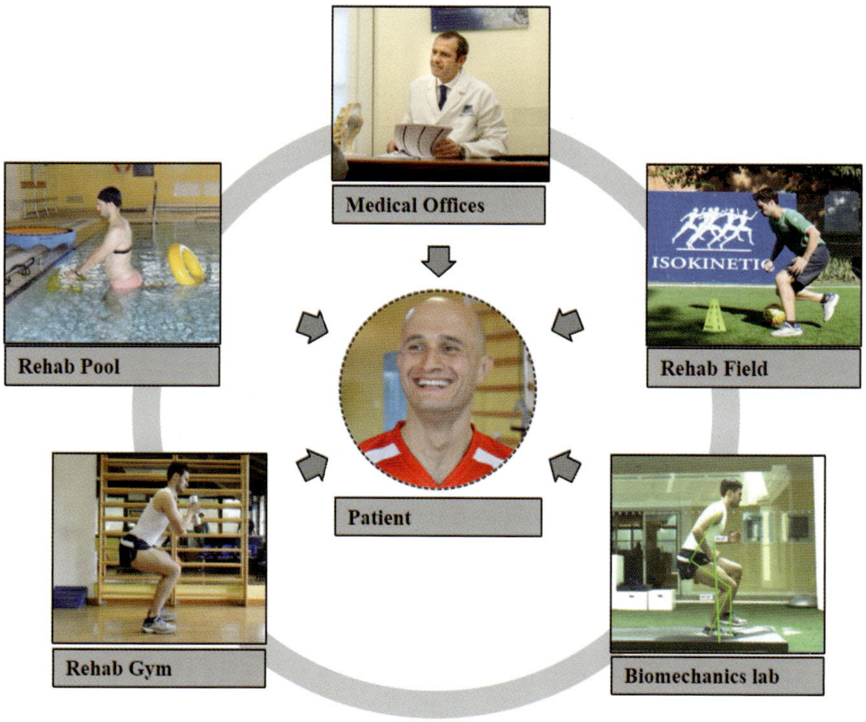

Figure 5 - Proper facilities. Ensuring the proper environment allows a customization of the protocol while progressing towards greater sport specificity in rehabilitation

may also be introduced initially and earlier in the pool, which again allows a better control of movements reducing the ground reaction forces, elicited during movements. Finally, this special environment allows earlier implementation of neuroplasticity exercises (e.g. kicking in water or headings on floating) that mimic sport-specific gestures, which will be performed subsequently in other environments (e.g. gym, field).

The rehabilitation gym remains the predominant environment in terms of total volume of therapeutic sessions, while the other spaces support specific clinical needs. The post-acute period as well the majority of the exercises for ROM recovery are undertaken in the gym. The crucial phase for the gym is the isolated strengthening period, which is often neglected but is crucial to develop the capability of the athlete to progress to targeted neuromuscular training and sport-specific gesture recovery. A combination of open kinetic chain (OKC) and closed kinetic chain (CKC), using both machines (e g. isokinetic dynamometers, leg press) and functional exercises are adopted to recover strength, tailored to the patient's specific responses.

The biomechanics lab (spaces dedicated to movements) is a relatively recent addition to the injury recovery process. It is suggested to consider not only isolated joint function and strength but the whole musculoskeletal (MSK) system and neuromuscular (NM) function. As such, re-integrating recently re-activated and strengthened muscles into proper and safe movement patterns is of paramount importance to allow long-term normal function and overall biomechanics. Especially in certain MSK conditions (e.g. PFP, patellofemoral pain, and ACL injury in young athletes) where biomechanical factors are well known determinants of injury risk, patients should be tested and carefully treated with personalized NM training to overcome deficits in dynamic lower limb control. Setting up a proper "movement" lab to test and train motor patterns should be one of the priorities in modern updated rehabilitation.

Sports fields are dedicated to OFR. OFR stands as the very last phase of functional recovery, to really bridge the gap between standard rehabilitation and return to the team. Practically, it consists of a step-wised five sub-phases program of progressive return to sport activity [8, 9, 10]. The possibility to deliver this kind of service is particularly important for high level athletes, but also applicable to all activity levels and sports. A multi-sports organization of this space is warranted to cover all the specific needs of the sports patients.

In order to deliver an updated, world class service of sports rehabilitation, correct facilities need to be in place. The structural advances can facilitate, but not replace a correct application of the key principles of rehabilitation. In lay terms, proper structures "do not treat or cure" the patients, but facilitate the team guiding the application of innovative, evidence based, soccer medicine intervention.

Proper method

The third and necessary concept is a common clinical method shared by the components of the Sports Medicine Team. The proposed strategy related to the general clinical method is based on three key aspects (fig. 6): (1) a leader of the team (Case Manager Concept), (2) an appropriate communication model and (3) an updated and evidence based clinical approach.

It is recommended to identify a leader within the Sports Medicine Team, that should guide the patient through the whole rehabilitation process after soccer injuries. Within all the people involved in the recovery, the Sports Physician should act as the leader of the group, taking full responsibility of the patient's outcome. Hence, in the Isokinetic Medical Group definition, the Case Manager is the treating physician in charge of the patient at 360°, taking precise tactical (e.g. little changes in the rehabilitation protocol) and strategical (e.g. surgical versus conservative approach) decisions together with the patient, in agreement with the rest of the team.

In the normal practice the injured soccer player generally sees many different professional figures with various titles and specializations, potentially giving very conflicting suggestions, creating chaos and confusion in the patient's mind. If you are familiar with sports medicine practice, you can easily understand the aforementioned statement. To minimize the risk of this, the concept of the Case Manager was introduced in the day by day practice. The Case Manager oversees the process from

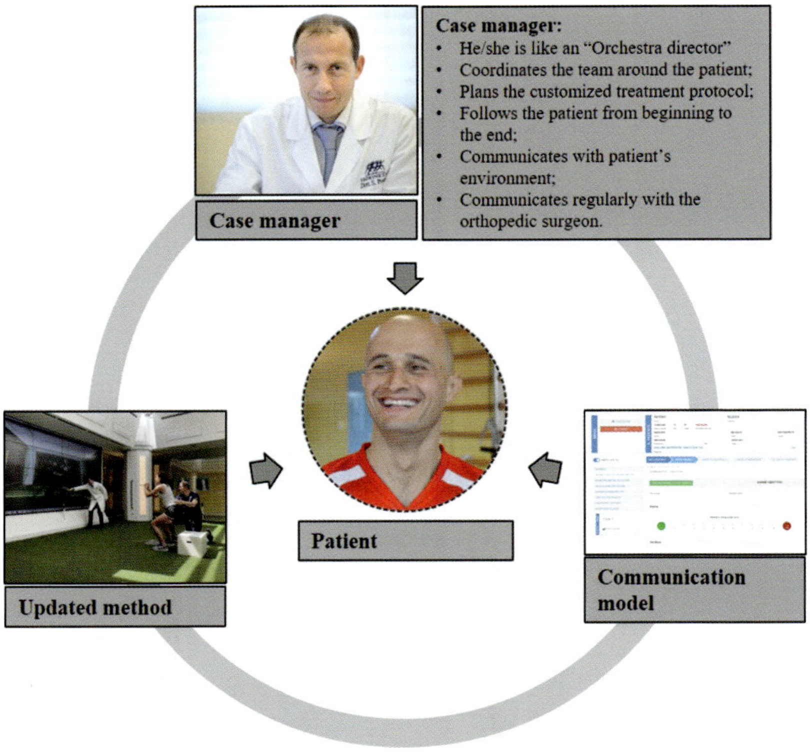

Figure 6 - Proper method. Pitfalls of having an appropriate clinical method in soccer player rehabilitation

the beginning to the end (fig. 5).

• He/she is the Doctor that consults on the patient for the initial consultation to the discharge consultation (plus all the control consultation needed in the middle).

• He/she plans the customized treatment protocol on the soccer player.

• He/she coordinates the Sports Medicine Team around the injured player.

• He/she takes care of the communication with the patient's environment (e.g. family, coach, agent, team's doctor).

• He/she communicates regularly with the orthopedic surgeon in the case of a surgical patient.

• He/she really feels the responsibility (together with the team) of the patient's outcome.

Secondly, the Case Manager and the whole Sports Medicine Team should use an appropriate communication model to be well informed on the patient's conditions. Using the clinical chart, having digital reports to be shared, organizing dedicated meetings are some formal communication hints. Beside these, informal communication is also important as it can strengthen the bonds between the caregivers. Each organization should look and decide for the most appropriate communication model, satisfying clinical needs (e.g. controlling the process around the patient).

Finally, in modern sports medicine we can no longer accept purely eminence-based approach, based on statements like "we have always done in this way, so we will carry on doing like this forever". Medicine is a complex practice based on experience and evidence. However, medicine is a constantly evolving practice, that can evolve only if we will be able to find the balance between research and clinical practice. Thus, we recommend applying an innovative and evidence-based approach and, when applicable, studying the results of the literature and those of your own patients to progress. New doesn't always mean good or bad. Incorporating changes and translating research concepts into practice is the optimal way to progress. In fact, as Charles H. Mayo stated back in 1931 about Medical Practice: "today the only thing that is permanent is change"; so what is true today was not yesterday and may not be tomorrow. Sports medicine practice will evolve embracing the required changes as evidence and sports evolve as well.

The clinical pitfalls concerning how a proper method should be applied are treated in the remaining sections of the chapter, where a suggested clinical approach to major soccer injuries is warranted.

The injury to recovery process: changing the status quo

In the recent years, there has been perhaps a stronger interest in late-phase than early-phase rehabilitation following long-term injuries [9, 10, 11]. This is an answer to an increasing need to really optimize neuromuscular function after soccer injuries. The paradigm is shifting from symptom resolution to a comprehensive recovery of soccer player's full potential. Hence, to change the status quo, we need to challenge the typical and outdated vision of sports injuries.

As medical doctors our focus is generally on the acute lesion (e.g. acute knee injury with ACL and MCL complete rupture): we want to fix it as soon as possible, removing critical patient's symptoms. This approach is completely right but may be reductionistic in nature. If we focus too much on the injured joint, we may lose the opportunity to plan a long-term recovery strategy. We propose to focus on the return to play (RTP) from the very beginning, focusing all the necessary steps that should be done in order to complete the recovery. We need to change the focus from the injured joint to the whole athlete (soccer player in this case) (fig. 7). In this way you have the real possibility to complete the functional recovery after soccer injuries. If not, the risk is applying only a short-term strategy.

Even if the paradigm is slowly changing, it is well established that there is a potential lack of control in the last phase of rehabilitation after long-term injuries, such as ACL injury (fig. 8). As a medical community, we often lose control over the last crucial phases of recovery, when the patient is generally symptom free but presenting multi-faceted functional deficits. This is exactly what we should control better to allow a successful and safe RTP.

Adopting a RTP philosophy is critical to visualize all the crucial modifiable variables that can be targeted to ameliorate patients outcome, such as:

1. recovery of muscles strength (full recovery);
2. cardiovascular fitness reconditioning;
3. movement pattern's restoration;
4. recovery of soccer player's profile through completion of OFR;
5. psychological readiness to RTP.

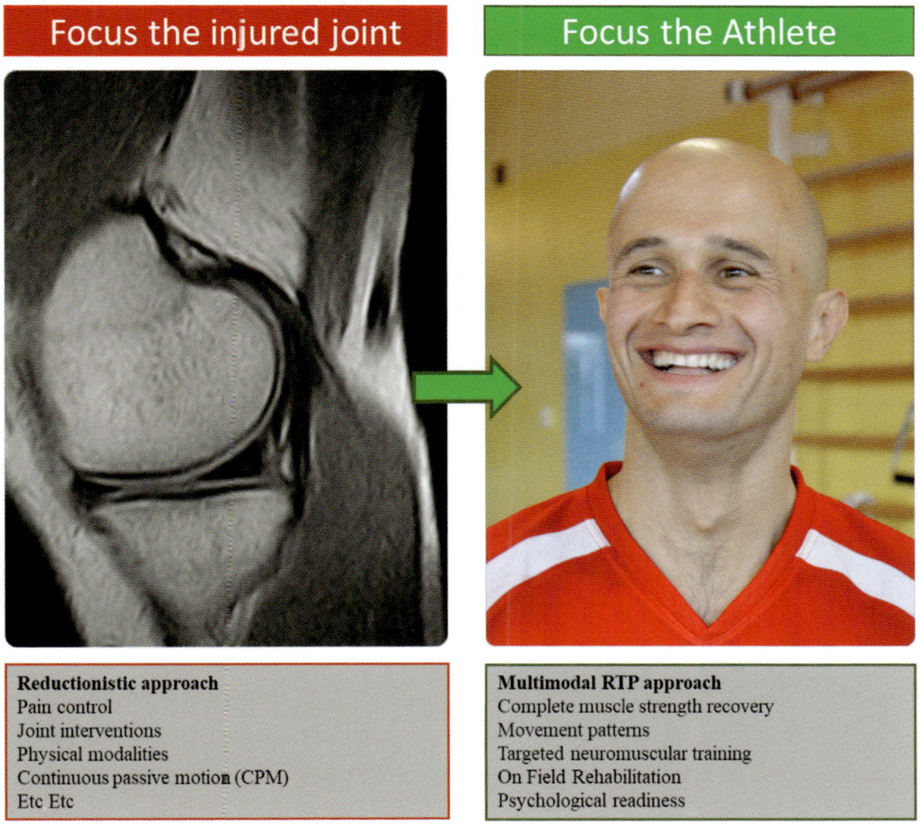

Figure 7 - Changing the status quo. Multimodal RTP approach versus reductionistic single joint focus. A focus on the whole athlete's recovery is recommended in the recovery after soccer injuries

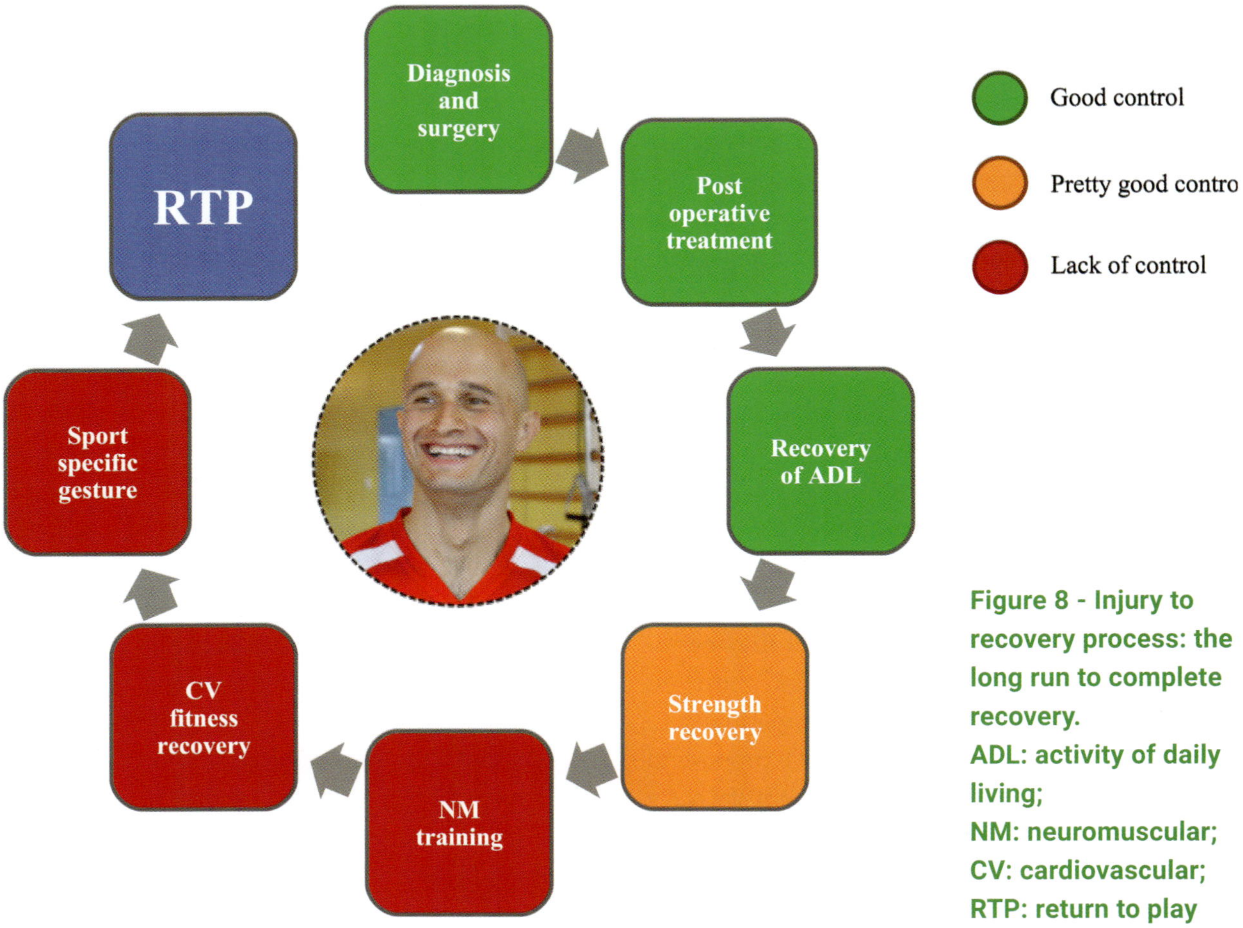

Figure 8 - Injury to recovery process: the long run to complete recovery.
ADL: activity of daily living;
NM: neuromuscular;
CV: cardiovascular;
RTP: return to play

The difficult balance between performance and health of the players/injury risk

An even bigger problem in high level competitive sports, such as soccer, is the difficult balance between performance and injury risk/health of the players. This is for example, an inner trait of elite soccer and, as medical professional, we should accept it, trying to balance the two aspects and considering that in athlete's mind the most important point is always performance. Firstly, performance and health do not always take an opposite direction. For instance, over the past few years, injury prevention (treated extensively later in this chapter) has received a lot of attention in soccer medicine. A link between a larger application of prevention (less injuries) and team ranking has been reported [12, 13]. Secondly, as a professional involved in soccer medicine, one should accept the substantial injury risk of soccer, which can be reduced but not eliminated. As health providers we should always aim to push for a "sustainable" (by the athlete) performance. This is true for uninjured as well as for injured players. An injury is often an opportunity to take care of the patient's health all round, but only if the correct mind-setting of long-term recovery is applied.

In the next sub-paragraph, the example of the ACL injured athlete is discussed in detail to better show a practical implication of the over-mentioned concept in rehabilitation.

The example of the ACL injured soccer player: RTP and second injury risk

When dealing with soccer injuries, a perfect example of a difficult balance in functional outcomes is the case of ACL injuries.

Results of the current care of the ACL injured athlete have been recently challenged. On one side there seems to be very good patient reported outcome (PRO) satisfaction at short to medium term follow up, but on the other hand an unsatisfactory RTP rate has been reported [14], together with a

high risk of second ACL injury in the young, active individuals [15].
We will concentrate our practical example on these two delicate outcomes: RTP at preinjury level on one side and risk of second ACL injury on the other (fig. 9).
RTP at the same pre-injury level is nothing but a very challenging outcome following ACLR. Many variables (baseline, surgical and rehabilitation factors) interact in a complex manner to determine the likelihood of a successful RTP. Just to cite a basic example, age and gender play a role, with youngest males being generally favored for a positive outcome [14]. However, modifiable factors, such as results of functional testing, can affect the RTP as well [16]. In other words, we can increase the RTP rate with our rehabilitation intervention. In our experience, based on large cohorts of patients, four main modifiable factors can be used to increase the rate of RTP: recovery of knee spanning muscle strength, recovery of cardio-vascular fitness, completion of OFR program, and general compliance to the proposed protocol. The fact that the around 30% of patients do not have RTP to pre-injury level may be explained in part by low adherence to rehabilitation protocol and residual symptoms/functional deficit. However, the main reasons to unsuccessful RTP following ACLR may lay in not-knee related life-decisions (finish of high school, wedding, change of work etc.) and psychological reasons (excessive fear of re-injury/movement or inner psychological traits).
On the other hand, avoiding a second ACL injury is the second main mid-term goal of the ACLR patient. Again, the causation of such an event is multi-factorial in nature, with baseline, surgical and rehabilitation factors to be considered. Within the baseline factors, young age and having a higher activity level are well known risk factors of secondary injuries. After ACLR a teenager can expect a 20%-30% re-injury rate (considering both ipsilateral graft injuries and contralateral native ACL injuries) with different results depending on time of follow-up [17, 18]. Within all the possible determinants of such a devastating outcome for the soccer player, biomechanical factors and neuromuscular control seem to be the key ones [19], as we will discuss subsequently.
Anyway, the first condition that should be met to allow a second injury to happen is the exposure to risk activity (e.g. RTP to the same soccer level). Simply, the higher the RTP rate, logically the higher the second ACL injury rate. This is the main dilemma of nowadays sport medicine practice.
In our opinion, this should not be considered a dilemma but a conditional status. Something we need to accept as clinician (and of course trying to control), considering that the inner biological variability of functional recovery will not allow to prevent every single second ACL rupture. Many

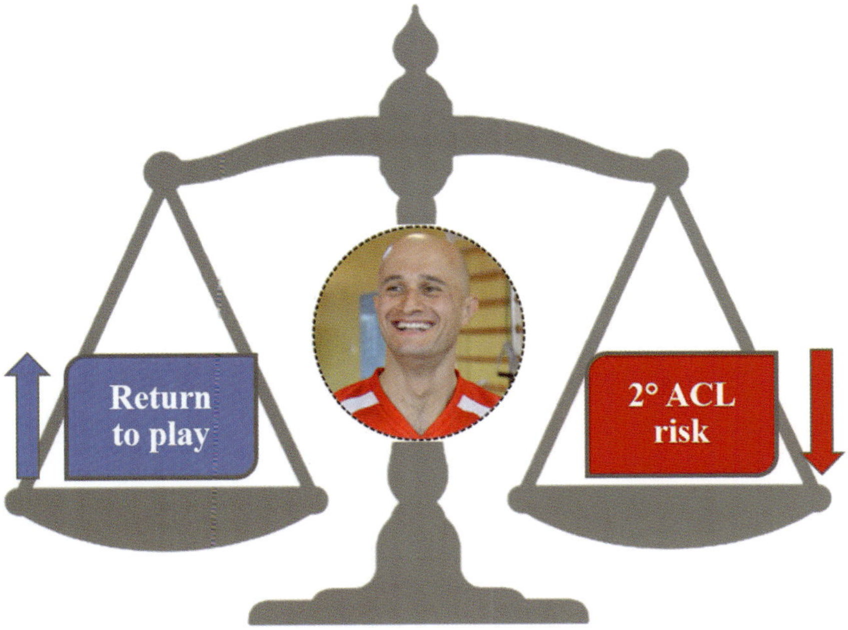

Figure 9 - Balance between RTP rate and second ACL injury risk after ACLR in the soccer player. Equilibrium between these two important outcomes should be pursued with every single case after ACLR, targeting the intervention based on patient's profile and desires non-modifiable factors, from genetic predisposition to bony morphology cannot be controlled, but of course we can ameliorate the dynamic lower limb control during high load tasks, concentrating on key biomechanical and NM control factors. Simply, we can really try to complete the recovery path, minimizing the risk (not to zero) because we also want them to RTP.

As RTP to personal activity level is also part of the normal participation in society, RTP is part of the World Health Organization (WHO) definition of health. We cannot focus merely on second ACL injury prevention, if we could not just prevent people to get back to previous activity level. Balance is needed and this balance should also be adapted on the single patient condition. The case of a 33 year old professional basketball player is very different from the case of a 15 year old recreational soccer player. Given the risk stratification (based on age), the Sport Medicine Team will increase the attention on second ACL reduction in the second case and on RTP in the first case.

All this sub-section is just an example on how measure of performance (exposure) can interact with primary or secondary injury risk. Indeed, balance is needed for our soccer patients. In the next section few points of such an approach will be treated separately in a precise way.

Evolving sport medicine: hot topics

As clearly stated above, sports (soccer) medicine is a constantly evolving branch of medicine. This practice is relatively young and is progressing faster than other more traditional medical fields. Several relatively new concepts have been highlighted over the last decade. In the next sub-sections four main principles will be discussed.

Criteria based progression

Nowadays, it is widely accepted that progression of rehabilitation after major soccer injuries (e.g. severe knee injuries or muscle injuries) should be criteria – rather than time – based. Despite this wide consensus among rehabilitation practitioners, the debate is still open regarding whether or not to incorporate time frames.

That said, the logical approach is using a customized clinical and functional criteria-based progression. The time, mostly related to tissue healing considerations (in greater part not well studied and neither proved) should be considered afterwards, being a secondary issue.

To cite a common example, 3 months after a structural severe hamstring injury a soccer player may be not ready to return to competition even if the globally considered "safe time threshold" has been passed.

The same concept of balancing RTP and recurrence risk should be always applied. In certain clinical situation rehabilitation may be accelerated (e.g. elite mature soccer player willing to be back for the last international competition), while in others may it be decelerated (e.g. young competitive soccer player with knee injury during the growth spurt). In all the cases the progression should be based on specific and stringent criteria. The protocol should be progressive and customized.

The delicate balance between RTP (e.g. fast and effective RTP) and risk of recurrence (e.g. second muscle or knee injury) should be pursued, also respecting patient's will, while counseling him/her with the appropriate number and risk stratification. A honest and careful discussion about this topic can allow to reach the best decision. Then, a "higher risk taker" population will adopt a slightly different approach than a "lower risk taker" population.

A Sports Medicine Team must always aim to complete the program. If the recovery will last over the expectations (based on criteria), this is part of normal variability and again it should be accepted. The application of clinical and functional criteria should be adopted to guide the rehabilitation process and should not be limited to clearing the patients to RTP. In short, it is not recommended to use only RTP criteria (fig. 10) but to use the same concept to progress during functional recovery. For this reason, we introduced the so-called "traffic lights concept". Pre-defined functional goals (e.g. walking without crutches or running etc.) are allowed only if specific clinical and functional criteria are previously satisfied. The example reported in figure 10 refers to the end stage traffic light for RTP (balanced for RTP probability and second ACL risk), but the same concept can be applied for every goal and in every clinical condition. We

published our approach as applied to RTP after ACLR in soccer players [8] and after cartilage procedures [20], but the same kind of protocol has been recently suggested for other clinical entities, as muscle injuries [21].
The most important aspect of such a way of thinking is that if the traffic light is red, hence you don't have the safe condition to proceed, you should remain in the previous phase to satisfy progression criteria. This easy mind-setting is hard to apply in the day-by-day practice.

Neuromuscular function: from activation to sport specific drills (IMG manual PPT)

The recent evidence suggests that complete recovery of NM function is warranted during rehabilitation following soccer injuries. This concept is more a mindset, rather than a predetermined rule as the recovery of proper function is really a continuum, without real borders between concepts and phases.
We suggest to begin thinking biomechanically and neurophysiologically from the very beginning of rehabilitation of an injured soccer player.
The theoretical framework to tackle NM function inside a rehabilitation setting is presented in figure 11 and follows this sequence:
1. re-activate the key muscles to overcome a specific deficit;
2. strengthen in isolation the key muscles to increase muscle size and function;
3. re-integrate the muscles into specific functional movement (aiming for perfect quality);
4. re-insert qualitative movement patterns into sport-specific movements.
In each of these different phases of activity a different mix of therapeutic exercises should be applied. In the muscle re-activation phase, it is important to target the activation of the specific muscle (e.g. gluteus maximus activation). In the strengthening

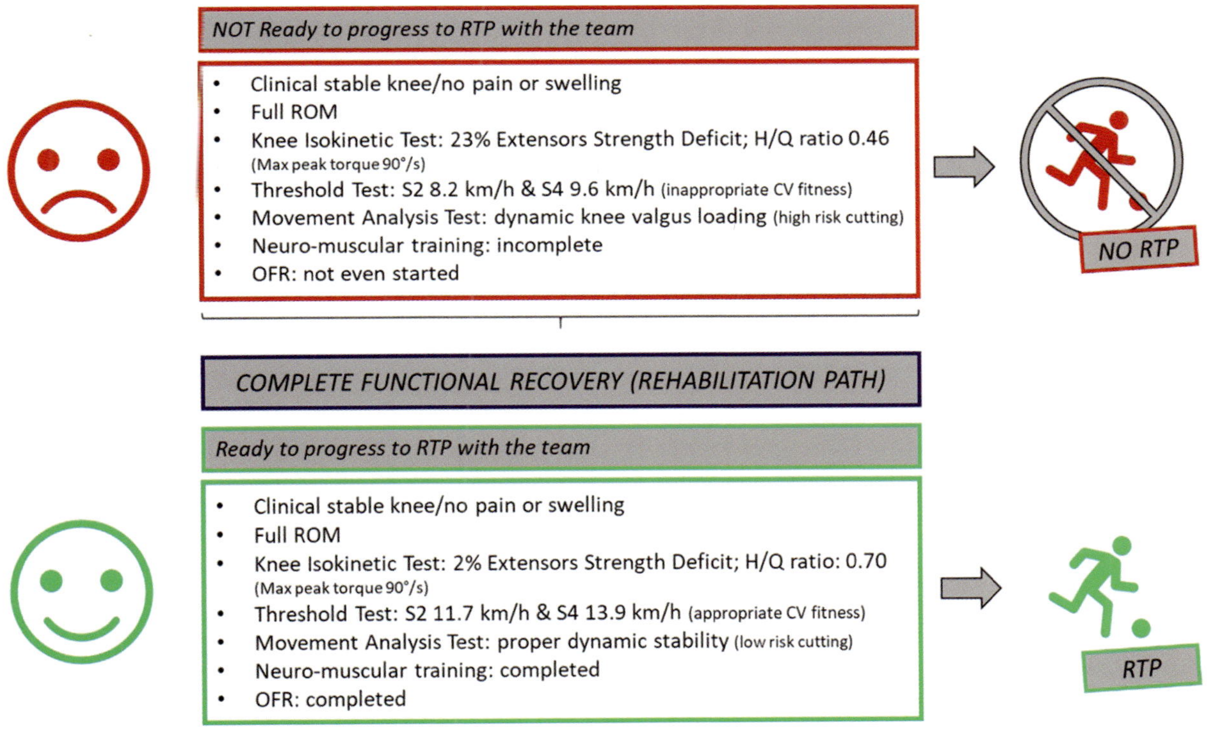

Figure 10 - To RTP or not to RTP, this is the dilemma. Progressing through rehabilitation (early, mid or late stage) should be based on objective criteria. Case 1 is a patient that should not be cleared to RTP basing on his/her functional status. Case 2 is a patient that may be cleared to RTP basing on his/her functional testing and completion of the program. This framework can be applied in every clinical scenario.
ROM: range of motion; S2: aerobic threshold at 2 mmol/L of blood lactate; S4: anaerobic threshold at 4 mmol/L of blood lactate; OFR: on field rehabilitation

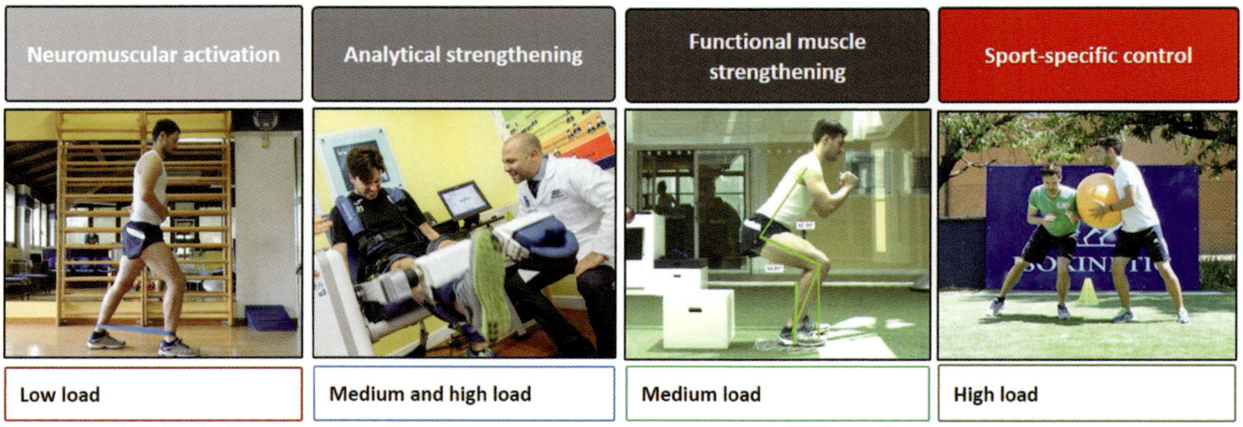

Figure 11 - From neuromuscular (re)activation to control in sport specific gesture. A correct addressing of neuromuscular function seems to be an important clinical principle in rehabilitation of soccer injuries

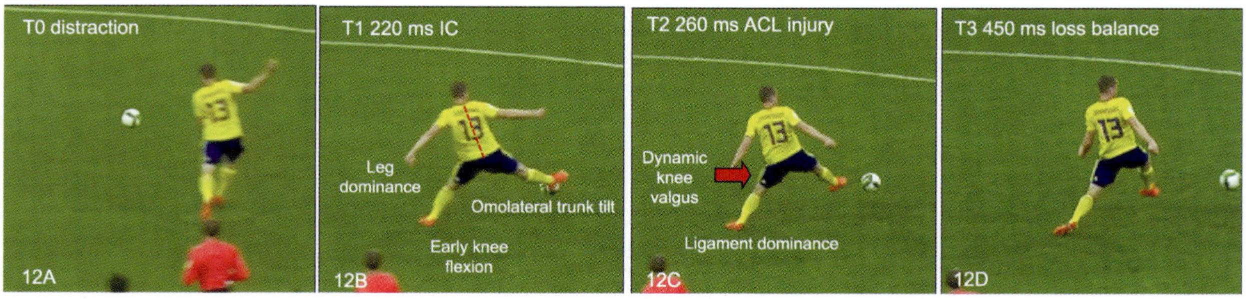

Figure 12 - Mechanism of ACL injury in a soccer player. The main risk factors are high-lighted IC: initial contact; ACL: anterior cruciate ligament; ms: milliseconds

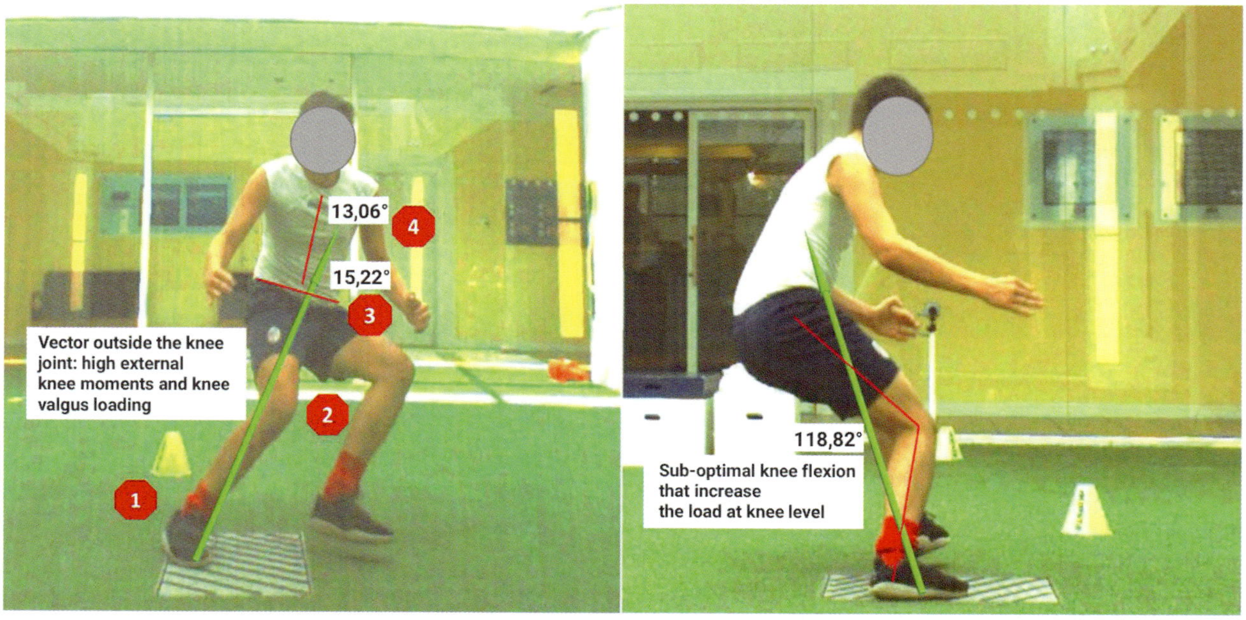

Figure 13 - Example of high-risk cutting tasks after ACLR. When a dynamic knee valgus loading (knee moving inwards) is applied the load on the ACL-graft may increase
1) foot-intrarotation; 2) dynamic knee valgus appearance; 3) contralateral pelvic drop; 4) trunk already rotated and tilted

phase the key is to apply medium to high load, with a combination of exercises to increase muscle strength. In the last two phases of activity the (1) activated and (2) strengthen muscles should be re-integrated in specific movements, with progression (from double leg squat to cutting and hopping tasks). Optimal movement quality is key in this third step. Finally, the reconstructed, high quality movement patterns (with activated and strong key muscles) should be gradually re-inserted into the sport specific gesture.

This theoretical framework of activity stands as an added key principle of rehabilitation of soccer injuries.

Movement quality as the new frontier?

Especially when dealing with lower limb injuries and more in detail knee issues, biomechanical and NM control factors appear to be new important additions to the treatment algorithm. The integration of measures of movement quantity (e.g. knee/hip muscles isokinetic or isometric test) with movement quality (e.g. frontal and lateral plane analysis of medium to high load movement pattern) can add important information to the best way to treat every patient.

Muscle strength gives to the patient the capability to move well, but it is generally not enough to allow safe movement patterns after major knee injuries. A qualitative movement evaluation may add important kinematic information. For example, a patient with very strong hip abductors can still have residual dynamic knee valgus loading because of repetitive movement pattern that was reinforced through the years. In this case, motor learning techniques should be applied in order to re-established safe motor control in dynamic tasks.

On one hand, studies about the mechanism of ACL injuries clearly showed that there are a few important and consistent factors that can be depicted: (1) ligament dominance (excessive valgus loading); (2) quadriceps dominance (low knee flexion); (3) leg dominance (all the load on one lower limb) and (4) trunk dominance (trunk dysfunction with omolateral tilt increasing the external knee abduction moment). These factors are highlighted in figure 12.

On the other hand, evidence suggests that an increase in dynamic knee valgus loading put the patients at increased risk of second ACL injury after ACLR [19, 22]. Even if few studies have been published on the topic, based on these two clues, we strongly encourage clinicians to think how mitigating high external load at knee level that could be detrimental in term of secondary injuries or overload problems, as the same patterns have been also linked to patellofemoral pain and general lower limb injuries in athletes.

An example of an at-risk dynamic knee valgus loading is reported in figure 13, where the information is coupled with a sub-optimal movement strategy on the lateral plane, exposing the patient to high external knee loads, threatening the ACL graft integrity.

Even if we use the example of the knee surgery patient, this kind of approach may be used for every clinical situation. An important concept about qualitative movement assessment is that if you don't perform this kind of tests, you don't really know if the soccer player displays high risk movement patterns. A key role of management and quality control says "inspect what you expect"; the information gives you the power to intervene with targeted NM training, applying biofeedback techniques [23] to overcome the high-risk movement patterns and decrease the re-injury risk. In our experience a minimum of 10-12 sessions of NMT are necessary to really modify a patient's motor patterning.

Even if of great importance in late-phase rehabilitation, movement quality is only one of the corner stone of the last and next paragraph concept we would like to introduce.

On field rehabilitation

The final part of recovery stands between "standard rehabilitation" and return to the team. This is a well-known risky and grey area of functional recovery after soccer injuries. As explained in the above chapter, the patient is generally symptom free but still presenting functional limitation.

In our experience, completing a careful and stepwise program of OFR is beneficial for a complete functional recovery, increasing the quality of the clinical results [8, 20, 24] and potentially increasing also the RTP rate. The process consists in a complex gradual resumption of soccer specific

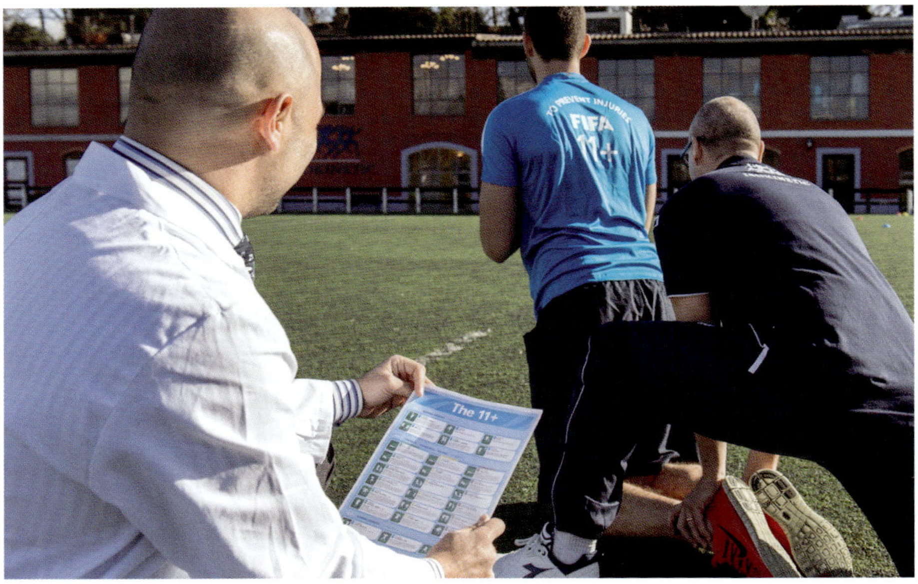

Figure 14 - Introducing the patient to neuromuscular prevention programs like the FIFA 11+ can be a powerful addition to increase the awareness of the soccer player to preventative measures

activities, based on four main pillars of activity [9]: (1) restoring movement quality, (2) physical conditioning, (3) restoring sport-specific skills, (4) progressively developing chronic training load. These main areas of activity progress through the five stages of OFR, as recently described in the literature [10].

The goal of this very specialized treatment is to progressively re-insert the patients in the specific soccer contest, while checking the reaction of the injured joints. In this context the use of global positioning system (GPS) to monitor different metrics of external player load is also warranted. A live feedback during each OFR sessions is very useful in controlling the increase (it should be gradual) of load week after week.

For a long-term injury, we recommend a minimum of five weeks for a total of 10-12 OFR sessions before the resumption of training with the team.

Beyond rehabilitation: prevention considerations

Beside the real focus of this chapter (soccer rehabilitation), it is worth underlining the role of primary and continuous prevention. Primary prevention for lower limb MSK injuries works [25, 26, 27]. About NMT programs (e.g. the FIFA 11+) authors demonstrated an injury reduction of 37% during matches and 29% during training sessions [28]. The same or even higher treatment effect regards also the very young athletes as the new FIFA 11+ kids is also effective cutting the 74 % of severe injuries and the 55% of lower limb injuries in very young soccer players [29].

In terms of ACL injuries there is now conclusive evidence that prevention programs reduced 67% (2/3) of ACL injuries in female athletes and 50% (1/2) of ACL injuries in all athletes [30]. The effectiveness of these programs is correlated with two main aspects: (1) the composition of the programs and the form (movement quality) of the preventative exercises and (2) the weekly frequency (compliance of the athlete), with 3 times/week being the optimal threshold.

The soccer medical practitioner (or better the soccer medicine team) should be aware of these findings, in order to suggest the athlete, once finished the recovery, to keep on going with specific and effective intervention on his/her health. Suggesting such programs and educating the patients to carry on therapeutic exercises (fig. 14) is a final and key addiction.

Conclusions

The principles of rehabilitation of the injured soccer player have been presented widely in this chapter. A combination of organizational and clinical pitfalls should be considered when designing a high-quality soccer rehabilitation service. As sport medicine and orthopedic rehabilitation is a young and fast evolving branch of medicine, modern clinical practice should be based on embracing changes and innovation in a constructive way, always aiming to improve patient's outcomes and health.

Bibliography

1. Kunz M. Big Count: 265 Million Playing Football. FIFA magazine 2007.
2. Ekstrand J, Hägglund M, Waldén M. Injury incidence and injury patterns in professional football: the UEFA injury study. Br J Sports Med. 2011 Jun;45(7):553-8.
3. Ekstrand J, Hägglund M, Waldén M. Epidemiology of muscle injuries in professional football (soccer). Am J Sports Med. 2011 Jun;39(6):1226-32.
4. Arnason A, Sigurdsson SB, Gudmundsson A et al. Risk factors for injuries in football. Am J Sports Med. 2004 Jan-Feb;32(1 Suppl):5S-16S.
5. Arundale AJH, Silvers-Granelli HJ, Snyder-Mackler L. Career length and injury incidence after anterior cruciate ligament reconstruction in Major League Soccer Players. Orthop J Sports Med. 2018 Jan 24;6(1): 1-8.
6. Lohmander LS, Englund M, Dahl LL et al. The long-term consequence of anterior cruciate ligament and meniscus injuries osteoarthritis. Am J Sports Med. 2007 Oct;35(10):1756-69.
7. Buckthorpe M, Pirotti E, Della Villa F. Benefits of water exercise for ACL rehabilitation – A clinical commentary. IJSPT 2019 (In press).
8. Della Villa S, Boldrini L, Ricci M et al. Clinical Outcomes and Return-to-Sports Participation of 50 Soccer Players After Anterior Cruciate Ligament Reconstruction Through a Sport-Specific Rehabilitation Protocol. Sports Health. 2012 Jan;4(1):17-24.
9. Buckthorpe M, Della Villa F, Della Villa S et al. On-field Rehabilitation Part 1: 4 Pillars of High-Quality On-field Rehabilitation Are Restoring Movement Quality, Physical Conditioning, Restoring Sport-Specific Skills, and Progressively Developing Chronic Training Load. J Orthop Sports Phys Ther. 2019 Jul 10:1-5.
10. Buckthorpe M, Della Villa F, Della Villa S et al. On-field Rehabilitation Part 2: A 5-Stage Program for the Soccer Player Focused on Linear Movements, Multidirectional Movements, Soccer-Specific Skills, Soccer-Specific Movements, and Modified Practice. J Orthop Sports Phys Ther. 2019 Jul 10:1-6.
11. Buckthorpe M. Optimising the Late-Stage Rehabilitation and Return-to-Sport Training and Testing Process After ACL Reconstruction. Sports Med. 2019 Jul;49(7):1043-58.
12. Eirale C, Tol JL, Farooq A et al. Low injury rate strongly correlates with team success in Qatari professional football. Br J Sports Med 2013 Aug;47(12):807–8.
13. Hägglund M, Waldén M, Magnusson H et al. Injuries affect team performance negatively in professional: football: an 11-year follow-up of the UEFA Champions League injury study. Br J Sports Med. 2013 Aug;47(12):738-42.
14. Ardern CL, Taylor NF, Feller, JA et al. Fifty-five per cent return to competitive sport following anterior cruciate ligament reconstruction surgery: an updated systematic review and meta-analysis including aspects of physical functioning and contextual factors. BJSM 2014 48(21), 1543-1552.
15. Wiggins AJ, Grandhi RK, Schneider DK, et al. Risk of Secondary Injury in Younger Athletes After Anterior Cruciate Ligament Reconstruction: A Systematic Review and Meta-analysis. Am J Sports Med. 2016 Jul;44(7):1861-76.
16. Nawasreh Z, Logerstedt D, Cummer K, et al. Functional performance 6 months after ACL reconstruction can predict return to participation in the same preinjury activity level 12 and 24 months after surgery. Br J Sports Med. 2018 Mar;52(6):375.
17. Paterno MV, Rauh MJ, Schmitt LC et al. Incidence of Second ACL Injuries 2 Years After Primary ACL Reconstruction and Return to Sport. Am J Sports Med. 2014 Jul;42(7):1567-73.
18. Webster KE, Feller JA. Exploring the High Reinjury Rate in Younger Patients Undergoing Anterior Cruciate Ligament Reconstruction. Am J Sports Med. 2016 Nov;44(11):2827-32.
19. Paterno MV, Schmitt LC, Ford KR et al. Biomechanical measures during landing and postural stability predict second anterior cruciate ligament injury after anterior cruciate ligament reconstruction and return to sport. Am J Sports Med. 2010 Oct;38(10):1968-78.
20. Della Villa S, Kon E, Filardo G et al. Does intensive rehabilitation permit early return to sport without compromising the clinical outcome after arthroscopic autologous chondrocyte implantation in highly competitive athletes? Am J Sports Med. 2010 Jan;38(1):68-77.
21. Heiderscheit BC, Sherry MA, Silder A et al Hamstring strain injuries: recommendations for diagnosis, rehabilitation, and injury prevention. J Orthop Sports Phys 2010 Ther 40(2):67–81.
22. Krosshaug T, Steffen K, Kristianslund E et al (2016). The Vertical Drop Jump Is a Poor Screening Test for ACL Injuries in Female Elite Soccer and Handball players: a prospective cohort study on 710 Athletes. Am J Sports Med 2016 Apr;44(4):874-83.
23. Gokeler A, Benjaminse A, Hewett TE et al. Feedback techniques to target functional deficits following anterior cruciate ligament reconstruction: implications for motor control and reduction of second injury risk. Sports Med. 2013 Nov;43(11):1065-74.
24. Della Villa F, Ricci M, Perdisa F et al. Anterior cruciate ligament reconstruction and rehabilitation: predictors of functional outcome. Joints. 2016 Jan 31;3(4):179-85.
25. Emery CA, Meeuwisse WH. The effectiveness of a neuromuscular prevention strategy to reduce injuries in youth soccer: a cluster-randomised controlled trial. Br J Sports Med. 2010 Jun;44(8):555-62.
26. Mandelbaum B, Silvers HJ, Watanabe DS et al. J Effectiveness of a neuromuscular and proprioceptive training program in preventing anterior cruciate ligament injuries in female athletes: 2-year follow-up. Am Sports Med. 2005 33(7):1003–10.
27. Walden M, Atroshi I, Magnusson H et al. Prevention of acute knee injuries in adolescent female football players: cluster randomized controlled trial. BMJ 2012 344:e3042.
28. Soligard T, Myklebust G, Steffen K et al. Comprehensive warm-up programme to prevent injuries in young female footballers: cluster randomised controlled trial. BMJ 2008 337:a2469.
29. Rössler R, Junge A, Bizzini M et al. A Multinational Cluster Randomised Controlled Trial to Assess the Efficacy of '11+ Kids': A Warm-Up Programme to Prevent Injuries in Children's Football. Sports Med. 2018 Jun;48(6):1493-1504.
30. Webster KE, Hewett TE. Meta-analysis of meta-analyses of anterior cruciate ligament injury reduction training programs. J Orthop Res. 2018 Oct;36(10):2696-2708.
31. Dye SF. The knee as a biologic transmission with an envelope of function: a theory. Clin Orthop Relat Res. 1996 Apr;(325):10-8.